Handbook of Dialysis

P9-ECS-442

Handbook of Dialysis

Fourth Edition

Edited by

John T. Daugirdas, MD
Clinical Professor of Medicine
University of Illinois at Chicago
Chicago, Illinois

Peter G. Blake, MB, FRCPC, FRCPI
Professor of Medicine
University of Western Ontario
Chair of Nephrology
London Health Sciences Centre
London, Canada

Todd S. Ing, MD
Professor Emeritus of Medicine
Department of Medicine
Stritch School of Medicine
Loyola University Chicago
Maywood, Illinois
Physician
Veterans Affairs Hospital
Hines, Illinois

Wolters Kluwer | Lippincott Williams & Wilkins
Health

Philadelphia · Baltimore · New York · London
Buenos Aires · Hong Kong · Sydney · Tokyo

Acquisitions Editor : Lisa McAllister
Managing Editor : Kerry B. Barrett
Project Manager : Nicole Walz
Marketing Manager : Kimberly Schonberger
Manufacturing Coordinator : Kathy Brown
Creative Director : Doug Smock
Cover Designer : Robert Dieters
Production Services : Techbooks
Printer : R.R. Donnelley, Crawfordsville

© 2007 by LIPPINCOTT WILLIAMS & WILKINS, a Wolters Kluwer business
© 2001 by LIPPINCOTT WILLIAMS & WILKINS, © 1994 and 1988 by J.B.
Lippincott
530 Walnut Street
Philadelphia, PA 19106 USA
LWW.com

Printed in the USA

Library of Congress Cataloging-in-Publication Data

Handbook of dialysis / [edited by] John T. Daugirdas, Peter G. Blake, Todd S. Ing. – 4th ed.
    p. ; cm.
  Includes bibliographical references and index.
  ISBN 13: 978-0-7817-5253-4
  ISBN 10: 0-7817-5253-1 (pbk. : alk. paper)
  1. Hemodialysis—Handbooks, manuals, etc. I. Daugirdas, John T.
II. Blake, Peter Gerard, 1956– III. Ing, Todd S.
  [DNLM: 1. Renal Dialysis—Handbooks. WJ 39 H2355 2007]
  RC901.7.H45H36 2001
  617.4′61059—dc22

                       2006028284

---

                    10 9 8 7 6 5 4 3 2

To Stasys Mačiulis, MD—a beloved grandfather never met who continues to guide and inspire.

(JTD)

To my wife Rose and to my sons, Matthew and Andrew—the three most important people in my life.

(PB)

To Oliver M. Wrong, MD, FRCP, my exemplary mentor.

(TSI)

Contents

Part III: Peritoneal Dialysis

Part IV. Clinical Problem Areas

Contributing Authors

Suhail Ahmad, MD *Associate Professor of Medicine, University of Washington; Medical Director, Scribner Kidney Center, Seattle, Washington*

Michael Allon, MD *Professor of Medicine, Department of Nephrology, University of Alabama at Birmingham; Medical Director of Dialysis, University of Alabama Hospital, Birmingham, Alabama*

Shubha Ananthakrishnan, MD *Fellow in Nephrology, Section of Nephrology, Kaiser Permanente Medical Center, San Francisco, California*

Stephen R. Ash, MD, FACP *Chairman and Director of Research and Development, HemoCleanse, Inc. and Ash Access Technologies, Lafayette, Indiana*

Joanne M. Bargman, MD, FRCPC *Professor of Medicine, University of Toronto; Staff Nephrologist and Director, Peritoneal Dialysis Unit, Department of Medicine, Division of Nephrology, University Health Network, Toronto, Ontario, Canada*

Robert L. Benz, MD, FACP *Clinical Professor of Medicine, Department of Internal Medicine and Nephrology, Thomas Jefferson Medical College, Philadelphia, Pennsylvania; Chief, Department of Nephrology, Lankenau Hospital and Main Line Hospitals, Wynnewood, Pennsylvania*

Anatole Besarab, MD *Wayne State University School of Medicine; Senior Staff, Department of Internal Medicine, Division of Nephrology, Henry Ford Hospital, Detroit, Michigan*

Peter G. Blake, MB, FRCPC, FRCPI *Professor of Medicine, University of Western Ontario; Chair of Nephrology, London Health Sciences Centre, London, Ontario, Canada*

Adin Boldur, MD *Attending Nephrologist, Kidney Specialists of Southern Nevada, Las Vegas, Nevada*

Juan P. Bosch, MD *Chief Medical Officer, Gambro AB, Stockholm, Sweden*

Neil Boudville, MBBS, FRACP *Senior Lecturer, School of Medicine and Pharmacology, University of Western Australia, Crawley WA; Nephrologist, Department of Renal Medicine, Sir Charles Gairdner Hospital, Perth WA, Australia*

Bernard Canaud, MD, PhD   *Professor of Nephrology,
Montpellier II University–School of Medicine; Head,
Nephrology, Dialysis and Intensive Care Unit, Lapeyronie
Hospital, Montpellier, France*

Joan P. Cannon, PharmD   *Assistant Professor, Department of
Pharmacy Practice, University of Illinois at Chicago, College
of Pharmacy, Chicago, Illinois; Infectious Disease Clinical
Pharmacist, Pharmacy Service 119, Edward Hines, Jr. VA
Hospital, Hines, Illinois*

Ralph J. Caruana, MD   *Professor, Department of Medicine,
Medical College of Georgia; Chief Medical Officer, Medical
Staff Office, MCG Health Inc., Augusta, Georgia*

Steven C. Cheng, MD   *Clinical Instructor, Department of
Nephrology, Washington University School of Medicine;
Attending Physician, Department of Nephrology,
Barnes-Jewish Hospital, St. Louis, Missouri*

Scott D. Cohen, MD   *Nephrology Fellow, Department of
Medicine, George Washington University; Nephrology Fellow,
Department of Medicine, George Washington University
Hospital, Washington, District of Columbia*

Daniel W. Coyne, MD   *Professor of Medicine, Department of
Medicine, Washington University; Staff Physician,
Barnes-Jewish Hospital, St. Louis, Missouri*

John T. Daugirdas, MD   *Clinical Professor of Medicine,
University of Illinois at Chicago, Chicago, Illinois*

Andrew Davenport, MD, FRCP   *Honorary Senior Lecturer
and Consultant Renal Physician, University College London
Center for Nephrology, Royal Free Hospital, London, United
Kingdom*

Marc E. De Broe, MD, PhD   *Professor Emeritus, Faculty of
Medicine, University of Antwerp, Wilrijk, Belgium*

James A. Delmez, MD   *Professor of Medicine, Renal Division,
Washington University School of Medicine; Physician, Renal
Division, Barnes-Jewish Hospital, St. Louis, Missouri*

Thomas Depner, MD   *Professor of Medicine, Department of
Internal Medicine, University of California, Davis; Director of
Dialysis Services, Department of Internal Medicine, University
of California Davis Medical Center, Sacramento,
California*

Patrick C. D'Haese, PhD   *Faculty of Medicine, University of
Antwerp, Wilrijk, Belgium*

Steven Fishbane, MD   *Professor of Medicine, State University of New York at Stony Brook, School of Medicine, Stony Brook, New York; Chief, Department of Nephrology, Winthrop University Hospital, Mineola, New York*

Michael J. Flanigan, MD   *Emeritus Professor of Medicine, Division of Nephrology, University of Iowa Carver College of Medicine, Iowa City, Iowa; Staff Physician, Division of Nephrology and Hypertension, Marshfield Clinic–Lakeland, Minocqua, Wisconsin*

Eli A. Friedman, MD, MACP   *Distinguished Teaching Professor of Medicine, Department of Medicine, Downstate Medical Center; Director, Division of Renal Disease, Department of Medicine, University Hospital of Brooklyn, Brooklyn, New York*

Susan Grossman, MD   *Associate Professor of Clinical Medicine, Department of Internal Medicine, New York College of Medicine, Valhalla, New York; Chief, Nephrology Division, Vice Chair, Department of Medicine, St. Vincent's Staten Island, Staten Island, New York*

Raymond M. Hakim, MD, PhD   *Adjunct Professor of Medicine, Vanderbilt University; Chief Medical Officer, Renal Care Group, Nashville, Tennessee*

Olof Heimbürger, MD, PhD   *Division of Renal Medicine, Department of Clinical Science, Intervention, and Technology, Karolinska Institute; Senior Physician and Director of Peritoneal Dialysis, Department of Renal Medicine, Karolinska University Hospital, Stockholm, Sweden*

Joachim Hertel, MD, FACP   *Attending Physician, Department of Medicine, University Hospital, Augusta, Georgia*

Nicholas Hoenich, PhD   *Lecturer, School of Clinical Medical Sciences, Newcastle University, Newcastle upon Tyne, United Kingdom*

Vicenzio Holder-Perkins, MD, MPH   *Assistant Clinical Professor, Department of Psychiatry and Behavioral Sciences, George Washington University, School of Medicine, Washington, District of Columbia; Assistant Clinical Professor, Department of Psychiatry, INOVA Fairfax Hospital, Falls Church, Virginia*

Susan Hou, MD   *Professor of Medicine, Department of Medicine, Stritch School of Medicine, Loyola University Chicago, Maywood, Illinois*

T. Alp Ikizler, MD   *Associate Professor of Medicine, Department of Medicine and Nephrology, Vanderbilt University Medical Center, Nashville, Tennessee*

Todd S. Ing, MD   *Professor Emeritus of Medicine, Department of Medicine, Stritch School of Medicine, Loyola University Chicago, Maywood, Illinois; Physician, Veterans Affairs Hospital, Hines, Illinois*

Nuhad Ismail, MD   *Associate Professor of Medicine, Department of Medicine, Division of General Internal Medicine, Vanderbilt University School of Medicine, Nashville, Tennessee*

Ravi Jayakaran, (MSc) B Tech (SA), B Ed, Pg DDT (Ind),   *Honorary Lecturer, Faculty of Health Sciences, Durban University of Technology, Durban, South Africa; Chief Clinical Technologist, Department of Nephrology, Johannesburg Hospital, Johannesburg, Gateng, South Africa*

Allen M. Kaufman, MD   *Associate Professor of Medicine, Albert Einstein College of Medicine, Bronx, New York; Attending Physician, Department of Medicine, Beth Israel Medical Center, New York, New York*

Jonathan Kay, MD   *Associate Clinical Professor of Medicine, Department of Medicine, Harvard Medical School; Director, Clinical Trials, Rheumatology Unit, Department of Medicine, Massachusetts General Hospital, Boston, Massachusetts*

D. Kayichian, MD   *Assistant Clinical Professor of Medicine, Department of Medicine, University of California at Irvine School of Medicine, Orange, California*

Paul L. Kimmel, MD   *Professor, Department of Medicine, George Washington University; Attending Physician, Department of Medicine, George Washington University Hospital, Washington, District of Columbia*

Dobri D. Kiprov, MD, HP   *Chief, Division of Immunotherapy, Department of Medicine, California Pacific Medical Center, San Francisco, California*

Petras V. Kisielius, MD, FACS   *Attending Physician, Department of Urology, Elmhurst Memorial Hospital, Elmhurst, Illinois*

Chagriya Kitiyakara, MD, BS, MRCP (UK)   *Associate Professor, Department of Medicine, Ramathibodi Hospital, Mahidol University, Bangkok, Thailand*

Stephen M. Korbet, MD   *Professor of Medicine, Department of Internal Medicine, Rush University Medical Center, Chicago, Illinois*

Detlef Krieter, MD *Senior Research Fellow, Department of Medicine, Division of Nephrology, University Hospital Würzburg; Nephrologist, Department of Medicine, Division of Nephrology, University Hospital Würzburg, Würzburg, Germany*

Victoria Kumar, MD *Associate Professor of Medicine, Department of Medicine, University of California Davis Medical Center, Davis, California*

Kar Neng Lai, MD, DSc *Yu Chiu Kwong Chair Professor of Medicine, Department of Medicine, University of Hong Kong; Chief of Medicine, Department of Medicine, Queen Mary Hospital, Hong Kong*

David J. Leehey, MD *Professor, Department of Medicine, Loyola University Medical Center, Maywood, Illinois; Staff Physician, Department of Medicine, Veterans Affairs Hospital, Hines, Illinois*

Joseph R. Lentino, MD, PhD *Professor, Department of Medicine, Loyola University Stritch School of Medicine, Maywood, Illinois; Chief, Infectious Diseases Section, Department of Medicine–Neurology Service, Veterans Affairs Hospital, Hines, Illinois*

Nathan W. Levin, MD *Professor of Clinical Medicine, Albert Einstein College of Medicine, Bronx, New York; Medical and Research Director, Department of Nephrology, Renal Research Institute, New York, New York*

Robert Levin *Corporate Technical Director, Renal Research Institute, New York, New York*

Susie Q. Lew, MD, FACP, FASN *Professor of Medicine, Department of Medicine, Geroge Washington University; Attending Physician, Department of Medicine, George Washington University, Washington, District of Columbia*

Philip Kam-Tao Li MD, FRCP, FACP *Professor, Department of Medicine and Therapeutics, Chinese University of Hong Kong; Chief of Nephrology and Consultant, Department of Medicine and Therapeutics, Prince of Wales Hospital, Shatin, Hong Kong*

Victoria S. Lim, MD *Professor, Department of Internal Medicine, College of Medicine; Staff Physician, Department of Internal Medicine, University of Iowa Hospitals and Clinics, Iowa City, Iowa*

Robert M. Lindsay, MD, FRCPC, FRCP (Edin), FRCP (Glasg), FACP *Professor of Medicine, Department of Medicine, University of Western Ontario School of Medicine, London, Ontario, Canada*

Susan R. Mendley, MD   *Associate Professor, Department of Pediatrics and Medicine, University of Maryland; Director, Department of Pediatric Nephrology, University of Maryland Hospital for Children, Baltimore, Maryland*

Jennifer S. Messer, CHT, OCDT, CCNT   *ICU Nephrology Technologist, Department of Nephrology and Hypertension, The Cleveland Clinic, Cleveland, Ohio*

Madhukar Misra, MD, FASN, FACP, FRCP (UK)   *Associate Professor, Department of Internal Medicine, Division of Nephrology, University of Missouri Columbia, Columbia, Missouri*

Gihad E. Nesrallah, MD, FRCPC, FACP   *Adjunct Professor of Medicine, University of Western Ontario, London, Ontario; Staff Nephrologist, Division of Nephrology, Humber River Regional Hospital, Toronto, Ontario, Canada*

Anthony J. Nicholls, MB, FRCP   *Honorary Professor of Medicine, Peninsula Medical School; Consultant Nephrologist, Kidney Unit, Royal Devon and Exeter Hospital, Exeter, United Kingdom*

Allen R. Nissenson, MD, FACP   *Professor of Medicine, Department of Nephrology, University of California, Los Angeles; Director, Dialysis Program, Department of Nephrology, David Geffen School of Medicine, Los Angeles, California*

Chima Oleru, MD   *Fellow in Nephrology, Division of Nephrology and Hypertension, Beth Israel Medical Center, New York, New York*

Emil P. Paganini, MD, FACP, FRCPC   *Professor of Medicine, Department of Nephrology and Hypertension; Section Head, Department of Dialysis and Extracorporeal Therapy, The Cleveland Clinic, Cleveland, Ohio*

Biff F. Palmer, MD   *Professor of Internal Medicine, Director, Renal Fellowship Program, Department of Internal Medicine, Division of Nephrology, University of Texas Southwestern Medical School, Dallas, Texas*

Shona Pendse, MD, MMSc   *Instructor in Medicine, Department of Medicine, Harvard Medical School; Associate Physician, Renal Division, Brigham and Women's Hospital, Boston, Massachusetts*

Andreas Pierratos, MD, FRCPC   *Associate Professor, Department of Medicine, University of Toronto, Toronto, Ontario; Nephrologist, Department of Nephrology, Humber River Regional Hospital, Weston, Ontario, Canada*

Mark R. Pressman, PhD   *Clinical Professor of Medicine, Department of Medicine, Jefferson Medical College, Philadelphia, Pennsylvania; Director, Sleep Medicine Services, Lankenau Hospital, Wynnewood, Pennsylvania*

Sarah S. Prichard, MD   *Vice President, Global Medical/Clinical Affairs and Research, Baxter Healthcare–Renal, McGaw Park, Illinois*

Michael V. Rocco, MD   *Professor, Department of Internal Medicine and Nephrology, Wake Forest University School of Medicine; Nephrologist, Department of Internal Medicine and Nephrology, North Carolina Baptist Hospital, Winston-Salem, North Carolina*

Edward A. Ross, MD   *Associate Professor, Division of Nephrology, Hypertension, and Transplantation, University of Florida; Director, End-Stage Renal Disease Program, Division of Nephrology, Hypertension, and Transplantation, University of Florida and Shands Hospital, Gainesville, Florida*

Mark J. Sarnak, MD, MS   *Associate Professor, Department of Medicine, Division of Nephrology, Tufts-New England Medical Center; Associate Director, Research Training Program, Tufts-New England Medical Center, Boston, Massachusetts*

Richard A. Sherman, MD   *Professor of Medicine, Department of Medicine, Division of Nephrology, UMDNJ-Robert Wood Johnson Medical School; Robert Wood Johnson University Hospital, New Brunswick, New Jersey*

Ajay Singh, MD, MB, MRCP   *Associate Professor of Medicine, Harvard Medical School; Clinical Chief and Physician, Renal Division, Brigham and Women's Hospital, Boston, Massachusetts*

Rita S. Suri, MD, FRCPC, FACP   *Assistant Professor, Department of Medicine, University of Western Ontario; Nephrologist, Department of Medicine, London Health Sciences Center, University of Western Ontario, London, Ontario, Canada*

Cheuk-Chun Szeto, MD, FRCP (Edin)   *Senior Lecturer, Department of Medicine and Therapeutics, The Chinese University of Hong Kong; Senior Lecturer, Department of Medicine and Therapeutics, Prince of Wales Hospital, Shatin, Hong Kong*

Boon Wee Teo, MD   *Assistant Professor, Department of Medicine, Yong Loo Lin School of Medicine, National University of Singapore; Associate Consultant, Department of Medicine, National University Hospital, Singapore*

Antonios H. Tzamaloukas, MD   *Professor, Department of Medicine, University of New Mexico School of Medicine; Chief, Renal Section, Medicine Service (111C), New Mexico Veterans Affairs Health Care System, Albuquerque, New Mexico*

N. D. Vaziri, MD, MACP   *Professor of Medicine, Physiology and Biophysics, Department of Medicine, University of California Irvine, Irvine, California; Chief, Division of Nephrology and Hypertension, Department of Medicine and Nephrology, University of California, Irvine Medical Center, Orange, California*

Richard A. Ward, PhD   *Kidney Disease Program, University of Louisville, Louisville, Kentucky*

Daniel E. Weiner, MD, MS   *Assistant Professor of Medicine, Tufts University School of Medicine; Nephrologist, Associate Medical Director, DCI-Boston, Division of Nephrology, Tufts-New England Medical Center, Boston, Massachusetts*

James F. Winchester, MD, FRCP (Glas), FACP   *Professor of Clinical Medicine, Department of Medicine, Albert Einstein College of Medicine, Bronx, New York; Chief, Division of Nephrology, Beth Israel Medical Center, New York, New York*

Jack Work, MD,   *Professor, Department of Medicine, Emory University, Atlanta, Georgia*

Edward T. Zawada, MD, MACP   *Professor Emeritus of Medicine, Department of Medicine, University of South Dakota School of Medicine, Sioux Falls, South Dakota*

Carmine Zoccali, MD, FASN   *Postgraduate Professor of Nephrology, Messina, Cataria and Palermo Universities; Director, Renal, Hypertension, and Transplant Unit, Reggio Cal Hospital; Research Group Leader, (Clinical Epidemiology and Pathophysiology of Renal Diseases and Hypertension, CNR-IBIM, National Research Council of Italy), Reggio Cal, Italy*

Preface

It has been 5 years since the third edition of the *Handbook of Dialysis* was first printed, and since that time, translations have appeared in many languages, including Chinese, Japanese, and Russian. We are particularly gratified by the strong international interest in this text. In putting together this fourth edition, we were most respectful of the concept that nephrology is now very much international. KDOQI guidelines are being incorporated into KDIGO, and practice patterns are becoming more uniform. Differences between US and international nephrology remain, but the international experience is enriching our knowledge and practice base. Given this strong international interest, in this fourth edition, all measurement values and examples were given both in English units and SI values. A chapter is included on hemodiafiltration, which remains a niche therapy for chronic treatment in the United States, but which is much more widely used in the rest of the developed world.

Since the third edition, progress in dialysis has been incremental. Much more attention is being paid to predialysis, stage 1-4, CKD (chronic kidney disease). Accordingly, this area is covered in more depth. In previous versions, issues pertaining to water treatment for dialysis had only been summarized. In this edition, particularly with suggestions that patient results improve with use of ultrapure dialysate, more extended discussion is provided. Much progress has also been made in the field of obtaining vascular access, especially in methods of assuring arteriovenous fistulas for patients who previously might have received either venous catheters or grafts. These sections were entirely rewritten, and access was divided into two separate chapters, one focusing on catheters and one on fistulas and grafts.

The use of continuous therapies has undergone much simplification due to availability of new machines. Some of the earlier, do-it-yourself approaches to CRRT were accordingly deleted. We added a chapter on how to provide short daily and long nocturnal dialysis, a requirement as more frequent dialysis schedules become more popular both in the United States and abroad. Advances in the area of peritoneal dialysis have been gradual since the appearance of the third edition. Providers have become perhaps less interested in quantification of dose and more concerned about glycemic load and ultrafiltration, and now new PD solutions using alternative osmotic agents are widely available. Our European colleagues were particularly helpful in reviewing this area. Knowledge of bone disease and methods to control both hyperphosphatemia and hyperparathyroidism has grown enormously since the third edition, and this new information, including the latest guidelines, is emphasized. In each chapter, we have tried to incorporate the latest information available and to include information in the 2006 KDOQI guideline updates. Web links at the end of many chapters will help ensure that the book remains current as new findings and treatments emerge in the years to come.

Although a flood of information has become available pertaining to all aspects of medicine, we have tried to maintain the unique character of the *Handbook of Dialysis*, explaining each area from the basics, but then progressing to an advanced level of understanding, and keeping the discussion at a practical level, realizing that texts like the *Handbook of Dialysis* are often relied upon by both new and experienced nephrology care providers to help them in their difficult job of providing the best care for our patients.

John T. Daugirdas, MD
Peter G. Blake, MB, FRCPC, FRCPI
Todd S. Ing, MD

Handbook of Dialysis

Chronic Kidney Disease Management

Approach to Patients with Chronic Kidney Disease, Stages 1–4

Shona S. Pendse and Ajay Singh

I. Why identify and treat patients with chronic kidney disease (CKD)? One may find a correctible cause. By mitigating one or more risk factors, one may be able to slow progression of renal disease or reduce cardiovascular risk.

II. Stages of CKD. The National Kidney Foundation's (NKF) Kidney Disease Outcome Quality Initiative (KDOQI) has suggested staging CKD from stage 1 (mildest) to stage 5 (most severe) based on the level of estimated glomerular filtration rate (GFR) normalized to body surface area. The two mildest stages—stages 1 and 2, in which the GFR is still above 60 mL per minute per 1.73 m^2—require evidence for kidney damage apart from reduced GFR. Kidney damage can be manifest as pathologic changes on kidney biopsy; abnormalities in the composition of the blood or urine, such as, for urine, proteinuria or changes in the urine sediment examination; or abnormalities in imaging tests. The more severe stages of CKD—stages 3, 4, and 5—are present by definition when the GFR is below 60, 30, and 15, respectively (Table 1-1).

III. Screening for CKD
Screening should include monitoring for the presence of proteinuria and measurement of kidney function.

A. Urinary protein measurement. The American Diabetes Association (ADA) recommends that an evaluation for microalbuminuria be performed in all type 2 diabetics at the time of diagnosis and in all type 1 diabetics 5 years after initial evaluation. Others who should be screened include patients with hypertension or heart failure, or those with any disease known to impact kidney function.

A urine dipstick examination should be performed on a random or "spot" urine. The dipstick used should be able to detect both albumin and evidence of blood or white cells. If the urine dipstick is positive for albumin, a spot protein-to-creatinine ratio on a urine sample should be measured. If the dipstick test suggests either blood or white cell activity, then a microscopic analysis should be performed of the urinary sediment.

B. Measuring GFR. The recommended approach to measuring GFR is to use an estimating equation based on the serum creatinine level.

1. Modification of Diet in Renal Disease (MDRD) equation: GFR = 186 × [SCr]$^{-1.154}$ × [Age]$^{-0.203}$ × [0.742 if patient is female] × [1.210 if patient is black]. This equation

Table 1-1.   Kidney disease outcomes quality initiative suggested stages of chronic kidney disease

Stage	Description	GFR[a]	Population	Prevalence
1	Kidney damage with normal or supranormal GFR	≥90	5,900,000	3.3%
2	Kidney damage with mild decrease in GFR	60–89	5,300,000	3.0%
3	Moderate decrease in GFR	30–59	7,600,000	4.3%
4	Severe decrease in GFR	15–29	400,000	0.2%
5	Kidney failure	<15	300,000	0.2%

GFR, glomerular filtration rate.
[a] GFR expressed in mL per minute per 1.73 m^2.

was derived from the MDRD trial and reports GFR normalized to body surface area. There are several more complex equations derived from the same study that contain additional variables, but consensus has emerged that this parsimonious equation is to be preferred. *In 2006 the National Kidney Disease Education Program (NKDEP) issued guidelines for standardizing serum creatinine methods based on isotope dilution mass spectrometry (IDMS). IDMS-standardized serum creatinines are slightly different than those values that were used to derive the MDRD equation (Levey et al., 2006). For laboratories using the new IDMS-standardized serum creatinine values, the "186" term in the equation above should be set to "175" instead. When serum creatinine is measured in SI units (mcmol/L), one needs to divide the creatinine value by 88.5, and then the equation with either the 186 or 175 multiplier can be used as listed.* The MDRD equation differs from the previously dominant Cockcroft and Gault formula, which, in its usual form, simply predicts the creatinine clearance not normalized to body surface area. The Cockcroft and Gault formula overestimates GFR in the lower range, due to increased tubular secretion of creatinine. A number of papers have suggested alternative methods for estimating GFR, including use of equations based on serum cystatin level, which is not confounded by muscle mass or dietary creatine intake. However, the MDRD equation is the most popular validated equation in current use.

2.   Urinary clearance measurements. There are some situations where a serum creatinine level is not reflective of GFR, and this includes patients who have markedly reduced creatinine generation rates due to muscle wasting and patients with cirrhosis (muscle wasting plus inability to determine ascites-free body weight for normalization). In such cases the serum creatinine can overestimate the GFR, and a 24-hour urine collection should be done if practical. There are difficulties with 24-hour urine creatinine measurements as well, however, and these include variations in urine collection (i.e., incorrect collections) and variations in the tubular secretion of creatinine.

Creatinine clearance overestimates GFR because creatinine is both filtered by the glomerulus and, to a lesser degree, secreted by the proximal tubule. On the other hand, urea clearance underestimates GFR since it is both filtered and reabsorbed. For this reason one can estimate GFR as the mean value of the creatinine and urea clearances at low (<15) values of GFR.

Another approach is to measure creatinine clearance but to perform the 24-hour urine collection after oral administration of **cimetidine,** an organic cation that competitively inhibits tubular secretion of creatinine.

C.   Ultrasound and serum electrolytes. In patients found to have CKD, one should image the kidneys, commonly by ultrasound, to look for structural abnormalities and possible obstruction and measure serum electrolytes (Na, K, Cl, HCO_3) to screen for metabolic acidosis and electrolyte disorders, the presence of which may give clues to an underlying renal disease.

IV.   Mitigating risk of progression of CKD and of cardiovascular disease. In CKD patients, risk factors for progression of renal disease are very similar to those associated with increased cardiovascular risk. One purpose of identifying CKD patients early on is to attempt to correct and/or mitigate such risk factors, in the hopes of both maintaining GFR and minimizing cardiovascular risk. The main risk factors include smoking, high blood pressure, hyperglycemia in diabetics (and perhaps in nondiabetics as well), elevated blood lipid levels, anemia, and elevated serum phosphorus levels. Urinary protein excretion and even microalbuminuria markedly increase both the risk of progression and cardiovascular complications. Levels of inflammatory mediators, notably C-reactive protein (CRP), are increased in CKD and are associated with increased atherosclerotic risk.

A.   Cessation of smoking. Smoking is a traditional cardiovascular risk factor, and cessation of smoking is important in terms of limiting cardiovascular risk. Recent evidence suggests that smoking markedly accelerates the rate of progression of renal disease, emphasizing the importance of stopping smoking by CKD patients.

B.   Control of blood pressure and proteinuria. The target blood pressure should be <130/80 for all patients with kidney disease, diabetics and nondiabetics, regardless of degree of proteinuria (according to the 2003 KDOQI). Whether or not hypertension is present, use of an angiotensin-converting enzyme inhibitor/angiotensin receptor blocker (ACE-I/ARB) is recommended to slow the rate of progression in patients with diabetic kidney disease as well as in nondiabetic CKD patients with proteinuria (spot urine protein-to-creatinine ratio of $\geq$200 mg/g). Thiazide diuretics are the diuretic of choice for mild CKD, when S_{Cr} is <1.8 mg/dL (<160 mcmol/L). When S_{Cr} is >1.8 mg/dL (>160 mcmol/L), a loop diuretic (twice-a-day dosing regimen) is recommended, due to presumed reduced efficacy of thiazides under those circumstances; however, lack of efficacy of thiazides in patients with reduced GFR has been challenged (Dussol et al., 2005).

Doses of ACE-Is/ARBs can be titrated up to minimize proteinuria, but blood pressure, potassium, and creatinine should be monitored after initiation of therapy and after each dose change. Sodium restriction and use of diuretics increase the antiproteinuric effects of ACE-I/ARB therapy. ACE-Is or ARBs are contraindicated in patients who are pregnant, particularly beyond the first trimester, and in patients with a history of angioedema. For patients with an estimated GFR >15 mL per minute per 1.73 m^2, one rarely needs to adjust the dose of antihypertensive drugs downward due to impaired renal excretion, although the plasma half-life of some classes of antihypertensives will be increased (see Chapter 31).

C. Beta-blockers and aspirin: Cardioprotective effects. The cardioprotective effects of beta-blockers are not diminished in CKD patients. Aspirin and beta-blocker cardioprotection after myocardial infarction is similar in CKD patients and in patients with normal renal function (Shlipak et al., 2002). Because most CKD patients, especially in stage 3 and higher, tend to have cardiac disease, a case can be made for routinely treating such patients with both aspirin and beta-blockers, although this is not widely practiced at all centers. Aspirin has been associated with GI bleeding in endstage renal disease (ESRD) patients. Whether an increased risk is present in stage 1 to 4 CKD patients is not well known.

D. Strict glycemic control in diabetics with CKD. The DCCT and UKPDS studies for type 1 and type 2 diabetics, respectively, have unequivocally demonstrated that tight glycemic control slows the development of microvascular and macrovascular disease. Tight glycemic control also slows the rate of progression of renal disease in diabetics with CKD. Interestingly, glycosylated hemoglobin is a predictor of mortality even in nondiabetic CKD patients. The goal of glycemic control should be a HbA1C of <7.0%.

E. Lipid-lowering therapy. Elevated levels of low-density lipoprotein cholesterol (LDL-C) and other lipid marker molecules are a traditional risk factor for cardiovascular disease, and the cardioprotective effects of statins in non-CKD patients, even when cholesterol levels are in the normal range, have been described in several studies. Also, data in animals suggest that high lipid levels and cholesterol loading may augment glomerular injury. Thus, treatment of CKD patients with statins to reduce lipids may both prevent progression and lower cardiovascular risk. Guidelines of when and how to treat elevated lipid levels in non-CKD patients (National Cholesterol Education Program/ATP III) recommend initiation of lifestyle changes and then pharmacologic therapy, based on different LDL-C levels stratified by level of cardiovascular risk; for patients with a high number of traditional cardiovascular risk factors, an LDL-C goal of <100 mg/dL (<2.6 mmol/L) is recommended. Drug therapy is recommended when LDL-C levels are >130 mg/dL (3.4 mmol/L) and is optional when LDL-C levels are between 100 and 130 mg/dL (2.6 and 3.4 mmol/L). Higher goal levels of LDL-C,

130 mg/dL or 160 mg/dL (3.4 or 4.2 mmol/L), are allowed in patients with more than two or less than two cardiovascular risk factors, respectively. CKD patients can logically be treated according to the same scheme; most of them will have a number of both traditional and nontraditional risk factors, and so target LDL-C levels should generally be <100 mg/dL (2.6 mmol/L). Additionally, fibrate therapy should be considered for isolated hypertriglyceridemia. For a more complete discussion of treatment of dyslipidemias in stage 5 (ESRD) patients, see Chapter 37.

   1. Statins: Cardioprotective effects. The cardioprotective effects of statins, well-documented in nonuremic patients, are controversial in CKD. It may depend on the level of renal failure. In diabetics, use of statins was cardioprotective in pre-ESRD patients (Collaborative Atorvastatin Diabetes Study [CARDS] trial: Colhoun et al., 2004; Tonelli et al., 2005) but had no benefit in patients already on dialysis (4D study: Wanner et al., 2004).

      a. Dose adjustment for renal insufficiency. Statins as a class have been associated with rhabdomyolysis, and dose reduction in severe renal impairment is recommended for some statins (e.g., rosuvastatin) or when statins are used in combination with fibrates (Chapter 37).

F. Correction of anemia. Anemia is common in stage 3 CKD patients. Many of these patients also have some degree of heart failure. Across the spectrum of CKD, the risk of left ventricular hypertrophy (LVH) increases progressively as renal function worsens. In patients with heart failure, anemia treatment markedly improves both laboratory and clinical measures of functioning. Whether or not early correction of anemia retards or prevents the development of LVH in CKD patients is not well settled at this time, but there are data to suggest that this may be the case. Furthermore, anemia treatment with erythropoietin may decrease the rate of progression of kidney disease (Gouva et al., 2004).

   1. When to treat and to what hemoglobin (Hb) level. Diagnosis and management of anemia is similar to that in ESRD patients, and is discussed in detail in Chapter 32. The NKF KDOQI guidelines recommend that erythropoietin therapy should be started when the hemoglobin falls below 10 g/dL (100 g/L). The goal of therapy should be to maintain the hemoglobin between 11 and 12 g/dL (110 and 120 g/L). Two recent randomized trials found either no benefit (Drüeke et al., 2006), or increased cardiovascular risk (Singh et al., 2006) when a Hb of greater than 13 g/dL (130 g/L) was targeted, and the United States FDA has issued an alert suggesting that Hb levels greater than 12 g/dL (120 g/L) should generally be avoided.

   2. Iron management. Evaluation of iron profile should be performed to ensure that the patient is iron replete, since exogenous erythropoietin will result in increased iron utilization. Routine measurement of erythropoietin levels is not recommended. One issue is whether CKD patients not yet on dialysis require IV iron. Such patients are not losing as much blood as ESRD patients on hemodialysis, given the absence of regular hemodialysis procedures, less frequent blood sampling, and perhaps less gastrointestinal (GI) irritation and GI blood loss. In one study of CKD patients (mean GFR 30 mL per minute, with percent transferrin saturation [TSAT] <25% and serum ferritin <300 ng/mL), use of IV iron was more effective in correcting anemia than use of oral iron (Van Wyck et al., 2005).

G. Control of serum phosphorus, vitamin D, and parathyroid hormone. The phosphorus–vitamin D–parathyroid axis should be monitored and, when needed, corrected in CKD patients, because derangements of these interacting measures can be associated with progression of cardiovascular disease (in terms of LVH and vascular calcification) as well as progression of renal disease. Also, left untreated, hyperphosphatemia and low levels of 1,25-dihydroxyvitamin D_3 (1,25-D) will lead to secondary hyperparathyroidism and associated bone disease. The management of serum phosphorus, vitamin D, and parathyroid hormone levels in dialysis patients is fully discussed in Chapter 35 and only issues pertinent to CKD will be discussed here.

1. Hyperphosphatemia. High serum phosphorus levels are a risk factor for mortality and adverse cardiovascular outcomes in both CKD and ESRD patients. Even in nonuremic patients, mild serum phosphorus elevations are associated with increased cardiovascular risk. Hyperphosphatemia is associated with increased risk of vascular calcification, and has been implicated in LVH in ESRD. In a number of experimental renal failure models, hyperphosphatemia accelerates progression of renal failure as well. Apart from all this, there is the well-documented stimulatory effect of hyperphosphatemia on the parathyroid gland growth and on parathyroid hormone secretion.

a. Dietary management. Management includes a careful dietary review to look for abnormally high consumption of foods rich in phosphate, including dairy products, certain colas, and processed meats. Phosphate intake should be restricted to 800–1,000 mg per day (26–32 mmol/L per day).

b. Target serum phosphorus levels. In patients with CKD stages 3 and 4 the target serum phosphorus should be maintained between 2.7 and 4.6 mg/dL (0.9 and 1.5 mmol/L). In patients with stage 5 CKD and those on dialysis, serum phosphorus should be maintained between 3.5 and 5.5 mg/dL (1.1 and 1.8 mmol/L). Serum phosphorus levels should be checked monthly upon initiation of phosphorus restriction.

c. Phosphorus binders. Phosphorus binders may need to be used. The choices are described in Chapter 35. It is prudent to restrict total calcium intake in CKD patients to about 1500 mg per day (37 mmol/L per day) (KDOQI guidelines are less restrictive, and suggest a ceiling of 2000 mg per day [50 mmol/L per day]), to minimize the risk of vascular calcification. This means that if calcium salts are used as phosphorus binders, they may need to be combined with either sevelamer, lanthanum, or, possibly, magnesium. Aluminum-containing phosphorus binders generally should not be used. Use of sevelamer as a phosphorus binder has been shown to perhaps stabilize the rate of vascular calcification in CKD patients and to improve outcomes, although studies are not definitive in this area. It has been argued that if there is a beneficial effect, it may be due partially to the lipid-lowering effects of sevelamer. This remains an active area of ongoing research.

2. Serum calcium levels and calcium × phosphorus product. In patients with CKD stages 3 and 4, corrected calcium levels should be maintained within the "normal" range for the laboratory being used. In patients with CKD stage 5, serum levels of total calcium should be maintained toward the lower values of the normal range of the laboratory being used (8.4–9.5 mg/dL [2.1–2.4 mmol/L]). The target calcium × phosphorus product is below 55 mg^2/dL^2 (4.4 mmol^2/L^2), although even lower may be better.

3. Serum parathyroid hormone levels. Control of serum parathyroid hormone (PTH) levels is important to minimize the degree of parathyroid gland hypertrophy (and the risk of developing large, nonsuppressible glands). Hyperparathyroidism is associated with bone disease, and PTH may also act as a uremic toxin with adverse effects on many different organ systems. The control of PTH secretion is detailed in Chapter 35. PTH secretion can be reduced by avoiding hyperphosphatemia. Previous recommendations to maintain serum calcium at the high end of the normal range to ensure PTH suppression have been replaced by a strategy of keeping serum calcium toward the middle or low range of normal, to minimize the risk of vascular calcification. 1,25-Vitamin D suppresses PTH, and one needs to make sure that CKD patients are vitamin D replete, with use of active vitamin D compounds in stage 4 and higher CKD. Calcium receptor sensitizers such as cinacalcet can suppress PTH secretion as well and may be useful as adjunctive therapy.

   a. Frequency of measurement. The 2003 NKF KDOQI clinical practice guidelines for bone metabolism and disease in CKD recommend measuring PTH levels, as well as serum calcium and phosphorus, in all patients with a GFR <60 mL per minute per 1.73 m^2. The frequency of these measurements should be every 12 months for normalized GFR values >30 mL per minute, and every 3 months when normalized GFR is between 15 and 30.

   b. Target range of PTH. The intact PTH assay has been available since 1990 and identifies both 1–84 and 7–84 PTH, and most bone biopsy studies have employed this assay. Bio-intact PTH, also known as biPTH or whole PTH, is a newer assay that detects only the 1–84 PTH, resulting in values about 50%–55% of intact PTH values. Either assay can be employed for diagnosis and treatment of hyperparathyroidism in CKD, but the target PTH

Table 1-2. Target PTH values for various stages of CKD

CKD Stage	GFR Range	Intact PTH	Bio-intact PTH	Intact PTH	Bio-intact PTH
	mL per minute per 1.73 m^2	pg/mL		pmol/L	
3	30–59	35–70	18–35	3.7–7.4	1.9–3.7
4	15–29	70–110	35–55	7.4–11.6	3.7–5.8
5	<15 or dialysis	150–300	80–160	16–32	8.4–17

range will depend on the assay employed. As CKD progresses, the bone becomes resistant to the actions of PTH; therefore, the target PTH range increases. The KDOQI recommendations for target PTH based on stage of CKD and type of PTH assay are shown in Table 1-2.

4.   Vitamin D. In CKD patients, 25-D levels are quite low, probably because of lack of sunlight exposure and low ingestion of vitamin D–containing foods. As CKD progresses, the rate of conversion of 25-D to 1,25-D by the 1-α-hydroxylase enzyme diminishes, and even with adequate 25-D levels, serum 1–25-D levels may be reduced and PTH suppression may be inadequate. Vitamin D affects multiple organ systems, most of these effects being beneficial, although excess vitamin D has been associated with vascular calcification and even accelerated renal failure. The 1-α-hydroxylase enzyme exists in various tissues, suggesting that it may be important to ensure proper levels of both 25-D and 1,25-D in the circulation for optimum health. Recently active vitamin D sterol administration has been linked to improved survival and improved cardiovascular outcomes in ESRD patients. The mechanism of this survival benefit is not clear, and these are observational studies that need to be confirmed.

a.   Target serum levels of 25-D in CKD. Serum levels of 25-D should be at least 30 ng/mL (75 nmol/L). Low serum levels of 25-D have been linked to severe muscle weakness in elderly nonuremic patients. Because CKD patients typically have very low levels of 25-D in the serum, for primary prevention, CKD patients should be supplemented with at least 800 IU of cholecalciferol per day. Cholecalciferol is available in the United States only as an over-the-counter vitamin supplement. This level of cholecalciferol supplementation does not affect GI absorption of calcium or phosphorus. To treat a low serum 25-D level, the KDOQI guidelines recommend using ergocalciferol, which is slightly less effective than cholecalciferol, but which is available in the United States as a formulary drug.

b.   When to use active vitamin D preparations. In the more severe stages of CKD, conversion of 25-D to 1,25-D in the kidney becomes suboptimal, and even with adequate stores of 25-D, the serum levels of 1,25-D may be low and PTH may not be adequately suppressed. In stage 3 and stage 4 CKD patients in whom serum PTH is above the target range despite adequate serum levels of 25-D, the use of an active vitamin D preparation is indicated. Choices and doses of active vitamin D preparations (e.g., calcitriol, paricalcitol, and doxercalciferol) are outlined in Chapter 35. As in ESRD patients, when active vitamin D sterols are being given, the dose should be held or reduced in the presence of hypercalcemia or hyperphosphatemia.

5. Cinacalcet. Cinacalcet is a calcimimetic drug that increases the sensitivity of calcium receptors on the parathyroid gland to calcium, resulting in a decrease in PTH secretion. One main advantage of cinacalcet is its use in patients with hyperparathyroidism and high serum calcium and/or phosphorus levels, where use of active vitamin D sterols to suppress PTH would be contraindicated (active vitamin D sterols increase GI absorption of phosphorus and may worsen hyperphosphatemia). Cinacalcet has been shown to lower PTH levels in stage 3 and 4 CKD patients (Charytan et al., 2005). The relative roles of cinacalcet versus active vitamin D sterols for PTH suppression in predialysis patients are not yet well defined, but there is no reason that cinacalcet should not be used in this population.

H. Protein restriction. One needs to apply judgment when restricting protein intake, especially in malnourished CKD patients. Patients who are malnourished at the start of dialysis have a poorer survival than their well-nourished counterparts, and restricting food choices always carries the risk of a worsening nutritional status. The evidence suggesting that protein restriction slows progression is there, but is not very strong. Recommendations do exist, however, to restrict protein intake to about 0.8 g/kg per day in all patients with CKD, with further restriction to 0.6 g/kg per day in those with a creatinine clearance <25 mL per minute (according to the KDOQI guidelines). Close follow-up for any evidence of malnutrition, either by clinical parameters or by serum albumin, is essential. Ideally a dietitian should be monitoring such patients carefully. The recommended caloric intake is 30–35 kcal/kg per day. In stage 4 and 5 patients, evidence of failing nutritional status is one key determinant in the decision to begin dialysis therapy.

I. Approach to obesity. One difficult question in CKD patients is how to approach obesity. In nonuremic patients obesity is associated with increased death rate, cardiovascular risk, and inflammatory mediator levels. Also, marked obesity per se may increase the degree of both proteinuria and accelerate the rate of progression of renal disease. In dialysis patients, probably due to a different risk environment, obesity does not appear to have much, if any, of an adverse effect on survival. So CKD patients with mildly increased levels of body mass index may not benefit from an aggressive weight loss reduction program. On the other hand, patients in the earlier stages of CKD, and especially those who are quite obese, should benefit from a lower weight.

J. Acidosis. Given that chronic metabolic acidosis results in increased resorption of bone, the use of sodium bicarbonate is recommended to maintain the serum bicarbonate level at ≥ 22 mmol/L. The usual amount of sodium bicarbonate to give is 0.5–1.0 mmol/L/kg per day.

K.   Microcrystalline charcoal. An avant-garde area of research suggests that certain toxins (e.g., indoles) that affect progression may derive from intestinal bacteria, and that absorbing such fibrogenic toxins, or else changing the bacterial flora so that less of these toxins are generated in the gut, might retard the rate of progression. Use of a microcrystalline charcoal adsorbent (Kremezin) has been shown to slow the rate of renal decline in humans in several small studies. In other, preliminary studies, use of certain bacteria to alter the gut microflora reduced the levels of indole-type compounds in the gut. Microcrystalline charcoal therapy is not currently available in the United States.

L.   Nephrology referral. Studies have also shown higher mortality rates among patients referred late compared to those referred early. It is not clear if these benefits are due to a selection bias, or if they are due to superior care provided by nephrologists. There are many potential treatment benefits associated with early referral to nephrology, including timely placement of vascular or peritoneal access, early institution of dietary counseling, and the early detection and management of hypertension, anemia, acidosis, and hyperphosphatemia. A multiple risk factor targeted disease management approach is recommended in CKD patients, irrespective of who is providing for their care.

M.   Management of later stages of CKD. Tasks here include preparation for dialysis; placement of vascular or peritoneal access; choosing the most appropriate mode and location of dialysis (i.e., peritoneal dialysis, outpatient hemodialysis center, home hemodialysis); vaccinations; continued nutritional management, particularly in terms of phosphorus control; and volume restriction. A key decision is when to initiate dialysis, and when, if appropriate, to do preemptive renal transplantation. These are discussed in the next chapter.

SELECTED READING

Charytan C, et al. Cinacalcet hydrochloride is an effective treatment for secondary hyperparathyroidism in patients with CKD not receiving dialysis. *Am J Kidney Dis* 2005;46(1):58–67.

Colhoun HM, et al. Primary prevention of cardiovascular disease with atorvastatin in type 2 diabetes in the Collaborative Atorvastatin Diabetes Study (CARDS): multicentre andomized placebo-controlled trial. *Lancet* 2004;364:685–696.

Coyne D, et al. Paricalcitol capsule for the treatment of secondary hyperparathyroidism in stages 3 and 4 CKD. *Am J Kidney Dis* 2006;47:263–276.

Drüeke TB, et al., for the CREATE Investigators. Normalization of Hemoglobin Level in Patients with Chronic Kidney Disease and Anemia. *N Engl J Med* 2006;355:2071–2084.

Dussol B, et al. A randomized trial of furosemide vs hydrochloro-thiazide in patients with chronic renal failure and hypertension. *Nephrol Dial Transplant* 2005;20(2):349–353.

Gouva C, et al. Treating anemia early in renal failure patients slows the decline of renal function: a randomized controlled trial. *Kidney Int* 2004;66(2):753–760.

LaClair RE, et al. Prevalence of calcidiol deficiency in CKD: a cross-sectional study across latitudes in the United States. *Am J Kidney Dis* 2006;45:1026–1033.

Levey AS, et al. Using standardized serum creatinine values in the modification of diet in renal disease study equation for estimating glomerular filtration rate. *Ann Intern Med* 2006;145(4):247–254.

Shlipak MG, et al. Association of renal insufficiency with treatment and outcomes after myocardial infarction in elderly patients. *Ann Intern Med* 2002;137(7):555–562.

Singh AK, et al., for the CHOIR Investigators. Correction of Ane-mia with Epoetin Alfa in Chronic Kidney Disease. *N Engl J Med* 2006;355:2085–2098.

Smith GL, et al. Serum urea nitrogen, creatinine, and estimators of renal function. Mortality in older patients with cardiovascular disease. *Arch Intern Med* 2006;166:1134–1142.

Stevens LA, et al. Assessing kidney function—measured and esti-mated glomerular filtration rate. *N Engl J Med* 2006;354:2473–2483.

Tonelli M, et al. Effect of pravastatin in people with diabetes and chronic kidney disease. *J Am Soc Nephrol* 2005;16(12):3748–3754.

Van Wyck DB, et al., for the United States Iron Sucrose (Venofer) Clinical Trials Group. A randomized, controlled trial comparing IV iron sucrose to oral iron in anemic patients with nondialysis-dependent CKD. *Kidney Int* 2005;68(6):2846–2856.

Wanner C, et al. Randomized controlled trial on the efficacy and safety of atorvastatin in patients with type 2 diabetes on hemodialysis (4D study): demographic and baseline characteristics. *Kidney Blood Press Res* 2004;27:259–266.

WEB REFERENCES

GFR clearance calculator: www.hdcn.com/calcf/gfr.htm

HDCN CKD channel: www.hdcn.com/ch/ckd/

Kidney Disease: Improving Global Outcomes (KDIGO): www.kdigo. org

U.S. National Kidney Foundation Kidney Disease Outcomes Quality Initiative (KDOQI): www.kdoqi.org

Initiation of Dialysis

Shona Pendse, Ajay Singh, and
Edward Zawada, Jr.

Once a patient has reached stage 4 chronic kidney disease (CKD) (estimated glomerular filtration rate [eGFR] of <30 mL per minute per 1.73 m^2), ideally he or she is under a nephrologist's care, and the risk factors associated with cardiovascular disease and progression described in Chapter 1 are being optimally managed. Survival of end-stage renal disease (ESRD) patients on dialysis depends to a large extent on their condition at the time dialysis was first initiated. Accordingly, it is important to pay attention to control of blood pressure, anemia, calcium/phosphorus intake, and nutrition during the predialysis period, as is timely insertion of an arteriovenous fistula if hemodialysis has been selected. When this is done using a multidisciplinary predialysis program that includes patient and family education, early choice of appropriate modality, and elective creation of dialysis access, the advantages have been fewer urgent dialyses, fewer hospital days in the first month after beginning dialysis, and substantial cost savings per patient at the time of commencing dialysis.

I. Choice of modality
A. Patient education. Of key importance is patient education about the various treatment options available in the event dialysis will become necessary. Would the patient best benefit from some form of dialysis, from pre-emptive transplantation, or from continued conservative management? In some cases, due to extreme patient debility or other reasons, dialysis may not be an appropriate option, and palliative care may be the best choice.
B. Options for renal replacement therapy
   1. Transplantation. It is clear that transplantation offers survival superior to the standard forms of dialysis being offered today. Transplantation may not be indicated, however, for a patient who has severe problems with compliance in terms of medications. Even if transplantation is decided upon as the best option, the question of timing remains. A short period of dialysis prior to transplantation does not adversely impact graft survival results (Goldfarb-Rumyantzev et al., 2005). Anecdotally, patients with immunologically mediated renal disease (e.g., vasculitis) sometimes benefit from a short period of dialysis prior to transplantation, presumably because an extended period of uremia serves to suppress the underlying autoimmune disease process.
   2. Dialysis: Home versus in-center therapy. Among the ESRD therapies, the choices made will depend on what is available in the local community. One of the main decisions to be made is whether the patient will be coming in

to a clinic for regular dialysis (hemodialysis in this case), or whether he or she would prefer the independence of dialyzing at home, using either a home hemodialysis system or peritoneal dialysis. Obviously transportation issues are very important here, as is the status of a patient's home, the amount of support available through interested family members who might assist as caregivers, and technical issues such as available water quality and electricity.

In observational studies, mortality rates are lower in home hemodialysis patients than in in-center hemodialysis patients, even after adjustments for common comorbidities. Some of this home dialysis advantage may be due to a patient selection bias. Mortality rates between in-center hemodialysis and peritoneal dialysis patients tend to be similar for the first few years, or mortality rates may even be a bit lower for peritoneal dialysis initially. After 2 years, mortality rates in peritoneal dialysis patients tend to be higher, especially for elderly diabetics and patients with cardiovascular comorbidities.

3. Short daily hemodialysis. Normally, whether done at home or in-center, hemodialysis therapy is offered three times per week, usually 3–4 hours per session. When the same amount of dialysis time is broken up into five or six sessions per week, a number of studies have shown a decrease in intradialytic symptoms, including hypotension and cramps. In some studies, nutritional and cardiovascular benefits also have been claimed, although there are very few randomized trials using substantial numbers of patients. The details of so-called short daily hemodialysis are discussed in Chapter 14. Usually this therapy is done at home, but sometimes it is offered in-center. Even though the dialysis session length is short, one needs to add machine setup and cleanup time, and for in-center treatment, one needs to also consider transportation and waiting time. Short daily hemodialysis is gaining in popularity, especially with the availability of machines dedicated to delivering such therapy in the home setting.

4. Long nocturnal hemodialysis. Whereas the number of hours spent per week on dialysis is usually similar or only slightly increased with short daily hemodialysis, with nocturnal dialysis, one enters another order of magnitude of dialysis hours per week. The nocturnal dialysis sessions are usually 8–10 hours in length. When given every other night, a therapy that can be delivered either at home or in-center, the weekly dialysis time is about 30 hours, compared to 12 hours in a usual three sessions × 4 hours dialysis schedule. Most patients on nocturnal hemodialysis dialyze 5–6 nights per week, giving 40–50 hours of treatment per week. Such frequent nocturnal dialysis is almost always done at home, and it is offered in a limited, if growing, number of locations across the United States.

5. Peritoneal dialysis. Due to its simplicity, peritoneal dialysis offers patients a home-based therapy with very little requirement for special water systems and simple equipment setup time. The percent of patients choosing peritoneal dialysis (PD) over hemodialysis is about 12% in the United States, and 20%–30% in Canada. There are two types of PD for a patient to consider: Continuous ambulatory peritoneal dialysis (CAPD), where a patient performs manual exchanges four or five times per day, and continuous cycling peritoneal dialysis (CCPD), where a patient hooks up to a machine at night and exchanges are carried out automatically while the patient sleeps. The relative benefits of each type of PD are discussed more fully in Chapters 19 and 22.

Patients for whom PD is often favored include:
1. Infants or very young children
2. Patients with severe cardiovascular disease
3. Patients with difficult vascular access (e.g., diabetics)
4. Patients who desire greater freedom to travel
5. Patients who wish to perform home dialysis but do not have a suitable partner to assist them

Contraindications include an unsuitable peritoneum due to presence of adhesions, fibrosis, or malignancy. Also, a substantial number of patients experience an increase in the membrane transport over time, resulting in either inadequate solute clearance or ultrafiltration. A consensus appears to be building that the glucose load supplied via PD may be excessive, particularly in diabetics, and diabetics tend to have a higher mortality when placed on PD versus hemodialysis. A major cause of abandonment of PD is the occurrence of frequent episodes of peritonitis, although patient burnout is also a factor.

PD tends to be less expensive than hemodialysis, particularly in developing countries. Also, it allows patients independence and freedom to travel and does not constrain patients to a fixed in-center dialysis schedule. On the other hand, PD may not be the best option for patients who don't have a "do-it-yourself" mentality, or who don't have the stability or social and family support at home to carry out a PD program. Some patients simply prefer a hemodialysis schedule of three or more well-defined periods per week during which they can get their dialysis "over with," leaving them free of any other dialysis responsibility.

There have been a number of improvements in peritoneal dialysis over the past several years, including better disconnect systems, resulting in decreased peritonitis rates. Also, with use of CCPD, there can be improved clearances. Finally, new PD solutions have become available, including glucose-based solutions with decreased amounts of glucose degradation products, as well as solutions using amino acids or icodextrin as the osmotic agent.

6. The option not to dialyze: Palliative care. There are no absolute contraindications to dialysis therapy. In some states legal precedent exists guaranteeing dialysis to anyone who desires it despite the severity of other medical problems. When a patient is unable to voice his or her own thoughts and when the family has divided opinions about the desirability of initiation of life support by dialysis, the hospital ethics committee may be of assistance.

The U.S. Renal Physicians Association has issued a clinical practice guideline for stopping or never beginning dialysis in certain patients, and relies upon shared decision making, informed consent or refusal, estimating prognosis, and a time-limited trial of dialysis where indicated.

Patients with advanced disease in an organ system other than the kidneys, or those with malignancy, have sometimes been excluded from chronic dialysis. For example, those with advanced liver disease might have ascites, encephalopathy, bleeding diathesis, and hypotension. These concomitant problems may make access difficult, and the dialysis treatments may create too much hypotension or fail to correct the accompanying fluid overload. In some such patients, dialysis may be futile. Futility is an ethical principle on which one can make a reasonable decision not to initiate dialysis. On the other hand, some such patients may achieve good quality of life and "remission" of failure of the other organ system with the fluid removal, electrolyte balance, and improved nutrition provided by the multidisciplinary support available through ESRD management.

C.   Elderly patients and dialysis. In the United States and elsewhere, the fastest growing age group presenting for dialysis is the "oldest old" (patients older than 80 years). Access placement in this group is not particularly difficult, and cuffed venous catheters have been used with success in difficult cases. Time constraints are not a problem, and these individuals often arrive eager for their treatments. Transportation is often available from assisted-living providers, retirement community staff, or municipal programs. A high rate of compliance with all aspects of treatment often offsets a higher prevalence of comorbid (cardiac, vascular, malignancies) conditions in achieving a good outcome. As a result, many elderly patients placed on dialysis continue to enjoy a good quality-of-life and benefit from documented improvement in a variety of health outcome measures.

II.   Dialysis access placement issues. For hemodialysis the preferred access is an arteriovenous (AV) fistula. It is sometimes difficult to get one of these to work, and hence a lead time of at least 6 months prior to anticipated dialysis is recommended to allow for correction of suboptimal flow or placement of a second fistula in the event that the initial fistula does not function properly. AV grafts should be placed at least 3–6 weeks prior to the anticipated start of dialysis to allow healing of the tissues around the graft to limit extravasation of blood, although some newer graft materials can be cannulated immediately after placement.

For peritoneal dialysis, a peritoneal catheter should be in place at least 2 weeks prior to anticipated start of dialysis. In the past, an AV fistula was recommended as a fall-back option for patients who are to be placed on peritoneal dialysis. This is no longer the norm.

III.   When to initiate dialysis.

A.   Uremic syndrome. The uremic syndrome consists of symptoms and signs that result from toxic effects of elevated levels of nitrogenous and other wastes in the blood.

1. **Symptoms.** Uremic patients commonly become nauseated and often vomit soon after awakening. They may lose their appetite such that the mere thought of eating makes them feel ill. They often feel fatigued, weak, and/or cold. Their mental status is altered; at first, only subtle changes in personality may appear, but eventually, the patients become confused and, ultimately, comatose.

2. **Signs.** The classic uremic physical findings of a sallow coloration of the skin due to accumulation of urochrome pigment (the pigment that gives urine its yellow color) and of an ammonia-like or urine-like odor to the breath are rarely seen unless the degree of uremia is severe. A pericardial friction rub or evidence of pericardial effusion with or without tamponade reflects uremic pericarditis, a condition that urgently requires dialysis treatment. Foot- or wrist-drop may be evidence of uremic motor neuropathy, a condition that also responds to dialysis. Tremor, asterixis, multifocal myoclonus, or seizures are signs of uremic encephalopathy. Prolongation of the bleeding time occurs and can be a problem in the patient requiring surgery.

3. **Signs and symptoms: Uremia versus anemia.** Several of the symptoms and signs previously ascribed exclusively to uremia may be partially due to the associated anemia. For example, when the anemia of dialysis patients is corrected with erythropoietin, they experience a marked decrease in fatigue and a concomitant increase in sense of well-being and exercise tolerance. The bleeding time may also improve, and there may be improvement in angina pectoris and a reduction in left ventricular hypertrophy. There are improvements in cognitive function as well.

4. **Relationship between uremic syndrome and eGFR.** The uremic syndrome commonly develops when the eGFR falls below 10 mL per minute per 1.73 m^2. Certain individuals, especially those with comorbidities, appear to be especially susceptible and may require earlier initiation of chronic dialysis (e.g., when the eGFR falls to 15 mL per minute per 1.73 m^2). However, in chronic renal failure, decreased spontaneous protein intake, anemia, and derangements in Ca/PO_4/parathyroid hormone (PTH) homeostasis are already demonstrable when clearance is still 30–40 mL per minute per 1.73 m^2.

B. **Indications for dialysis in the chronic setting.** Usually dialysis is initiated in adult patients when the eGFR decreases to about 10 mL per minute per 1.73 m^2. However, evaluation of the need for dialysis should begin at a higher eGFR level, probably somewhere around 15–20 mL per minute per 1.73 m^2. Problems with criteria that are limited to clearance measures occur in patients with renal impairment who have problems with fluid overload, hyperkalemia, or "failure to thrive" that are out of proportion to their eGFR. For example, patients with advanced age and cognitive impairment may be poorly compliant with taking high-dose diuretics or potassium-lowering agents. Patients with advanced cardiac disease and borderline eGFRs may have trouble with refractory fluid retention. Patients without financial resources or insurance may have trouble paying for high-dose diuretics and antihypertensives to achieve good fluid and potassium control. Such patients may present frequently to emergency facilities with pulmonary edema, hyperkalemia, and worsening azotemia, which improve after short hospitalization or even after several hours in the emergency room and treatment with appropriate medications. Once these patients are initiated on dialysis, frequent dialysis therapy prevents fluid and potassium problems, and the emergency room visits and hospital admissions often decrease markedly or cease altogether. Delay in initiation of dialysis for such patients until their eGFRs fall into a specified range may have an adverse effect on their long-term survival.

Conditions that may argue for relatively early initiation of dialysis are listed in Table 2-1.

It should be noted that pericarditis or pleuritis without other cause is an indication for urgent dialysis, particularly pericarditis, where the risk of rapidly developing pericardial effusion and cardiac tamponade is present. Neurologic dysfunction, especially signs of encephalopathy (manifested by asterixis) or uremic neuropathy, is also cause for prompt dialysis, as is prolongation of the bleeding time, which could lead to gastrointestinal or other bleeding. Most of these urgent indications are found in patients who appear with acute on chronic renal failure. Additional indications for acute dialysis are more fully discussed in Chapter 8.

1. Concept of early or "timely" initiation of dialysis. The rationale for this approach was that ultimate survival on dialysis depends greatly on nutritional status and serum albumin status at the time dialysis is initiated. Patients started early on dialysis (at higher eGFR levels) have

Table 2-1. Complications that may prompt initiation of kidney replacement therapy[a]

Intractable extracellular volume overload and/or hypertension

Hyperkalemia refractory to dietary restriction and pharmacologic treatment

Metabolic acidosis refractory to bicarbonate treatment

Hyperphosphatemia refractory to dietary counseling and to treatment with phosphorus binders

Anemia refractory to erythropoietin and iron treatment

Otherwise unexplained decline in functioning or well-being

Recent weight loss or deterioration of nutritional status, especially if accompanied by nausea, vomiting, or other evidence of gastroduodenitis

Urgent Indications

Neurologic dysfunction (e.g., neuropathy, encephalopathy, psychiatric disturbance)

Pleuritis or pericarditis without other explanation

Bleeding diathesis manifested by prolonged bleeding time

---

[a]Modified from the National Kidney Foundation's 2006 Kidney Disease Outcomes Quality Initiative (KDOQI) hemodialysis adequacy guidelines.

higher serum albumin levels. Furthermore, spontaneous protein intake begins to fall early in chronic renal insufficiency (when eGFR is still above 25 mL per minute per 1.73 m^2). Several studies have claimed that early initiation of dialysis results in decrease in mortality and hospitalization rates.

Survival, however, may mistakenly appear to be prolonged in patients who initiate dialysis early if measurement of survival is from the time of initiation of dialysis. This statistical error is known as **lead time bias.** More recent thinking is based on studies such as those by Korevaar et al. (2001) and Traynor et al. (2002), which suggested that when lead time bias is eliminated by measuring survival from a specific level of renal function (irrespective of dialysis initiation), there was no benefit to earlier start of dialysis. Whether early start will improve hard outcomes such as hospitalization or mortality remains an open question, however, as proper randomized trials have yet to be done.

2.   Postponing dialysis in combination with dietary management. Investigators from Brescia, Italy (Brunori et al., 2003) have studied an old approach to uremic management, namely delaying dialysis and managing patients aggressively with an ultralow (0.3 g/kg per day) protein diet supplemented with essential amino acids plus keto-analogs of amino acids. In a randomized, prospective trial, patients over 70 with an eGFR of 5–7 mL per minute per 1.73 m^2 were assigned to dialysis or dietary intervention. Patients with poor cardiac function were excluded. Hospitalization rate was lower in the conservatively treated patients, and survival was at least as good as those treated with dialysis, with a strong trend for improved survival. The dietary approach delayed dialysis by an average of 9 months. This approach is opposite to the conventional wisdom of initiating dialysis early, but is supported by one of the few randomized, prospective trials of this question that have been performed.

SELECTED READINGS

Brunori GF, et al. Efficacy and safety of a very low protein diet in postponing dialysis in the elderly: a prospective randomized multicenter controlled study. *Nephrol Dial Transplant* 2003; 18(Suppl 4):440, abs T501.

Goldfarb-Rumyantzev AS, et al. The role of pretransplantation renal replacement therapy modality in kidney allograft and recipient survival. *Am J Kidney Dis* 2005;46(3):537–549.

Goovaerts T, Jadoul M, Goffin E. Influence of a pre-dialysis education programme (PDEP) on the mode of renal replacement therapy. *Nephrol Dial Transplant* 2005;20(9):1842–1847.

Korevaar JC, et al. When to initiate dialysis: effect of proposed US guidelines on survival. *Lancet* 2001;358(9287):1046–1050.

Marron B, et al., for the Spanish Group for CKD. Analysis of patient flow into dialysis: role of education in choice of dialysis modality. *Perit Dial Int* 2005;25(Suppl 3):S56–S59.

Mehrotra R, et al. Patient education and access of ESRD patients to renal replacement therapies beyond in-center hemodialysis. *Kidney Int* 2005;68(1):378–390.

Shih YC, et al. Impact of initial dialysis modality and modality switches on Medicare expenditures of end-stage renal disease patients. *Kidney Int* 2005;68(1):319–329.

Traynor JP, et al. Early initiation of dialysis fails to prolong survival in patients with end-stage renal failure. *J Am Soc Nephrol* 2002;13(8):2125–2132.

WEB REFERENCES

European and other national dialysis guidelines: www.kdigo.org

NKF KDOQI hemodialysis and peritoneal dialysis adequacy guidelines: www.kdoqi.org

Blood-based Therapies

Physiologic Principles and Urea Kinetic Modeling

John T. Daugirdas

Dialysis is a process whereby the solute composition of a solution, A, is altered by exposing solution A to a second solution, B, through a semipermeable membrane. Conceptually, one can view the semipermeable membrane as a sheet perforated by holes or pores. Water molecules and low molecular weight solutes in the two solutions can pass through the membrane pores and intermingle, but larger solutes (such as proteins) cannot pass through the semipermeable barrier, and the quantities of high molecular weight solutes on either side of the membrane will remain unchanged.

I. **Mechanisms of solute transport.** Solutes that can pass through the membrane pores are transported by two different mechanisms: Diffusion and ultrafiltration (convection).
A. **Diffusion** (Fig. 3-1). The movement of solutes by diffusion is the result of random molecular motion. The larger the molecular weight of a solute, the slower will be its rate of transport across a semipermeable membrane. Small molecules, moving about at high velocity, will collide with the membrane often, and their rate of diffusive transport through the membrane will be high. Large molecules, even those that can fit easily through the membrane pores, will diffuse through the membrane slowly because they will be moving about at low velocity and colliding with the membrane infrequently.
B. **Ultrafiltration.** The second mechanism of solute transport across semipermeable membranes is ultrafiltration (convective transport). Water molecules are extremely small and can pass through all semipermeable membranes. Ultrafiltration occurs when water driven by either a hydrostatic or an osmotic force is pushed through the membrane (Fig. 3-1). (Analogous processes are wind in the atmosphere and current in the ocean.) Those solutes that can pass easily through the membrane pores are swept along with the water (a process called "solvent drag"). The water being pushed through the membrane is accompanied by such solutes at close to their original concentrations. Larger solutes, especially those that are larger than the membrane pores, are held back. For such large solutes, the membrane acts as a sieve.
1. **Hydrostatic ultrafiltration**
a. **Transmembrane pressure.** During hemodialysis, water (along with small solutes) moves from the blood to dialysate in the dialyzer as a result of a hydrostatic pressure gradient between the blood and dialysate compartments. The rate of ultrafiltration will depend on the total pressure difference across the membrane (calculated as

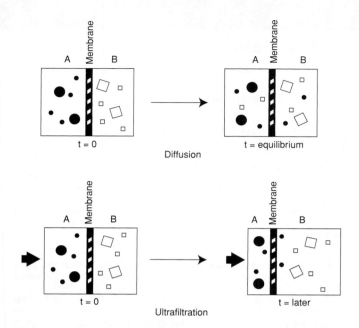

Figure 3-1.   The processes of diffusion (*top*) and ultrafiltration (*bottom*). As shown, in both processes, low molecular weight solutes can cross the semipermeable membrane, whereas larger solutes are held back.

the pressure in the blood compartment minus the pressure in the dialysate compartment).

b.   Ultrafiltration coefficient (K_{Uf}). The permeability of dialyzer membranes to water, though high, can vary considerably and is a function of membrane thickness and pore size. The permeability of a membrane to water is indicated by its ultrafiltration coefficient, K_{Uf}. K_{Uf} is defined as the number of milliliters of fluid per hour that will be transferred across the membrane per mm Hg pressure gradient across the membrane.

2.   Osmotic ultrafiltration. Osmotic ultrafiltration is described in Chapter 18.

3.   Implications of ultrafiltration on solute clearance
a.   Hemofiltration and hemodiafiltration. Whereas diffusive removal of a solute depends on its size, all ultrafiltered solutes below the membrane pore size are removed at approximately the same rate. This principle has led to use of a technique called *hemofiltration,* whereby a large amount of ultrafiltration (more than is required to restore euvolemia) is coupled with infusion of a replacement fluid in order to remove solutes. Although hemodialysis and hemofiltration often have comparable

removal of small solutes such as urea (MW 60), hemofiltration can effect much higher removal of larger, poorly diffusible solutes, such as inulin (MW 5,200). Sometimes hemodialysis and hemofiltration are combined. The procedure is then called *hemodiafiltration*.

C. Removal of protein-bound compounds. The normal kidney detoxifies protein-bound organic acids and bases. Being protein bound, they are filtered to only a small extent and so bypass the glomerulus. However, in the peritubular capillary network, these substances are removed from albumin and taken up by proximal tubular cells. Then they are secreted into the tubular lumen, to be excreted in the urine. Other protein-bound compounds (bound to albumin and small proteins) are filtered into the glomerulus along with their carrier proteins. In the proximal tubule, the filtered proteins are catabolized along with their bound compounds.

Some of the derangements associated with uremia may be due to accumulation of protein-bound compounds. Removal of protein-bound compounds by hemodialysis depends on the percentage of the "free" fraction of the compound in plasma (the fraction that is exposed to dialysis). Also, removal depends on how quickly the free fraction is replenished by the protein-bound pool. Substances that are tightly bound to proteins with a low free fraction in the plasma will be removed to only a negligible extent by hemodialysis. Use of charcoal hemoperfusion is quite effective in lowering the blood concentration of protein-bound compounds but is not being done on a routine long-term basis to treat uremia.

II. Solute removal from the dialyzer perspective

A. Diffusion

   1. Hemodialysis circuit. In clinical use, the box containing two solutions in Figure 3-1 becomes the dialyzer, containing blood and dialysis solution. The latter consists of highly purified water into which sodium, potassium, calcium, magnesium, chloride, bicarbonate, and dextrose have been introduced. The low molecular weight waste products that accumulate in uremic blood are absent from the dialysis solution. For this reason, when uremic blood is exposed to dialysis solution, the flux rate of these solutes from blood to dialysate is initially much greater than the back-flux from dialysate to blood. Eventually, if the blood and dialysate were left in static contact with each other via the membrane, the concentration of permeable waste products in the dialysate would become equal to that in the blood, and no further net removal of waste products would occur. Transport back and forth across the membrane would continue, but the rates of transport and back-transport would be equal. In practice, during dialysis, concentration equilibrium is prevented, and the concentration gradient between blood and dialysate is maximized, by continuously refilling the dialysate compartment with fresh dialysis solution and by replacing dialyzed blood with undialyzed blood. Normally, the direction of dialysis solution flow is opposite to the direction of blood flow (Fig. 3-2). The purpose of "countercurrent" flow is to

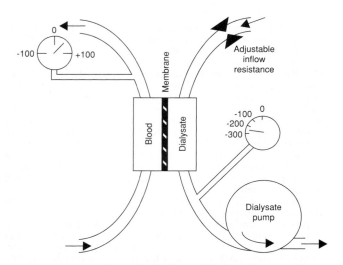

**Figure 3-2.   A dialyzer with blood flowing in one direction and
dialysis solution flowing in the opposite direction. Hydrostatic
pressure across the membrane (and ultrafiltration) is adjusted by
varying the resistance to inflow of dialysis solution. The position of
the gauges monitoring pressure at the blood and dialysate outflow
ports is also shown, along with typical operating pressures for a
low-flux membrane. In this case, the transmembrane pressure is
about 300 mm Hg (+50 mm Hg at the blood outlet, –[–250 mm Hg] at
the dialysate outlet).**

maximize the concentration difference of waste products
between blood and dialysate in all parts of the dialyzer.

2.   Dialyzer whole-blood clearance. The blood leaving
the dialyzer has a lower concentration of waste products
than the blood entering the dialyzer. For example, if the
plasma urea nitrogen level at the dialyzer inlet is 100 mg/dL
(36 mmol/L), at the dialyzer outlet the level may be 25 mg/dL
(9 mmol/L). However, the "work" that the dialyzer is doing
is not well represented by the extent to which it reduces the
blood concentration of a given waste product. If the blood
flow is slow, then very little urea is being removed. To better characterize dialyzer work, the percentage reduction in
the blood concentration of a given waste product is multiplied by the blood flow rate through the dialyzer to obtain a
hypothetical volume of blood that is being totally "cleared"
of that waste product each minute. In the above example,
the reduction in plasma urea nitrogen concentration from
100 to 25 mg/dL (36–9 mmol/L) translates to a 75% reduction. If the blood flow is 200 mL per minute, then 150 mL
per minute of blood (0.75 × 200) is being totally cleared of
urea.

One strength of the clearance concept is its independence from the concentration of the waste product in the

inflowing blood. For example, if the inflowing urea concentration is decreased to 50 mg/dL (18 mmol/L), the urea concentration in the out-flowing blood will decrease proportionately, from 25 to 12.5 mg/dL (9–4.5 mmol/L). The percentage removal, however, will still be 75 [100 × (50–12.5)/50], and the urea clearance will remain 150 mL per minute.

a. **Effect of erythrocytes.** In the concept of clearance described above, the blood was treated as a simple fluid. However, this is not the case. A blood flow of 200 mL per minute is really a plasma flow rate of 140 mL per minute and an erythrocyte flow rate of 60 mL per minute (at a hematocrit of 30%). What is measured at the dialyzer inlet and outlet are the plasma levels of a given waste product.

For urea, the presence of erythrocytes is not a major problem because urea diffuses into and out of erythrocytes quickly. For example, if the outlet plasma urea nitrogen level is 25 mg/dL (9 mmol/L), the urea concentration in erythrocytes will have been reduced to about that level also.

For creatinine and many other solutes, the problem is more complex because these substances do not equilibrate quickly between plasma and erythrocytes. Many other substances, such as phosphate, are present in different concentrations in plasma and erythrocytes. For such substances, the whole-blood clearance method using plasma levels is not a good approximation of removal rate during dialysis.

(1) **Computing the blood water urea clearance.** Urea is dissolved in erythrocytes and plasma water. Approximately 93% of plasma is water (depending on its protein concentration), and about 72% of an erythrocyte is water. However, because some urea associates with the nonwater portion of erythrocytes, one normally considers urea to be dissolved in a volume equal to 80% of the erythrocyte volume.

The correction for blood water becomes important when using the dialyzer clearance to compute how much urea is being removed during a dialysis session. Generally, not making the blood water correction will cause overestimation of the amount of urea removal by about 10%. The correction commonly used to account for blood water content of both plasma and erythrocytes together is to multiply the whole-blood clearance by 0.894 (see Table A-1).

(2) **Effect of hematocrit on blood water urea clearance.** Increasing the hematocrit (e.g., from 20%–40%) causes only a trivial reduction of the blood water urea clearance because the effective urea distribution volume in erythrocytes is similar to that in plasma.

(3) **Effect of hematocrit on clearance of creatinine and phosphorus.** Increasing the hematocrit will cause a reduction in the dialyzer clearances of creatinine and phosphorus. Creatinine may not be removed from erythrocytes to the same extent as from

the plasma during passage through the dialyzer. As the hematocrit is increased from 20% to 40%, creatinine removal decreases by about 8%. For phosphorus, the reduction will be about 13% because the amount of phosphorus available for transport out of red cells is smaller than the amount in plasma, and also because the rate of transport of phosphorus out of red cells during their passage through the dialyzer is slow.

3.   **Factors affecting the blood water urea clearance (_K_).** The principal determinants of the blood water clearance during dialysis are the blood flow rate, the dialysis solution flow rate, and the efficiency of the dialyzer used.

   a.   **Effect of the blood flow rate.** One might think that the blood clearance increases in direct proportion to the blood flow rate, given that clearance is computed as the blood flow rate times percentage reduction across the dialyzer in the plasma urea nitrogen level. This is only partially true. As the blood flow rate increases, the dialyzer is unable to remove urea with the same degree of efficiency. As a result, the plasma urea nitrogen level at the dialyzer outlet rises.

   Consider an example where the blood flow rate is 200 mL per minute, the inlet plasma urea nitrogen level is 100 mg/dL, and the outlet level is 25 mg/dL (36 and 9 mmol/L, respectively). The clearance is 200 mL × (100–25)/100 = 150 mL per minute. If the blood flow rate is now increased to 400 mL per minute, the outlet plasma urea nitrogen level will increase (how much depends on the efficiency of the dialyzer), typically from 25 to about 50 mg/dL (from 9–18 mmol/L). Now the clearance is 400 × (100 – 50)/100 = 200 mL per minute. Thus, a 100% increase in the blood flow rate (from 200–400 mL per minute) will have raised the blood urea clearance by only 33%, from 150 to 200 mL per minute.

   For dialysis of normal-size adults, the blood flow rate is usually set between 200 and 600 mL per minute, with flow rates of 350 to 500 mL per minute being used for most patients in the United States (many European countries prefer to use a lower average blood flow rate).

   b.   **Effect of dialysis solution flow rate.** Clearance of urea depends on the dialysis solution flow rate as well. A faster dialysis solution flow rate increases the efficiency of diffusion of urea from blood to dialysate; however, the effect is usually not large. The usual dialysis solution flow rate is 500 mL per minute. A flow rate of 800 mL per minute will increase urea clearance by about 12% when a high-efficiency dialyzer is used and when the blood flow rate is greater than 350 mL per minute. On the other hand, in some daily, nocturnal, or intensive care unit (ICU)–based applications, dialysate flow rate is markedly lower than 500 mL per minute. Such a reduced dialysate flow rate can cause substantial reduction in dialyzer clearance.

   c.   **Effect of dialyzer efficiency.** A high-efficiency dialyzer with a thin, large-surface-area membrane, wide pores, and a design that maximizes contact between blood and dialysate will remove a higher percentage of waste products than a low-efficiency dialyzer. For example, at a blood flow rate of 200 mL per minute, the blood entering a high-efficiency dialyzer may have an inlet concentration of 100 mg/dL and an outlet concentration of only 5 mg/dL (inlet = 36 mmol/L, outlet = 1.8 mmol/L). So the extraction percentage will be 95% instead of 75%, and the dialyzer urea clearance will be $0.95 \times 200 = 190$ mL per minute (not corrected for blood water).

(1) The dialyzer mass transfer area coefficient, K_0A. The efficiency of a given dialyzer in removing any solute can be described by a constant referred to as K_0A. This constant determines the height of the curve relating blood and dialysate flow rates to clearance (Fig. 3-3).

One can think of the K_0A, which is measured in milliliters per minute, as the maximum possible clearance of a given dialyzer at infinitely large blood and dialysate flow rates. Dialyzers of usual efficiency have in vitro K_0A values for urea of 500–700 mL per minute; high-efficiency dialyzers have K_0A values >700 mL per minute. In practice, these maximum clearance levels are never achieved because it is not possible to

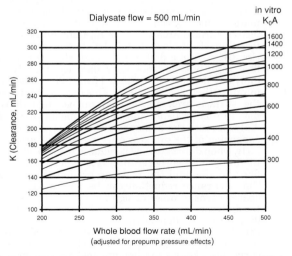

Figure 3-3.   Relationship between nominal blood flow rate (Q_B) and blood water urea clearance (K) as a function of dialyzer efficiency (K_0A). K was computed as per the equations in Table A-1. Clearance values from this nomogram will still overestimate true in vivo clearances slightly, but will correspond to urea volumes estimated by anthropometric equations.

approach the large blood and dialysate flow rates that
would be necessary.

Once the K_0A of a dialyzer is known, a nomogram
(see Fig. 3-3) or an equation (Table A-1) can be used
to predict the blood water urea clearance (K) at any
combination of blood (Q_B) and dialysate (Q_D) flow
rates.

EXAMPLE:

K_0A	$Q_B 200$	K $Q_B 400$	% Change in K
400	137	173	+26%
800	166	235	+42%

If a low-K_0A dialyzer is used (K_0A = 400 mL per
minute, row 1), doubling the blood flow rate from 200 to
400 will only increase the blood water urea clearance
(K) by 173/137, or 26%. However, with a higher-K_0A
dialyzer (K_0A = 800), K will increase by 235/166, or
42%. The clinical point is that one needs to use a high-
efficiency dialyzer to obtain a substantial increase in
clearance with a higher blood flow rate. A formal set
of equations to compute K from Q_B, Q_D, K_0A, and the
ultrafiltration rate is given in Table A-1.

(2)   **Effect of dialysate flow rate on K_0A.** In theory, the K_0A (maximum dialyzer clearance) depends
only on the permeability constant of the membrane
material for a given solute (K_0) multiplied by the effective surface area (A). The K_0A should be constant
for all levels of blood and dialysate flow rate. In practice, the K_0A of a dialyzer does not change with blood
flow rate, but the K_0A does increase slightly when
dialysate flow rate is increased from 500 to 800 mL per
minute (Cheung et al., 1997). This apparent increase in
the surface area of the dialyzer at high dialysate
flow rate is probably due to better penetration of the
dialysate into the hollow-fiber bundle, resulting in an
expansion of the dialyzer effective surface area. Similarly, when dialysate flow is reduced (e.g., to 300 mL per
minute), there is poorer dialysate penetration into the
fiber bundle, and the K_0A can be markedly reduced.
This clearance reduction can be mitigated by use of
spacer yarns or other design features that ensure better dialysate flow into the fiber bundle, and so is very
dialyzer design dependent.

(3)   **Computing the dialyzer K_0A** The K_0A urea is
the maximum height of the urea clearance curve. The
curve has a known mathematical shape, which is similar for all dialyzers. Thus, if one knows the actual clearance at any given blood and dialysate flow rates, one can
mathematically compute the peak height of the clearance curve, or the K_0A. A calculator to compute K_0A is
available on the Internet (see "Web References").

d. Effect of molecular weight on diffusive clearance. Because high molecular weight solutes move slowly through solutions, they diffuse poorly through the membrane. As a result, whereas urea (MW 60) may be removed from blood with an efficiency of 75% (e.g., concentration of outflow blood of 25 mg/dL [9 mmol/L], with inflow blood of 100 mg/dL [36 mmol/L]), creatinine (MW 113) may be removed with an extraction efficiency of only 60%; that is, if the inflow blood level of creatinine is 10 mg/dL, the outflow level may be as high as 4 mg/dL (inflow 885 mcmol/L, outflow 354 mcmol/L). Thus, the clearance for creatinine at 200 mL per minute blood flow may be only $0.6 \times 200 = 120$ mL per minute.

For even larger solutes, such as vitamin B_{12} (MW 1,355), the solute level at the blood outlet might be 75% of the level at the blood inlet. Thus, the percentage removed is 25%, and the clearance at 200 mL per minute blood flow would be $0.25 \times 200 = 50$ mL per minute. With vitamin B_{12}, the dialyzer clearance limits are reached early, and raising the blood flow rate above 200 mL per minute has only a modest effect on increasing clearance of such larger molecules.

e. Very large molecules. Very large molecules, such as β_2-microglobulin (MW 11,800), cannot get through the pores of standard (low-flux) dialysis membranes at all. Thus, dialyzer clearance of β_2-microglobulin will be zero! However, "high-flux" membranes have pores of sufficient size to pass this molecule. Also, some dialysis membranes remove β_2-microglobulin by adsorption.

B. Ultrafiltration
  1. Need for fluid removal. Ultrafiltration during dialysis is performed for the purpose of removing water accumulated either by ingestion of fluid or by metabolism of food during the interdialytic period. Typically, a patient being dialyzed thrice weekly will gain 1–4 kg of weight between treatments (most of it water), which will need to be removed during a 3- to 4-hour period of dialysis. Patients with acute fluid overload may need more rapid fluid removal. Thus, the clinical need for ultrafiltration usually ranges from 0.5–1.5 L per hour.

III. Solute removal from the patient perspective
A. Importance of urea. Solute removal during hemodialysis focuses on urea. Urea is manufactured by the liver from amino acid nitrogen via ammonia and is the principal way in which nitrogenous waste products are excreted from the body. Urea is a small molecule, with a molecular weight of 60. It is only slightly toxic. Urea generation occurs in proportion to protein breakdown, or the protein nitrogen appearance rate (PNA). In stable patients, the PNA is proportional to dietary protein intake. Using a mathematical model known as urea kinetics, one can compute both the rate of removal and production of urea. The extent of urea removal gives us a measure of the adequacy of dialysis, whereas the amount of urea nitrogen generation gives an estimate of dietary protein intake.

B.   The weekly serum urea nitrogen (SUN) profile. As a result of dialysis, the predialysis SUN level is typically reduced by about 70%, so that postdialysis SUN is 30% of the predialysis value. During the subsequent interdialytic period (assuming a thrice-weekly dialysis schedule), the SUN will rise to almost the same level as that seen prior to the first treatment. The result is a sawtooth pattern. The time-averaged SUN (TAC) level can be computed mathematically as the area under the sawtooth curve divided by time. Both the predialysis SUN and TAC SUN levels reflect the balance between urea production and removal. For a given level of dialysis therapy, predialysis SUN and TAC SUN will rise if urea nitrogen generation (g) is increased or will fall if g is decreased. Also, for any given rate of urea nitrogen generation, predialysis SUN and TAC SUN levels will rise if the amount of dialysis is decreased or will fall if the amount of dialysis is increased.

C.   Pitfalls in analyzing the predialysis SUN or TAC SUN. Early attempts to model dialysis adequacy focused on predialysis SUN or on the TAC SUN. Therapy was thought to be adequate as long as predialysis or TAC SUN was appropriately low. However, low predialysis or TAC SUN levels were found to be associated with a high mortality rate and were found to most often reflect inadequate protein intake rather than adequate dialysis.

D.   Indices of urea removal

1.   Urea reduction ratio (URR). The current primary measure of dialysis adequacy is the treatment-related urea reduction ratio, or URR. This is computed as follows: Assume that predialysis SUN is 60 mg/dL and postdialysis SUN is 18 mg/dL. The relative reduction in SUN (or urea) level is $(60 - 18)/60 = 42/60 = 0.70$. By convention, URR often is expressed as a percentage, so the value of the URR in this example would be 70%.

SI units: Assume that predialysis serum urea is 21 mmol/L and postdialysis is 6.4 mmol/L. The relative reduction in SUN (or urea) level is $(21 - 6.4)/21 = 14.6/21 = 0.70$. By convention, URR often is expressed as a percentage, so the value of the URR in this example would be 70%.

2.   Definition of sp*Kt/V* (single-pool *Kt/V*). Most published studies of dialysis adequacy have used the sp*Kt/V* ratio as a measure of urea removal. The sp*Kt/V* was popularized by Gotch and Sargent in their reanalysis of the National Cooperative Dialysis Study (1985). In that study, an sp*Kt/V* value <0.8 was found to be associated with a high likelihood of morbidity and/or treatment failure. Since that time, a number of additional studies have been published or presented suggesting that the delivered sp*Kt/V* is related to mortality in dialysis patients.

The sp*Kt/V* is a dimensionless ratio representing volume of plasma cleared (*Kt*) divided by the urea distribution volume (*V*). *K* is the dialyzer blood water urea clearance (L per hour), *t* is dialysis session length (hours, hr), and *V* is the distribution volume of urea (liters, L).

$K \times t = L/\text{hr} \times \text{hr} = L$

$V = \text{L}$

$(K \times t)/V = \text{L/L} =$ dimensionless ratio

If we deliver an spKt/V of 1.0, this implies that $K \times t$, or the total volume of blood cleared during the dialysis session, is equal to V, the urea distribution volume.

3. **How URR is related to spKt/V**

   a. **Holding tank model.** To understand how the URR is related to Kt/V, one first needs to consider the hypothetical example of fluid flowing through a dialyzer that completely clears the fluid of waste solute in a single pass (Fig. 3-4A). In such a case, the clearance "K" of this perfect dialyzer will be equal to the fluid flow through the device because the dialyzer outlet solute concentration is zero, and the extraction ratio will be 100%. Cleared fluid leaving the dialyzer is temporarily collected in a holding tank outside of the "body" until dialysis stops. At the end of dialysis, the dialyzed fluid in the holding tank is mixed back with any remaining fluid in the body that has not yet passed through the dialyzer.

   Because the dialyzed fluid is not routed back to the body until the end of dialysis, the inlet SUN concentration (80 mg/dL or ~28 mmol/L in this example) will remain constant throughout dialysis (Fig. 3-4B). The dialyzer outlet SUN concentration will always be zero. The volume of fluid cleared by the dialyzer and collected in the holding tank will be $K \times t$. If we assume that V is 40 L and that K is 10 L per hour, then $K \times t$ will be 40 L when 4 hours has elapsed. At that time, a volume $(K \times t)$ equal to the body water (V) will have passed through the dialyzer. $K \times t$ will be equal to V, and hence $K \times t$ divided by V, or Kt/V, will be equal to 1.0. When $Kt/V = 1.0$, the total-body water will have been completely cleared of waste solutes, and the urea reduction ratio, this time expressed as a fraction, and not as a percentage (URR = 1 – post-SUN/pre-SUN) will be URR = 1 – 0/80 = 1.0. In this idealized situation, a Kt/V of 1.0, thus represents a "perfect" dialysis, impossible to improve upon.

   At Kt/V values <1.0, the URR will be linearly related to Kt/V. For example, after only 2 hours at a K of 10 L per hour, $K \times t$ will be 20 L, and the Kt/V ratio will be 20:40 = 0.5. At that time, one-half of the total V will have been cleared of waste solute by passing through this ideal dialyzer. Because 20 L will have been cleared (SUN = 0 mg/dL) and 20 L will remain (SUN = 80 mg/dL [28 mmol/L]), on mixing these volumes at the end of dialysis, the postdialysis SUN will be 40 mg/dL (14 mmol/L), and the URR (1 – 40/80 or 1 – 14/28) will be 0.50. Similarly, Kt/V values of 0.25 and 0.75 will result in URR values of 0.25 and 0.75, respectively. Thus, when the dialyzer outlet is routed to a holding tank during dialysis, $Kt/V =$ URR. This relationship is shown graphically by the solid circles in Figure 3-4C.

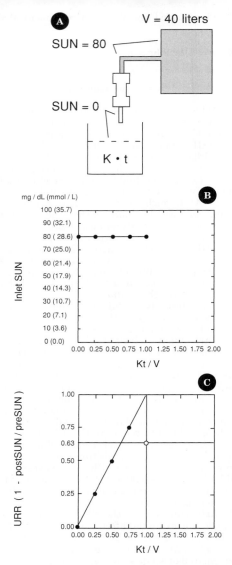

Figure 3-4. A: A fixed-volume model of urea removal (no urea generation) in which fluid from the dialyzer is routed to a holding tank and is mixed with the source "body" tank only at the end of dialysis. In this cartoon, blood flow rate = dialyzer clearance as we are assuming a perfect dialyzer. B: The dialyzer inlet serum urea nitrogen (SUN) (i.e., blood urea nitrogen [BUN]) remains constant (80 mg/dL [~28 mmol/L] in this example) throughout dialysis. C: In this model, Kt/V = urea reduction ratio (URR) and Kt/V = 1.0 represents a perfect dialysis (all toxins removed). (Reproduced with permission from Daugirdas JT. Urea kinetic modeling tutorial. *Hypertens Dial Clin Nephrol.* Available at: http://www.hdcn.com.)

b. Dialyzer outlet fluid returned continually during dialysis. In practice, there is no holding tank, and fluid leaving the dialyzer outlet is continually returned to the body or source tank throughout the dialysis session (Fig. 3-5A). As a result, the inlet SUN does not stay constant as in Figure 3-4B but falls continually during dialysis, as shown in Figure 3-5B. Dialyzer clearance (K) remains the same (i.e., equal to flow through the dialyzer). However, less urea is removed because the amount of urea in the blood that is being presented to the dialyzer now decreases as dialysis progresses. For this reason, the system with continuous fluid return is far less efficient than when fluid is kept in a holding tank until the end of dialysis. With this new arrangement, even after running all 40 L through our ideal dialyzer ($Kt/V = 1.0$), even though the outlet SUN has been zero, there still will be urea left in the tank. As shown by the hollow circles in Figure 3-5C, the URR will be 0.63 instead of 1.0 at a Kt/V value of 1.0. Even if we run all 40 L through a second ($Kt/V = 2.0$) and a third ($Kt/V = 3.0$) time, the postdialysis SUN still will not be zero (Fig. 3-5C). The SUN in the body will decline in an exponential fashion as a function of Kt/V (which can be thought of as the number of "passes" through an ideal dialyzer). The mathematical equation expressing the relationship between Kt/V and URR (i.e., $1 - $ post-SUN/pre-SUN) is:

$$Kt/V = \ln(1 - \text{URR})$$

where ln represents a function called the "natural logarithm."

If the URR is 0.63, then

$$Kt/V = -\ln(1 - 0.63)$$
$$= -\ln(0.37)$$
$$= 1.0$$

as shown in Figure 3-5C. This means that if the URR is 0.63, the entire volume of the "tank" will have been passed through an ideal dialyzer, and $Kt/V = 1.0$. From this point on, we will be using spKt/V where "sp" signifies "single-pool."

c. spKt/V versus URR: Correction for urea generation (g). In fact, there is a small amount of urea generated during dialysis, such that if you dialyze to a spKt/V of 1.0, the postdialysis SUN will drop from 100 mg/dL to only about 40 instead of from 100 to 37 (or will drop from 36 mmol/L to only 14.3 instead of 13.2), and the URR at sp$Kt/V = 1.0$ will be 0.60 rather than 0.63 (see top two nomogram lines in Fig. 3-6). The 0.03 shortfall in the expected URR is due to urea generated during the treatment.

d. spKt/V versus URR: Correction for ultrafiltrate volume removed. At any given URR, ultrafiltration during dialysis increases the amount of urea removed because by convention, spKt/V is based on a postdialysis

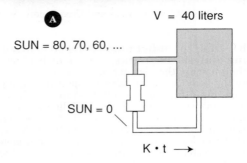

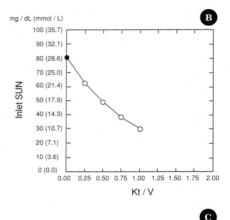

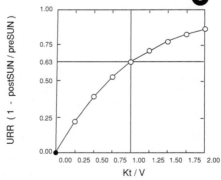

Figure 3-5. A: Another fixed-volume model, except this time the dialyzer outlet fluid is continually returned to the source tank throughout dialysis. As shown in B, the inlet serum urea nitrogen (SUN) now falls exponentially during dialysis, reducing dialysis efficiency. C: With continuous outlet return a urea reduction ratio (URR) of only 0.63 is reached when the total tank volume (V) is passed through the dialyzer, making $Kt/V = 1.0$. BUN, blood urea nitrogen. (Reproduced with permission from Daugirdas JT. Urea kinetic modeling. *Hypertens Dial Clin Nephrol.* Available at: http://www.hdcn.com.)

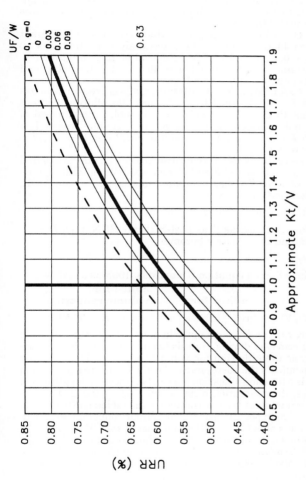

Figure 3-6. Actual relationship between *Kt/V* and urea reduction ratio (URR), taking into account urea generation and the effects of volume contraction. We now see that a *Kt/V* of 1.0 corresponds to a URR of 0.60 instead of 0.63, due to urea generation. In fact, depending on how much fluid is removed as a percent of the body weight, a *Kt/V* of 1.0 can be attained with URR values as low as 0.52, with an average URR of 0.57 (*heavy line* represents the usual UF/W of 3%). (Reproduced with permission from Daugirdas JT. Urea kinetic modeling. *Hypertens Dial Clin Nephrol*. Available at: http://www.hdcn.com.)

value for V. Assume two patients. Both have a pre- and post-SUN levels of 100 and 40 mg/dL (36 and 14.3 mmol/L), and both have postdialysis values for V of 40 L. However, patient A had 10% of body weight removed during dialysis. Predialysis V was therefore 44 L, ultrafiltration (UF) volume was 4 L, and UF/V was 4/40 = 0.10. In patient B, UF was zero. It is obvious that although URR was 0.60 for both patients, more urea nitrogen was removed from patient A.

Calculation in mg/dL units: Predialysis UN content was 44 L × 1 g/L = 44 g; postdialysis content was 40 L × 0.4 g/L = 16 g, for a removal of 28 g. In patient B, predialysis UN content was 40 L × 1 g/L = 40 g and removal was 40 − 16 = 24 g.

Calculation in SI units: Predialysis urea content was 44 L × 35.7 mmol/L = 1.57 mol. Postdialysis content was 40 L × 14.3 mmol/L = 0.57 mol, for a removal of 1 mol. In patient B, predialysis urea content was 40 L × 35.7 mmol/L = 1.43 mol, and removal was 1.43 − 0.57 = 0.86 mol.

4.   **Deriving spKt/V from the URR.** The effects of g and UF on the basic relation between spKt/V and URR can be corrected for. The basic equation linking spKt/V and URR, as described above, was

$$\text{sp}Kt/V = -\ln(1 - \text{URR})$$

Now, if we define R as post-SUN/pre-SUN, then $R = 1-$URR, and the equation becomes:

$$\text{sp}Kt/V = -\ln(R)$$

The adjusted equation (Daugirdas, 1995) is as follows:

$$\text{sp}(Kt/V) = \underbrace{-\ln(R - 0.008 \times t)}_{\text{adjust for } g} + \underbrace{(4 - 3.5 \times R) \times 0.55\ \text{UF}/V}_{\substack{\text{adjust for} \\ \text{volume reduction}}}$$

where t is the session length (in hours), UF is the volume of fluid removed during dialysis (in liters), and V is the postdialysis urea distribution volume (in liters). The $0.008 \times t$ term adjusts the post-/pre-SUN ratio, R, for urea generation and is a function of session length. For a session length of 3–4 hours, the generation term is about 0.024–0.032. The second adjustment term accounts for the added spKt/V due to reduction in postdialysis V. The volume reduction term usually adds about 10% to the unadjusted spKt/V term. If V is not known, an anthropometric estimate can be used (see Table A-2) or, alternatively, V can be assumed to be 55% of the postdialysis weight (W). The expression then simplifies to

$$\text{sp}(KtV) = -\ln(R - 0.008 \times t) + (4 - 3.5 \times R) \times \text{UF}/W$$

as 0.55 × UF/V is approximately equal to UF/W. A nomogram based on this equation is shown in Figure 3-6. From this nomogram, it is apparent that to reach an spKt/V of 1.0, the URR must be about 60% when no fluid is removed, but the URR need be only 52% when 9% of the postdialysis weight (UF/W = 0.09) is removed during dialysis. The lower URR reflects the added urea removal associated with volume contraction. Similarly, a URR of 0.60, which corresponds to an spKt/V of 1.0 when no fluid is removed, corresponds to an spKt/V of >1.2 when a large amount of fluid is removed during dialysis.

Thus, both the URR and spKt/V are mathematically linked, and both are determined primarily from the pre- and postdialysis SUN levels. The spKt/V also takes into account ultrafiltration and urea generation. Neither is superior to the other as a measure of outcome (Held et al., 1996).

5. Multipool models, urea inbound, and rebound. The model shown in Figure 3-5 assumes that urea is contained in a single body compartment. This assumption leads to a monoexponential decline in the SUN during dialysis, as per hollow circles in Figure 3-5B, and to a minimal rebound after dialysis has been discontinued. In fact, the SUN profile during dialysis deviates from the exponential decrease shown in Figure 3-5B, usually being lower than expected (Fig. 3-7). Also, following dialysis, SUN rebounds to levels that cannot be explained on the basis of urea generation (Fig. 3-7). These observations suggest that urea is being sequestered somewhere during dialysis, as shown in Figure 3-7. Because urea is being removed from a smaller apparent volume during the early part of dialysis, the SUN during the initial part of dialysis falls more quickly than expected. We have designated this unexpected fall in intradialytic SUN as urea **inbound**. Toward the end of dialysis, as a concentration gradient develops between the sequestered compartment and the accessible compartment, the fall in SUN slows. After dialysis is complete, continued movement of urea from the sequestered to the accessible compartment causes the postdialysis urea **rebound** (Fig. 3-7).

a. Regional blood flow model. An idea in vogue until recently was that urea sequestration occurred primarily intracellularly. It has now been shown that urea is sequestered during dialysis in tissues, primarily muscle, that contain a high percentage of total-body water, and hence urea, but receive a low percentage of the cardiac output. Because of the low ratio of blood flow through these tissues to their urea content, the transfer rate of urea from these tissues to the blood during dialysis is slow, causing urea sequestration.

b. Implications of urea inbound and rebound on measures of adequacy

(1) Single-pool urea kinetics overestimates amount of urea removal. Why is this so? Urea kinetics can be used to compute the amount of urea removed during dialysis. This is just an application of the basic clearance equation. If we know the SUN and the volume of plasma cleared, amount of urea removed is equal to the time-averaged SUN during the dialysis session multiplied by the liters of plasma cleared.

Example: Assuming that the predialysis SUN is 100 mg/dL and postdialysis SUN is 30, the single-pool

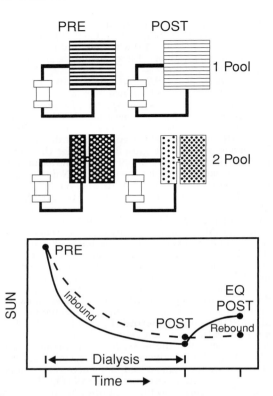

Figure 3-7. The effects of urea sequestration on the intradialytic fall in serum urea nitrogen (SUN; urea inbound) and the postdialysis increase in SUN (rebound). When there is sequestration, the intradialytic SUN level falls more quickly than expected (inbound) due to initial removal from a smaller apparent space. However, after dialysis is complete, continued entry of urea from the sequestered space to the proximal space causes urea rebound to occur. (Reproduced with permission from Daugirdas JT. Urea kinetic modeling. *Hypertens Dial Clin Nephrol.* Available at: http://www.hdcn.com.)

urea kinetic equations PREDICT that the intradialytic time-averaged SUN will be about 55 mg/dL. [For reasons beyond the scope of this handbook, this value of 55 is less than the arithmetic mean (65) of 100 and 30, the pre- and postdialysis SUN]. Urea nitrogen removed can then be estimated as liters of plasma cleared × Predicted intradialytic SUN.

Example in SI units: Assuming that the predialysis serum urea is 36 mmol/L and postdialysis urea is 11 mmol/L, the single-pool urea kinetic equations PREDICT that the intradialytic time-averaged serum urea will be about 20 mmol/L. [For reasons beyond the scope of this handbook, this value of 20 is less than the arithmetic mean (23.5) of 36 and 11, the pre- and postdialysis SUN]. Urea nitrogen removed can then be estimated as liters of plasma cleared × Predicted intradialytic SUN.

Problem: Assume that 57 liters of plasma are cleared during this dialysis treatment (e.g., 238 mL per minute × 240 minutes): How much urea nitrogen should be removed using the single-pool model?

Solution using mg/dL: We first convert all quantities to grams and liters, so predicted time-averaged intradialytic SUN = 0.55 g/L, and urea nitrogen removed = 57 L × 0.55 g/L = 32 g.

Solution in SI units: Serum urea = 20 mmol/L, and urea nitrogen removed = 57 L × 20 mmol/L = 1.14 mol.

Blood versus dialysate side urea discrepancy: However, if one collects the dialysate, and if one then multiplies the dialysate urea nitrogen concentration × volume of dialysate to compute the amount of urea nitrogen in the spent dialysate, one may find only 28 g of urea nitrogen (or 1.0 mol) in the tank, despite the fact that the blood-sided analysis predicted that 32 g (or 1.14 mol) should have been recovered. Why the discrepancy?

One reason for the error in computations is due to urea inbound. Due to urea sequestration during dialysis, the actual time-averaged intradialytic SUN was substantially lower than the predicted value of 55 mg/dL. Measurement of the SUN levels during dialysis would show that the true time-averaged intradialytic SUN was closer to 50 instead of 55 mg/dL. Therefore, the correct amount of removal is 50 mg/dL × 57 liters cleared, or 28 g per treatment—the same value as was obtained by dialysate recovery. In SI units, the intradialytic serum urea level was closer to 18 mmol/L than the expected 20, so for removal we get 18 mmol/L × 57 liters cleared, or 1.0 mol per treatment, the same value as obtained from dialysate recovery. *So single-pool urea kinetics overestimates the amount of urea removed, because it overestimates the intradialytic time-averaged value of the SUN.*

(2) The concept of equilibrated *Kt/V* (e*Kt/V*). After dialysis, urea diffuses back from sequestered tissue sites into the blood to cause a postdialysis rebound, which is largely complete by 30–60 minutes. One can measure the postdialysis SUN at this time and compute a "true" or equilibrated URR, which will be less than the URR based on an immediate postdialysis sample. The equilibrated URR can be translated into an equilibrated *Kt/V*. One can use the equilibrated post-SUN to compute R_{eq}, or the equilibrated post-/pre-SUN ratio. To do this, simply use R_{eq} instead of R in the *Kt/V* equation:

Example: Pre-SUN 100 mg/dL, post-SUN = 35, equilibrated post-SUN = 44.

In SI units: Pre-SUN = 35.7 mmol/L, post-SUN = 12.5, and equilibrated post-SUN = 15.7.

$$t = 3 \text{ hours, } UF/V = 0.06 \text{ (e.g., 3 kg removed from a patient with } V = 50 \text{ L}$$
$$R = 35/100 = 12.5/35.7 = 0.35$$
$$R_{eq} = 44/100 = 15.7/35.7 = 0.44$$

$$
\begin{aligned}
\mathbf{sp}Kt/V &= -\ln{(R - 0.008 \times t)} \\
&\quad + (4 - 3.5 \times R) \times 0.55 \times UF/V \\
&= -\ln{(0.35 \times 0.008 \times 3)} \\
&\quad + (4 - 3.5 \times 0.35) \times 0.55 \times 0.06 \\
&= 1.12 + 0.091 \\
&= \mathbf{1.21}
\end{aligned}
$$

$$
\begin{aligned}
\mathbf{e}Kt/V &= -\ln{(R_{eq} - 0.008 \times t)} \\
&\quad + (4 - 3.5 \times R_{eq}) \times 0.55 \times UF/V \\
&= -\ln{(0.44 \times 0.008 \times 3)} \\
&\quad + (4 - 3.5 \times 0.44) \times 0.55 \times 0.06 \\
&= 0.877 + 0.081 \\
&= \mathbf{0.96}
\end{aligned}
$$

So the equilibrated Kt/V, or eKt/V, is 0.96 instead of 1.21. In fact, eKt/V is typically about 0.2 Kt/V unit lower than the $spKt/V$. The amount by which it is lower depends on the efficiency, or rate of dialysis, as discussed below.

We can subtract eKt/V from $spKt/V$ to calculate the postdialysis rebound in terms of Kt/V:

$$eKt/V = spKt/V - \text{rebound}$$

Note that, in the above example, rebound was 1.21–0.96 = 0.25 Kt/V units.

(3)   Predicting postdialysis urea rebound. The amount of urea rebound depends on the intensity or rate of dialysis that was given. The rate of dialysis can be expressed as the number of Kt/V units per hour, or (Kt/V) divided by t in hours. A formula has been designed and validated that can predict the amount of rebound based on the rate of dialysis. This "rate equation" avoids the requirement of having to draw a postdialysis SUN level 30–60 minutes after the completion of dialysis. The rate equation (Daugirdas and Schneditz, 1997) predicts that:

$$\text{Rebound} = 0.6 \times \text{rate of dialysis} - 0.03 \text{ (arterial access)}$$

$$\text{Rebound} = 0.47 \times \text{rate of dialysis} - 0.02 \text{ (venous access)}$$

Substituting $(\text{sp}Kt/V)/t$ for (rate of dialysis), we have:

$$\text{e}Kt/V = \text{sp}Kt/V - 0.6 \times (\text{sp}Kt/V)/t + 0.03 \text{ (arterial access)}$$
$$\text{e}Kt/V = \text{sp}Kt/V - 0.47 \times (\text{sp}Kt/V)/t + 0.02 \text{ (venous access)}$$

In these equations, t is in hours, and $\text{sp}Kt/V$ divided by t simplifies to K/V (expressed as hr^{-1}). For example, if a $\text{sp}Kt/V$ of 1.2 is being delivered using an arterial access over 6, 3, or 2 hours:

$\text{sp}Kt/V$	t(hr)	$\text{sp}Kt/V$ per hr	Rebound	$\text{e}Kt/V$
1.2	6	0.2	0.09	1.11
1.2	3	0.4	0.21	0.99
1.2	2	0.6	0.33	0.87

then $\text{e}Kt/V$ will be about 1.1, 1.0, or 0.9, depending on whether these 1.2 $\text{sp}Kt/V$ units were delivered over 6, 3, or 2 hours.

(a) Why two formulas for $\text{e}Kt/V$ for arterial versus venous access? During dialysis an arteriovenous (AV) gradient for urea develops in the following fashion: Once dialysis is begun, the dialyzer returns dialyzed blood to the heart, which mixes in the heart with blood returning from tissues, diluting it and lowering the arterial urea level. Subsequently, as the arterial blood passes through the tissues, its urea level again increases, setting up the AV gradient. Usually, the magnitude of this AV gradient is on the order of 5% to 10%. Once dialysis is stopped, the AV urea gradient rapidly begins to close because the dialyzer is no longer feeding dialyzed blood to the heart.

Postdialysis urea rebound computed using the $(0.6 \times \text{rate of dialysis} - 0.03)$ equation above is based on total rebound from a postdialysis **arterial** blood sample. About 30% of the total postdialysis urea rebound is due to rapid closure of the AV gradient. If venous blood is sampled postdialysis, then 30% of the total rebound will have been accounted for, and the AV urea gradient must be subtracted from the total urea rebound. For this reason, there are two formulas to estimate $\text{e}Kt/V$: One for arterial postdialysis blood and one for venous postdialysis blood.

(b) Problems with the rate equation for ultra-short dialysis. These rate equations were derived from simulations done for 2.5- to 4-hour dialysis sessions. For very short dialysis sessions (2 hours or less), the rate equations don't predict rebound very accurately, and an alternative equation is more accurate (Tattersall equation). This alternative equation is discussed in more detail in Appendix A.

6. Access recirculation
  a. Definition. Normally blood flow through an AV access averages about 1 L per minute. The blood pump,

which normally routes a portion of this flow through the dialyzer, usually is set to take a flow of 350–500 mL per minute. Because flow through the vascular access normally exceeds the demand of the blood pump, usually all of the blood coming into the blood pump is coming from the access upstream to the needle insertion site. The urea concentration of blood entering the dialyzer is the same as that in the upstream access, and there is no AR (assuming, of course, that the access needles have not been placed too close to one another, and that the arterial and venous needle positions have not been inadvertently reversed). Now, in a failing AV graft or fistula, flow through the access can decrease markedly, say, to 350–500 mL per minute. In such circumstances, part of the flow leaving the dialyzer reverses flow through the access and re-enters the dialyzer. Then the dialyzer inlet blood becomes admixed, or "diluted," with dialyzer outlet blood. This phenomenon is called access recirculation (AR).

b.   Impact of AR on dialysis adequacy. When AR occurs, the urea concentration in the blood entering the dialyzer may be reduced by 5%–40% or more. The amount of urea removed in the dialyzer is equal to the volume of blood cleared × dialyzer inflow urea concentration. Although dialyzer clearance remains unchanged, the amount of urea removed is reduced because of the reduced urea concentration at the dialyzer inlet throughout dialysis.

c.   Impact of AR on apparent URR or spKt/V. In patients with AR, if blood at the end of dialysis is drawn from the dialyzer inlet blood line, the urea level in this blood will be lower than that in the patient's upstream blood, the latter representing the true postdialysis SUN concentration. Hence, the apparent postdialysis SUN will be artifactually low, and the URR and, consequently, the spKt/V both will be overestimated.

d.   Avoiding the impact of AR on URR or spKt/V by slowing the blood flow or by stopping dialysate flow at the end of dialysis prior to blood sampling. To ensure that blood being sampled reflects patient blood, one needs to slow the blood pump to a flow rate (e.g., 100 mL per minute) that is assuredly below the access flow rate for a short period of time (10–20 seconds). Lowering the blood flow stops the backward flow of blood from the dialyzer outlet to inlet and now all blood entering the arterial needle is upstream blood. The length of the slow-flow period depends on the dead space between the tip of the arterial needle and the sampling port (usually about 9 mL in most adult blood lines). A 10- to 20-second period of 100 mL per minute flow should be sufficient to allow the column of nonadmixed blood to reach the sampling port in most blood lines. A flow of 100 mL per minute = 100/60 = 1.7 mL per second; so in a 10- to 20-second slow-flow period, "upstream" blood will have advanced by 17–34 mL into the arterial blood line. Postdialysis blood should always be drawn after a short slow-flow period for this reason. It should be understood that merely stopping the blood pump prior to drawing the sample at the end of dialysis does not prevent this problem, as the admixed blood in the inlet blood line is simply "frozen" in place. A sample taken from the inlet blood line after stopping the pump still reflects admixed blood.

   (1) Stop dialysate flow method. Another clever method of avoiding this problem is to just shut off the dialysate flow for 3 minutes at the end of dialysis (or put dialysate flow into bypass) while letting the blood flow go full tilt. After 3 minutes, the SUN level in the blood leaving the dialyzer is similar to that going in, and so the inlet SUN level now reflects the SUN level in the patient's blood (see the 2006 National Kidney Foundation's [NKF] Kidney Disease Outcome Quality Initiative [KDOQI] adequacy guidelines).

7. Cardiopulmonary recirculation
   a. Definition. A recirculation can be defined broadly to occur whenever blood leaving the dialyzer outlet returns to the inlet without first having traversed the peripheral urea-rich tissues. In AR, the recirculation occurs via the short access segment between the venous and arterial needles. Cardiopulmonary recirculation occurs through the heart and lungs (which contain negligible amounts of urea) when the dialyzer is fed from the arterial circulation (e.g., via an AV access). During dialysis, cleared blood from the dialyzer outlet returns to the heart. In the aorta, the cleared blood is partitioned; some of it gets routed to the nonaccess arteries that lead it to the tissues to pick up more urea, but a fraction goes directly back through the access to the dialyzer without having traversed a peripheral capillary bed. When a dialyzer is fed from a venous access, cardiopulmonary recirculation cannot occur. Although an AV urea gradient is still present, all of the blood leaving the dialyzer must go through the peripheral capillary bed before it sees the dialyzer again.

   b. Impact of cardiopulmonary recirculation on dialysis adequacy. During dialysis using either an AV or venous access, there is an AV gradient for urea that is established. With an AV access, the dialyzer "rides" the arterial intradialytic urea nitrogen concentration curve, which is 5%–10% lower than the venous intradialytic urea nitrogen concentration curve. Hence, dialysis with an AV access is inherently less efficient (by about 5%–10%) than that using a venous access. This effect usually is outweighed by the lower blood flow rates achievable with venous accesses and the higher associated access (catheter) recirculation rate.

8. Urea modeling of urea distribution volume
   a. Definitions. Urea modeling can be used to determine the patient's apparent urea space, V. The principle is straightforward. Using blood-sided modeling, a value of spKt/V is determined from the URR and the degree of volume contraction, UF/V or UF/W (Fig. 3-6). Then an estimate is made for dialyzer blood water clearance, K (from

the dialyzer K_0A, blood flow rate, and dialysate flow rate, as per Fig. 3-3) or Table A-1. spKt/V is known, and now t and K are known, so V can be computed algebraically.

Problem: URR is 60% with UF/W = 0. t is 4 hours. Dialyzer K_0A is 800 mL per minute. Dialysate flow rate is 500 mL per minute. Blood flow rate is 450 mL per minute. What is V?

Solution: From Figure 3-6, spKt/V is 1.0. From the equations in Table A-1 or the nomogram in Figure 3-3, K is 250 mL per minute (15 L per hour). So by algebra, we know that K (15 L per hour) $\times t$ (4 hours) divided by V (L) is 1.0. V then is equal to $K \times t$ or to $15 \times 4 = 60,000$ mL, or 60 L.

b.   Use of modeled volume (V). Initially, the modeled V can be compared to expected values (usually 55% of body weight in men and 50% of body weight in women). An anthropometric estimate (Watson or Hume Weyers) of V can also be used (Table A-2). The modeled volume should be within about 25% of the anthropometric value for V. A more powerful use of V is to follow the modeled value over time. Although values for V have a substantial variation from treatment to treatment, a large change in V may reflect an error in blood sampling technique, an unrecorded change in the amount of dialysis ($K \times t$) given, or the presence of AR.

(1) V much smaller than usual. In this case, the URR is higher than expected, as is the spKt/V. Because the modeling program is told that K and t have not changed, the high spKt/V causes the program to conclude that the patient must have shrunk, as a smaller than usual value for V is calculated. Most often, if the V is reduced by about 100%, the problem is that the postdialysis blood sample was drawn from the outlet line instead of the inlet. Other potential causes are discussed in Chapter 6.

(2) V much larger than normal. The URR and spKt/V are lower than expected, and so the program concludes that if K and t are unchanged, then the patient must have somehow expanded to account for such a low URR. In fact, the real problem is that either K or t is lower than recorded. Most common problems include treatment interruption (full duration not given), lowering of blood flow rate due to technical problems (K lower than expected), or some sort of dialyzer performance problem resulting in reduced dialyzer clearance. AR can also cause this because the inflow blood urea level is lower than upstream blood, reducing effective access clearance. One caveat: The effects of AR on V will *only* be seen if blood is drawn properly (e.g., after a slow-flow period). If admixed blood is drawn postdialysis, then the URR will be artifactually increased. The expected lowering of URR due to AR then may not be seen, and modeled V may be unchanged!

(3)   Effect of URR on V. The V computed using single-pool modeling does not take into account all phases of rebound, especially compartment effects. By a mathematical coincidence, the single-pool V approximates the true V at a URR of about 65%–70%. At lower levels of URR, single-pool V is lower than the true V, and at higher levels of URR, single-pool V is greater than true V. Unless one is using very low levels of URR (e.g., for daily hemodialysis), this error in V is usually trivial, on the order of <5%, and not usually detectable in individual patients (Daugirdas and Smye, 1997).

9. **Urea nitrogen generation rate and the nPNA**

   a. **Utility of nPNA.** One of the benefits of urea modeling is that the generation rate of urea nitrogen (g) can be estimated from the urea nitrogen removal rate and the time-averaged plasma level. Because urea production comes from protein breakdown, a regression estimate can be used to derive the protein nitrogen appearance rate normalized to modeled V (nPNA) based on g. The actual clinical utility of g or nPNA is debatable. nPNA is not a very robust predictor of mortality (once serum albumin and creatinine are controlled for). Generally, outcome is poor when nPNA is low, as this usually reflects poor dietary intake. Before one can make the assumption that a low nPNA reflects a low dietary protein intake, one needs to make sure that other sources of urea loss such as residual renal clearance have been properly accounted for. Rarely, a patient with a low nPNA will be that way because he or she is getting better; there is marked anabolism and so the urea nitrogen is going into building muscle and not "appearing" in the blood. A high nPNA is not always due to a high protein intake; it may be due to increased appearance of urea due to tissue breakdown (i.e., hypercatabolism).

   b. **Methods of computing g (and thereby nPNA).** In standard urea kinetic modeling, there are two approaches to calculating g or nPNA: The three-point method and the two-point method.

      (1) **Three-point method.** The three-point method is more useful in an acute situation, as it does not depend on any steady-state assumptions. One simply measures the SUN before dialysis, after dialysis, and at some third point during the interdialytic interval (usually 44–68 hours later). Once V is known (estimated from Kt/V, K, and t during dialysis), one knows (a) the size of the box and (b) the increase in concentration of urea nitrogen during some or all of the interdialytic interval. It is simple algebra to compute how much material must be added to a box of size V to result in an increase in concentration from value 1 to value 2. The actual computation is a bit more complex because the value for g affects the URR, and this has a small effect on spKt/V and therefore on the initial estimate of V. Therefore, in practice, an iterative (going back and forth) mathematical approach is used to first estimate V assuming a g of about 6 mg per minute (0.214 mmol per minute); then, based on the first estimate of V and two interdialytic

SUN values, one computes a second, better estimate for
g. Then one goes back using this more accurate estimate
for g to compute a better estimate for V, and so on, until going back and forth no longer changes the answer.
Fluid gain during the interdialytic interval dampens
the increase in SUN, and this factor is also taken into
consideration in urea kinetic modeling programs.

Problem: Postdialysis V is 60 L and postdialysis
SUN is 30 mg/dL. A SUN value measured 48 hours
later is 78 mg/dL. What is g?

**Solution (simplified calculation neglecting vol-
ume changes):** $78 - 30 = 48$ mg/dL increase in SUN
over 48 hours = 1 mg/dL per hour. This is 10 mg/L per
hour × 60 L = 600 mg of urea nitrogen generated per
hour = 10 mg urea nitrogen per minute. $g = 10$ mg per
minute.

Solution in SI units: Posturea = 11 mmol/L and
next preurea = 28. So $28 - 11 = 17$ mmol/L increase in
urea over 48 hours = 0.35 mmol/L increase per hour.
To get g, multiply by the volume of 60 L to get 21 mmol
per hour or 0.35 mmol per minute.

(2) Two-point method. In the two-point modeling
method, a predialysis and postdialysis SUN only are obtained. There is no third SUN sample taken during the
interdialytic interval prior to the next dialysis. However, a value for g (and therefore nPNA) is computed.
How can this be done?

(a) Analogy to creatinine clearance. With urea
kinetics, we can ask the computer to generate a
weekly sawtooth SUN plasma profile, from which
we can compute a time-averaged SUN. This is analogous to the serum creatinine level. With creatinine
clearance, we know the creatinine generation rate
(from a 24-hour urine collection), and we use this
plus the serum creatinine level to compute clearance.
In urea kinetic modeling, we go the other way. We
know the urea clearance (from the dialysis session
spKt/V and residual renal urea clearance), and we
know the time-averaged urea level. From these two
quantities, the urea nitrogen generation rate can be
computed. The relationships between urea removal
(spKt/V), the predialysis SUN, and the urea generation rate (expressed as PNA rate normalized to V, or
nPNA), are shown in Figure 3-8. For any level of urea
removal (spKt/V and K_{ru}), there will be a direct linear relationship between urea generation (expressed
as nPNA) and the predialysis SUN.

**(b) How a two-point urea modeling program
computes the nPNA.** The computer generates a series of sawtooth SUN patterns based on the measured spKt/V and various hypothetical values of g.
As the values for g are increased, the height of the
sawteeth will rise. The computer then compares the
estimated predialysis SUN with the actual measured
value. If the value is too high, the computer inputs

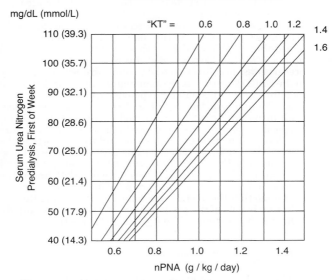

Figure 3-8. The relationship between nPNA, the first-of-week predialysis serum urea nitrogen (SUN), and Kt/V for patients undergoing dialysis three times per week. Similar nomograms have been devised for midweek (see Fig. A-3) and end-of-week predialysis SUN, and for twice-weekly schedules. "KT" = Kt/V adjusted for residual renal function (see Fig. A-3). (Reproduced with permission from Daugirdas JT. Urea kinetic modeling. *Hypertens Dial Clin Nephrol.* Available at: http://www.hdcn.com.)

a lower value of g and redoes the computation. The computer keeps adjusting the value for g until the predicted predialysis SUN value matches the actual value. For example, in Figure 3.8, identify the line where spKt/V = 1.2. If the nPNA is only 0.6 g/kg per day, then the height of the sawtooth (pre-SUN) at the first dialysis day of the week (after the 2-day interval) will only be 41 mg/dL (14.6 mmol/L). If the nPNA increases to 1.2 g/kg per day, then the height of the first-of-week pre-SUN sawtooth will stabilize at about 90 mg/dL (32 mmol/L) (Fig. 3-8).

(c) Formulas to obtain nPNA from spKt/V and predialysis SUN. These are given in Depner and Daugirdas (1996). A formal computation can be made by a urea kinetic modeling program. One such program is available through the Internet (see Web References).

10. Residual renal function. Residual renal function in end-stage renal disease (ESRD) patients can be approximated as the average of the creatinine and urea clearances. Urea clearance (K_{ru}) underestimates the glomerular filtration rate (GFR) due to proximal tubular urea reabsorption, whereas creatinine clearance (K_{rc}) overestimates GFR because of tubular secretion. It is well established that ESRD patients with substantial residual renal function (K_r) live longer, and so it is important to attempt to preserve residual function and to minimize potential injury to the ESRD kidney (e.g., by avoiding nephrotoxic drugs and by minimizing intradialytic hypotension).

a.   Measuring the K_{ru}. For this, one needs to collect all urine during a 24-hour period of the interdialytic interval. Usually, the patient starts the collection 24 hours before coming to the dialysis unit and then reports to the unit with the urine container and gives a sample of blood to measure the SUN. If the patient is receiving a usual amount of dialysis (three times a week only!), and if the collection interval is 24 hours prior to dialysis, one can assume that the average serum urea level during the collection is 90% of the predialysis SUN (Daugirdas, unpublished observations). The K_{ru} calculation is then:

$$K_{ru} = \frac{UUN}{SUN} \times \text{urine flow rate (mL/min)}$$

where UUN is the urine urea nitrogen concentration.

The units for the UUN and SUN do not matter, but they must be the same, as they cancel each other out. Typically, K_{ru} values of 0–8 mL per minute will be obtained.

Problem: If urine flow rate is 0.33 mL per minute, or 20 mL per hour, over 24 hours one would collect 480 mL of urine. Assume that the urine urea concentration is about 800 mg/dL (285 mmol/L) and that the collection was during the 24-hour interval immediately preceding a dialysis. Predialysis SUN for that dialysis is 56 mg/dL (20 mmol/L). What is the K_{ru}?

Solution in mg/dL units: First, compute the estimated mean SUN during the 24-hour collection interval. As discussed above, the estimated mean SUN during the collection period is 90% of the predialysis SUN, or $0.9 \times 56 = 50$ mg/dL. So $K_{ru} = (800$ mg/dL $\times 0.33$ mL per minute)/50 mg/dL $= 5.3$ mL per minute.

Solution in SI units: First, compute the estimated mean SUN during the 24-hour collection interval. As discussed above, the estimated mean SUN during the collection period is 90% of the predialysis SUN, or $0.9 \times 20 = 18$ mmol/L. So $K_{ru} = (0.285$ mmol/mL $\times 0.33$ mL per minute)/0.018 mmol/mL $= 5.3$ mL per minute.

b.   Adding the residual renal urea clearance to Kt/V-urea in peritoneal dialysis and in hemodialysis

(1)   In peritoneal dialysis, K_{ru} and Kt from Kt/V are additive. In peritoneal dialysis patients, as both residual renal urea clearance (K_{ru}) and peritoneal urea clearance (K_{pu}) are operative during a steady-state situation, K_{ru} and K_{pu} can be simply added. One milliliter per minute of K_{ru} mathematically approximates 10.08 L of urea clearance per week, as there as 10,080 minutes in a week. This is discussed further in the peritoneal dialysis physiology chapter.

(2) **In hemodialysis, K_{ru} cannot be simply added to Kt/V.** For hemodialysis, one cannot add dialyzer urea clearance (K_{totw} in Table A-1) and residual urea clearance (K_{ru}), as the dialyzer urea clearance is operative during a period of changing SUN and hence is less efficient in terms of urea removal than K_{ru}.

c. **The concept of equivalent urea clearance (eK_{ru}).** One can compute the equivalent clearance for any given dialysis regimen using the same principle as computing a creatinine clearance: If one knows the generation rate (24-hour collection in the case of creatinine) and the mean plasma level, one can compute clearance as a ratio of the two. Using any of a number of computer programs or a simplified equation (Depner and Daugirdas, 1997), one can compute both the urea nitrogen generation rate (g) and the time-averaged urea nitrogen level (TAC urea) and compute the ratio of the two to get an equivalent renal clearance.

$$Cr_{el} = \frac{UV}{P}$$

$$eK_{ru} = \frac{g}{TAC}$$

where Cr_{cl} is creatinine clearance (see Chapter 1) and eK_{ru} is the equivalent urea clearance, g is the urea nitrogen generation rate, and TAC is the time-averaged urea nitrogen level. This basic approach was first popularized by Casino and Lopez (1996).

Problem: The recommended minimum spKt/V for thrice-weekly dialysis is 1.2 per session. What is the equivalent renal urea clearance?

Solution: Assume this is given over 3 hours. Rebound using the rate equation (see above) will be about 0.2 Kt/V units. So eKt/V will be 1.0 per session. Using the Casino and Lopez nomogram (see their paper), this translates to an eK_{ru} of about 11 mL per minute.

d. **Going from eK_{ru} (in mL per minute) to weekly Kt/V.** Theoretically, one can take any hemodialysis prescription, compute g and TAC using a modeling program, and then convert it to eK_{ru}. This value can be added to the measured residual renal urea clearance. The resulting eK_{ru} can be expressed either in milliliters per minute or in liters per week. When expressed as liters per week, eK_{ru}, which is now equivalent to ($K \times t$), or volume of plasma cleared during the week, can be further divided by V to arrive at a weekly Kt/V-urea.

Problem: In a patient with $V = 35$ L, eK_{ru} is 11 mL per minute. What is the weekly Kt/V-urea?

Solution: 11 mL per minute × 10,080 mL per week divided by 1,000 to convert milliliters to liters gives a weekly volume of plasma cleared of 110 L per week. This is the $K \times t$ term of Kt/V. Dividing by $V = 35$, we get weekly Kt/V urea = 3.14.

e.   Problems with the Casino-Lopez eK_{ru} and its resultant weekly Kt/V-urea. One problem with this approach is that, as shown above in sections c and d, a thrice-weekly spKt/V of 1.2, or an eKt/V of 1.0, translates into an eK_{ru} of about 11 mL per minute, or a weekly $K \times t$ of about 110 L, or a weekly Kt/V of about 110/35, assuming $V = 35$ L, or 3.1. This suggests that a weekly Kt/V-urea of 3.1 is required as a minimum standard in patients being treated with intermittent hemodialysis. But we know from the peritoneal dialysis outcomes literature that a weekly Kt/V-urea (derived as the sum of residual renal and peritoneal urea clearance) of about 2.0–2.2 is a reasonable minimum target level of adequacy.

So the Casino-Lopez-derived eK_{ru} does not appear to be equivalent to either peritoneal dialysis Kt/V-urea or to residual renal urea clearance in terms of outcome.

The reasons for this difference in weekly Kt/V-urea targets between hemodialysis and peritoneal dialysis are speculative. One explanation is that urea may be less compartmentalized than other low molecular weight solutes. In such a case, equivalent amounts of urea removal where one therapy is highly intermittent may not represent equivalent therapy.

f.   The Gotch adjusted eK_{ru}. Gotch has proposed a new equation for eK_{ru} for hemodialysis regimens to correct this problem (National Kidney Foundation, 1997). Whereas the Casino-Lopez idea is to divide g by the time-averaged urea level (TAC urea), Gotch computes an adjusted eK_{ru} as being equal to g divided by the mean weekly predialysis plasma urea level.

Example   (mg   per   dL   units): Thrice-weekly hemodialysis schedule: $g = 6$ mg per minute per 35 L; TAC urea = 40 mg/dL; peak urea values for Mon., Wed., and Fri. = 65, 60, and 55 mg/dL, respectively; mean predialysis urea = (65 + 60 + 55)/3 = 60 mg/dL. In this case, we can see that the Gotch adjusted eK_{ru} will be about one-third lower than the Casino-Lopez eK_{ru}:

$$\text{e}K_{ru} \text{ (Casino-Lopez)} = g/\text{TAC-SUN}$$

$$= (6 \text{ mg per minute})/$$

$$(40 \text{ mg/dL})$$

$$= 0.15 \text{ dL per minute}$$

$$= 15 \text{ mL per minute}$$

$$\text{e}K_{ru}(\text{Gotch})\ g/(\text{mean pre-SUN}) = 6/60$$

$$= 0.10 \text{ dL per minute}$$

$$= 10 \text{ mL per minute}$$

Example (SI units): Thrice-weekly hemodialysis schedule: $g = 0.214$ mmol per minute per 35 L; TAC urea $= 14.3$ mmol/L; peak urea values for Mon., Wed., and Fri. $= 23$, 21, and 20 mmol/L, respectively; mean predialysis urea $= (23 + 21 + 20)/3 = 21.4$ mmol/L. In this case, we can see that the Gotch adjusted eK_{ru} will be about one-third lower than the Casino-Lopez eK_{ru}:

eK_{ru} (Casino-Lopez) $= g$/TAC-SUN

$$= (0.214 \text{ mmol per minute})/$$
$$(14.3 \text{ mmol/L})$$
$$= 0.015 \text{ L per minute}$$
$$= 15 \text{ mL per minute}$$

eK_{ru} (Gotch) g/(mean pre-SUN) $= 0.214/21.4$

$$= 0.010 \text{ L per minute}$$
$$= 10 \text{ mL per minute}$$

(1) Going from eK_{ru}-Gotch to standard Kt/V. Using the Gotch approach, a typical thrice-weekly hemodialysis regimen (sp$Kt/V = 1.2$) will yield an eK_{ru} of about 7 mL per minute, or 70 L per week, which in a person with $V = 35$ L translates into a weekly Kt/V urea of about 2.0. Thus, the Gotch modification of the eK_{ru} allows consistency and perhaps additivity among hemodialysis, peritoneal dialysis, and residual renal urea continuous-clearance equivalents.

It should be emphasized that the Gotch eK_{ru} is an intentionally down-regulated number and that it cannot be used directly in the computation of nPNA. For that purpose, the Casino-Lopez eK_{ru}(g/TAC) must be used.

11. Issues relating to normalizing by V. Normalizing Kt to V is convenient, because the Kt/V is directly related to the urea reduction ratio, as discussed above. However, because V represents largely muscle mass, it is not entirely clear that someone with 10% more muscle needs 10% more dialysis. In fact, dosing dialysis by Kt/V may disadvantage smaller people, with less muscle mass, as well as women, who have a lower level of V for any given level of height and weight compared to men. Although it is clear that some adjustment for body size should be made, a 1:1 ratio of dialysis to body weight may not be the best factor. An alternative approach is to scale the dialysis dose ($K \times t$) by body surface area. Several equations that do this are given in Appendix A. What would be the clinical implications of scaling dialysis dose by body surface area? Relatively more dialysis for smaller people, and relatively less dialysis for larger patients. Also, a 10% higher target dialysis dose in women, because V/BSA (body surface area) is different by this amount in men versus women (after rescaling to $V^{2/3}$). Some observational data support use of such an alternative, BSA scaling approach (see Lowrie et al., 2005). If one is using a Kt/V target, one should keep in mind the concept of using slightly higher (e.g., 15%) targets for smaller patients and again, for women, and perhaps not to be so concerned about accepting a slightly lower target in large patients with a large amount of muscle mass. These issues are discussed more completely in the 2006 NKF's KDOQI adequacy guidelines.

12. Estimating dialyzer clearance by pulsing dialysate with sodium and analyzing resulting changes in dialysate conductivity. Measuring adequacy using urea is time consuming and involves the use of needles, exposure of staff and patient to blood, and considerable effort in processing and analyzing blood samples. The most useful alternative approach being considered is to measure the clearance of the dialyzer online by causing a step increase in dialysate sodium and then measuring the conductivity of the dialysate flowing into the dialyzer and comparing this to the dialysate exiting the dialyzer over a short period of time. Many of the technical issues have been solved, and conductivity-based clearances reflect actual urea clearances quite well. An advantage of this method is that clearances can be computed multiple times throughout a dialysis session. One disadvantage is that conductivity-based clearances measure what happens on the machine side, but not so much on the patient side. Correlations with urea Kt/V are reasonable, despite substantial intrapatient variability. The conductivity approach to adequacy is expected to gain in popularity. See Gotch et al. (2004) and McIntyre et al. (2003) for a more complete analysis of these issues.

IV.   Acid–base aspects

A.   Acid–base balance. Acid production is a function of PNA (protein intake in noncatabolic patients). In nonuremic patients, acid production rate can be estimated at 0.77 [×] PNA and is about 60 mmol per day (420 mmol per week) for a 70-kg patient. One study suggests that acid production in hemodialysis patients is reduced to the range of 28 mmol per day for reasons that are not completely clear (Uribarri et al., 1998).

B.   Predialysis HCO₃ level. Metabolic acidosis has been linked to adverse effects on protein metabolism. However, outcome studies do not show an adverse effect of acidosis until the predialysis serum HCO₃ level decreases to <16 mmol/L. Attempts to maintain hemodialysis patients at predialysis HCO₃ levels in the mid-20s instead of 20 or less have yielded some benefit in terms of increases in serum albumin or in anthropometric measures of muscle mass, but this is controversial. The most recent KDOQI guidelines recommend a predialysis serum bicarbonate target of 22 mmol/L.

C.   Proper dialysate bicarbonate level. During hemodialysis, alkali is delivered to the patient from the dialysis solution in the form of bicarbonate. The usual dialysis solution bicarbonate level is 35–38 mM. Once predialysis acidosis has been largely corrected, further use of dialysis solution with a bicarbonate concentration of 38 mM may cause postdialysis alkalemia; postdialysis plasma bicarbonate levels of >30 mmol/L with pH values >7.55 have been reported. For this reason, the postdialysis plasma bicarbonate level should be monitored, and the dialysis solution bicarbonate concentration should be reduced if necessary; a reasonable target value for the postdialysis plasma bicarbonate level would be in the vicinity of 27 mmol/L. Not all machines are capable of easily delivering a lower than standard (35–38 mM) bicarbonate dialysate.

1. **Effect of ultrafiltration and interdialytic weight gain.** The amount of bicarbonate transfer to the patient is reduced at high ultrafiltration rates. For this reason, higher than usual dialysis solution bicarbonate levels often must be used in patients with large interdialytic weight gains. Another reason for this is that such patients often are found to have a high PNA. Whether this is due to high dietary protein intake or to negative nitrogen balance has not been ascertained. However, the high PNA per se engenders increased generation of acid equivalents.

2. **Effect of dialysis adequacy.** Dialyzer bicarbonate uptake generally is proportional to urea clearance (Kt/V). For this reason, underdialysis, as reflected by a poor Kt/V urea, usually results in predialysis acidosis as well.

3. **Effect of dialysis duration and frequency.** In the setting of frequent dialysis (more than three times a week) or long-session dialysis (i.e., nocturnal hemodialysis), the dialysis bicarbonate level may need to be reduced in order to keep serum HCO_3 level from becoming excessively high.

ACKNOWLEDGMENT

The urea kinetic modeling update of this chapter has been adapted from the urea kinetic modeling tutorial on *Hypertens Dial Clin Nephrol,* with permission.

SELECTED READINGS

Casino FG, Lopez T. The equivalent renal urea clearance. A new parameter to assess dialysis dose. *Nephrol Dial Transplant* 1996;11: 1574–1581.

Daugirdas JT. Simplified equations for monitoring Kt/V, PCRn, eKt/V, and ePCRn. *Adv Ren Replace Ther* 1995;2:295–304.

Daugirdas JT, Schneditz D. Overestimation of hemodialysis dose depends on dialysis efficiency by regional blood flow but not by conventional two pool urea kinetic analysis. *ASAIO J* 1995;41: M719–M724.

Daugirdas JT, et al, for the Hemodialysis Study Group. Factors that affect postdialysis rebound in serum urea concentration, including the rate of dialysis: results from the HEMO Study. *J Am Soc Nephrol* 2004;15(1):194–203.

Depner TA, Daugirdas JT. Equations for normalized protein catabolic rate based on two-point modeling of hemodialysis urea kinetics. *J Am Soc Nephrol* 1996;7:780–785.

Depner TA, et al. Dialyzer performance in the HEMO study: in vivo K_0A and true blood flow determined from a model of cross-dialyzer urea extraction. *ASAIO J* 2004;50(1):85–93.

Gotch FA. Abstract. Evolution of the single-pool urea kinetic model. *Semin Dial* 2001;14(4):252–256.

Gotch FA, et al. Mechanisms determining the ratio of conductivity clearance to urea clearance. *Kidney Int Suppl* 2004;(89):S3–S24.

Leypoldt JK, Jaber BL, Zimmerman DL. Predicting treatment dose for novel therapies using urea standard *Kt/V*. *Semin Dial* 2004;17(2):142–145.

Leypoldt JK, et al. Hemodialyzer mass transfer-area coefficients for urea increase at high dialysate flow rates. The Hemodialysis (HEMO) study. *Kidney Int* 1997;51:2013–2017.

Lowrie EG, et al. The online measurement of hemodialysis dose (Kt): clinical outcome as a function of body surface area. *Kidney Int* 2005;68(3):1344–1354.

McIntyre CW, et al. Assessment of haemodialysis adequacy by ionic dialysance: intra-patient variability of delivered treatment. *Nephrol Dial Transplant* 2003;18(3):559–563.

Schneditz D, et al. Cardiopulmonary recirculation during dialysis. *Kidney Int* 1992;42:1450.

Uribarri J, et al. Acid production in chronic hemodialysis patients. *J Am Soc Nephrol* 1998;9:114–120.

WEB REFERENCES

KDOQI Hemodialysis Adequacy guidelines 2006: http://www.kidney.org

Urea kinetic modeling calculators: http://www.hdcn.com/calcf/gfr.htm

Urea kinetic modeling channel: http://www.hdcn.com/ch/adeq/

Urea kinetic modeling tutorial/questions: http://www.hdcn.com/hd/ukmtutor.htm

Hemodialysis Apparatus

Suhail Ahmad, Madhukar Misra, Nicholas Hoenich, and John T. Daugirdas

Hemodialysis (HD) apparatus can be broadly divided into a blood circuit and a dialysis solution circuit, which meet at the dialyzer. The blood circuit begins at the vascular access. From there blood is pumped through an "arterial blood line" to the dialyzer. Blood is returned from the dialyzer to the patient via a "venous blood line." These terms are used even though often only venous blood is being accessed (such as when using a venous catheter). More precise would be to term these the "inflow" blood line and "outflow" blood line, but as often is the case, the more correct terms are rarely used. Various chambers, side ports, and monitors are attached to the inflow and outflow blood lines, and are used to infuse saline or heparin, to measure pressures and to detect any entrance of air. The dialysis solution circuit includes the dialysis solution supply system, which makes dialysis solution online from purified water and concentrate, and then pumps the solution through a different compartment of the dialyzer. The dialysis solution circuit includes various monitors that make sure that the dialysis solution is at the right temperature, has a safe concentration of dissolved salts, and is not being exposed to blood (due to a leak in the dialyzer membrane).

I. **The blood circuit.** The inflow (arterial) blood line connects the vascular access to the dialyzer, and the outflow (venous) blood line runs from the dialyzer back to the vascular access. Pumping is done by a blood pump, usually a spring-loaded roller pump that completely occludes the blood tubing during normal operation, and works like milking a straw along its length. Even though the pressure in an arteriovenous vascular access is often positive (greater than atmospheric), because the roller pump is pumping fairly fast (200–600 mL per minute) and because there is some resistance at the vascular access catheter or needle, the pressure in the blood line upstream to the roller pump is always negative (below zero), and often substantially so. How negative is a function of the blood flow rate, the blood viscosity (which increases with hematocrit), the size of the "arterial" needle or catheter lumen, and whether or not the end of the arterial needle or catheter is up against any sort of obstruction.

A. **Inflow blood line: Prepump segment.** Here we have a sampling port, on some lines a "prepump" pressure monitor (see P1 in Fig. 4-1), and a saline infusion line.

The sampling port is used to sample blood from the line. The saline "T" line is used to prime the dialyzer circuit, and also for rinse-back at the end of the procedure. Because all three of these elements (sampling port, monitor, and saline "T") are

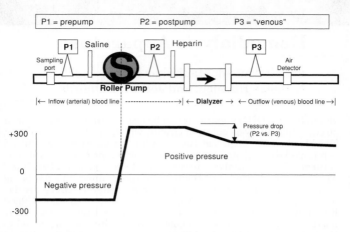

Figure 4-1. Pressure monitors (P1, P2, and P3) and pressures in blood circuit.

located in the negative pressure portion of the blood line, if a connection is broken here, air can quickly enter the blood line. Microbubbles of air can get trapped in the hollow fibers of the dialyzer, reducing efficiency of dialysis, and can also lead to clotting of the circuit. If enough air gets into the extracorporeal circuit undetected, it can enter the patient's blood stream and air embolism can result, with potentially fatal complications.

It is best to use blood lines with a prepump pressure monitor (P1), although not all blood lines have this. The actual monitor is usually a small "T" tubing attached to the line, which is usually kept filled with air, and which then is attached to an air chamber that communicates through a filter to a pressure transducer. This monitor should be configured to stop the pump in the event of inadvertent blood line disconnection. For example, a sudden line disconnection will lower the amount of suction in the prepump blood line, since it is much easier for the pump to draw in air instead of relatively viscous blood through a small-bore needle or catheter via the access. The operator sets one pressure cutoff limit for the prepump monitor that is slightly above the normal operating, negative pressure. If this cutoff is exceeded, then the blood pump shuts off and visual and audible alarms are sounded. The other cutoff limit is set more negative than the operating pressure; this other limit guards against excessive suction on the vascular access site.

B. Roller pump. The blood flow through the dialyzer is a function of roller pump rotation rate and the diameter and length of the blood line pump segment. In effect,

BFR = rpm (revolutions per minute)

$\times$ bloodline pump segment volume ($\pi r^2 \times$ length)

where BFR equals the blood flow rate.

The technician must set the roller pump to completely occlude the tubing during normal operation to ensure that the full "stroke volume" is being delivered with each pass of the roller. With some blood lines the tubing can flatten a bit at high (very negative) prepump pressures. This reduces the "stroke volume" of the blood line and can reduce the effective blood flow rate. Recent, more rigid blood tubings have solved this problem.

C. Inflow (arterial) blood line: Postpump segment. This contains a "T" for heparin infusion, and also, in some lines, a small "T" connected to a postpump (P2 in Fig. 4-1) pressure monitor. The pressure reading in this segment is always positive (above atmospheric). The pressure at P2 can be combined with the reading at the venous pressure monitor, P3, to estimate the average pressure in the blood compartment of the dialyzer. In some machines, this, in combination with pressure measured in the dialysis solution compartment, is used to calculate how much ultrafiltration is taking place during dialysis. The pressure at the postpump monitor is normally quite high, and depends on the blood flow rate, blood flow viscosity, and downstream resistance at the dialyzer and beyond. A sudden rise in the pressure at the P2 monitor is often a sign of impending clotting of the blood line and dialyzer.

D. Outflow (venous) blood line: Air trap and pressure monitor. This blood line contains a venous "drip chamber" that allows easy removal of any accumulated air from the line, a so-called "venous" pressure monitor (P3 in Fig. 4-1), and an air detector. The venous pressure can be used to monitor the state of coagulation. Incipient clotting of the blood circuit will usually first take place at the venous drip chamber, and clotting will cause a progressive rise in pressures at both P3 and P2. Venous pressure during dialysis is a function of blood flow rate, blood viscosity, and access (needle or catheter) resistance. In patients with AV access, trends in venous pressure from dialysis to dialysis, measured at a standard, low blood flow rate, and corrected for patient blood pressure and needle size, have been used to predict the occurrence of stenosis of the downstream vascular access (see Chapter 7). During dialysis, pressure cutoff limits are set so that if there is a sudden kink in the line (pressure shoots up over the limit), the blood pump will cut off. A sudden line disconnection ideally lowers the pressure below a properly set cutoff limit, again shutting down the machine and limiting the extent of blood loss. However, if the venous needle pulls out inadvertently, this may not change the outflow pressure much, since most of the outflow resistance is in the venous needle; in such instances the blood pump continues to operate, and catastrophic hemorrhage has been reported (Sandroni, 2005).

The venous air trap and detector are very important for patient safety. The chamber traps any air that may have entered the blood line before the blood is returned to the patient. Usually some type of level/air detector is placed around the top of the drip chamber; any increase in air (resulting in the drop of blood level) triggers an alarm. The power supply to the pump is cut off and dialysis stops. An additional safety device is a powerful clamp below the drip chamber that shuts off the blood flow by closing off the venous blood line, preventing any advance of blood from the drip chamber into the patient.

Additional practical information about the interpretation and use of pressure monitors during dialysis is given in Chapter 8.

II. Dialysis solution circuit. The dialysis solution circuit can be broadly divided into the following components: (a) water purification system, (b) concentrate and delivery system, (c) monitors and alarms, (d) ultrafiltration control, and (e) advanced control options.

A. Water purification system. Patients are exposed to about 120 to 200 L of water during each dialysis treatment. All small molecular weight substances present in the water can pass across the dialyzer and into the patient's bloodstream. For this reason, it is very important that the purity of the water used for dialysis be monitored and controlled. The Association for the Advancement of Medical Instrumentation (AAMI) has developed minimum standards for the purity of water used in hemodialysis. These and the methods of purifying water for dialysis are discussed in detail in Chapter 5.

B. Concentrate and delivery system. The basics of making dialysis solution are discussed in Chapter 5. To summarize, dialysis machines mix concentrated electrolyte solutions or powders with purified water to make a final dialysis solution that is delivered to the dialyzer. The final dialysis solution must be delivered at an appropriate temperature and it must be free of excessive dissolved air. This requires additional features, including monitors and alarms.

    1. Central versus individual proportioning. These are the two major types of dialysis solution delivery systems. With the central delivery system, all of the solution used for the dialysis unit is produced by a single apparatus that mixes concentrates with purified water and the final dialysis solution is pumped through pipes to each dialysis machine. With the individual system, each dialysis machine proportions its own dialysis solution concentrate with purified water. The central delivery system has the advantages of a lower initial equipment cost and reduced labor costs. However, it doesn't permit variations in the composition of dialysis solution for individual patients, and any error in the system exposes large numbers of patients to potentially grave complications.

C. Heating and degassing. Dialysis solution must be delivered to the dialyzer at the proper temperature (usually 35–38°C). Water obtained from a city water supply is below room temperature and must be heated; on heating the dissolved gases expand and bubble out. The dialysis machine must remove this air from the water before use. Degassing is usually done by exposing the heated water to a negative pressure.

D. Monitors and alarms. Several monitors and alarms are placed in the dialysis solution circuit to ensure safety.

    1. Conductivity. If the proportioning system that dilutes the concentrate with water malfunctions, an excessively dilute or concentrated dialysis solution can be produced. Exposure of blood to a severely hyperosmolar dialysis solution can lead to hypernatremia and other electrolyte disturbances. Exposure to a severely hypo-osmolar dialysis solution can result in rapid hemolysis or hyponatremia. Because the primary solutes in dialysis solution are electrolytes, the degree of concentration of dialysis solution will be reflected by its electrical conductivity, and proper proportioning of concentrate to water can be monitored by a meter that continuously measures the conductivity of the product dialysis solution as it is being fed to the dialyzer. The normal range is 12–16 mS/cm. Problems with conductivity out of range include:

    a. Empty concentrate container
    b. Concentrate line connector not plugged in
    c. Low water inlet pressure
    d. Water leaks or puddles beneath the mixing chambers

2. Temperature. Malfunction of the heating element in the dialysis machine can result in the production of excessively cool or hot dialysis solution. Use of cool dialysis solution (down to 35°C) is not dangerous unless the patient is unconscious, in which case hypothermia can occur. A conscious patient will complain of the cold and shiver. On the other hand, use of a dialysis solution heated to >42°C can lead to blood protein denaturation and, ultimately, to hemolysis. A temperature sensor in the machine continuously monitors dialysis solution temperature.

3. Bypass valve. If either the dialysis solution conductivity or temperature is found to be out of limits, a bypass valve is activated to divert the dialysis solution around the dialyzer directly to the drain.

4. Blood leak detector. The blood leak detector is placed in the dialysis solution outflow line. If this detector senses blood, as occurs when a leak develops through the dialyzer membrane, the appropriate alarm is activated.

5. Dialysate outflow pressure monitor. In machines that do not have special pumps and circuitry to control the ultrafiltration (UF) rate directly, the pressure at this location can be used in conjunction with the pressure at the blood outflow line to calculate the dialyzer transmembrane pressure (TMP) and thereby estimate the UF rate.

E. Ultrafiltration control. With the use of high-flux/high-efficiency dialyzers it is necessary to have machines that can be programmed for and control the UF rate throughout the treatment. There are several different methods by which the ultrafiltration rate can be precisely controlled. The hydraulics involved are often complex and beyond the scope of this manual. Suffice it to say that precise ultrafiltration control is a desirable feature for a dialysis machine to have and that manual efforts to determine the ultrafiltration rate by estimating the TMP are fraught with potential errors.

The most advanced method of ultrafiltration control is the so-called volumetric method. Such volumetric circuitry is incorporated into many advanced dialysis machines. With these machines, even dialyzers that are very water permeable (K_{Uf}

>10 mL per hour per mm Hg) can be used safely. Such systems have methods of tracking the dialysis solution inflow and matching it with the dialysis solution outflow either by having balancing chambers or double gear systems. This ensures that the volume of fluid delivered to the dialyzer is equal to that removed from the dialyzer. A separate line from the dialysate outflow line goes through a UF pump, which sets the UF rate. The pump is controlled by a central computer processor, which tracks the desired UF and the total UF and adjusts the UF pump speed accordingly. The line from the UF pump rejoins the dialysis solution outflow before it goes to the drain.

In simpler, older dialysis machines, the amount of fluid removed is estimated based on the water permeability (K_{Uf}) of the dialyzer and the pressures measured across the dialyzer membrane, using data from pressure sensors in the blood line and in the dialysis solution line.

F. **Advanced control options**

1. **Adjustable bicarbonate.** Machines with a variable bicarbonate option can alter the proportioning of bicarbonate concentrate to water. They allow delivery of final bicarbonate concentrations as low as 20 mM and as high as 40 mM. Such machines are very useful to treat acidotic patients or patients either with frank alkalemia or who are at high risk of developing respiratory alkalosis. However, the concentrations of other electrolytes must be closely monitored.

2. **Variable sodium.** This option permits rapid alteration of the dialysis solution sodium concentration by simply turning a dial. The sodium concentration is usually altered by changing the proportions of "acid concentrate" and water. Changing the dialysis solution sodium level in this manner will also change the concentration of all other solutes present in the "acid concentrate." The variable sodium option allows for the individualization of the dialysis solution sodium concentration on a patient-by-patient basis and also allows for the sodium concentration to be changed during the dialysis procedure.

3. **Programmable ultrafiltration.** Normally, ultrafiltration is performed at the same rate throughout the dialysis session. Some believe that a constant rate of fluid removal is not necessarily the best approach, especially when the sodium concentration is being varied during the dialysis session. Some dialysis machines allow for the bulk of the ultrafiltration to be performed during the initial portion of a dialysis session and also allow the operator to devise any form of ultrafiltration profile desired. The clinical benefits of programmable ultrafiltration have not been demonstrated by controlled studies.

4. **Dialysate urea sensor (online *Kt/V* monitor).** At least two manufacturers have developed urea sensors that measure urea concentration in the spent dialysate at multiple time points during dialysis. The sensors use this information to calculate the amount of urea removed per treatment and also can generate a dialysate side equivalent to the equilibrated Kt/V discussed in Chapter 3.

5. Online sodium clearance monitors. Because sodium clearance is similar to urea clearance, it can be used to estimate the urea clearance of a dialyzer just prior to use and also during dialysis. Typically, the machine, by acutely changing the concentrate:water proportioning ratio, initiates a momentary change in the sodium concentration of the dialysis solution flowing into the dialyzer. A conductivity sensor then estimates the resultant change in sodium of the dialysis solution leaving the dialyzer. This is a useful method of ensuring, at the point of dialysis, that the urea clearance of a reused dialyzer is still in the clinically acceptable range, and is increasingly being used to monitor adequacy from treatment to treatment.

6. Blood temperature control module. This module monitors the temperature of incoming and exiting blood, as well as of dialysis solution. It allows for control of thermal balance during dialysis. One can set the machine to add or remove heat from the patient during dialysis or to keep the body temperature constant. This module is particularly useful in providing low-temperature dialysis solutions for increased hemodynamic stability. The module may also be used to measure access recirculation or blood flow as described below.

7. Modules to measure access recirculation or access blood flow. These all work on the dilution principle (Fig. 4-2). The composition of the blood leaving the dialyzer is quickly altered by (a) injecting 5 mL of isotonic or hypertonic saline, (b) acutely changing the dialyzer ultrafiltration rate to promote hemoconcentration, or (c) acutely changing the dialysis solution temperature to cool the returning blood. A sensor attached to the blood inflow line seeks to detect the resulting change in conductivity, hematocrit, or temperature. If there is access recirculation, the perturbation

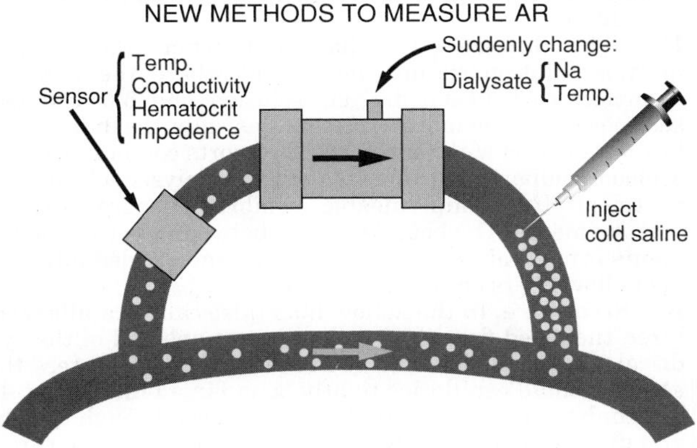

Figure 4-2. Principles of measuring access recirculation (AR). (Reproduced from Daugirdas JT. *Hypertens Dial Clin Nephrol* 1997. Available at: http://www.hdcn.com.)

caused in the outflow line will almost immediately be detected in the inflow line sensor, and the magnitude of the perturbation will reflect the degree of recirculation. To measure access flow, the lines are deliberately reversed, such that the inflow (arterial) needle is drawing blood from the access "downstream" to the outflow (venous) needle. In this manner, access recirculation is induced. The degree of recirculation is then measured as above. The degree of recirculation is proportional to the ratio of flows in the extracorporeal circuit and access. Once the degree of recirculation has been measured, the extracorporeal blood flow is known, and the rate of access blood flow can be calculated (Krivitski, 1995).

8.   Blood volume monitors. These use an ultrasonic or optical sensor operating on the inflow blood line to detect changes in hematocrit during dialysis. Normally, in the course of fluid removal, the hematocrit increases, and the amount of increase reflects the degree of plasma volume reduction. One claimed feature of such monitors is to be able to anticipate and prevent a hypotensive episode by reducing ultrafiltration whenever a limiting increase in hematocrit during dialysis has occurred or when a "crash crit," identified during previous sessions, is being approached. Another potential use is to identify patients with covert fluid overload by recognizing that such patients tend to have only a minimal, or no, increase in hematocrit during dialysis despite fluid removal.

9.   Single blood pathway ("single-needle") devices. Most hemodialysis treatments are performed using two separate blood pathways: One to obtain blood from the patient and another to return blood to the patient. Several systems allow dialysis to be performed using a Y-shaped single blood pathway. Description and discussion of single-needle devices is beyond the scope of this book as they are used only rarely in the United States; their use is increasing in the context of home dialysis and, especially, home nocturnal dialysis.

III.   The dialyzer. The dialyzer is where the blood and dialysis solution circuits meet, and where the movement of molecules between dialysis solution and blood across a semipermeable membrane occurs. Basically, the dialyzer shell is a box or tube with four ports. Two ports communicate with a blood compartment and two with a dialysis solution compartment. The semipermeable membrane separates the two compartments. The boundary area between the two compartments is maximized by using a membrane divided into multiple hollow fibers or parallel plates.

A.   Structure. In the hollow-fiber (also called capillary) dialyzer, the blood flows into a chamber at one end of the cylindrical shell, called a *header*. From there, blood enters thousands of small capillaries tightly bound in a bundle (Fig. 4-3). The dialyzer is designed so that blood flows through the fibers and dialysis solution flows around the outside. Once through the capillaries, the blood collects in a chamber at the other end of the cylindrical shell, the second header, and is then routed back to the patient through the venous tubing and

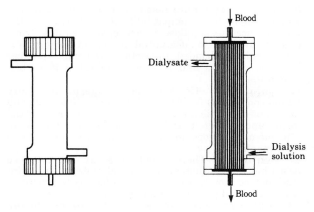

Hollow-fiber dialyzer

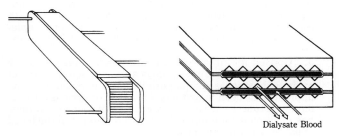

Parallel-plate dialyzer

Figure 4-3. Blood and dialysis solution flow pathways through a hollow-fiber and parallel-plate dialyzer. (Modified from Man NK, Jungers P. Hemodialysis equipment. In: Hamburger J, Crosnier J, Grunfeld JP, eds. *Nephrology.* New York: Wiley, 1979:1206, 1207.)

venous access device. In parallel-plate dialyzers, now rarely used in the United States, the blood is routed between sheets of membranes laid on top of one another. The dialyzer is configured so that blood and dialysis solution pass through alternate spaces between the membrane sheets.

    1. Membranes. Four types of membranes are currently used in dialyzers: cellulose, "substituted" cellulose, cellulosynthetic, and synthetic.

    a. Cellulose. The cellulose is obtained from processed cotton. Cellulose membranes go by various names, such as regenerated cellulose, cuprammonium cellulose (Cuprophane), cuprammonium rayon, and saponified cellulose ester.

    b. Substituted cellulose. The cellulose polymer has a large number of free hydroxyl groups at its surface. These free hydroxyl group are responsible for blood cell activation causing bio-incompatibility of the dialyzer. In the cellulose acetate, cellulose diacetate, and cellulose triacetate membranes, a substantial number of these groups are chemically bonded to acetate, reducing the free hydroxyl moieties and making membranes more biocompatible.

c. **Cellulosynthetic.** A synthetic material (a tertiary amino compound) is added to liquefied cellulose during formation of the membrane. As a result, the surface of the membrane is altered, and biocompatibility is increased. This membrane goes under the trade names of Cellosyn or Hemophan.

d. **Synthetics.** These membranes are not cellulose based but are synthetic plastics, and materials used include polyacrylonitrile (PAN), polysulfone, polycarbonate, polyamide, and polymethyl-methacrylate (PMMA).

2. **Complement activation with different membrane materials.** During dialysis using membranes made from unsubstituted cellulose, the free hydroxyl groups on the membrane surface activate the complement system in blood flowing through the dialyzer. Complement activation occurs to a much lesser extent with substituted cellulose or cellulosynthetic membranes, and least of all with the synthetic membranes. The consequences of complement activation during dialysis are discussed in Chapter 10.

3. **Coated membranes.** Much research is ongoing to try to limit the effect of hemodialysis on increasing levels of oxidant substances and potentially harmful cytokines. One approach has been to coat membranes with various antioxidant substances such as vitamin E. Use of such membranes has resulted in an improved antioxidant profile in the blood of patients using the device.

4. **Membrane permeability to solutes and to water.** The permeability to solutes and water of each of the four membrane types can be altered markedly by adjusting the thickness of the membrane and the pore size.

5. **Membrane efficiency versus flux.** The ability of a dialyzer to remove small molecular weight solutes, such as urea, is primarily a function of its membrane surface area (plus a minor component due to dialyzer and membrane design). A high-efficiency dialyzer is basically a big dialyzer that by virtue of its larger surface area has a high ability to remove urea. High-efficiency dialyzers can have small or large pores, and thus can have either high or low clearance for larger molecular weight solutes, such as β_2-microglobulin (MW 11,800). High-flux membranes have large pores that are capable of passing larger molecules, such as β_2-microglobulin. Usually, β_2-microglobulin clearances are not reported in standard dialyzer specification charts. High-flux membranes also have high water permeability, with coefficient of ultrafiltration (K_{Uf}) values >10 mL per hour per mm Hg, and usually >20 mL per hour per mm Hg.

B. Interpreting a dialyzer specification sheet (Table 4-1). Information usually provided about dialyzers includes K_{Uf}; clearance of solutes such as urea, creatinine, vitamin B_{12}, and phosphate (and occasionally β_2-microglobulin); membrane surface area; priming volume; fiber length; and fiber wall thickness.

1. K_{Uf}. The ultrafiltration coefficient, as defined in Chapter 3, is the volume of plasma water filtered in milliliters per hour for each mm Hg of transmembrane pressure (TMP). Thus, the ultrafiltration rate per hour is the product of K_{Uf} and TMP; a K_{Uf} of 2.0 is considered to be a low value. To remove 1,000 mL per hour, 500 mm Hg TMP will be needed. If the K_{Uf} is 4.0, the permeability to water is moderate, and the required TMP will be only 250 mm Hg. If the K_{Uf} is 8.0, the TMP will have to be only 125 mm Hg. Certain synthetic membranes are noted for their extremely high permeability to water, with K_{Uf} values in the range of 10–60 mL per hour per mm Hg. When the K_{Uf} is high, small errors in setting the TMP will result in large errors in the amount of ultrafiltrate removed. For this reason, dialyzers with a $K_{Uf} > 6.0$ (certainly those with a $K_{Uf} > 8.0$) should be used only with dialysis machines that contain special pumps and circuits that directly control the ultrafiltration rate.

The K_{Uf} values reported by dialyzer companies are usually in vitro values. In practice, the in vivo K_{Uf} is often somewhat lower (5%–30%). Some companies publish both an in vitro K_{Uf} and an "expected in vivo" K_{Uf} value. The numbers listed in Table 4-1 are mostly in vitro values.

2. Clearance. Similar to the native kidney, the solute removal efficiency can be expressed in terms of clearance. It can be defined as the volume of blood (plasma) from which a solute is removed per unit time during its transit through the dialyzer. Clearance can be expressed as:

$$K_s = Q_B \frac{(C_{bi} - C_{bo})}{C_{bi}}$$

where K_s = clearance of solute s, C_{bi} = blood concentration of s at dialyzer inlet (arterial), and C_{bo} = blood concentration of s at dialyzer outlet (venous). Q_B = blood flow rate.

a. Mass transfer area coefficient (K_0A). The K_0A is the maximum theoretical clearance of the dialyzer in milliliters per minute for a given solute at infinite blood and dialysis solution flow rates. For any given membrane, K_0A will be proportional to the surface area of the membrane in the dialyzer, although there is a drop-off in the gain in K_0A as membrane surface area becomes very large. The dialyzer mass transfer area coefficient for urea, K_0A, is a measure of dialyzer efficiency in clearing urea and solutes of similar molecular weight.

Dialyzers with K_0A values <500 should be used only for "low-efficiency" dialysis or for small patients. Dialyzers with K_0A values of 500–700 represent moderate-efficiency dialyzers, useful for routine therapy. Dialyzers with K_0A values >700 are used for "high-efficiency" dialysis.

Table 4-1. Specifications of selected dialyzers and hemofilters

Manufacturer	Model		Surface Area (m²)	Membrane	Sterilization	Performance					
						K_{UF} mL per Hour per mm Hg	Urea Cl Q_B = 200 mL per Minute	Urea Cl Q_B = 300 mL per Minute	K_0A mL per minute	Priming Volume mL	Use
ASAHI	PAN	65DX	1.3	Polyacrylonitrile	ETO	29.0	181	231	635	100	HD
		85DX	1.7	Polyacrylonitrile	ETO	38.0	190	251	839	124	HD
		110DX	2.2	Polyacrylonitrile	ETO	49.0	193	260	955	161	HD
	APS	550S	1.1	Polysulfone	Gamma	50.0	180	226	619	66	HD
		650S	1.3	Polysulfone	Gamma	57.0	186	240	731	80	HD
		900S	1.8	Polysulfone	Gamma	68.0	192	258	911	105	HD
		1050S	2.1	Polysulfone	Gamma	75.0	193	261	955	114	HD
	Rexeed	15R	1.5	Polysulfone	Gamma	63.0	196		1,138	82	HD
		18R	1.8	Polysulfone	Gamma	71.0	198		1,367	95	HD
		21R	2.1	Polysulfone	Gamma	74.0	199		1,597	112	HD
		25R	2.5	Polysulfone	Gamma	80.0	199		1,597	128	HD
		25S	2.5	Polysulfone	Gamma	80.0	199		1,597	128	HD
	ViE	13	1.3	Polysulfone-vitamin E	Gamma	37.0	183		670	80	HD
		15	1.5	Polysulfone-vitamin E	Gamma	40.0	187		755	90	HD
		18	1.8	Polysulfone-vitamin E	Gamma	43.0	190		839	105	HD
		21	2.1	Polysulfone-vitamin E	Gamma	45.0	192		911	114	HD
B BRAUN SCHIWA	Diacap	PS10 Low	1.0	Polysulfone	Gamma	6.8	176	217	562	58	HD
		PS12 Low	1.2	Polysulfone	Gamma	7.9	183	233	670	68	HD
		PS15 Low	1.5	Polysulfone	Gamma	9.8	189	240	809	90	HD
		PS18 Low	1.8	Polysulfone	Gamma	12.3	192	253	911	104	HD
		PS20 Low	2.0	Polysulfone	Gamma	13.7	194	258	1,005	113	HD
		PS10 High	1.0	Polysulfone	Gamma	34.0	180	223	619	58	HD/HF/HDF
		PS12 High	1.2	Polysulfone	Gamma	42.0	186	238	731	68	HD/HF/HDF
		PS15 High	1.5	Polysulfone	Gamma	50.0	190	245	839	90	HD/HF/HDF
		PS18 High	1.8	Polysulfone	Gamma	55.0	192	250	911	110	HD/HF/HDF

BAXTER	PSN	PS20 High		Membrane	Sterilization						HD/HF/HDF
		120	2.0	Polysulfone	Gamma	58.0	194	253	1,005	121	HD
		140	1.2	Polysynthane	ETO	6.7	180	228	619	75	HD
		110	1.4	Polysynthane	ETO	7.6	184	237	689	84	HD
	CA	110	1.1	Cellulose acetate	ETO or Gamma	5.3	176	215	562	74	HD
		130	1.3	Cellulose acetate	ETO or Gamma	5.6	179	229	604	85	HD
		150	1.5	Cellulose acetate	ETO or Gamma	7.2	185	238	709	98	HD
		170	1.7	Cellulose acetate	ETO or Gamma	7.6	194	247	1,005	110	HD
		190	1.9	Cellulose acetate	ETO or Gamma	10.1	198		1,367	133	HD
	CA-HP	90	0.9	Cellulose diacetate	ETO	7.3	172	213	515	60	HD
		110	1.1	Cellulose diacetate	ETO	7.7	177	227	575	70	HD
		130	1.3	Cellulose diacetate	ETO	9.1	186	240	731	80	HD
		150	1.5	Cellulose diacetate	ETO	10.2	187	245	755	95	HD
		170	1.7	Cellulose diacetate	ETO	10.0	192	259	911	105	HD
		210	2.1	Cellulose diacetate	ETO	13.2	194	266	1,005	125	HD
		90G	0.8	Cellulose diacetate	ETO or Gamma	6.8	173	214	526	60	HD
	DICEA	110G	1.1	Cellulose diacetate	ETO or Gamma	8.4	179	229	604	70	HD
		130G	1.3	Cellulose diacetate	ETO or Gamma	10.0	186	239	731	80	HD
		150G	1.5	Cellulose diacetate	ETO or Gamma	11.4	189	248	809	95	HD
		170G	1.7	Cellulose diacetate	ETO or Gamma	12.5	191	260	873	105	HD
		210G	2.1	Cellulose diacetate	ETO or Gamma	15.5	196	268	1,138	125	HD

continued

Table 4-1. *Continued.*

Manufacturer	Model	Surface Area (m²)	Membrane	Sterilization	K_{Uf} per Hour per mm Hg	Urea Cl Q_B = 200 mL per Minute	Urea Cl Q_B = 300 mL per Minute	K_0A mL per minute	Priming Volume mL	Use
TRICEA	110G	1.1	Cellulose triacetate	Gamma	25.0	188	259	781	65	HD/HF/HDF
EXELTRA	150G	1.5	Cellulose triacetate	Gamma	29.0	197	278	1,233	90	HD/HF/HDF
	190G	1.9	Cellulose triacetate	Gamma	37.0	198	284	1,367	115	HD/HF/HDF
	210G	2.1	Cellulose triacetate	Gamma	39.0	199	287	1,597	125	HD/HF/HDF
	150	1.5	Cellulose triacetate	Gamma	31.0	193	262	955	95	HD/HF/HDF
	170	1.7	Cellulose triacetate	Gamma	34.0	196	268	1,138	105	HD/HF/HDF
	190	1.9	Cellulose triacetate	Gamma	36.0	197	273	1,233	115	HD/HF/HDF
	210Plus	2.1	Cellulose triacetate	Gamma	47.0	199		1,597	125	HD/HF/HDF
SYNTRA	120	1.2	Polyethersulfone	Gamma	58.0	185	238	709	87	HD/HF/HDF
	160	1.6	Polyethersulfone	Gamma	73.0	190	253	839	117	HD/HF/HDF
BELLCO-SORIN BLS	512	1.3	Polyethersulfone	Gamma or Heat	10.0		226	599	77	HD/HF/HDF
	514	1.4	Polyethersulfone	Gamma or Heat	12.0		229	621	85	HD/HF/HDF
	517	1.7	Polyethersulfone	Gamma or Heat	17.0		234	662	99	HD/HF/HDF
	812	1.2	Polyethersulfone	Gamma or Heat	51.0		241	726	73	HD/HF/HDF
	814	1.4	Polyethersulfone	Gamma or Heat	61.0		246	778	85	HD/HF/HDF
	816	1.6	Polyethersulfone	Gamma or Heat	68.0		250	824	94	HD/HF/HDF
	819	1.9	Polyethersulfone	Gamma or Heat	80.0		255	888	109	HD/HF/HDF

Manufacturer	Series	Model		Membrane	Sterilization						
FRESENIUS	F	4HPS	0.8	Polysulfone	Steam	8.0	170	190	494	51	HD
		5HPS	1.0	Polysulfone	Steam	10.0	179	217	604	63	HD
		6HPS	1.3	Polysulfone	Steam	13.0	186	237	731	78	HD
		7HPS	1.6	Polysulfone	Steam	16.0	188	240	781	96	HD
		8HPS	1.8	Polysulfone	Steam	18.0		252	849	113	HD
		10HPS	2.1	Polysulfone	Steam	21.0		259	945	132	HD
	Optiflux F	160NR	1.5	Polysulfone	Steam	45.0		266	1,064	84	HD/HF/HDF
		180A	1.8	Polysulfone	Steam	55.0		274	1,239	105	HD/HF/HDF
		200A	2.0	Polysulfone	Steam	56.0		277	1,321	113	HD/HF/HDF
		200NR	2.0	Polysulfone	Steam	56.0		277	1,321	113	HD/HF/HDF
	F	50S	1.0	Polysulfone	Steam	30.0	178		589	63	HD/HDF
		60S	1.3	Polysulfone	Steam	40.0	185		709	82	HD/HDF
		70S	1.6	Polysulfone	Steam	50.0	190		839	98	HD/HDF
	FX	40	0.6	Polysulfone	Steam	20.0	170		494	32	HD/HF/HDF
		50	1.0	Polysulfone	Steam	33.0	189		809	53	HD/HF/HDF
		60	1.4	Polysulfone	Steam	46.0	193		955	74	HD/HF/HDF
		80	1.8	Polysulfone	Steam	59.0		276	1,292	95	HD/HF/HDF
		100	2.2	Polysulfone	Steam	73.0		278	1,351	116	HD/HF/HDF
GAMBRO	Polyflux	14S	1.4	Polyamide blend	Steam	62.0	186	242	731	102	HD
		17S	1.7	Polyamide blend	Steam	71.0	191	254	873	121	HD
		21S	2.1	Polyamide blend	Steam	83.0		267	1,083	152	HD
		24S	2.4	Polyamide blend	Steam	60.0		274	1,239	165	HD
		140H	1.4	Polyamide blend	Steam	52.0	193	261	955	75	HD/HF/HDF
		170H	1.7	Polyamide blend	Steam	65.0	195	268	1,065	94	HD/HF/HDF
		210H	2.1	Polyamide blend	Steam	78.0		282	1,487	120	HD/HF/HDF
		17R	1.7	Polyamide blend	Steam	71.0		254	874	121	HD/HF/HDF
		21R	2.1	Polyamide blend	Steam	83.0		267	1,083	152	HD/HF/HDF
		24R	2.4	Polyamide blend	Steam	77.0		274	1,239	165	HD/HF/HDF
		14L	1.4	Polyamide blend	Steam	10.0		252	849	81	HD

continued

Table 4-1. *Continued.*

Manufacturer	Model	Surface Area (m²)	Membrane	Sterilization	Performance					Use
					K_{Uf} mL per Hour per mm Hg	Urea Cl Q_B = 200 mL per Minute	Urea Cl Q_B = 300 mL per Minute	K_oA mL per minute	Priming Volume mL	
HOSPAL	17L	1.7	Polyamide blend	Steam	12.5		264	1,027	104	HD
	21L	2.1	Polyamide blend	Steam	15.0		275	1,265	123	HD
	6L/6LR	1.4	Polyamide blend	Steam	8.6		242	736	115	HD
	8L/8LR	1.7	Polyamide blend	Steam	11.3		253	861	125	HD
	10L/10LR	2.1	Polyamide blend	Steam	14.0		263	1,010	156	HD
	Nephral ST 200	1.1	Polyacrylonitrile	Gamma	33.0	173	216	526	64	HD/HF/HDF
	300	1.3	Polyacrylonitrile	Gamma	40.0	181	231	635	81	HD/HF/HDF
	400	1.7	Polyacrylonitrile	Gamma	50.0	189	250	809	98	HD/HF/HDF
	500	2.2	Polyacrylonitrile	Gamma	65	195		1,065	126	HD/HF/HDF
IDEMSA	MHP 120	1.2	Polyethersulfone	Gamma	29.0	180	220	619	71	HD/HF/HDF
	140	1.4	Polyethersulfone	Gamma	33.0	182	224	652	81	HD/HF/HDF
	160	1.6	Polyethersulfone	Gamma	37.0	186	233	731	88	HD/HF/HDF
	180	1.8	Polyethersulfone	Gamma	44.0	193	245	955	104	HD/HF/HDF
	200	2.0	Polyethersulfone	Gamma	50.0	195	251	1,065	112	HD/HF/HDF
NIPRO	Surelyzer PES 110DH	1.1	Polyethersulfone	Gamma	32	187		755	68	HD/HDF
	150DH	1.5	Polyethersulfone	Gamma	43	195	249	1,065	93	HD/HDF

Brand	Model		Material	Sterilization							Type
Sureflux	190DH	1.9	Polyethersulfone	Gamma	55	198		1,367	118	HD/HDF
	150L	1.5	Cellulose triacetate	Gamma	12.8		249	812	90	HD
	150E	1.5	Cellulose triacetate	Gamma	20.5		250	824	90	HD
FB	150U	1.5	Cellulose triacetate	Gamma	29.8		263	1,010	90	HD/HF/HDF
	150UH	1.5	Cellulose triacetate	Gamma	50.1		270	1,145	90	HD/HF/HDF
	150DL	1.5	Polyethersulfone	Gamma	16		231	637	90	HD
Surelyzer PES										
NIKKISO FLX	15GW	1.5	Polyester polymer alloy	Gamma	39	193		955	92	HD/HDF
	18GW	1.8	Polyester polymer alloy	Gamma	47	197		1,233	108	HD/HDF
FDX	150GW	1.5	Polyester polymer alloy	Gamma	50	190		839	91	HD/HDF
	180GW	1.8	Polyester polymer alloy	Gamma	57	192		911	108	HD/HDF
FDY	150GW	1.5	Polyester polymer alloy	Gamma	52	191		873	91	HD/HDF
	180GW	1.8	Polyester polymer alloy	Gamma	59	193		955	108	HD/HDF

continued

Table 4-1. Continued.

Manufacturer	Model		Surface Area (m²)	Membrane	Sterilization	K_{UF} mL per Hour per mm Hg	Urea Cl Q_B = 200 mL per Minute	Urea Cl Q_B = 300 mL per Minute	K_0A mL per minute	Priming Volume mL	Use
							Performance				
NEPHROS	OLpur MD	190	1.9	Polyethersulfone	E-beam	90	283[a]		1,527	140	HDF
		220	2.2	Polyethersulfone	E-beam	105	291[a]		1,976	155	HDF
TORAY	B1-H		1.0	PMMA	Gamma	9	169		484	73	HD
			1.3	PMMA	Gamma	12	180		619	86	HD
			1.6	PMMA	Gamma	14	187		755	98	HD
	B3		1.0	PMMA	Gamma	7	175		550	61	HD
			1.3	PMMA	Gamma	8.8	184		689	76	HD
			1.6	PMMA	Gamma	8.7	188		781	95	HD
			2.0	PMMA	Gamma	11	193		955	118	HD
	BK-P		1.3	PMMA	Gamma	26	182		652	76	HD/HDF
			1.6	PMMA	Gamma	33	189		809	94	HD/HDF
			2.1	PMMA	Gamma	41	194		1,005	126	HD/HDF
	BS		1.3	Polysulfone	Gamma	47	192		911	81	HD/HF/HDF
			1.6	Polysulfone	Gamma	50.0	194		1,005	102	HD/HF/HDF
			1.8	Polysulfone	Gamma	52.0	197		1,233	116	HD/HF/HDF

N.B. Apart from those made of cellulose material in the form of polysynthane and of various acetate salts of cellulose, all of the above filters are fashioned from synthetic material. All the filters above listed consist of hollow fibers. K_{UF}, ultrafiltration coefficient; Cl, clearance; Q_B, blood flow rate; K_0A, mass transfer area coefficient for urea; ETO, ethylene oxide; Gamma, gamma irradiation; E-beam, electron-beam; PMMA, polymethylmethacrylate; HD, hemodialysis; HF, hemofiltration; HDF, hemodiafiltration; Qs, substitution fluid administration rate.
[a]Cl/K_0A data at Qs = 200 mL per minute.

b. Obtaining the dialyzer K_0A. The K_0A, or maximum theoretical clearance of any dialyzer, can be computed from the urea clearances on a dialyzer specification sheet, according to Figure A-5. A more exact computation is given in Table A-3.

Once the dialyzer K_0A is known, Figure A-1a can be used to estimate the in vivo urea clearance at any given blood flow rate when the dialysis solution flow rate is 500 mL per minute. For more precise values, and when Q_D (dialysis solution flow rate) is other than 500 mL per minute, use the equations in Table A-1.

(1) Urea. The clearance values provided by the manufacturer for urea (MW 60) are those measured in vitro. Clearances are usually reported at "blood" flow rates of 200, 300, and 400 mL per minute. The values in the specification sheet for urea clearance are usually higher than those obtained during actual dialysis but are useful for comparing dialyzers.

(2) Creatinine. Some manufacturers provide creatinine (MW 113) clearance values. The dialyzer creatinine clearance is usually about 80% of the urea clearance and provides no clinically useful additional information, as the clearances for the two molecules are almost always proportional, regardless of membrane or dialyzer type.

(3) Vitamin B_{12} and β_2-microglobulin. In vitro clearance of vitamin B_{12} (MW 1,355) is an indication of how well the membrane allows the passage of larger molecular weight solutes. Recently, it has become customary to consider the clearance of β_2-microglobulin (MW 11,800) rather than vitamin B_{12} to characterize the flux of a dialyzer. In vitro measures of β_2-microglobulin are problematic and are not usually reported. One problem with making dialyzers very permeable to increase β_2-microglobulin removal has been increased loss of albumin. It turns out that much of this problem is due to nonuniformity of pore size in such membranes. New "nanotechnology" approaches to manufacturing high-flux membranes have resulted in relatively high β_2-microglobulin removal rates with very acceptable (low) levels of albumin loss.

(4) Phosphate clearance. Because of the growing interest in prevention of hyperphosphatemia to improve outcome, some dialyzer manufacturers have begun to optimize the phosphate clearance of their dialyzers. This is often reported on dialyzer spec sheets. The main barrier to phosphate removal is the rather quick fall in serum Pi that occurs early during dialysis. Because of this, only slight improvements in Pi removal with such optimized membranes are to be expected.

(5) Protein-losing membranes. Because some uremic toxins are tightly bound to albumin, one school of thought has been to use membranes with a high albumin permeability deliberately. Such protein-losing membranes are not widely used.

3.   Surface area. The membrane surface area of most dialyzers ranges between 0.8–2.1 m². Large surface area dialyzers normally have high urea clearances, although dialyzer design and thickness of the membrane are also important. With an unsubstituted cellulose membrane, a large membrane surface area is undesirable because the degree of complement activation is proportional to the membrane surface area. Surface area is not as important an issue with more biocompatible membranes such as synthetic membranes with regard to complement activation since their complement activation per unit area is quite low to begin with.

4.   Priming volume. The priming volume of most of dialyzers is usually 60–120 mL and is related to the membrane surface area. It should be remembered that the priming volume of the blood lines is about 100–150 mL. Hence, total extracorporeal circuit volume will be 160–270 mL. In the typical adult patient, the presence of 10 or 20 mL more or less in the dialyzer is of little clinical importance, but priming volume could be important in pediatric or very small patients.

5.   Fiber length and thickness. This information is of little clinical usefulness. Both membrane thickness and fiber length influence dialyzer efficiency.

6.   Mode of sterilization. The three primary methods of sterilization are by use of γ-irradiation, steam autoclaving, or ethylene oxide gas. The use of ethylene oxide has lost popularity because of the rare but serious occurrence of anaphylactic reactions during dialysis in occasional patients who are allergic to ethylene oxide.

SELECTED READINGS

Core curriculum for the dialysis technician. Medical Media Publishing, 2006.

Krivitski NM. Theory and validation of access flow measurement by dilution technique during hemodialysis. *Kidney Int* 1995;48:244–250.

Misra M. Core curriculum. The basics of hemodialysis equipment. *Hemodial Int* 2005;9:30–36.

Sandroni S. Venous needle dislodgement during hemodialysis: an unresolved risk of catastrophic hemorrhage (abstract). *Hemodial Int* 2005;9:102–103.

WEB REFERENCES

Dialyzer K_0A calculator: www.hdcn.com/calc.htm
Expanded dialyzer clearance table: www.hdcn.com/calc.htm

Product Water and Hemodialysis Solution Preparation

Richard A. Ward and Todd S. Ing

I. Product water for hemodialysis. Patients are exposed to 120–200 L of dialysis solution during each dialysis treatment. Any small molecular weight contaminants in the dialysis solution can enter the blood unimpeded and accumulate in the body in the absence of renal excretion. Therefore, the chemical and microbiologic purity of dialysis solution is important if patient injury is to be avoided. Dialysis solution is prepared from purified water (product water) and concentrates, the latter containing the electrolytes necessary to provide dialysis solution of the prescribed composition. Most concentrates are obtained from commercial sources and their purity is subject to regulatory oversight. The purity of the water used to prepare dialysis solution, or to reconstitute concentrates from powder at a dialysis facility, is the responsibility of the dialysis facility. Some substances added to municipal water supplies for public health reasons pose no threat to healthy individuals at the concentrations used, but can cause injury to renal failure patients if these substances are allowed to remain in the water used for dialysis. Therefore, all municipal water supplies should be assumed to contain substances harmful to dialysis patients and all dialysis facilities require a system for purifying municipal water before it is used to prepare dialysis solution.

A. Water contaminants harmful to dialysis patients. What follows is a list of the most common offending substances. Please see the Suggested Readings for a more complete discussion of the others.

1. Aluminum is added as a flocculating agent by many municipal water systems (aluminum sulfate is used to remove nonfilterable suspended particles). Aluminum causes bone disease, a progressive and often fatal neurologic deterioration known as the dialysis encephalopathy syndrome, and anemia.

2. Chloramine is added to water to prevent bacterial proliferation. Chloramine causes hemolytic anemia.

3. Fluoride. This is added to water supplies to reduce tooth decay. Large amounts of **fluoride** can elute from an exhausted deionizer and cause severe pruritus, nausea, and fatal ventricular fibrillation.

4. Copper and zinc. These can leach from metal pipes and fittings and cause hemolytic anemia. Lead, also, as well as aluminum, can enter the water stream in a similar fashion.

5.   Bacteria and endotoxin. Because the substances added to municipal water to suppress bacterial proliferation are removed by a dialysis facility's water purification system, both the water used to prepare dialysis solution and the final dialysis solution are susceptible to microbiologic contamination by bacteria and their endotoxins. Endotoxins, endotoxin fragments, and other bacterial products, such as short bacterial DNA fragments, some of which can be as small as 1,250 daltons, can cross the dialyzer membranes and enter the bloodstream to produce pyrogenic reactions and other untoward effects.

B.   Water and dialysis solution quality requirements

1.   AAMI versus European Pharmacopoeia. The Association for the Advancement of Medical Instrumentation (AAMI) has developed minimum standards for the purity of the water used to prepare dialysis solution and also has made recommendations concerning the purity of the final dialysis solution produced. The European Pharmacopoeia has developed more stringent recommendations for microbiological contaminants. These standards and recommendations set maximum levels for chemicals known to be toxic to hemodialysis patients, for chemicals known to be toxic to the general population, and for bacteria and their endotoxins.

Current AAMI recommendations are that product water used to prepare dialysis solution, and the resultant dialysis solution, should contain **<200 colony-forming units (CFU)/mL** of bacteria and **<2.0 endotoxin units (EU)/mL** of endotoxin. The values for product water recommended by the European Pharmacopoeia are **<100 CFU/mL** and **<0.25 EU/mL,** respectively (no values for dialysis solution are recommended by the European Pharmacopoeia). Pyrogenic reactions do not occur when levels of bacteria and endotoxins in the dialysis solution are maintained below these limits.

2.   Low concentration of endotoxin fragments and ultrapure dialysis solution. Recently, it has become apparent that low levels of endotoxins and endotoxin fragments in dialysis solution, while not causing pyrogenic reactions, may contribute to a chronic inflammatory response that may be associated with long-term morbidity in dialysis patients. In observational studies, the use of very pure dialysis solution has been suggested to reduce the plasma levels of C-reactive protein and interleukin-6; to improve the response of anemia to erythropoietin therapy; to promote better nutrition as evidenced by increases in plasma albumin value, estimated dry body weight, midarm muscle circumference, and urea nitrogen appearance rate; to reduce plasma levels of β_2-microglobulin and pentosidine (a surrogate marker of carbonyl stress); to slow the loss of residual renal function; and to lower cardiovascular morbidity.

3.   When is ultrapure dialysis solution indicated? Although not all of the above benefits have been fully confirmed, some authorities believe that "ultrapure dialysis solution," which is characterized by a **bacteria level below 0.1 CFU/mL** and **endotoxin level below 0.03 EU/mL,**

should be used routinely. Use of ultrapure dialysis solution is thus highly desirable for hemodialysis, and is a requirement for online convective therapies, such as hemofiltration and hemodiafiltration (see Chapter 15).

C. Methods of purifying water for hemodialysis. Systems used to purify water for dialysis consist of three parts: **Pretreatment, primary purification, and distribution** to the point of use.

    1. Pretreatment. These components usually include a valve to blend hot and cold water to a constant temperature, some form of preliminary filtration, softening, and adsorption with activated carbon. This cascade is designed to prepare the water for optimal operation of the primary purification process. Correction of pH (using injection of hydrochloric acid) is sometimes needed to correct excessive alkalinity, which can impede functioning of carbon adsorption beds as well as of the reverse osmosis (RO) membrane.

        a. Water softener. A water softener is used to remove calcium and magnesium from water by ionic exchange with sodium that has been affixed to a resin bed. The resin exchanges two Na^+ ions for Ca^{++} and Mg^{++} as well as other cations such as iron and manganese. The water softener protects the RO membrane downstream, as calcium and magnesium can form scale or mineral deposits on these membranes and foul them, sometimes very quickly. Water softener resins need to be regenerated on a routine basis using a concentrated sodium chloride solution (brine). During regeneration, water is drawn into the softener in a reverse direction (backwashing) and then the brine solution is introduced to regenerate the resin, replacing the adsorbed Ca^{++} and Mg^{++} with sodium ion.

        b. Carbon adsorption. Adsorption by activated carbon is utilized to remove chlorine and chloramines, which are not removed by reverse osmosis, and which can damage the RO membrane. Chloramines can cause hemolytic anemia. Chloramines take a longer time to be adsorbed by the carbon than chlorine, and so when municipalities change over from using chlorine to chloramines (chlorine in the water can combine with organic contaminants to form potentially cancer-causing compounds), outbreaks of hemolytic anemia have been reported. Carbon adsorption also removes other small organic compounds that may be in the water. Two carbon adsorption beds are used in series to permit sequential replacement as the upstream bed becomes exhausted. Optimal removal of chloramines by carbon adsorption may require adjustment of the pH of the feed water. Even with pH adjustment, carbon adsorption may provide inadequate removal of chloramines if the water contains corrosion inhibitors or other substances that prevent chloramine molecules from reaching the surface of the carbon. In these situations it may be necessary to use alternative methods of chloramine removal such as injection of sodium metabisulfite.

    2. Primary purification process. The primary purification process is almost always reverse osmosis. A filter is normally set in place just upstream to the RO membrane to catch any carbon particles and resin beads that may have been inadvertently released from the pretreatment system.

a.   Reverse osmosis. This is achieved by high pressure filtration of water (using a powerful pump) through a semipermeable membrane that will hold back the dissolved solutes. Reverse osmosis will remove more than 95% of ionic contaminants and nonionic contaminants as small as glucose. In addition, it provides an effective barrier against bacteria and endotoxins. In many cases, reverse osmosis will provide water of sufficient quality for the preparation of dialysis solution without further purification.

b.   Deionization. Deionization may be used as an alternative to reverse osmosis, but is more frequently used to further purify water following processing by reverse osmosis. Deionizers do not remove nonionic contaminants, bacteria, or endotoxins. A solid-phase deionizer contains either two beds (one for the cationic resin and the other for the anionic resin) or one bed (containing a mixture of both resins). Cationic resins contain sulfuric radicals and these exchange hydrogen ions for other cations such as sodium, calcium, and aluminum. Anionic resins contain ammonium radicals, which exchange hydroxyl ions for other anions such as chloride, phosphate, and fluoride. The exchanged hydrogen and hydroxyl ions then combine to become water. By the time the water has reached the deionizer, all bacteriostatic substances such as chlorine and chloramines will have been removed, and so the bacterial contamination level of water flowing through deionizer tanks is subject to increase. For this reason, deionizers are usually followed by an **ultrafilter.** Some centers also prefer to destroy bacteria (whether in a vegetative or a sporulated state) with **ultraviolet radiation.** However, the process increases the lipopolysaccharide and peptidoglycan content of the treated water due to bacterial death.

3.   Distribution of purified water. Purified water intended for the preparation of dialysis solution must be distributed to the individual dialysis machines to produce dialysis solution that remains free of contaminants. Chemical contaminants are avoided by using inert materials, such as plastics, for all components that contact the purified water and dialysis solution. Microbiologic contamination is avoided by using appropriately designed and constructed piping systems in combination with regular disinfection. The water distribution system is configured in a loop without multiple branches or dead ends. If the distribution system includes a storage tank (ideally, the use of a storage tank should be avoided), the tank is of the minimum required size, has a tight-fitting lid, and is designed for ease of disinfection.

Water storage and distribution systems are disinfected on a regular schedule to prevent bacterial colonization of the system and minimize the formation of biofilm, which, once established, is very difficult to remove. When chemical germicides are used, disinfection is generally performed at least monthly. Distribution systems are now available that can be disinfected with hot water. These systems allow more frequent disinfection because there is no need to rinse the system free of residual germicide. Water and dialysis solution cultures and endotoxin tests are performed to demonstrate the adequacy of disinfection.

Bicarbonate concentrate mixing and distribution systems, including containers used to distribute centrally prepared concentrate to individual dialysis machines, are disinfected frequently because bicarbonate concentrates are particularly susceptible to bacterial contamination.

4. Safety standards. Careful procedures and documentation of the functioning of each part of the water supply system must be done. Both AAMI and the European Best Practices Group have developed standards for equipment used to purify water for dialysis that are designed to maximize patient safety. These include chemical purity monitoring of water and dialysis solution. Chloramines are checked for at least daily. Absence of other chronic toxic components from the feed water must be verified on a regular basis. Both water and dialysis fluid must be checked using high-sensitivity methods for bacterial growth and presence of endotoxin. Finally, the patients themselves must be monitored, being always alert for evidence of unexplained clusters of hemolytic, pyrogenic, or other unusual reactions. In addition, patients' blood aluminum levels are followed as described in Chapter 43.

II. Dialysis solution preparation

A. Proportioning machines. To reduce bulk and shipping costs, dialysis fluid is manufactured in concentrated form and machines proportion it with water before delivering it to the dialyzer. The dialysis machine incorporates pumps and one-way valve systems that make the final dialysis solution by taking fixed volumes of dialysate concentrates and mixing them with a fixed volume of heated purified water, or by using conductivity-based servocontrol systems to mix the concentrates and water. As discussed in the previous chapter, the ionic composition of the final dialysis solution is checked by conductivity, which is kept in a very tight range. As long as the solution remains in the target conductivity range, the dialysis solution is allowed to pass on to the dialyzer. If conductivity gets outside the range, an alarm sounds and dialysis stops.

B. Dual-concentrate system for bicarbonate-based solutions. Almost all dialysis solution used today is bicarbonate based, and this engenders a solubility issue. When making a bicarbonate solution of about 30 mM, the pH will be close to 8.0. At this pH, calcium and magnesium will precipitate out from solution, reducing their diffusible concentration and also contributing to scaling on dialysis machine lines and passages. To circumvent the problem of calcium and magnesium precipitation, a bicarbonate-based dialysis solution–generating system utilizes two concentrates, a "bicarbonate" concentrate and an "acid" concentrate. The "acid" concentrate contains a small amount of acetic or citric acid plus sodium, potassium (as needed), calcium, magnesium, chloride, and dextrose (optional). Its low pH keeps the calcium and magnesium in solution.

Specially designed double proportioning systems mix the two concentrates sequentially with purified water to make the final dialysis solution. During mixing, the small amount of organic acid in the "acid" concentrate (about 2–4 mM) reacts with an equimolar amount of bicarbonate in the "bicarbonate" concentrate to generate carbon dioxide. The carbon dioxide generated forms carbonic acid, which lowers the pH of the final bicarbonate-containing solution to approximately 7.0–7.4. At this pH range, the calcium and magnesium in the dialysis solution remain dissolved. The ratio of "acid" concentrate:"base" concentrate:water in the various proportioning systems available depends on the machine manufacturer. Liquid "acid" concentrates are available between 35 times to 45 times concentrated, and the corresponding liquid "bicarbonate" concentrates are also concentrated differently.

C.   Dry concentrates

    1.   Bicarbonate. In some machines, a cartridge containing dry sodium bicarbonate is used in place of a liquid "bicarbonate" concentrate. Use of dry bicarbonate cartridges obviates the problem of bacterial growth in "bicarbonate" concentrate and the concern of subsequent contamination of the final dialysis solutions.

    2.   Acid (citric acid or sodium diacetate). While acetic acid is a liquid, dry "acid" concentrates can be made using either citric acid or sodium diacetate. The low concentration of citrate generated in citric acid–based dialysis solution may chelate plasma calcium that is adjacent to the dialysis membrane, impeding coagulation, improving dialyzer clearance slightly, and increasing the dialyzer reuse number. Sodium diacetate is a compound containing acetic acid and sodium acetate. Acid concentrates formulated with sodium diacetate typically contain a higher concentration of organic anions than traditional acid concentrates. It is important to take the higher concentration of acetate, which generates bicarbonate as it is metabolized, into account when selecting a bicarbonate concentration for the final dialysis solution.

D.   Final dialysis solution composition. The composition range of typically used dialysis solutions is given in Table 5-1. The concentrations of sodium, potassium, and calcium can be varied by choosing different "acid" concentrates or by adding powders containing salts of these cations to the appropriate "acid" concentrates prior to use. In addition, some dialysis machines allow the concentration of sodium in the dialysis solution to be varied during the course of an individual treatment—a practice known as sodium profiling. Sodium profiling may help reduce the tendency to intradialytic hypotension and the postdialysis washed-out feeling in some patients, but whenever the average dialysis solution sodium level is increased, this may predispose to increased thirst, excessive fluid intake, and hypertension (see Chapter 10). Some dialysis

Table 5-1. Composition of a standard hemodialysis solution

Component	Concentration (mM)
Sodium	135–145
Potassium	0–4
Calcium	1.25–1.75
	(2.5–3.5 mEq/L)
Magnesium	0.25–0.375
	(0.5–0.75 mEq/L)
Chloride	98–124
Acetate or citrate[a]	2–4
Bicarbonate	30–40
Glucose	0–11
PCO_2	40–110 (mm Hg)
pH	7.1–7.3 (units)

[a]The acetate or citrate is added in the form of acetic or citric acid to the "acid concentrate." When mixed with the "bicarbonate concentrate," the hydrogen ion from either of these acids reacts with bicarbonate to form CO_2 (i.e., carbonic acid) to establish a buffer system.

machines also allow the bicarbonate level to be varied without changing to a different concentrate by altering the proportioning pump ratio. This allows use of dialysis solution bicarbonate levels from 20–40 mM, and such a feature is particularly useful when more frequent dialysis is employed, when dialyzing nonuremic patients (e.g., to treat poisoning), or to treat alkalemic patients.

E. Disinfection of dialysis machines. Dialysis machines are disinfected according to the manufacturer's recommendations. The water inlet lines to the dialysis machines are disinfected at the same time as the water distribution system. Dialysis machines are now available that incorporate a bacteria- and endotoxin-retentive ultrafilter in the dialysis solution line immediately before the dialyzer. These filters, which are rated for a certain number of treatments or months of operation, are disinfected when the dialysis machine is disinfected. Such ultrafilters also facilitate the routine preparation of "ultrapure dialysis solutions."

SELECTED READINGS

Amato RL. Water treatment for hemodialysis—updated to include the latest AAMI standards for dialysate (RD52:2004). *Nephrol Nurs J* 2005;332(2):151–167.

Association for the Advancement of Medical Instrumentation. *Dialysate for hemodialysis, ANSI/AAMI RD52:2004.* Arlington, VA: Association for the Advancement of Medical Instrumentation, 2004.

Association for the Advancement of Medical Instrumentation. *Water treatment equipment for hemodialysis applications, ANSI/AAMI RD62:2001.* Arlington, VA: Association for the Advancement of Medical Instrumentation, 2001.

Canaud B, et al. Microbiologic purity of dialysate: rationale and technical aspects. *Blood Purif* 2000;18:200–213.

European Renal Association—European Dialysis and Transplantation Association. European best practice guidelines for haemodialysis, section IV—dialysis fluid purity. *Nephrol Dial Transplant* 2002;17(Suppl 7):45–62.

Ledebo I. Ultrapure dialysis fluid—direct and indirect benefits in dialysis therapy. *Blood Purif* 2004;22(Suppl 2):20–25.

Monograph 1167:1997 (corrected 2000). Haemodialysis solutions, concentrated, water for diluting. European Pharmacopoeia Supplement 2001.

Sam R, et al. Composition and clinical use of hemodialysates. *Hemodial Int* 2006;10:15–28.

Schindler R, et al. Short bacterial DNA fragments: detection in dialysate and induction of cytokines. *J Am Soc Nephrol* 2004;15:3207–3214.

Ward RA. Ultrapure dialysate. *Semin Dial* 2004;17:489–497.

Ward RA. Water processing for hemodialysis. Part I. A historical perspective. *Semin Dial* 1997;10:26–31.

Venous Catheter Access for Hemodialysis

Michael Allon and Jack Work

I. General comments. The necessity for vascular access in patients with renal failure can be temporary or permanent. The necessity for temporary access may vary from several hours (single dialysis) to a few months (if used to dialyze while waiting for an arteriovenous [AV] fistula to mature). Temporary access is established by the percutaneous insertion of a catheter into a large vein (internal jugular, femoral, or, less desirably, subclavian). Construction of a permanent vascular access permits repeated angioaccess for months to years.

An ideal permanent access delivers a flow adequate for the dialysis prescription, lasts a long time, and has a low complication rate. The autologous AV fistula comes closest to satisfying these criteria because it has the best 5-year patency rate and during this period requires many fewer interventions than other access methods. Prosthetic accesses (AV grafts) are constructed by the insertion of a subcutaneous tube in a straight, curved, or loop configuration between an extremity artery and vein. Placement of a cuffed tunneled double-lumen catheter into an internal jugular vein for long-term access is also done in selected circumstances.

Although the autologous AV fistula is clearly the desired access for patients initiating hemodialysis, there is disproportionate use of AV grafts in the United States and an excessive dependence on cuffed indwelling central venous catheters. Guidelines developed by the National Kidney Foundation Dialysis Outcomes Quality Improvement initiative (KDOQI and Fistula First) promote the increased use of AV fistulas and earlier referral of patients to nephrologists, permitting earlier patient evaluation and construction of either an AV fistula or graft, thereby minimizing the use of venous catheter access (see Web References).

This chapter will deal with the use of venous catheter access for hemodialysis. Although it clearly is the least desirable form of access, it often is the initial access that patients requiring acute or otherwise unplanned dialysis are exposed to. Chapter 7 will describe arteriovenous access.

II. Venous access

A. Indications

    1. Short term. Venous catheters are commonly used for acute angioaccess in the following patients: (a) those with acute renal failure; (b) those requiring hemodialysis or hemoperfusion for overdose or intoxication; (c) those with end-stage renal failure needing urgent hemodialysis but without available mature access; (d) those on maintenance hemodialysis who have lost effective use of their permanent access and require temporary access until permanent access function can be re-established; (e) patients requiring plasmapheresis; (f) peritoneal dialysis patients whose abdomens are being rested prior to new peritoneal catheter placement (usually for severe peritonitis that required peritoneal dialysis catheter removal); and (g) transplant recipients needing temporary hemodialysis during severe rejection episodes.

2.   Longer term. Venous catheters are utilized as a long-term vascular access for patients in whom an AV access cannot be readily created. Such patients include small children, some diabetic patients with severe vascular disease, patients who are morbidly obese, and patients who have undergone multiple AV access insertions and in whom additional sites for AV access insertion are not available. Additional indications include patients with cardiomyopathy unable to sustain adequate blood pressures or access flows. Whereas catheters were initially favored for more frequent dialysis, there has been good recent experience with nocturnal dialysis and short daily dialysis using AV fistulas or grafts.

3.   Outcomes. Patients being dialyzed with venous catheters don't do as well as those using an arteriovenous access. Catheter patients develop infections more often, they have higher levels of inflammatory markers such as C-reactive protein, and they die more frequently. It is unclear if these associative risks reflect a different patient population receiving catheters, some risk factor that occurs when AV accesses fail and a catheter must be placed, or if they are due completely to some property of catheter use per se. Probably all three are important.

Survival rates for catheters are about 60% at 6 months and 40% at 1 year if revisions are included. Inadequate blood flow through venous catheters remains a significant problem. Nominal flow >400 mL per minute (actual flow 350 mL per minute) can rarely be obtained, and usually flow is limited to a range closer to 300 mL per minute. This limits use of venous catheters in larger patients and results in a lower than average urea reduction ratio (URR) or fractional urea clearance *(Kt/V)*.

B.   Catheter types and design

1.   Cuffed versus uncuffed. Use of an uncuffed catheter for periods of time beyond several weeks results in a relatively high rate of infection and is not recommended. Dacron or felt cuffs bonded to the catheter reduce the incidence of line-related infection and of catheter migration and must be used whenever a longer-term use of the catheter is anticipated, or when it is anticipated that a patient will be discharged from the hospital with a catheter remaining in place.

2.   Design issues. Dual-lumen venous catheters are available in a "double-D" configuration or where the two lumens are in some related, side-by-side configuration. Coaxial catheters are now less frequently used. A side-by-side port design permits the intravenous portion of the catheter to be split into two parts close to the termination point. This results in a softer, more pliable catheter end, a greater separation of inlet and outlet ports, and perhaps a lower recirculation rate.

A new "palindrome" symmetrical tip configuration (Philibert et al., 2005) has been reported to greatly reduce or eliminate recirculation when the normal flow through the catheter is reversed (line reversal is sometimes required as a stopgap measure when using dysfunctional catheters). The Tesio catheter system consists of two completely separate catheters, one for inflow and one for outflow. One touted advantage of the Tesio catheters is that they are made of softer, silicone material.

3. Antiseptic impregnation. Venous catheters for non-dialysis use have been impregnated with antiseptic or silver-based coatings in an attempt to inhibit bacterial growth and infection rate, and some studies show success with this approach. Sometimes the cuff alone is impregnated with such material. At the present time there are no studies using such antiseptic-bonded catheters for dialysis that demonstrate improved outcomes.

C. Insertion location. The optimal insertion site is the **right internal jugular vein.** The subclavian site should generally be avoided because it is associated with a higher incidence of insertion-related complications (pneumothorax, hemothorax, subclavian artery perforation, brachial plexus injury) and, more importantly, a higher incidence (up to 40%) of central venous stenosis. Catheterization of the femoral vein is a good choice when the need for hemodialysis (or hemoperfusion or plasmapheresis) is expected to be short (<1 week). The femoral approach is useful for performing the initial hemodialysis treatment in patients who present with acute pulmonary edema because the patient's head and chest can be elevated during insertion. Although some have used cuffed femoral catheters in ambulatory patients (usually when few or no other access option is easily available), this is not recommended, and almost all femoral catheters used are inserted into hospitalized, bedridden patients. When femoral catheters are used, the length must be sufficiently long (usually at least 20 cm) so that the tip is in the inferior vena cava to permit better flow and to minimize recirculation.

D. Insertion technique

    1. Ultrasound guidance. Use of an ultrasound monitor to guide insertion is highly desirable, and portable, bedside monitors are available. The central veins of the neck exhibit anatomic variability, and occasionally one of them may be absent. Atypical or ectatic carotid arteries are also a problem (Fig. 6-1). With the use of ultrasound guidance, the rate of successful internal jugular puncture on first attempt increases markedly and the rate of carotid artery punctures is greatly reduced.

    2. Initial preparation and how to position the ultrasound probe. The catheter should be inserted using an aseptic technique, with the operator wearing a sterile

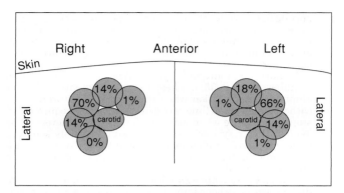

Figure 6-1.   Anatomic variability of internal jugular vein as viewed using ultrasound localization. (Modified from Caridi JG et al: Sonographic guidance when using the right internal jugular vein for central vein access. *Am J Roentgenol* 1998;171:1259–1263, with permission.)

surgical gown and gloves in a maximum barrier protection environment. Prior to surgical scrub, it is helpful to examine the selected site using an ultrasound to ensure that the patient has a suitable vein in the selected location. The insertion site and surrounding areas should be cleansed with surgical scrub and draped appropriately (include shoulder and chest wall if a cuffed tunneled catheter is to be inserted). The ultrasound probe should be covered with a sterile sheath. The ultrasound probe may be placed parallel to the long axis of the vessel and the cannulation needle inserted adjacent to the end or short axis of the probe. Alternatively, the probe may be placed perpendicular to the long axis of the vessel. This approach gives the vein the more typical appearance of a circle but limits the visualization of the needle. The vein typically collapses with gentle pressure of the probe, whereas the artery does not. For right internal jugular vein cannulation as an example, the ultrasound probe is placed parallel and superior to the clavicle, over the groove between the sternal and clavicular heads of the sternocleidomastoid muscle. It is important to avoid inserting the catheter through the muscle, as this is uncomfortable for the patient.

3.   Initial insertion of the guidewire through a 21-gauge needle. The site for insertion is infiltrated with local anesthesia. Using real-time ultrasound guidance, a 21-gauge micropuncture needle with an attached syringe is inserted into the vein. The small needle limits potential complications if the carotid artery is inadvertently punctured compared to a larger 18-gauge needle, which is usually included in commercially available dialysis catheter trays. Under direct visualization, the vein will be seen to gently push in before penetrating the anterior vein wall. The syringe is removed, and a 0.018" guidewire is inserted through the needle. The guidewire is advanced. The position of the guidewire is confirmed using fluoroscopy.

4. **Insertion of the dilator over the guidewire.** The needle is then removed and a coaxial 5-French dilator is then advanced over the guidewire. The guidewire and 3-French inner translational dilator are removed, leaving the 5-French outer dilator in place. A flow switch or stopcock is attached to the dilator to prevent the possibility of an air embolism.

a. **Uncuffed catheter insertion.** The next step depends on whether one is placing a noncuffed temporary or cuffed tunneled catheter. For temporary catheter placement, a standard 0.035" guidewire is advanced into the vein and then the 5-French dilator is removed, leaving the guidewire. In stepwise fashion, dilators of increasing size are passed over the guidewire to progressively dilate the soft tissue and venous tract; the dilator should move freely on the guidewire. The dilator should not be forcefully advanced, as it is possible for the dilator to get off axis and impinge on the guidewire and perforate the vein and/or the mediastinum. If there is any doubt as to location of the dilator or if there is hesitancy or difficulty in dilating the tract, fluoroscopy should be used to assist in placement. The last dilator is then exchanged for the temporary catheter, which is advanced over the guidewire into position. After securing the catheter in place, a chest radiograph should be obtained for confirmation of correct positioning and to check for any complications, if a fluoroscope was not available during insertion. If the patient requires long-term dialysis support, the temporary noncuffed catheter, when located in the internal jugular vein, may be safely converted to a cuffed tunneled catheter if there is no evidence of an exit site infection.

b. **Cuffed catheter insertion**

(1) **Creating the skin exit site and tunnel.** For cuffed tunneled catheter insertion, a small skin incision is made from the 5-French dilator extending laterally. The subcutaneous tissue is then exposed with blunt dissection, creating a subcutaneous pocket so that the catheter bend will be kink free. Further dissection is made to ensure that the soft tissue around the 5-French dilator is free. The catheter exit site is then identified. This may be accomplished by using the fourth rib interspace landmark technique, or the catheter length may be determined more precisely by using a guidewire to measure the distance from the insertion site to the midright atrium. Using this measurement as a guide, the length of tunnel may then be determined, so that the cuff is within the tunnel approximately 1–2 cm from the exit site.

(2) **Inserting the catheter through the skin exit site.** Once the exit site for the catheter is identified, the area is infiltrated with local anesthesia; a puncture is made through the skin using a number 11 knife blade

inserted parallel to the skin. The knife is inserted to
the widest point of the blade; this incision accommo-
dates most dual-lumen catheters. A long needle is used
to infiltrate the tunnel tract with local anesthesia extending from the exit site to the venotomy insertion
site. The catheter is mounted on the end of the tunneling device and the tunneling device is pulled from the
exit site subcutaneously to the insertion site. The cuff of
the catheter is pulled into the tunnel and the tunneling
device is then removed from the catheter.

(3)   Dilating the deep tissues and venous tract. A
guidewire such as a Benson or angled guidewire is now
passed through the dilator into the inferior vena cava.
Placement of the guidewire into the inferior vena cava
decreases the likelihood of cardiac arrhythmias. The
guidewire provided with most catheter trays may also
be used. The 5-French dilator is then removed, and in
stepwise fashion, dilators of increasing size are passed
over the guidewire in order to progressively dilate the
soft tissue and venous tract. The dilator should move
freely on the guidewire. It is possible for the dilator to
get off axis and impinge on the guidewire and perforate
the vein and/or the mediastinum. If there is any doubt
as to the location of the dilator or if there is hesitancy
or difficulty in dilating the tract, the fluoroscope should
be used to verify proper positioning.

(4)   Completing catheter insertion. After the final
dilation, the dilator is inserted with peel-away sheath.
As one inserts the sheath, a resistance is felt as the
sheath goes through the soft tissue and then a final resistance as it enters the vein. The dilator and
sheath are then removed and the catheter threaded
over the guidewire without using the sheath and advanced through the venous tract into final position.
One may need to slightly torque the catheter in order to advance it through the tract. This maneuver decreases the possibility of air embolism and may result
in both a smaller venotomy and in less postprocedure
bleeding.

Alternatively, if the peel-away sheath is used, the
sheath is advanced slightly and the dilator removed
while occluding the sheath, leaving the guidewire in
place to ensure access is available if there are any difficulties. The sheath should be grasped between the
finger and thumb of one's hand in order to occlude
the sheath. This prevents bleeding and/or aspiration
of air while leaving enough length of the sheath to insert the catheter. Once the dilator and guidewire have
been removed, the catheter is threaded over the wire
and advanced into the opening of the sheath in such
a way as to avoid twisting the catheter. The catheter
is fed through the sheath. The catheter is pushed far-
ther into the sheath and the sheath is peeled downward
toward the skin. As soon as the catheter is advanced

maximally, the sheath is pulled out and then peeled down outside of the venotomy. This avoids the sheath creating a larger venous tract.

(5) Setting and securing the catheter cuff. Once the sheath has been completely removed, the catheter is pulled back into the tunnel so that the cuff now is approximately 1–2 cm from the exit site. The catheter is now checked to ensure that it is functioning properly. A 10-mL syringe should be able to rapidly pull back blood without any shuttering if the catheter is to deliver a blood flow >300 mL per minute.

The venotomy insertion site is closed using appropriate suture after confirmation of adequate flow. The exit site is closed using a pursestring suture wrapped around the catheter to provide a harness for the catheter at the skin surface. Additional suture is used to hold the catheter at the hub. Using "air knots" to secure the catheter hub increases patient comfort and decreases the likelihood of skin necrosis. Topical antibiotic ointment may be applied to the incisions and needle puncture sites, and a gauze dressing is applied.

E. Insertion-related complications. These are listed in Table 6-1 and include arterial puncture, pneumothorax, hemothorax, air embolism, mediastinal hemorrhage, pericardial tamponade, and brachial plexus injury. Arrhythmias can also occur as a result of endocardial irritation, especially when the catheter or guidewire has been advanced too deeply. Rarely, erosion of the superior vena cava can occur. The sum of all early major complications should not exceed 5% of all central venous catheter placements.

Table 6-1. Complications of central venous catheterization

Immediate Complications
Arterial puncture
Pneumothorax
Hemothorax
Arrhythmias
Air embolism
Perforation of vein or cardiac chamber
Pericardial tamponade

Delayed Complications
Thrombosis
Infection
Vascular stricture
Arteriovenous fistula

Injury to Adjacent Structures
Brachial plexus
Trachea
Recurrent laryngeal nerve

F.   Care and use of venous catheters

   1.   Dressings. During catheter connect and disconnect procedures, both dialysis staff and patient should wear surgical masks. A face shield should not be used without a surgical mask because the shield tends to focus the wearer's breath directly on the exposed catheter hub. The lumen and catheter tips should never remain open to air. A cap or syringe should always be placed on or in the catheter lumen while maintaining a clean field under the catheter connectors. Catheter lumens must be kept sterile: Interdialytic infusions through the catheter are forbidden.

   After each dialysis, catheter hubs or blood line connectors should be soaked in povidone–iodine for 3–5 minutes, then dried prior to separation. The catheter should be covered with a sterile dry dressing. Nonbreathable or nonporous transparent film dressings should be avoided as they pose a greater threat of exit site colonization than dry dressings.

   2.   Catheter locks

      a.   Heparin. After each dialysis session, the dead space of each lumen is filled with heparin through the catheter injection ports using 1,000–5,000 units/mL. There is no evidence that the higher concentration of heparin is of any benefit in preventing catheter thrombosis. Any lock solution will leak out to the level of the most proximal side hole of the catheter. Thus, use of higher heparin concentration may result in significant systemic anticoagulation. The dead space of each catheter lumen varies among manufacturers and length of catheter. The required volume of heparin is usually labeled on the catheter hub. It is important to record this information on the patient's chart so it is readily available to the dialysis staff. Injection of a volume of heparin solution larger than necessary should be avoided as it results in some degree of systemic anticoagulation that may be hazardous to patients at risk for bleeding. Prior to each dialysis, the heparin in each lumen is aspirated, the catheter flushed with heparinized saline (100 units/mL), and hemodialysis initiated.

      b.   Citrate. Citrate can be used as an anticoagulant because it chelates calcium, which is essential for clotting to occur. Citrate can also be used with a wider range of antibiotic solutions when an antibiotic-containing lock is desired (see below). Despite some initial enthusiasm, the efficacy of citrate locks to maintain catheter patency has not been shown to be better than heparin, although it may result in a cost savings in some countries (Weijmer et al., 2005) but not in others. It is prudent to use the lowest effective concentration (4% citrate). Very high concentrations of citrate should not be used because of the risk of inadvertently injecting concentrated citrate into the left atrium, acutely lowering the ionized calcium level, and precipitating a cardiac arrhythmia.

   3.   Bathing and showering. The exit site should never be immersed in bath water. Showering is best avoided, but if the patient showers it should be done prior to coming to the dialysis unit, where a new dressing and antibacterial ointment will be promptly applied. Showering should be done only after the exit site sinus tract has become established.

G. Infection. Infection is the leading cause of catheter loss and increases morbidity and mortality. Infection may arise from the migration of the patient's own skin flora through the puncture site and onto the outer catheter surface. More frequently, infection may result from contamination of the catheter connectors, lumen contamination during dialysis, or infused solutions. Catheters can also become colonized from more remote sites during bacteremia. Gram-positive bacteria (usually *Staphylococcus* species) are the most common culprits.

    1. Prevention

      a. Aseptic insertion and handling of the catheters. This was discussed above in F 1.

      b. Minimize duration of catheter use. This is a most important factor. The incidence of infection of central uncuffed catheters is generally under 8% at 2 weeks. By 1 month, 25% of uncuffed central catheters will have become infected, and this figure doubles by the end of the second month (Oliver, 2000). Catheter-related septicemia may occur in 2%–20% of catheters. Patients should not be discharged from the hospital with an uncuffed nontunneled catheter; these catheters may easily be converted to a cuffed tunneled catheter.

        (1) Limitations on use of femoral catheters. Uncuffed femoral catheters, especially if used in patients who are moving from bed to chair or who are ambulating, should be removed after 2–4 days of use. Cuffed femoral catheters can be left in place for longer periods, but should not be viewed as "permanent" vascular access unless all other possible access options have been exhausted.

      c. Prophylactic antibiotics. Systemic antibiotics are not given routinely prior to cuffed catheter insertion. **Mupirocin treatment of the catheter exit site** to lower *Staphylococcus* colonization has been shown to reduce the catheter infection rate and to increase the survival rate (e.g., Johnson DW et al., 2002). However, these usually have been short (3–4-month) studies, and the long-term emergence of mupirocin resistance remains a concern.

    2. Diagnosis and treatment

      a. Uncuffed catheters

        (1) Localized exit site infection. If there is erythema and/or crust but no purulent discharge, one can usually treat with appropriate antibiotics for up to 2 weeks. The catheter must be removed if systemic signs of infection develop (leukocytosis or temperature >38°C), if pus can be expressed from the tract of the catheter, or if the infection persists or recurs after an initial course of antibiotics. If blood cultures are positive, then the catheter should be removed.

(2)   Systemic infection. The initial presentation is typically with fever and leukocytosis. The degree of fever may increase during dialysis, and this is not necessarily a sign of pyrogenic reaction. Signs of exit site infection are common but on occasion may be absent. In some patients, another source for infection will be present (e.g., pneumonia, urinary tract infection, wound infection). In such cases, the distant infection can be treated, and the catheter may be left in place cautiously with close continued surveillance. On the other hand, if initial history, physical examination, or radiologic studies show no other apparent source, catheter infection should be presumed, and the catheter should be promptly removed. Blood cultures should be obtained from a peripheral vein and through the catheter prior to removal. On removal, the catheter tip should be cultured (Table 6-2). The duration of antibiotic treatment depends on clinical response. In general, antibiotic therapy should be continued for a minimum of 2–3 weeks.

(3)   Placement of a new catheter. A new catheter may be inserted at another site, ideally after several days when blood cultures have turned negative.

Table 6-2.   General recommendations for the diagnosis and management of catheter-related infections[a]

Culture of Catheters

1. Culture of catheters should be done only when catheter-related bloodstream infection is suspected (B-II).
2. Quantitative or semiquantitative cultures of catheters are recommended (A-II).
3. When culturing a central venous catheter segment, either the catheter tip or a subcutaneous segment should be submitted for culture (B-III).
4. If available, acridine orange leukocyte cytospin should be considered for rapid diagnosis of central venous catheter infection (B-II).

Culture of Blood Samples

1. Two sets of blood samples for culture, with at least one drawn percutaneously, should be obtained from all patients with a new episode of suspected central venous catheter-related bloodstream infection (A-II).
2. Paired quantitative blood cultures or paired qualitative blood cultures with a continuously monitored differential time to positivity are recommended for the diagnosis of catheter-related infection, especially when the long-term catheter cannot be removed (A-II).

[a]A and B level recommendations (highest strength) only.
From Mermel, et al. *Clin Infect Dis* 2001;32:1249–1272.

b. Cuffed tunneled catheters

(1) Exit site infection is a localized infection of the skin and soft tissue around the catheter exit site. The tunnel is not involved and evidence of systemic infection is absent. The site should be cleaned with appropriate antimicrobial agents, a sterile dressing applied, and systemic or oral antibiotics given. If the exit site infection persists, catheter revision with a new exit site away from the infected area may be required.

(2) Tunnel infection is infection along the subcutaneous tunnel extending proximal to the cuff toward the insertion site and venotomy. Typically, there is marked tenderness, swelling, and erythema along the catheter tract in association with purulent drainage from the exit site. Tunnel infection requires the immediate removal of the catheter.

(3) Catheter-related bacteremia is a common complication of cuffed tunneled catheters with an incidence of 2–5 episodes per 1,000 catheter days (Allon, 2004). Patients present with signs and symptoms of systemic infection, which may be severe or minimal. Milder cases present with fever or chills, whereas more severe cases exhibit hemodynamic instability. Patients may develop septic symptoms after initiation of dialysis, suggesting systemic release of bacteria and/or endotoxin from the catheter. Gram-positive organisms, primarily *Staphylococcus* species, are the most common, but Gram-negative organisms may be isolated in up to 40% of cases.

Treatment of catheter-related bacteremia requires consideration of choice and duration of antibiotic, and management of the catheter (Fig. 6-2). In catheter-dependent patients with fever or chills, bacteremia is confirmed in 59%–81% of cases (Allon, 2004). For this reason, it is imperative to initiate systemic antibiotics promptly after obtaining blood cultures. The initial antibiotic regimen should include coverage for both Gram-positive and Gram-negative bacteria. If methicillin-resistant *Staphylococcus* is known to be common in the local hemodialysis population, the initial therapy should include vancomycin, rather than a first-generation cephalosporin. Adequate empiric Gram-negative coverage can be provided with either an aminoglycoside or a third-generation cephalosporin. To minimize the selection for antibiotic-resistant pathogens, it is imperative to track the blood culture results. Antibiotics should be discontinued promptly if the blood cultures had no growth, and the antibiotic regimen adjusted once the bacterial sensitivities are available. A 2- to 3-week course of systemic antibiotics is adequate in uncomplicated cases of catheter-related bacteremia. A longer course (6 weeks) is indicated if there is a metastatic infection, such as endocarditis or osteomyelitis. Finally, it is imperative to obtain

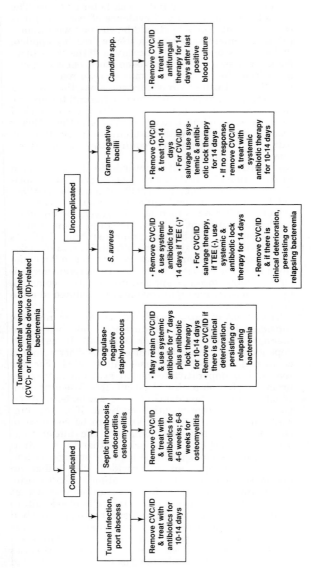

Figure 6-2.   Approach to the management of a patient with a tunneled central vein catheter (CVC)–related bloodstream infection. *TEE, transesophageal echocardiography. (Reproduced with permission from Mermel LA et al. Guidelines for the management of intravascular catheter-related infections. *Clin Infect Dis* 2001;32:1249–1272.)

surveillance blood cultures 1 week after completing the course of antibiotics.

From an infectious disease perspective, the catheter should be removed. However, since the patient will continue to require dialysis support, placement of a temporary catheter becomes necessary. Thus, the decision to remove the catheter should be individualized based on the severity of sepsis and alternative venous access sites. If the patient is clinically septic and unstable despite administration of systemic antibiotics, the catheter should be removed as soon as possible. Attempts to maintain the same catheter by treating through the infection have not been successful, with a success rate of <30% and with the risk of metastatic infections. Several studies support the use of guidewire exchange, reporting a >80% salvage and cure (Saad, 1999; Beathard, 1999). Thus, removing the infected catheter and with it presumably the biofilm harboring the bacteria and replacing it with a new catheter through the same venotomy preserves the venous access site while curing the infection.

Another approach to treatment of patients with catheter-related bacteremia is to instill a concentrated antibiotic-heparin lock ("antibiotic-lock") into the catheter lumen at the end of each dialysis session, as an adjunct to systemic antibiotics (Fig. 6-3). The antibiotic lock is used only for the duration of systemic antibiotics, after which a standard heparin lock is resumed. In about two thirds of cases, the antibiotic lock successfully sterilizes the catheter biofilm, thereby permitting successful treatment of the bacteremia while salvaging the infected catheter. In the remaining one third of cases, the patient has persistent fever or positive surveillance cultures, in which case prompt catheter replacement is indicated. The antibiotic lock protocol is most commonly successful in catheter-related bacteremia due to *Staphylococcus epidermidis* (75%) or Gram-negative infections (87%), and less often successful in *Staphylococcus aureus* infections (40%) (Allon, 2004; Poole, 2004).

c. Complications of catheter infection. Delay in therapy or prolonged attempts to salvage an infected cuffed catheter can lead to serious complications, including endocarditis, osteomyelitis, suppurative thrombophlebitis, and spinal epidural abscess. The last is a rare but serious neurologic complication in hemodialysis patients. In one series, 50% of cases were associated with attempted salvage of an infected cuffed venous catheter (Kovalik, 1996). Presenting complaints are fever, backache, local spinal tenderness, leg pain and weakness, sphincter dysfunction, paresis, and/or paralysis. For diagnosis, magnetic resonance imaging appears to be less sensitive (80%) than computed tomography-myelography. Plain computed tomographic scanning without myelography has low sensitivity and

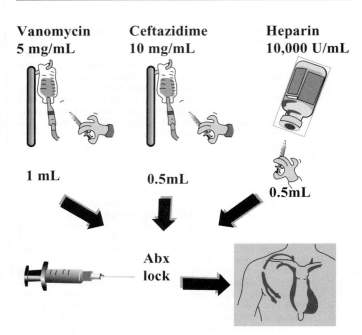

Vanomycin
5 mg/mL

Ceftazidime
10 mg/mL

Heparin
10,000 U/mL

1 mL

0.5mL

0.5mL

Abx
lock

Figure 6-3.   Preparation of the antibiotic lock. Aliquots from the antibiotic solutions prepared for intravenous infusion and of heparin are mixed in a single syringe and instilled into each catheter lumen at the end of each hemodialysis session. Once the course of intravenous antibiotics has been completed, standard heparin locks are resumed. (Adapted from Poole CV, et al. Treatment of catheter-related bacteremia with an antibiotic lock protocol: effect of bacterial pathogen. *Nephrol Dial Transplant* 2004;19:1237–1244.)

can give misleading results (e.g., disc protrusion). Early (immediate) decompressive surgery usually is advised, although rarely patients can be treated with antibiotics only.

Endocarditis should be suspected in patients in whom fever and bacteremia persist despite appropriate antibiotics and catheter removal. This complication is seen most commonly in the setting of *S. aureus* bacteremia. The patients frequently develop symptomatic heart failure and a new heart murmur. A transthoracic or transesophageal echocardiogram confirms a valvular vegetation and insufficiency.

H.   Catheter dysfunction

1.   Early. Initial dysfunction of a cuffed tunneled catheter is due to improper placement with either malposition, kinking, or intracatheter thrombosis. Many dysfunctional catheters exhibit positional occlusion during dialysis. Early

Table 6-3.   Dosing of tissue plasminogen activator (tPA) for occluded catheters

Catheter Lock and Aspirate Technique

Alteplase (1 mg/mL): Infuse 2 mg or volume of catheter into each catheter lumen as needed. For catheter lumen volumes >2 mL, after 2 mL of tPA is injected, inject sufficient normal saline to fill the catheter. For example, a 40-cm catheter with 2.6 mL volume per lumen: alteplase 2 mL injected (1 mg/mL), then 0.6 mL normal saline.

After initial administration, let the thrombolytic dwell for 30 minutes and then aspirate. If there is no blood return, let the thrombolytic dwell for another 30 minutes. If there is still no blood return, repeat the dose and aspirate again at 30 and 60 minutes.

If a catheter is "occluded" and the thrombolytic cannot be injected, connect a three-way stopcock to the occluded catheter hub, and with a 20-mL nonfilled syringe aspirate on the catheter. The remaining port of the three-way stopcock should have the volume of thrombolytic in a syringe. With negative pressure on the catheter turn the stopcock so it is now open to the catheter and the thrombolytic. The negative pressure will be transferred to the thrombolytic syringe; aspirating its contents into the catheter.

Infusion Technique

When the dwell technique is unsuccessful, attempt a short-term infusion.

Begin by loading the catheter with tPA 2 mL per lumen. The concentration of tPA is 1 mg/mL. Once loaded, an infusion of tPA, 1 mg per lumen per hour, is run for 2–4 hours and then rechecked.

The amount of thrombolytic utilized with infusion is probably not of sufficient amount to cause bleeding complications, but absolute and relative contraindications should be considered, and then risk versus benefit.

Locking catheters as well as biweekly or monthly instillations of thrombolytics have reportedly reduced catheter occlusions.

Adapted with permission from www.venousaccess.com. For additional thrombolytic protocols see Lok et al., 2006.

failures usually require catheter repositioning or replacement under fluoroscopy.

    a. Intracatheter thrombosis. Most simple thromboses will respond to intraluminal thrombolytic injection of tissue plasminogen activator (tPA) as described in Table 6-3.

  2. Late dysfunction

    a. Fibrin sleeves and mural thrombi. In addition to malposition and simple intracatheter or catheter tip thrombus, formation of a fibrin sleeve or a mural thrombus may be the cause of "late" catheter dysfunction. Almost all catheters inserted into a central vein develop a fibrin sleeve within 1 to several weeks after insertion.

Such fibrin sleeves are initially clinically silent until they obstruct the ports at the distal end of the catheter. Generally, saline infuses into a port but aspiration is difficult, the so-called *ball-valve* effect. Fibrin sleeves may serve as a nidus for infection as well. A catheter venogram should be performed to confirm the diagnosis. The following methods can be used to deal with fibrin sheaths.

b. Systemic thrombolytics. Several tPA protocols have been described (Savader et al., 2001; Clase et al., 2001).

c. Snare catheter stripping. This procedure requires cannulation of the femoral vein and advancement of the snare up the inferior vena cava to the occluded catheter. The operator then pulls away the adherent fibrin sleeve/thrombus from the catheter, after which the removed material embolizes to the lung. Clinically evident pulmonary embolism has been reported to result from this procedure but is unusual. The potential delayed effects of multiple iatrogenic pulmonary embolizations on long-term pulmonary function are of theoretical concern. The fibrin sheath tends to reoccur rapidly after this procedure and the cost of the special snare catheter is several times the cost of a new catheter.

d. Exchange of the catheter over a guidewire. This will solve many problems and has been shown to be as effective as snare catheter stripping in the case of fibrin sleeve formation. However, the new catheter frequently is advanced into the fibrin sheath, leading to the same problem.

e. Exchange of the catheter over a guidewire with disruption of the sheath with an angioplasty balloon. This procedure appears to be the most effective. The existing catheter is freed up and pulled back and contrast injected to demonstrate the presence of a sheath. If present, the catheter is removed over a guidewire and an angioplasty balloon advanced over the wire and dilated to disrupt the fibrin sheath. A new catheter is then advanced over the wire, and contrast injected to document disruption of the sheath.

3. Prevention. The incidence of early dysfunction due to malposition may be strongly dependent on the experience of the person performing the insertion. Tesio-type silicone catheters may have a lower incidence of positional dysfunction due to the spiral winding of their exit holes around the distal 3.5 cm of each catheter. Also, fibrin formation may be less around silicone catheters.

The use of warfarin or other anticoagulants on a chronic basis has not been shown to limit fibrin sleeve formation or catheter thrombus formation (Mokrzycki, 2001).

I. Embolic complications. Large clots adherent to the end of the catheter or to the vessel wall can be clinically silent or can give rise to embolic events. Large mural thrombi also can proceed to stenosis and central vein thrombosis as described below. Treatment options for a ball thrombus or a catheter-associated right atrial thrombus include simple catheter removal, systemic or catheter fibrinolytic therapy, and, rarely, thoracotomy with thrombectomy.

J. Central vein stenosis, thrombosis, stricture

    1. Incidence. Central venous stenosis arises from endothelial injury at the site of catheter–endothelial contact through the release of a variety of growth factors. The incidence increases with the use of stiff, nonsilicone catheters; with the use of the subclavian approach (presumably because of higher angular stresses on the catheter in the subclavian position); and in patients with previous catheter-related infections.

    2. Presentation/diagnosis. A stenosis may be asymptomatic and clinically silent until unmasked by the creation of an AV fistula. Symptoms are invariably those of gross edema (often explosive) of the entire arm and in extreme cases the development of venous skin ulcers. When the stenosis develops after an access has been placed, development of the edema may be slower.

    3. Treatment. Ligation of the vascular access produces the most rapid improvement but sacrifices the access. Initial anticoagulation (with heparin followed by warfarin) and elevation may ameliorate the symptoms and signs if thrombosis is present, but more definitive therapy can be avoided in only a minority of such cases. Balloon angioplasty has been used for stenosis, but the lesion tends to recur. Stent placement combined with angioplasty is indicated in elastic central vein lesions or if the stenosis recurs within a 3-month period. However, stent placement rarely solves the problem long term with stenosis reoccurring in the stent. Some patients may be candidates for surgical axillary–internal jugular bypass of the affected subclavian vein.

SELECTED READINGS

Allon M. Dialysis catheter-related bacteremia: treatment and prophylaxis. *Am J Kidney Dis* 2004;44:779–791.

Allon M. Saving infected catheters: why and how. *Blood Purif* 2005;23:23–28.

Asif A, et al. Conversion of tunneled hemodialysis catheter-consigned patients to arteriovenous fistula. *Kidney Int* 2005;67:2399–2406.

Beathard GA. Management of bacteremia associated with tunneled-cuffed hemodialysis catheters. *J Am Soc Nephrol* 1999;10:1045–1049.

Clase CM, et al. Thrombolysis for restoration of patency to hemodialysis central venous catheters: a systematic review. *J Thromb Thrombolysis* 2001;11(2):127–136.

Frankel A. Temporary access and central venous catheters. *Eur J Vasc Endovasc Surg* 2006;31(4):417–422.

Haymond J, et al. Efficacy of low-dose alteplase for treatment of hemodialysis catheter occlusions. *J Vasc Access* 2005;6:76–82.

Johnson DW, et al. A randomized controlled trial of topical exit site mupirocin application in patients with tunnelled, cuffed haemodialysis catheters. *Nephrol Dial Transplant* 2002;17:1802–1807.

Kovalik EC, et al. A clustering of epidural abscesses in chronic hemodialysis patients: risks of salvaging access catheters in cases of infection. *J Am Soc Nephrol* 1996;7:2264–2267.

Lee T, Barker J, Allon M. Tunneled catheters in hemodialysis patients: reasons and subsequent outcomes. *Am J Kidney Dis* 2005;46:501–508.

Little MA, Walshe JJ. A longitudinal study of the repeated use of alteplase as therapy for tunneled hemodialysis dysfunction. *Am J Kidney Dis* 2002;39:86–91.

Lok CE, et al. A patient-focused approach to thrombolytic use in the management of catheter malfunction. *Semin Dial* 2006;19:381–390.

Maya ID, Allon M. Outcomes of tunneled femoral hemodialysis catheters: comparison with internal jugular vein catheters. *Kidney Int* 2005;68:2886–2889.

Mermel LA, et al. Guidelines for the management of intravascular catheter-related infections. *Clin Infect Dis* 2001;32:1249–1272.

Mokrzycki MH, et al. A randomized trial of minidose warfarin for the prevention of late malfunction in tunneled, cuffed hemodialysis catheters. *Kidney Int* 2001;59:1935–1942.

Oliver MJ, et al. Risk of bacteremia from temporary hemodialysis catheters by site of insertion and duration of use: A prospective study. *Kidney Int* 2000;58:2543–2545.

Philibert D, et al. Clinical experience with a chronic hemodialysis catheter with symmetrical tip configuration (Palindrome TM). *J Am Soc Nephrol* 2005;16:455A.

Poole CV, et al. Treatment of catheter-related bacteremia with an antibiotic lock protocol: effect of bacterial pathogen. *Nephrol Dial Transplant* 2004;19:1237–1244.

Saad TF. Bacteremia associated with tunneled, cuffed hemodialysis catheters. *Am J Kidney Dis* 1999;34:1114–1124.

Savader SJ, et al. Treatment of hemodialysis catheter-associated fibrin sheaths by rt-PA infusion: critical analysis of 124 procedures. *J Vasc Interv Radiol* 2001;12(6):711–715.

Weijmer MC, et al. Randomized, clinical trial comparison of trisodium citrate 30% and heparin as catheter-locking solution in hemodialysis patients. *J Am Soc Nephrol* 2005;16:2769–2777.

WEB REFERENCES

KDOQI 2005–2006 access guidelines: http://www.kidney.org

Vascular Access Society guidelines: http://www.vascularaccesssociety.com/guidelines/index.htm

American Society of Diagnostic and Interventional Nephrology: http://www.asdin.org/

HDCN vascular access channel: http://www.hdcn.com/ch/access/

CDC guidelines for prevention of intravascular catheter-related infections: http://www.cdc.gov/ncidod/dhqp/gl_intravascular.html

Joint Infectious Disease Society of North America, American Society of Critical Care Medicine, Society of Critical Care Medicine, and Society of Healthcare Epidemiology of America guidelines for management of catheter-related infections: http://www.hdcn.com/ch/access/

Arteriovenous Access for Hemodialysis

Victoria Kumar, Thomas Depner,
Anatole Besarab, and
Shubha Ananthakrishnan

I. Two types of arteriovenous (AV) access: Fistulas and grafts. An AV fistula is formed by subcutaneous anastomosis of an artery to an adjacent native vein, allowing flow directly from the artery to the vein. Traditionally the anastomosis is made at the wrist between the radial artery and the cephalic vein, although there are many variations possible, with anastomoses in the snuffbox, in the forearm area, or at the elbow or upper arm. An AV graft is similar, except that the distance between the feeding artery and vein is bridged by a tube made of prosthetic material. An AV fistula cannot be used immediately. One must wait approximately 6 weeks (sometimes less, sometimes more) for the feeding artery and vein to dilate. During this interval the flow in the fistula increases and the vein wall thickens. During actual use of an AV fistula, both dialysis needles are inserted into the native vein, whereas during use of AV grafts, both needles are inserted into the prosthetic tube linking the artery and vein. AV grafts can be used earlier than fistulas, but a delay of 1–3 weeks is recommended to allow healing to occur around the graft, minimizing the potential for tracking of extravasated blood after the needles are removed. Some varieties of early-use grafts have self-sealing properties, allowing their use sooner after implantation.

A. Why AV fistulas are better than grafts. In general, an AV graft is a much less desirable access option than an AV fistula because grafts almost invariably promote hyperplasia of the venous intima at or downstream from the graft–vein anastomosis, causing stenosis and eventual obstruction. The intimal hyperplasia is probably caused by turbulence at the anastomosis and possibly by the compliance mismatch between the graft and the vein. Other possible causes include periodic exposure to activated blood exiting the dialyzer, although AV grafts can develop stenoses even when left unused. AV fistulas are much less prone to develop venous neointimal hyperplasia so fistulas may remain patent for years, sometimes for decades. In addition to higher long-term patency rates, AV fistulas have fewer infections than grafts, probably because there is no implanted foreign material.

Although an AV graft is a worse access option than an AV fistula, it is far superior to a central vein catheter. Patients with AV grafts have less serious infections, lower morbidity, and higher survival rates than patients managed with venous catheters.

B. Guidelines targeting increased use of AV fistulas. Guidelines developed by the National Kidney Foundation's Kidney Disease Outcomes Quality Initiative (KDOQI) and the "Fistula First" initiative (see Web References) promote construction of AV fistulas, targeting at least 60% use of AV fistulas in patients beginning dialysis and 50% fistula use in prevalent patients. Some U.S. centers and many European centers achieve much higher percentages (90% or higher). Early referral of patients to nephrologists, permitting early access evaluation and construction of an AV access, avoids the risks of a central vein catheter that is usually required when the patient is referred late in the course of their chronic kidney disease (CKD). Other important factors include availability and use of preoperative imaging of the arterial and venous systems to maximize successful creation of a functioning AV fistula and the availability of a dedicated and trained access surgeon functioning as part of a vascular access team.

II. Anticipating the need for AV access. In patients with progressive renal failure, the veins of both arms must be protected, anticipating their possible use for vascular access. Accordingly, one should minimize venipunctures and placement of catheters into the forearm veins, especially the cephalic veins of either arm. The dorsum of the hand should be used when venipuncture cannot be avoided. Because of the risk of central vein stenosis, the subclavian vein should not be cannulated unless absolutely necessary and percutaneously inserted central catheter (PICC) lines should be avoided.

Patients with a glomerular filtration rate (GFR) of <30 mL per minute per 1.73 m^2 should be educated about all renal replacement modality options including peritoneal dialysis and renal transplantation. For those choosing hemodialysis, an AV fistula should be placed at least 6 months prior to the initiation of dialysis, as anticipated from serial estimates of GFR using methods described in Chapter 1. In patients planning to start peritoneal dialysis, creation of an AV fistula is optional. Backup AV fistulas were sometimes created in peritoneal dialysis patients to avoid the risks associated with central vein catheters when peritoneal dialysis must be stopped for a time, for example, to replace the catheter because of malfunction or severe peritonitis. However, peritonitis rates are much lower now than in the past, so most centers no longer create backup AV fistulas in their peritoneal dialysis patients. Patients who are planning to receive a live donor kidney in the near future but who need dialysis for a short time can be managed without an AV access. In such patients short-term use (<6 months) of a cuffed venous catheter for access is appropriate unless the patient has a contraindication to venous catheter use (such as cardiac valvular disease, which might predispose to endocarditis, etc.).

A. Preoperative evaluation

    1. Patient history. A thorough history is required, querying about previous episodes of central vein cannulations or intravenous pacemaker implantation, prior use of PICC lines, or prior vascular surgery. Comorbid conditions such as congestive heart failure, diabetes mellitus, or peripheral vascular disease may limit options for access construction.

Patients with severe heart failure may not tolerate the additional cardiac output required to circulate blood through the access. Patients with severe vascular disease due to atherosclerosis or diabetes or patients with extensive damage to their arm veins due to prior needle sticks may not have adequate blood vessels to support creation of an AV access, although even in such patients an AV fistula often can be created in the upper arm area.

2. Physical examination. In both arms, measurements should include arm girth, blood pressure, and an Allen test of radial and ulnar blood flow. The patient should be examined for evidence of previous central or venous catheterization and for signs of trauma or surgery of the arm, chest, or neck, including previous AV access surgery. The presence of arm edema, collateral veins, or differential extremity size should prompt an evaluation of the central veins.

3. Imaging studies. Routine preoperative mapping of the arm to evaluate veins and arteries helps with selection of the most appropriate vein and the best location of the access. Use of imaging studies has been shown to increase both the rate of fistula placements and the success rate in obtaining a functioning access.

   a. Doppler ultrasonography. Doppler ultrasonography, which can measure flow velocity as well as the inner diameter of the brachial and radial arteries and peripheral veins, should be performed in nearly all patients to detect central vein stenosis and to identify suitable arteries and veins for fistula or graft placement.

   (1) Minimal vein and artery size. Controversy exists about the minimum size of the feeding artery and target vein for a successful fistula. One study suggested that the minimum vein lumen diameter should be about 2.5 mm for successful surgical anastomosis (Silva et al., 1998) and minimal arterial diameter should be 2.0 mm. However, smaller, "borderline" vessels down to 1.5 mm (for both artery and vein) have been used to create successful fistulas, although this may require a surgeon experienced with manipulating such small vessels. More important may be the ability of the artery and vein to dilate after anastomosis, to allow an increase in flow.

   (2) Vein dilation test. During the Doppler study the proximal vein is occluded and the increase in size is recorded. An average increase in internal diameter of 50% has been associated with a good fistula outcome (Malovrh et al., 2002).

   (3) Arterial dilation test. During the Doppler study the pulse contour of the artery is examined. The pulse contour of the artery is normally triphasic, due to high peripheral resistance. The patient is asked to clench the fist for 2 minutes, and then to open the hand; the resulting hyperemic response normally converts the triphasic arterial pulse contour to a biphasic pattern in patients capable of a healthy dilation.

   (4) Brachial artery flow. Flow in the brachial artery is measured at the axilla. A brachial artery flow >80 mL per minute predicts successful maturation of an AV fistula.

(5) Mapping. The cephalic and ulnar venous systems should also be evaluated for continuity and absence of strictures. Some surgeons perform venous mapping with a proximal tourniquet in place to distend and better identify veins suitable for fistula construction.

b. Venography. Venography should be reserved for selected patients, including those with a history of transvenous pacemaker placement, physical findings of upper extremity edema, collateral veins around the shoulder or on the chest wall, and/or unequal extremity size. If venography is performed, 30 mL or less of diluted low-dose contrast (low ionic strength, low osmolality contrast diluted 1:4) should be used to avoid nephrotoxicity. Full-strength contrast is usually not required for venography.

c. Arteriography. Arteriography is indicated when pulses in the desired access location are markedly diminished or absent or there is a >20 mm Hg difference in mean arterial pressure (MAP) between the two arms.

d. Magnetic resonance. Magnetic resonance imaging may also identify suitable veins for AV construction.

III. AV Fistulas

A. Location. At least nine potential sites for AV fistulas can be found in an upper extremity. A wrist radiocephalic or Brescia-Cimino fistula (Fig. 7-1) placed in the nondominant arm is the preferred access. Other forearm AV fistulas, such as the snuff-box or ulnar–basilic fistula, should be considered when a radiocephalic fistula is not an option. If a forearm fistula is not possible, especially in diabetic or elderly patients with atherosclerosis, then an elbow brachial–cephalic or a transposed brachiobasilic fistula is a good option. Less commonly used options are the Gracz fistula (which uses a perforating vein that arterializes both upper arm cephalic and basilic veins) and the brachial bidirectional cephalic

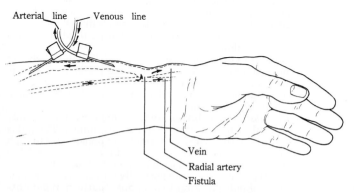

Figure 7-1.   The radiocephalic arteriovenous (AV) fistula, showing blood flow and the usual position of the access needles.

fistula (which arterializes both forearm and upper arm cephalic veins). When all sites in the nondominant arm have been exhausted, the dominant arm can be used.

B. Construction. Fistula surgery is usually performed in the operating room under regional anesthesia. The anastomosis can be either side of artery to side of vein or side of artery to end of vein. In both instances, distal blood flow through the artery is preserved. With the side-to-side method (Fig. 7-1), higher pressures may sometimes be transmitted to the veins in the hand, causing swelling. The side-of-artery–to–end-of-vein anastomosis prevents venous hypertension in the hand because the distal vein is tied. The details of the operative techniques are beyond the scope of this book. It is important to emphasize that AV fistula placement is not something that can be relegated to a junior or inexperienced vascular surgeon, but is best done by a surgeon with both experience and interest in performing these sometimes complex and demanding procedures.

C. Perioperative care and maturation. Some centers prepare the patient for AV fistula surgery by having the patient perform arm exercises for several weeks prior to surgery. Following surgery, the arm should initially be kept elevated and tight circumferential dressings should be avoided. The fistula blood flow should be checked daily (more frequently initially) by feeling for a thrill at the anastomotic site and by listening for an associated bruit. This examination can be performed by a physician, nurse, dialysis technician, or, preferably, the educated patient. The fistula should never be used for venipuncture. Hand exercises (e.g., squeezing a rubber ball, possibly with a light tourniquet applied on the arm above the fistula) may help increase blood flow and pressure, respectively, thereby accelerating maturation.

The maturation process generally requires at least 1 month, but may require up to 6 months. At the time of intended use, the vein diameter should be at least 4 mm. An AV fistula must be allowed to mature because premature cannulation is associated with infiltration, compression of the vessel, and permanent loss of the fistula. Failure to mature the superficial veins of the fistula may result from poor brachial artery inflow, an inadequate anastomosis, or an inability of the artery and/or vein to dilate due to vessel damage or sclerosis. One remediable cause is the presence of multiple tributary branches in the vein draining the AV fistula. These branches siphon off the increased venous flow, lessening the flow-induced increase in fistula pressure that induces maturation of the main venous channel. Often ligation of side branches can bring about or hasten maturation.

If a fistula cannot be cannulated or delivers a blood flow <350 mL per minute 6 or more weeks after placement, an imaging fistulogram should be obtained to determine the source of the problem.

IV. AV grafts

A. General. When an adequate AV fistula cannot be created, an AV connection using a graft tube made from biologic or synthetic material is the next preferred type of vascular access.

As described at the outset of this chapter, AV grafts are much less desirable than AV fistulas, primarily because of their lower long-term patency rates. However, AV grafts do have some advantages, including (a) a large surface area for needle placement, (b) easy cannulation, (c) short maturation time, and (d) easy surgical handling characteristics.

B. Characteristics. Most AV grafts placed in the United States are composed of expanded polytetrafluoroethylene (PTFE). The choice of synthetic or biologic material should be based on the surgeon's preference and experience. Use of cryopreserved vein grafts, especially those placed in the thigh, is associated with a high risk of infection. Short grafts have no advantage over long grafts in terms of patency and longevity. Tapered grafts, externally supported grafts, or elastic grafts do not provide results better than standard PTFE grafts. Modification of the distal anastomosis of PTFE grafts with a venous cuff may decrease venous stenosis and increase graft patency.

C. Configuration and location. Grafts may be placed in straight, looped, or curved configurations (Fig. 7-2). The most

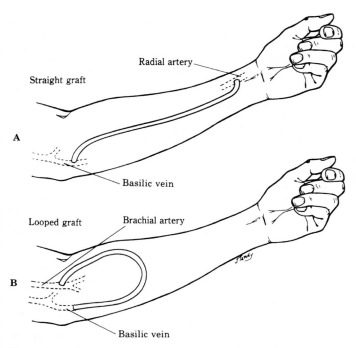

Figure 7-2. The two most common types of AV grafts. A: The straight graft between the radial artery and basilic vein. B: The loop graft between the brachial artery and basilic vein. (Modifed from Larson E, et al. *Development of the clinical nephrology practitioner.* St. Louis: Mosby, 1982.)

common initial sites for AV graft placement are a straight graft from the radial artery at the wrist to the basilic vein (Fig. 7-2A); a loop graft in the forearm from the brachial artery to the basilic vein (Fig. 7-2B); or an upper arm graft from brachial artery to axillary vein. Patient-specific features and projected time on dialysis help determine location, but a distal graft in the nondominant arm is generally preferred initially. While this approach preserves proximal arm sites for future placement of a fistula, distal grafts are associated with more frequent episodes of thrombosis and may be unnecessary in patients whose dependence on hemodialysis is expected to be short lived. A distal graft (e.g., straight forearm graft from radial artery to an antecubital fossa vein) can sometimes be used to mature a proximal downstream vein for future AV fistula construction.

1. When the usual access sites have been expended. The axillary artery can be used as the source of a loop graft in the upper extremity. The graft can extend from the arm to the internal jugular vein to bypass a subclavian vein stenosis on the same side. Grafts can also be placed in the thigh, but with a higher associated complication rate. Chest wall axilloaxillary (necklace) grafts are another option.

2. Surgical placement. AV grafts should be placed in the operating room under regional anesthesia (with general anesthesia backup) by a surgeon skilled in performing vascular anastomoses. Prophylactic antibiotics are often administered just prior to the operation.

The anastomosis should be made between the end of the graft and the side of the vein or artery to minimize interference with blood flow through the native vessels. Some studies suggest that nonpenetrating clips may be superior to conventional sutures by avoiding endothelial penetration. A clip should be placed at the arterial and venous anastomoses for identification during subsequent angiography.

3. Postoperative care. This is the same for grafts as for fistulas. The extremity is kept elevated for several days, and graft function is checked regularly by assessing for venous pulsation, thrill, and bruit. Most graft surgery is now performed in outpatient clinics.

4. Maturation

    a. How soon to cannulate. Although some advocate immediate use of an AV graft for dialysis, adhesion between the graft and the subcutaneous tunnel to prevent hematoma formation requires at least 2–3 weeks. A PTFE graft should not be cannulated for at least 2 weeks after placement and is considered mature when edema and erythema have resolved and the graft course is easily palpable. Cannulation of a graft that cannot be easily palpated or is edematous invites inaccurate needle insertion, leading to hematoma formation or frank laceration. Patients with persistent arm edema that does not respond to elevation should have an imaging study to evaluate the central veins.

    b. Early-use grafts. Several early-use grafts have been introduced for immediate postoperative access to avoid risks from temporary catheters. The performance of a multilayered, self-sealing polyurethane graft is comparable to that of a conventional PTFE graft and allows for early access. Its placement requires more skill than conventional PTFE to avoid graft kinking and twisting within the tunnel. Composite grafts should not be cannulated for at least 24 hours after placement, and not until swelling has resolved and the graft can be easily palpated. A self-sealing graft composed of heparin-bonded polycarbonate that is immediately available for puncture has been developed.

V. General issues relating to both AV fistulas and grafts

A. Cannulation

1. Skin preparation. An aseptic technique must be used for all cannulation procedures.

2. Anesthesia. In pain-sensitive patients, a topical anesthetic cream can be applied to the skin about 30 minutes prior to puncture, but this is rarely required. Most patients, especially those with new accesses, require subcutaneously injected lidocaine prior to needle cannulation. Injected anesthetic is especially helpful when manipulation of the needle is anticipated. Patients with established needle tracts often tolerate direct puncture without anesthesia and some find the anesthetic injection more painful than a direct stick.

3. Use of tourniquets for AV fistulas. A tourniquet or blood pressure cuff should be used to enlarge and stabilize the vein for easier cannulation of AV fistulas. A tourniquet should not be used during the dialysis treatment; improvement in pumped blood flow with a tourniquet suggests an inflow stenosis that requires further investigation. If a tourniquet is not required for cannulation and the fistula does not soften with arm elevation, a downstream (outflow) stenosis may be present and should be searched for using imaging studies.

4. Needle size. During the initial use of a permanent vascular access, some nephrologists recommend the use of small (16- to 17-gauge) needles and low blood flow rates, particularly in AV fistulas. In mature accesses, larger (15-gauge) needles are needed to support the required blood flow rates (>350 mL per minute) for high-efficiency dialysis.

5. Needle position and orientation. Two needles are placed into the dilated vein(s) of the fistula or into the graft. The needle leading to the dialyzer blood inlet is always placed in the more upstream segment but at least 3 cm away from the arterial anastomotic site. This upstream or "arterial" needle may point either upstream or downstream. Pointing the upstream needle in a downstream direction is popular in some countries, the rationale being that the "flap" left behind when the needle is withdrawn tends to close more naturally with the flow of blood. However, there is no controlled evidence to suggest that this is the case. The downstream (outlet or "venous") needle should be inserted pointing downstream, approximately 5 cm downstream to the upstream (arterial) needle (to minimize recirculation). Some caregivers rotate each needle 180 degrees along the needle axis after insertion to prevent potential injury to the deep wall of the vessel by the needle point. This issue has not been systematically studied.

   a. Risk of inflow/outflow needle reversal. Special care must be taken when cannulating forearm loop grafts. In more than 80% of such grafts, the arterial limb will be medial (ulnar), but in the remainder the arterial limb may lie on the radial side of the forearm (as in Fig. 7-2). For reference, a "road map" of the access from the surgeon is very useful. Reversal of needle placement may occur unless the dialysis clinic staff knows that blood in this particular graft flows in the opposite-to-usual direction. Reverse needle placement substantially increases the amount of recirculation (to >20%) and can result in inadequate delivery of dialysis. This happens more commonly than one would expect, as patients may have access surgery at another center and a diagram of the inserted access might not be readily available. When in doubt, a careful physical examination with transient occlusion of the access and palpation on either side of the occluding finger for pulsations will reveal the direction of blood flow in most cases.

6. Repeated punctures: Needle rotation, buttonhole technique. The manner in which needles are inserted affects the long-term patency and survival of accesses, particularly of AV fistulas. The "ladder" or rotational approach uses the entire length of the access without localizing needle sticks to any two areas. Grouping needle sticks in one or two specific areas weakens the wall, producing an aneurysm. In AV fistulas, a less commonly used alternative is the "buttonhole" method. With this method, the AV fistula is always punctured through a limited number of sites, the use of which may be rotated. The needle must be placed precisely through the same needle tract used previously. Ideally, after the buttonhole has been developed using sharp needles, special "dulled" needles are used to minimize laceration of the buttonhole tract. There is no published experience with the buttonhole method in AV grafts, and it should not be tried in AV grafts without further study.

7. Hemostasis postdialysis. Following needle removal, direct pressure over the site, usually with the tip of one or two fingers pushed firmly but not so hard as to occlude flow, is the best method for achieving hemostasis. One must prevent hematoma formation at the access site while controlling bleeding at the skin exit site. Pressure must be held for at least 10 minutes before checking the needle site for bleeding. Prolonged bleeding (>20 minutes) may indicate increased intra-access pressure due to an unsuspected outflow stenosis. Bleeding also is common in patients receiving therapeutic doses of anticoagulants such as warfarin. Adhesive bandages should not be applied until complete hemostasis has been achieved.

B.   Complications. Complications related to vascular access are a common reason for hospitalization in chronic dialysis patients. In the United States, access failure is the most common cause for hospitalization and in some centers accounts for the largest number of hospital days in end-stage renal disease patients.

   1.   Stenosis. Vascular access stenosis is a harbinger of thrombosis, reduces access blood flow, and can lead to underdialysis. The most common cause of stenosis in AV grafts is myointimal hyperplasia, which usually occurs at or just distal to the graft–vein anastomosis. In AV fistulas, the location and cause of stenosis is more varied and may be due to turbulence or needle stick injury causing fibrosis, abscess, or pseudoaneurysm formation. Because access patency is much worse after thrombectomy than after elective angioplasty, current KDOQI guidelines recommend prospective monitoring and surveillance of AV fistulas and grafts for hemodynamically significant stenosis.

   a.   Clinical indicators. Recurrent clotting (twice a month or more), difficult needle placement (strictures), difficulty with hemostasis on needle withdrawal (intra-access hypertension), a persistently swollen arm, and a reduction in the urea reduction ratio (URR) or Kt/V are all suggestive of stenosis but are generally very late manifestations of access dysfunction. Physical examination is an important tool for detection of access dysfunction and should include inspection for swelling and palpation for a pulse and a thrill along the entire length of the graft or fistula vein, with special attention paid to the regions both beyond and between the vascular anastomoses. A continuous, soft, low-pitched bruit should be present over a well-functioning access site. Stenosis is suggested by an increase in intensity of the thrill or the pitch of the bruit as one moves the finger or stethoscope along the midportion of the graft or along the draining fistula vein. The predictive value of clinical monitoring for access stenosis is about 70% in grafts according to a recent study.

   Other methods for predicting stenosis include measurement of access flow by ultrasound dilution, Doppler ultrasound, or magnetic resonance angiography, and by serial measurements of intra-access pressure (P_{IA}).

   b.   Access flow measurements and surveillance. To what extent low access flow reflects stenosis and the risk of thrombosis depends on the type of access. Flow through a native AV fistula commonly averages 500–800 mL per minute, and in grafts, flow is somewhat higher, about 1,000 mL per minute (but may be 3,000 mL per minute or higher). Native AV fistulas may maintain patency at flows as low as 200 mL per minute, whereas AV grafts begin to clot at access flows between 600 and 800 mL per minute— flows that often provide adequate dialysis but offer few clinical premonitory signs that the access is at risk for thrombosis. The current KDOQI recommendations are to intervene (i.e., have the patient referred for fistulogram) if access flow is <600 mL per minute or if the access flow is <1,000 mL per minute and has decreased by >25% over the preceding 4 months. While regular surveillance of vascular access for stenosis has been shown to decrease thrombosis rates when compared to historical controls, recent prospective studies have not shown conclusively that detection of stenosis and correction with angioplasty improves graft survival.

(1) Direct measurement of access flow

    (a) Indicator dilution. This method for measuring access blood flow during hemodialysis treatments was pioneered by Krivitski, who used ultrasound velocity to detect dilution of the blood by a bolus of saline. Other indicators have been used such as dyes and heat as well as detectors of light transmission and heat (thermistor), but ultrasound has been most widely tested and is now the preferred method for measuring access flow during dialysis. The system consists of a control box, two matched flow/dilutions sensors, a laptop computer, a data analysis software package, and a rolling stand that can be easily moved between patients (Fig. 7-3). To measure flow in the graft or fistula, the blood pump is stopped and the blood lines are reversed at the needle tubing-to-blood line connections. If available, an inline clamp or twister device can be activated, which reverses the pathway between the needle tubings and blood lines by clamping lines or twisting a valve without having to make any disconnection/reconnection. The blood

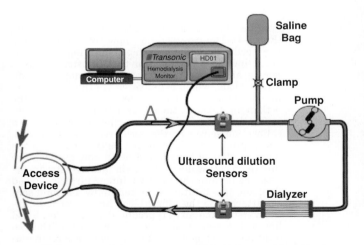

Figure 7-3. Measurement of access recirculation by saline dilution using ultrasound detection. See text for description of the setup and method. (Reproduced with permission from Transonic Systems, Inc., Ithaca, NY.)

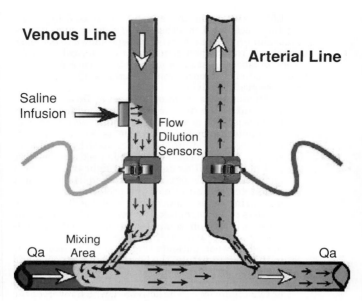

Figure 7-4. Measurement of access flow by saline dilution showing blood line reversal and position of blood line sensors See text for details of the method. (Reproduced with permission from Transonic Systems, Inc., Ithaca, NY.)

pump is then restarted at 250–300 mL per minute (Fig. 7-4). The reversed flow now creates an obligatory recirculation because blood entering the inflow blood line is now coming from the downstream access needle, and so part of this flow now is composed of dialyzed blood, which is delivered via the outlet blood line to the upstream access needle. A bolus of saline is then injected into the dialyzer outlet blood line, diluting the blood. This dilution effect is detected by a calibration sensor on the outlet (venous) blood line, which produces a dilution versus time curve on the monitor. Part of the diluted blood now goes via the upstream access needle back via the downstream access needle into the dialyzer inflow (arterial) blood line, and this dilution is picked up by a second sensor attached to the inflow blood line. A second dilution versus time curve is produced at the inflow blood line by this sensor, and the relative areas of the two dilution curves is a measure of the access recirculation (AR) that the line reversal has caused. The extent of this recirculation is proportional to the ratio of flow through the extracorporeal circuit (which is simply the blood pump speed, Qb) to flow through the access. Since AR and Qb are known, the third variable, access blood flow, can be easily calculated.

(b) Doppler. Doppler ultrasonography, though usually used to detect stenotic lesions directly, can also be used to measure the rate of flow through a vascular access. A variety of machines and several different flow velocity algorithms have been used. There is systematic underestimation or overestimation of flow by some machines. Flow measurement by Doppler depends on an accurate measurement of both velocity and vessel diameter. This may be difficult when flow is turbulent in an access and the diameter is not uniform. Because of these confounders, flow is better measured at the brachial artery, where the vessel is a smooth cylinder of blood and flow is nonturbulent. Almost all of the flow in the brachial artery (apart from about 60–80 mL per minute nutrient flow) flows through the vascular access, and brachial artery flow correlates very well with access flow rate.

(c) Magnetic resonance angiography can be used to measure access flow quite accurately, but is too expensive for routine use.

(2) Indirect measurement of access flow.

(a) Intra-access pressure (P_{IA}) and access flow. Flow, pressure, and resistance are mathematically related. In an AV graft, the P_{IA} is usually <50% of MAP. Most of this pressure drop occurs at the arterial anastomosis, unless there is intragraft stenosis. When outflow stenosis develops (e.g., due to neointimal hyperplasia at or downstream from the graft–vein anastomosis), P_{IA} rises and flow decreases. When P_{IA} rises above 50% of the MAP (P_{IA}/MAP >0.50), graft flow commonly has decreased into the thrombosis-prone range of 600–800 mL per minute, and the presence of stenosis is likely. In AV fistulas, blood entering the venous system returns via multiple collateral veins. As a consequence, P_{IA} in an AV fistula, which is on average lower than in an AV graft, may not increase with outlet stenosis, and is therefore less valuable as a surveillance tool for stenosis in fistulas. If a stenosis develops in the body of an AV graft between the areas used for arterial and venous limb cannulation, P_{IA} at the venous needle remains normal or can even decrease, despite increasing stenosis. Stenosis at the arterial anastomosis of both grafts and fistulas causes P_{IA} to decrease and a widely patent arterial anastomosis causes high basal P_{IA} in the absence of stenosis.

One study (Spergel et al., 2004) found little relationship between access flow and the static venous pressure–to–MAP ratio. Recently, an engineering flow model (White et al., 2005) showed that the ability of this ratio to predict flow was greatly reduced when the arterial diameter was greater than

Table 7-1. Measuring the EQP_{IA}/MAP ratio

Example:
1. Measure MAP: Assume that BP is 190/100. MAP is diastolic plus one third of pulse pressure, or 130 mm Hg.
2. Measure static intra-access pressure:
   a. With the blood pump off and the blood line upstream to the venous drip chamber clamped, the venous drip chamber pressure is 60 mm Hg.
   b. Compute offset using equation: offset (mm Hg) = $-1.6 + 0.74 \times H$ (cm), where H is the height between the access and middle of the drip chamber. Assume H is 35 cm. Then offset = $3.4 + 25.9 = 29.3$ mm Hg.
   c. Add offset to compute EQP_{IA}: $EQP_{IA} = 60 + 29.3 = 89.3$ mm Hg.
   d. Compute the EQP_{IA}/MAP ratio. In this case, $89/130 = 0.68$, which is >0.5. This access is at risk for stenosis.

EQP_{IA}, equivalent intra-access pressure; MAP, mean arterial pressure; BP, blood pressure.

that of the draining vein. Because of these pressure and arterial size confounders, serial measurements of pressure in each patient are more valuable than isolated measurements of either P_{IA} or the P_{IA}/MAP ratio. Details of how to compute this ratio are given in Table 7-1.

(b) Static venous pressure. Pressures in the drip chamber of the venous return line in the absence of extracorporeal blood flow (static venous pressure) are preferred over dynamic venous pressure (see below), but are time consuming. A rise in static venous pressure over time in an individual patient is highly predictive of the presence of venous stenosis.

(c) Dynamic venous pressure or equivalent P_{IA}. Dynamic venous pressures are measured during routine hemodialysis in the presence of extracorporeal blood flow. The advantage of this method is that these pressures are recorded routinely during dialysis and can be read off the dialysis machine with the blood pump running. However, measurements are meaningful only if taken at the beginning of dialysis with low blood flow rates (200–225 mL per minute) because at high blood flow rates, much of the resistance to flow is from the needle and not the vascular access. A baseline value should be established when the access is first used. The threshold pressure that triggers further evaluation depends on the size of the needle; for 15-gauge needles, it is >115–120 mm Hg; for 16-gauge needles, it is >150 mm Hg. The threshold pressure must be exceeded three times in succession to be significant. The measurement of dynamic venous pressure is less sensitive and specific than direct measurements of access flow rates and prone to error. However, improved accuracy has been reported when measurements are made repeatedly at very low blood flow rates (Vasc-Alert system) and are adjusted for needle size as well as hematocrit. In such cases, a diagnosis of impending access failure depends more on the trend of the pressures than on the actual measured pressures themselves.

c. **Access recirculation.** Recirculation of dialyzed blood across the access device immediately back through the dialysis circuit does not appear until access flow decreases to a level near to or less than flow in the extracorporeal circuit. Thus, barring inadvertent needle reversal or improper needle placement, access recirculation will not be present until access flow falls to the range of 350–500 mL per minute. At this range of flow, AV grafts are already at high risk for thrombosis, so if true recirculation is detected in an AV graft, it is an urgent indication to image the graft and correct the stenosis. On the other hand, in AV fistulas, continued patency is likely even when recirculation is present (flow in the 350–500 mL per minute range). The benefits of screening AV fistulas for access recirculation are relatively small in terms of preventing thrombosis, but screening for recirculation is useful to prevent underdialysis.

Both urea-based and non–urea-based (e.g., ultrasound dilution) techniques have been used to detect recirculation. The urea-based methods have been described in Chapter 3. The ultrasound dilution technique described earlier can be used to measure recirculation. In this case the blood lines are not reversed. If venous blood is recirculating through the access, the injected bolus of saline will be detected by the arterial sensor soon after injection.

Measurement of access recirculation by thermal dilution using a blood temperature monitor (BTM) yields results similar to those obtained by the ultrasound dilution technique. During a routine dialysis treatment, a bolus of cold saline is injected into the venous line and the temperature drop is measured in the arterial blood line. Since currently available BTM recirculation methods include a component related to cardiopulmonary recirculation, they only detect recirculation in AV accesses when it is greater than about 15%.

It is important to note that access stenosis between the needles will not cause recirculation but may markedly reduce access flow to thrombosis-prone levels. Stenosis in this location should be suspected when access flows are measured to be below the blood pump flow rate, but recirculation is not detectable. Recirculation exceeding 10% using the recommended two-needle urea-based method, 5% using the ultrasound dilution method, or 15% using the thermal dilution method should prompt investigation.

d. **Imaging the vascular access**

(1) **Doppler ultrasonography.** This noninvasive technique allows direct imaging of the flow pattern in AV grafts and fistulas. It has been useful for detecting

stenoses and for mapping aneurysms. Doppler flow measurements are prohibitively expensive for routine assessment. Their chief role is in the evaluation of flow and anatomy in accesses that have been screened by other techniques.

(2) **Venography.** Most centers refer patients with a high probability of stenosis as determined by low-cost methods directly for angiography and balloon angioplasty, bypassing Doppler altogether.

e. **Intervention after access stenosis had been identified.** Once a stenosis >50% is detected, percutaneous transluminal catheter angioplasty (PTCA) or surgical revision of the lesion should be performed if one or more of the following are present: (a) abnormal physical examination; (b) previous history of thrombosis; (c) decreasing access flow; and (d) elevated or increasing measured static intra-access pressures (normalized to MAP). The expertise at each institution should determine which procedure is to be performed. If repeated angioplasties have been required within a short period for the same lesion, surgical revision should be considered. Although endovascular stents have been employed for the treatment of venous stenoses, they offer no particular advantage over PTCA for the treatment of routine lesions. Residual stenosis, elastic recoil, and extravasation of blood from the lesion are all indications for stent placement.

f. **Flow measurements immediately after access revision.** Sometimes radiographic correction of an apparent stenosis does not result in improvement in the access blood flow rate. At other times, access blood flow initially increases, but then falls back to pretreatment levels within a day or two of the procedure. Measurement of access flow immediately after a revision or angioplasty is helpful in terms of determining the likelihood that the access will remain open for a clinically useful period.

2. **Thrombosis**

a. **Predisposing factors.** An increasingly recognized number of dialysis patients have subtle accentuations of hemostasis, including high fibrinogen levels, reduced levels of protein S or C, factor V Leiden mutation, lupus anticoagulant, or elevated hematocrit levels due to erythropoietin therapy. Whether or not these conditions are associated with increased access thrombosis is controversial. Warfarin may be indicated for some of these patients, although in patients with protein S or C deficiency, use of warfarin may precipitate skin necrosis, and in patients with lupus anticoagulant, the prothrombin time is an unreliable measure of anticoagulation.

b. **Prevention.** Anticoagulants and antiplatelet drugs may help prevent AV access thrombosis, but most studies published thus far do not support their routine use. Separate randomized clinical trials (RCTs) of both low-dose warfarin (target international normalized ratio [INR] 1.4–1.9) and clopidogrel plus aspirin versus placebo in patients with PTFE grafts failed to demonstrate a reduction in thrombotic events or prolongation of graft survival. Both studies showed clinically and statistically significant bleeding complications in the treated patients. However, another RCT found a decrease in the relative risk of thrombosis in patients with new PTFE grafts treated with dipyridamole. Use of angiotensin-converting enzyme inhibitors and daily fish oil supplementation may prevent venous stenosis and graft thrombosis in newly constructed AV grafts. At the present time, implant irradiation (brachytherapy) has been found to be ineffective in preventing intimal hyperplasia/thrombosis in grafts.

c. **Treatment**

(1) **In AV fistulas.** Thrombosis of the fistula occurs either soon after its construction or as a late event. Patients should be taught to monitor their fistula daily, when possible. Early thrombosis results from technical factors and almost always requires surgical revision, although there may be inadvertent compression while sleeping. Poor flow precedes late thrombosis in most cases, but hypotension or hypercoagulability may also precipitate thrombosis in the absence of downward flow trends. Treatment of thrombosis can be difficult but should be performed using either PTCA or surgical thrombectomy, depending on the expertise of each institution.

(2) **In AV grafts.** Thrombosis can be managed by surgical thrombectomy or by mechanical or pharmacomechanical thrombolysis, again depending on the expertise of the medical center. However, it is essential that the following be considered: Treatment should be performed urgently to avoid the need for temporary access. The entire access circuit should be thoroughly evaluated during the procedure by imaging. Residual stenosis exceeding 85% should be retreated by balloon angioplasty or surgical revision. The role of antiplatelet drugs or warfarin in patients with recurrent thrombosis is unknown. Patients who clot with intra-access flows >1,000 mL per minute should be educated to avoid external access compression, evaluated for hypercoagulability, and/or examined for presence of delayed hypotension after dialysis. Routine monitoring and surveillance of the graft should resume shortly after successful treatment. For patients with failed thrombectomy and thrombolysis, surgical efforts should be focused on creating a secondary fistula from the venous drainage of the graft. Such fistulas are possible because of the venous enlargement and thickening caused by the previous graft, and have the advantage of being usable much sooner after creation of the fistula. KDOQI guidelines recommend that every patient should be evaluated for a secondary fistula after each episode of graft failure.

(3) Silent infection in thrombosed AV grafts. Old thrombosed grafts may become infected with few local signs, suggesting that perhaps such grafts should be electively removed soon after they are abandoned. However, because surgical removal often requires extensive tissue dissection, this area needs further study before a blanket recommendation can be made.

(4) Role of the interventional nephrologist. In most institutions, vascular access–related procedures are performed by surgeons and interventional radiologists. Numerous centers in the United States now offer the nephrologist formal training in techniques including percutaneous balloon angioplasty, thrombectomy, and insertion of tunneled hemodialysis catheters. Because nephrologists have a different clinical perspective of patients and their access-related problems, they may be better suited to help minimize delays and to decrease hospitalizations, costs, and patient frustrations.

3. Ischemia in a limb bearing an AV access. All patients, especially diabetics and elderly patients with atherosclerosis, should be monitored for the development of limb ischemia following AV access construction.

a. Detection. Patients with an established fistula should be assessed monthly by interval history and physical examination. Ischemia distal to an AV access can occur at any time (hours to months) following access construction. Subjective complaints include pain, coldness, numbness, tingling, and impairment of motor function. Objective findings include changes in skin temperature and/or color; loss of sensation, motor function, or distal arterial pulses; and the development of edema in the hand or arm when compared to the contralateral side.

b. Management. Mild ischemia manifested by coldness or paresthesias but without sensory or motor loss can be managed expectantly. Pain of the hand on exercise due to a "steal" effect (or in extreme instances, pain at rest) or the appearance of nonhealing ulcers usually requires surgical intervention. Severe ischemia with nerve injury is a surgical emergency. With the usual radiocephalic side-to-side fistula, the radial artery anastomosis regularly steals blood flow from the ulnar artery system. Converting the side-of-artery to an end-of-artery anastomosis can sometimes be used to treat ischemia due to steal. Severe cases of steal syndrome require ligation of the AV fistula, but distal revascularization interval ligation (DRIL) can be used to treat ischemia while preserving fistula patency. The DRIL technique requires ligation of the artery immediately distal to the origin of the AV fistula and construction of a reversed saphenous vein bypass from the artery proximal to the origin of the fistula to the artery distal to the site of ligation. Treatment of hand edema after placement of an AV fistula consists of converting the anastomosis from a side-of-vein to an end-of-vein opening or by selectively tying off affected veins. A small increase in circumference (2–3 cm) of the arm bearing the access is common after placement of AV grafts, but larger increases indicate venous hypertension usually due to stenosis of the central veins.

4. **Pseudoaneurysm**
   a. **AV fistula.** Pseudoaneurysm in the draining vein is much more common than a true aneurysm. It results from inadequate hemostasis and extravasation of blood following dialysis needle removal. Most pseudoaneurysms and true aneurysms are treated by observation only and by avoiding puncture of the fistula in the area of the aneurysm site. When marked enlargement and compromise of the overlying skin develops, rupture may develop, producing hemorrhage. Large aneurysms can prevent adequate needle placement and limit potential puncture sites.
   b. **AV graft.** These should be treated by resection and insertion of an interposition graft if they are (a) rapidly expanding, (b) >12 mm in diameter, and (c) threatening viability of the overlying skin. AV grafts should also be revised if pseudoaneurysm formation limits the number of puncture sites available or for persistent symptoms (pain, throbbing).

5. **Infections**
   a. **AV fistula.** Infections are rare and usually caused by staphylococci; they should be treated in the same manner as subacute endocarditis with 6 weeks of antibiotics. Diagnosis is based on local signs of inflammation. Prompt therapy with antistaphylococcal antimicrobials, after local and blood cultures have been obtained, is often curative. Only septic embolus during therapy warrants removal of the fistula.
   b. **AV graft.** Graft infection occurs eventually in 5%–20% of grafts placed, although thigh grafts have a higher rate of infection. Prophylactic antimicrobials should be used when patients with vascular grafts undergo procedures capable of inducing bacteremia, such as dental extraction or genitourinary manipulation. Most graft infections are staphylococcal, but rarely Gram-negative organisms such as *Escherichia coli* may be cultured. Initial antibiotic treatment should include drugs active against Gram-negative and Gram-positive organisms as well as against *Enterococcus*. Local infection of a graft can be treated with antibiotics (based on culture results) and by incision/resection of the infected portion. Extensive infection requires complete excision/removal.

   Septicemia may occur without local signs. In such cases, a technetium-labeled leukocyte scan may help reveal a graft infection, but care must be taken to remove any blood-soaked dressings prior to scanning, as they may lead to a falsely positive result. Hemorrhage may occur due to rupture of an infected graft. A graft placed within 30 days that becomes infected should be removed.

6. **Congestive heart failure.** Blood flow rate through an AV fistula or graft can vary from barely adequate (400 mL per minute) to >3,000 mL per minute. Wrist and forearm

accesses have lower flows than upper arm accesses. Accesses in the leg often have the highest flow rates. Congestive heart failure is unusual with a forearm access but may occur in patients with upper arm or femoral fistulas, particularly if there is coexistent heart disease. Long-term cardiac function is generally unaffected by the presence of an AV access. Surgical narrowing or banding should be done only after cardiac studies have shown marked changes in cardiac output following transient occlusion of the fistula. In patients with unexplained high cardiac output states, one should always first consider and correct any anemia that may be present. Use of vasodilators such as minoxidil or hydralazine without concomitant beta-blockade is another common, correctable cause of high cardiac output.

C. **Clinical outcome goals and monitoring**

1. **Establishment of a vascular access team and continuous quality improvement (CQI).** Establishment of a vascular access team that includes nephrologists, surgeons, interventionists, a vascular access coordinator, and dialysis personnel is essential to ensuring good vascular access outcomes. Ideally the vascular access team should meet regularly to review data and provide a measurement of performance based on established KDOQI guidelines. Data collected should include number and type of vascular accesses, infection and thrombosis rates, number and type of interventions performed, and time to access failure. Centers should monitor outcome results after thrombosis and set minimum goals for both immediate and long-term patency. Trends should be analyzed and feedback provided to all members of the team. This approach fosters preemptive action and salvage rather than replacement of AV accesses. It also helps ensure delivery of an adequate dialysis dose.

2. **Maximizing AV fistula placement.** Dialysis centers should strive to construct an AV fistula in at least 60% of all patients new to hemodialysis. The long-term rate of thrombosis of AV fistulas should be <0.25 episodes per patient year at risk.

3. **Goals for AV graft placement.** Primary access failure rates (failure within the first 30 days after surgery) of newly placed AV grafts should not be >15% for forearm straight grafts, 10% for forearm loop grafts, and 5% for upper arm grafts, as per KDOQI guidelines. The cumulative patency rates of all AV grafts should be at least 70% at 1 year, 60% at 2 years, and 50% at 3 years. The rate of graft thrombosis should not exceed 0.5 thrombotic episodes per patient year at risk.

4. **Goals for limiting use of venous catheters.** Ideally, <10% of chronic hemodialysis patients should be using catheters as their permanent access, but this number may be higher in new centers or centers with many new patients; in centers serving patients with reduced access to health care; in centers with high comorbidity prevalence, especially vascular disease; in centers where extra efforts are employed to place AV fistulas (longer maturation time); in centers where, because of longer patient survival,

potential sites for AV access are exhausted; or, especially, when combinations of these circumstances exist.

SELECTED READINGS

Ayus AC, Sheikh-Hamad D. Silent infections in clotted hemodialysis access grafts. *J Am Soc Nephrol* 1998;9:1314–1317.

Besarab A, et al. Simplified measurement of intra-access pressure. *ASAIO J* 1996;42:M682–M687.

Besarab A, et al. The utility of intra-access monitoring in detecting and correcting venous outlet stenoses prior to thrombosis. *Kidney Int* 1995;47:1364–1373.

Besarab A, Sherman R. The relationship of recirculation to access blood flow. *Am J Kidney Dis* 1997;29:223–229.

Campos RP, et al. Stenosis in hemodialysis arteriovenous fistula: evaluation and treatment. *Hemodial Int* 2006;10(2):152–161.

Chemla ES, et al. Complex bypasses and fistulas for difficult hemodialysis access: a prospective, single-center experience. *Semin Dial* 2006;19(3):246–250.

Chin AI, et al. Intra-access blood flow in patients with newly created upper-arm arteriovenous native fistulas for hemodialysis access. *Am J Kidney Dis* 2004;44(5):850–858.

Crowther MA, et al. Low-intensity warfarin is ineffective for prevention of PTFE graft failure in patients on hemodialysis: a randomized controlled trial. *Am J Soc Nephrol* 2002;13(9):2331–2337.

Depner TA, Krivitsky NM, MacGibbon D. Hemodialysis access recirculation measured by ultrasound dilution. *ASAIO J* 1995;41:M749–M753.

Gradzki R, et al. Use of ACE inhibitors is associated with prolonged survival of arteriovenous grafts. *Am J Kidney Dis* 2001;38(6):1240–1244.

Huijbregts HJ, Blankestijn PJ. Dialysis access—guidelines for current practice. *Eur J Vasc Endovasc Surg* 2006;31(3):284–287.

Kaufman JS, et al. Randomized controlled trial of clopidogrel plus aspirin to prevent hemodialysis access graft thrombosis. *J Am Soc Nephrol* 2003;14(9):2313–2321.

Krivitski NM. Theory and validation of access flow measurement by dilution technique during hemodialysis. *Kidney Int* 1995;48:244–250.

Lok CE, et al. Reducing vascular access morbidity: a comparative trial of two vascular access monitoring strategies. *Nephrol Dial Transplant* 2003;18(6):1174–1180.

Malovrh M. Native arteriovenous fistula. Preoperative evaluation. *Am J Kidney Dis* 2002;39:1218–1225.

Maya ID, et al. Vascular access stenosis: comparison of arteriovenous grafts and fistulas. *Am J Kidney Dis* 2004;44(5):859–865.

Oakes DD, et al. Surgical salvage of failed radiocephalic arteriovenous fistulas: techniques and results in 29 patients. *Kidney Int* 1998;53:480–487.

Ohira S, Kon T, Imura T. Evaluation of primary failure in native AV-fistulae (early fistula failure). *Hemodial Int* 2006;10(2):173–179.

Ortega T, et al. The timely construction of arteriovenous fistulas: a key to reducing morbidity and mortality and to improving cost management. *Nephrol Dial Transplant* 2005;20(3):598–603.

Rayner HC, et al. Vascular access results from the Dialysis Outcomes and Practice Patterns Study (DOPPS): performance against Kidney Disease Outcomes Quality Initiative (K/DOQI) Clinical Practice guidelines. *Am J Kidney Dis* 2004;44(5 Suppl 3):22–26.

Saran R, et al. Association between vascular access failures and the use of specific drugs: the Dialysis Outcomes and Practice Patterns Study (DOPPS). *Am J Kidney Dis* 2002;40(6):1255–1263.

Sessa C, et al. Treatment of hand ischemia following angioaccess surgery using the distal revascularization interval-ligation technique with preservation of vascular access: description of an 18-case series. *Ann Vasc Surg* 2004;18(6):685–694.

Silva MB Jr, et al. A strategy for increasing use of autogenous hemodialysis access procedures: impact of preoperative noninvasive evaluation. *J Vasc Surg* 1998;27(2):302–307.

White JJ, et al. Paulson relation between static venous pressure (VP), hemodialysis graft blood flow (Q), and stenosis: analysis by fluid mechanics model [Abstract]. *J Am Soc Nephrol* 2005;F-PO531.

Xue JL, et al. The association of initial hemodialysis access type with mortality outcomes in elderly Medicare ESRD patients. *Am J Kidney Dis* 2003;42(5):1013–1019.

WEB REFERENCES

KDOQI guidelines for vascular access: http://www.kidney.org

Fistula First initiative: http://www.fistulafirst.org

American Society of Diagnostic and Interventional Radiology: http://www.asdin.org/

Vascular Web: http://www.vascularweb.org/

HDCN Vascular Access Channel: http://www.hdcn.com/ch/access/

8

Acute Hemodialysis Prescription

John T. Daugirdas, Edward A. Ross, and
Allen R. Nissenson

I. The hemodialysis prescription. All patients are different, and the circumstances eventuating in the need for acute hemodialysis vary widely. The prescription for hemodialysis will change accordingly. As a teaching tool only, we present a "typical" prescription for an acute hemodialysis in a 70-kg adult.

R_x: **Acute hemodialysis (not for initial treatment)**
Session length: Perform hemodialysis for 4 hours
Blood flow rate: 350 mL per minute
Dialyzer:
Dialyzer membrane: your choice
Dialyzer K_{Uf}: your choice
Dialyzer efficiency: usually a dialyzer with a K_0A of 500–800 is used
Dialysis solution composition (variable):
Base: bicarbonate 25 mM
Sodium: 145 mM
Potassium: 3.5 mM
Calcium: 1.75 mM (3.5 mEq/L)
Magnesium: 0.375 mM (0.75 mEq/L)
Dextrose: 11 mM (200 mg/dL)
Phosphate: none
Dialysis solution flow rate: 500 mL per minute
Dialysis solution temperature: 35–36°C
Fluid removal orders:
Use ultrafiltration control device
Remove 2.2 L over 4 hours at a constant rate
Anticoagulation orders:
See Chapter 12

A. Determining dialysis session length and blood flow rate. The dialysis session length together with the blood flow rate are the most important determinants of the amount of dialysis to be given (dialyzer efficiency is also a factor).

1. Reduce the amount of dialysis for the initial one or two sessions. For the initial treatment, especially when the predialysis serum urea nitrogen (SUN) level is very high (e.g., >125 mg/dL [44 mmol/L]), the dialysis session length and blood flow rate should both be reduced. A urea reduction ratio of <40% should be targeted. This usually means using a blood flow rate of only 250 mL per minute (200 mL per minute in small patients) for adults along with a 2-hour treatment time. A longer initial dialysis session or use of excessively high blood flow rates in the acute setting may result in the so-called **disequilibrium syndrome,** described more fully in Chapter 10. This neurologic syndrome, which includes the appearance of obtundation, or even seizures and coma, during or after dialysis, has been associated with excessively rapid removal of blood solutes. The risk of disequilibrium syndrome is increased when the predialysis serum urea nitrogen level is high. After the initial dialysis session, the patient can be re-evaluated and should generally be dialyzed again the following day. The length of the second dialysis session can usually be increased to 3 hours, provided that the predialysis serum urea nitrogen level is <100 mg/dL (36 mmol/L). Subsequent dialysis sessions can be as long as needed. The length of a single dialysis treatment rarely exceeds 6 hours unless the purpose of dialysis is treatment of drug overdose. Slow low-efficiency hemodialysis (SLED) uses low blood and dialysis solution flow rates and longer treatment sessions in order to more safely remove fluid. SLED is described in Chapter 13.

2.   Dialysis frequency and dose for subsequent treatments and dialysis adequacy. It is difficult to deliver a large amount of dialysis in the acute setting. Most intensive care unit patients are fluid overloaded, and urea distribution volume is often much greater than 50%–60% of body weight. True delivered blood flow rate through a venous catheter rarely exceeds 350 mL per minute and often is substantially lower. Recirculation occurs in venous catheters and is greatest with catheters in the femoral position due to the low pericatheter venous flow rate. Often the treatment is interrupted due to hypotension. Furthermore, the degree of urea sequestration in muscle may be increased, as such patients often are on pressors, reducing blood flow to muscle and skin, which contain a substantial portion of urea and other dissolved waste products. Concomitant intravenous infusions, which often are given to patients in an acute setting, dilute the urea level in the blood and reduce further the efficiency of dialysis.

A typical 3- to 4-hour acute-dialysis session will deliver a single-pool Kt/V of only 0.9, with an equilibrated Kt/V of 0.7. Dialysate-side urea removal may be even lower (Evanson et al., 1999). This low level of Kt/V, if given three times per week, is associated with a high mortality in chronic, stable patients. One option is to dialyze sick patients with acute renal failure on a daily (six or seven times per week) basis. Each treatment is then approximately 3–4 hours in length. Data by Schiffl et al. (2002) suggest that mortality is reduced in patients with acute renal failure dialyzed six times per week as opposed to those receiving dialysis every other day. If every-other-day dialysis is to be given, the treatment length should probably be set at 4–6 hours, to deliver a single-pool Kt/V of at least 1.2–1.3, as recommended for chronic therapy.

The amount of dialysis may need to be adjusted upward in hypercatabolic patients. A low predialysis SUN level should not be used as a justification to reduce the amount of dialysis unless substantial residual renal urea clearance is documented; many acute renal failure patients tend to have decreased urea generation rates due to lack of protein ingestion and/or to impairment of urea synthesis by the liver. Therefore, in such patients a low SUN does not necessarily reflect low levels of other uremic toxins.

B. Choosing a dialyzer

　1. Membrane material. The differences among dialyzer membranes are discussed in Chapter 4.

　　Unsubstituted cellulose membranes activate complement to a greater degree than do substituted cellulose membranes or synthetic membranes. Several studies initially suggested that use of unsubstituted cellulose membranes for acute dialysis might prolong the course of acute renal failure and increase the risk of oliguria; the hypothesis was that complement-activated neutrophils might migrate to injured glomeruli and cause further damage by generating reactive oxygen compounds. However, subsequent randomized studies failed to find any deleterious effects of using unsubstituted cellulose membranes for acute dialysis. One study (Herrero et al., 2002) did find that patients dialyzed with bioincompatible membranes had a lower pulmonary diffusing capacity. A meta-analysis of studies done up until the year 2002 suggested that unsubstituted cellulose membranes should not be used for acute dialysis (Subramanian et al., 2002). A Cochrane report, however, recently suggested that no firm conclusions could be drawn as of 2006 regarding the benefits of any one group of dialysis membranes over another for acute or chronic dialysis. The best dialyzer to select for acute dialysis, therefore, remains unclear.

　　No recommendation favoring use of high-flux membranes for acute dialysis can be made at this time, as membrane flux has not been studied as a separate factor in any randomized study of acute dialysis.

　　a. Anaphylactoid reactions. These can occur and depend on both membrane material and sterilization mode. See Chapter 10 for details.

　2. Ultrafiltration coefficient (K_{Uf}). Ultrafiltration controllers are now available on most dialysis machines, and these accurately control the ultrafiltration rate by means of special pumps and circuits. By and large, most of the machines with volumetric ultrafiltration controllers are designed to use dialyzers of high water permeability (e.g., K_{Uf} >6.0) and may lose accuracy if a high fluid removal rate is attempted using a dialyzer that is relatively impermeable to water.

　　If a dialysis machine with an ultrafiltration controller is not available, then a membrane with a relatively low water permeability (K_{Uf}) should be chosen, so that the transmembrane pressure (TMP) will have to be set at a relatively high level to remove the amount of fluid desired; then the inevitable errors in maintaining the desired TMP will have less impact on the rate of fluid removal. When close monitoring of the fluid removal rate is required and a machine with advanced ultrafiltration control circuitry is not available, the fluid removal rate can be monitored by placing the patient on an electronic bed or chair scale and continuously following the weight during dialysis.

3. Dialyzer urea clearance. For the first couple of dialysis sessions, it is best to avoid using very high-efficiency dialyzers, although these can be used as long as the blood flow is low. A dialyzer with an in vitro $K_0 A$ urea of about 500 mL per minute is recommended for the initial session to minimize the risk of inadvertent overdialysis and of developing the disequilibrium syndrome. Also, when heparin-free dialysis is used, there is less risk (theoretically) of clotting when a lower blood flow rate is used with a smaller dialyzer, as the blood velocity through a small fiber bundle will be higher. After the initial one or two sessions, particularly if a high blood flow rate is being used, the largest dialyzer that can economically be used should be chosen.

C. Choosing the dialysis solution. In our example, we have chosen a bicarbonate level of 25 mM, with a sodium level of 145 mM, a potassium level of 3.5 mM, a calcium level of 1.75 mM (3.5 mEq/L), a magnesium level of 0.375 mM (0.75 mEq/L), a dextrose level of 11 mmol/L (200 mg/dL), and no phosphorus. Depending on the circumstances, this prescription may have to be altered in a given patient. It is important to recognize that for acute patients the dialysis solution composition should be tailored. The "standard" composition designed for acidotic, hyperphosphatemic, hyperkalemic, chronic dialysis patients is often inappropriate in an acute setting.

1. Dialysis solution bicarbonate concentration. In the sample prescription above, we have chosen to use a 25 mM bicarbonate level. Intensive care unit patients often are relatively alkalotic for reasons described below, and so prescriptions for "standard" bicarbonate dialysis solution, containing 35–38 mM, should not be used without first carefully evaluating the patient's acid–base status.

If the predialysis plasma bicarbonate level is 28 mM or higher, or if the patient has respiratory alkalosis, a custom dialysis solution containing an appropriately lower bicarbonate level (e.g., 20–28 mM, depending on the degree of alkalosis) should be used.

a. Dangers of metabolic alkalosis. A dialysis patient with even a mild metabolic alkalosis (e.g., plasma bicarbonate level of 30 mmol/L) requires very little hyperventilation to increase blood pH to dangerous levels. In many respects, alkalemia (blood pH >7.50) is more dangerous than acidemia. Dangers of alkalemia include soft tissue calcification and cardiac arrhythmia (sometimes with sudden death). Alkalemia also has been associated with such adverse symptoms as nausea, lethargy, and headache.

In dialysis patients, the most common causes of metabolic alkalosis are a reduced intake of protein, intensive dialysis for any reason (e.g., daily dialysis), and vomiting or nasogastric suction. Another common cause is administered lactate or acetate with total parenteral nutrition (TPN) solutions, or citrate due to citrate antico-agulation.

One uncommon cause is the coadministration of aluminum hydroxide with sodium polystyrene sulfonate resin. This combination can cause alkalosis because the resin binds aluminum, and the latter can no longer bind to and sequester bicarbonate secreted by the pancreas. The bicarbonate is reabsorbed, causing the alkalosis (Madias and Levey, 1983).

b. Predialysis respiratory alkalosis. Many patients who are candidates for acute dialysis have pre-existing respiratory alkalosis. The causes of respiratory alkalosis are the same as in patients with normal renal function and include pulmonary disease (pneumonia, edema, embolus), hepatic failure, and central nervous system disorders. Normally, compensation for respiratory alkalosis is twofold. There is an acute decrease in the plasma bicarbonate level due to release of hydrogen ions from body buffer stores. In patients with normal renal function, there is a further delayed (2–3 days) compensatory fall in the plasma bicarbonate level due to excretion of bicarbonate in the urine. Renal bicarbonate excretion obviously cannot occur in dialysis patients.

The therapeutic goal should always be to normalize the pH rather than the plasma bicarbonate level. In patients with respiratory alkalosis, the plasma bicarbonate level at which the blood pH will be normal may be as low as 17–20 mmol/L; the dialysis solution to use should contain less than the usual amount of bicarbonate to achieve a postdialysis plasma bicarbonate level in the desired subnormal range.

c. Achieving an appropriately low dialysis solution bicarbonate level. In certain machines, the proportioning ratio of concentrate to product water is fixed, and as a result the dialysis solution bicarbonate level can be reduced only by changing the concentrate bicarbonate level. With such machines the bicarbonate cannot be reduced below about 32 mM. In machines where the concentrate:product water ratio can be changed, bicarbonate levels as low as 20 mM usually can be delivered, but not lower. A low-base dialysis solution can be made using a batch system (i.e., mixing the solution from its component chemicals in a large tank). The problems of batch-mixing bicarbonate-containing dialysis solution (loss of PCO_2 and calcium and magnesium precipitation) are discussed in Chapter 4.

d. Patients with severe predialysis acidosis

(1) Dangers of excessive correction of metabolic acidosis. Excessive correction of severe metabolic acidosis (starting plasma bicarbonate level <10 mmol/L) can have adverse consequences, including paradoxical acidification of the cerebrospinal fluid and an increase in the tissue production rate of lactic acid. Initial therapy should aim for only partial correction of the plasma bicarbonate level; a target postdialysis plasma bicarbonate value of 15–20 mmol/L is generally appropriate; and for such severely acidotic patients, a dialysis solution bicarbonate level of 20–25 mM is normally used.

(2) Respiratory acidosis. The normal compensation to respiratory acidosis is an acute buffer response, which can increase the plasma bicarbonate level by 2–4 mmol/L, followed by a delayed (3–4 days) increase in renal bicarbonate generation. Because the second response is obviated in dialysis patients, respiratory acidosis will have a more pronounced effect on blood pH than in patients with normal renal function. For such patients, dialysis solution bicarbonate levels should be at the higher range, targeted to keep their pH in the normal range.

2. Dialysis solution sodium level. The dialysis solution sodium level in the sample prescription is 145 mM. This level is generally acceptable for patients who have normal or slightly reduced predialysis serum sodium concentrations. If marked predialysis hypernatremia or hyponatremia is present, the dialysis solution sodium level will have to be adjusted accordingly.

a. Hyponatremia. Hyponatremia is common in seriously ill patients requiring acute dialysis, primarily because such patients often have received large amounts of hyponatric intravenous solutions with their medications and parenteral nutrition. Hyponatremia is frequently seen accompanying severe hyperglycemia in diabetic dialysis patients. For every increase of 100 mg/dL (5.5 mmol/L) in the serum glucose concentration, there is a corresponding initial decrease of 1.3 mmol/L in the serum sodium concentration due to osmotic shift of water from the intracellular to the extracellular compartment. Because osmotic diuresis secondary to the hyperglycemia does not occur, the excess plasma water is not excreted and hyponatremia is maintained. Correction of hyperglycemia by insulin administration reverses the initial water shift and thereby corrects the hyponatremia.

(1) Predialysis serum sodium level >130 mmol/L. If the patient is to undergo an average-efficiency, 4-hour dialysis, then a postdialysis serum sodium level of 140 mmol/L can usually be achieved by setting the dialysis solution sodium concentration to 140 + (140 − predialysis serum sodium value). For example, if the predialysis serum sodium level is 130 mmol/L, to attain normonatremia the dialysis solution sodium concentration should be 150 mM (140 + [140 − 130]). Overcorrection or undercorrection of the serum sodium level results if an unusually intense or mild dialysis treatment, respectively, is administered (e.g., by virtue of altered treatment length or blood flow).

(2) Predialysis serum sodium level <130 mmol/L. When the degree of predialysis hyponatremia is moderate to severe, and especially if the hyponatremia is of long duration, it may be dangerous to achieve normonatremia quickly. Rapid correction of hyponatremia has been linked to a potentially fatal neurologic syndrome known as osmotic demyelination syndrome. The maximum safe rate of correction of the serum sodium concentration in severely hyponatremic patients is controversial. At this stage of incomplete knowledge, it seems prudent when treating patients with severe, longstanding hyponatremia to set the dialysis solution sodium level no higher than 15–20 mM above the plasma level, with the goal of correcting hyponatremia during multiple dialysis treatments performed over several days.

b. **Hypernatremia.** Hypernatremia is less common than hyponatremia in a hemodialysis setting but does occur, usually in a context of dehydration, osmotic diuresis, and failure to give sufficient electrolyte-free water. It is somewhat dangerous to attempt to correct hypernatremia by hemodialyzing against a low-sodium dialysis solution. Whenever the dialysis solution sodium level is more than 3–5 mM lower than the plasma value, three complications of dialysis occur with increased incidence:

(1) Osmotic contraction of the plasma volume occurs as water shifts from the dialyzed blood (containing less sodium than before) to the relatively hyperosmotic interstitium, causing hypotension.

(2) The propensity to develop muscle cramps is increased.

(3) Water from the dialyzed, relatively hyponatremic blood enters cells, causing cerebral edema and exacerbating the disequilibrium syndrome.

The risk of disequilibrium syndrome is the most important one; use of low-sodium dialysis solution should certainly be avoided in situations in which the predialysis SUN level is high (e.g., >100 mg/dL [36 mmol/L]). The safest approach is to first dialyze a patient with a dialysis solution sodium level close (within 2 mM) to that of plasma and then correct the hypernatremia by slow administration of slightly hyponatric fluids.

3. **Dialysis solution potassium level.** The usual dialysis solution potassium concentration for acute dialysis ranges from 2.0–4.5 mM. An important number of patients requiring acute dialysis will have a plasma potassium value in the normal or even the subnormal range, especially in patients with nonoliguric acute renal failure and in oliguric patients if food intake is poor. Hypokalemia is also a complication of total parenteral nutrition. Correction of severe acidosis during dialysis causes a shift of potassium into cells, lowering the plasma potassium level further. Hypokalemia and arrhythmia can result.

Whenever the predialysis serum potassium level is <4.0 mmol/L, the dialysis solution potassium level should be 4.0 mM or higher.

In patients with a predialysis plasma potassium level >5.5 mmol/L, a dialysis solution potassium level of 2.0 is usually appropriate in stable patients, but the dialysis solution potassium concentration should be raised to 2.5 or 3.0 in patients at risk for arrhythmia or in those receiving digitalis. If the potassium level is >7.0, some nephrologists will use a dialysis solution potassium level below 2.0 mM. However, the plasma potassium level must be monitored hourly, and there is considerable danger of precipitating arrhythmia if the plasma potassium concentration is lowered too rapidly.

    a. Potassium rebound. There is a marked rebound increase in the serum potassium level within 1–2 hours after dialysis. One should resist the temptation to treat a postdialysis hypokalemia with potassium supplements unless there are extenuating circumstances.

    b. Acute hyperkalemia. Patients with very severe hyperkalemia present with alterations on the electrocardiogram (low P waves, peaked T waves, widening of the QRS, cardiac standstill), along with weakness and lethargy. Such patients should be treated immediately with intravenous infusion of calcium chloride or calcium gluconate and/or intravenous glucose plus insulin while arrangements for emergency hemodialysis are being made. The response to intravenous sodium bicarbonate in dialysis patients is suboptimal. Another therapy is intravenous or inhaled albuterol.

    c. Subacute hyperkalemia. Initial treatment should always be a careful review of the diet for high-potassium foods. The majority of patients respond to reduced alimentary potassium intake. If this fails, then oral administration of a sodium–potassium exchange resin (e.g., sodium polystyrene sulfonate) can be tried. The resin usually is given orally with sorbitol to prevent constipation or mixed with sorbitol as an enema. However, several reports of intestinal necrosis associated with sorbitol and oral sodium polystyrene sulfonate have been published (e.g., Gardiner, 1997).

    d. Potassium removal and dialysis solution glucose. Potassium removal during dialysis using glucose-free dialysis solution may be 30% greater than potassium removal using a 200 mg/dL (11 mmol/L) glucose solution because with glucose-free dialysis solution there may be decreased intradialytic translocation of potassium into cells (Ward et al., 1987). Use of a dialysis solution containing 100 mg/dL (5.5 mmol/L) glucose may be the best option.

4. Dialysis solution calcium levels. The normal level for acute dialysis is 1.5–1.75 mM (3.0–3.5 mEq/L). There is some evidence that dialysis solution calcium levels <1.5 mM (3.0 mEq/L) predispose to hypotension during dialysis (van der Sande et al., 1998). In patients with predialysis hypocalcemia, unless a sufficiently high dialysis solution calcium level is used, correction of acidosis can result in further lowering of the ionized plasma calcium level (with possible precipitation of seizures). One study showed that QTc dispersion increased (potentially promoting arrhythmias) when a low calcium dialysis solution was used (Nappi et al., 2000). Routine use of 1.25 mM (2.5 mEq/L) calcium dialysis solution (now standard for treatment of chronic dialysis patients taking calcium-containing phosphorus binders) is conceptually inappropriate in the acute setting, where a decline in the ionized calcium concentration is usually undesirable.

   a. Dialytic treatment of acute hypercalcemia. Hemodialysis can be effective in lowering the serum calcium concentration in hypercalcemic patients. In most commercially prepared hemodialysis solutions, the calcium concentration ranges from 1.25 to 1.75 mM (2.5–3.5 mEq/L). We prefer to add at least 1.25 mM (2.5 mEq/L) calcium to the hemodialysis solution to minimize the possibility of an overly rapid decrease in the serum ionized calcium (which can cause tetany or seizures). Frequent measurement of the serum ionized calcium concentration and physical examination of the patient should be performed during dialysis to avoid these complications.

5. Dialysis solution magnesium levels. The usual dialysis solution magnesium level ranges from 0.25 to 0.75 mM (0.5–1.5 mEq/L). Magnesium is a vasodilator, and in acute dialysis one preliminary report suggests that blood pressure is better maintained when a dialysis solution magnesium level of 0.375 mM (0.75 mEq/L) was used versus dialysis solution containing 0.75 mM (1.5 mEq/L) magnesium (Roy and Danziger, 1996). In another paper (Kyriazis et al., 2004), a higher dialysis solution magnesium was found to be of benefit. So the best dialysis solution magnesium level to use for acute dialysis in terms of blood pressure maintenance remains unknown.

   a. Hypomagnesemia. Hypomagnesemia occurs in malnourished dialysis patients and in dialysis patients receiving TPN (due to shifting of magnesium into cells during anabolism). Hypomagnesemia can cause cardiac arrhythmia and can impair the release and action of parathyroid hormone. Serum magnesium values should be carefully monitored in dialysis patients during TPN, and TPN fluids should be supplemented routinely with magnesium unless the serum magnesium level is high.

   b. Hypermagnesemia. Hypermagnesemia is usually caused by accidental or covert use of magnesium-containing laxatives, enemas, or antacids. Manifestations of hypermagnesemia include hypotension, weakness, and bradyarrhythmias. Treatment is cessation of ingestion of magnesium-containing compounds. Hemodialysis also is effective in lowering the serum magnesium level.

6. Dialysis solution dextrose level. Dialysis solution for acute dialysis should always contain dextrose (100–200 mg/dL; 5.5–11 mmol/L). Septic patients, diabetics, and patients receiving beta-blockers are at risk of developing severe hypoglycemia during dialysis. Addition of dextrose to the dialysis solution reduces the risk of hypoglycemia and may also result in a lower incidence of dialysis-related side effects. The interaction between dialysis solution glucose and potassium has been discussed above.

7. Dialysis solution phosphate levels. Phosphate is normally absent from the dialysis solution, and justifiably so, as patients in renal failure typically have elevated serum phosphate values. Use of a large-surface-area dialyzer and provision of a longer dialysis session increase the amount of phosphate removed during dialysis.

    a. Hypophosphatemia. Malnourished patients and patients receiving hyperalimentation may have low or low-normal predialysis serum phosphate levels. Predialysis hypophosphatemia may also be present in patients being intensively dialyzed for any purpose. In such patients, hypophosphatemia can be aggravated by dialysis against a zero-phosphate bath. Severe hypophosphatemia can cause respiratory muscle weakness and alterations in hemoglobin oxygen affinity. This can lead to respiratory arrest during dialysis. For patients at risk, phosphate can be added to the dialysis solution. Alternatively, phosphate can be given intravenously, although this must be done carefully to avoid overcorrection and hypocalcemia.

    b. Adding phosphorus to bicarbonate-containing dialysis solutions. For prevention of hypophosphatemia the phosphorus concentration in the final dialysis solution should be about 1.3 mmol/L (4 mg/dL).

Phosphorus cannot be added to concentrate for acetate-containing dialysis solutions because of Ca-Mg-PO$_4$ solubility problems. Phosphorus can be added to the bicarbonate component of the concentrate (which does not contain calcium or magnesium).

    (1) Phosphosoda-buffered saline laxative (designed for oral consumption, manufactured by C. B. Fleet Co., Inc., Lynchburg, VA) is an inexpensive source of phosphorus. This product contains 0.48 g of sodium biphosphate (NaH$_2$PO$_4$· H$_2$O) and 0.18 g of sodium phosphate (Na$_2$HPO$_4$· 7H$_2$O) per mL, totaling 4.8 mmol/mL sodium and 4.2 mmol/mL phosphorus.

    (2) The amount added to the bicarbonate component of the concentrate depends on the dilution ratio. In most machines, the bicarbonate component is diluted 1:20. If such is the case, then addition of 60 mL of the above product to 9.5 L of bicarbonate component concentrate (the amount required to generate 190 L of final dialysis solution) results in a phosphorus level in the final dialysis solution of 1.3 mmol/L. (Additional information is given in Yu et al., 1992.) This use is not Food and Drug Administration–approved, and information about Fleet's phosphosoda content of aluminum and other trace elements is not available at this time.

    (3) An alternative method, using phosphate designed for IV injection, has been described (Hussain et al., 2005).

D. Choosing the dialysis solution flow rates. For acute dialysis, the usual dialysis solution flow rate is 500 mL per minute.

E. Dialysis solution temperature. This is usually 35–37°C. The lower range should be used in hypotension-prone patients (see Chapter 10).

F. Ultrafiltration orders. Fluid removal needs can range from 0–5 kg per dialysis session.

　　1. Guidelines for ultrafiltration orders. Some guidelines to gauge the total amount of fluid that needs to be removed are as follows:

　　　　a. Even patients who are quite edematous and in pulmonary edema rarely need removal of more than 4 L of fluid during the initial session. Remaining excess fluid is best removed during a second session the following day.

　　　　b. If the patient does not have pedal edema or anasarca, in the absence of pulmonary congestion, it is unusual to need to remove >2–3 L over the dialysis session. In fact, the fluid removal requirement may be zero in patients with little or no jugular venous distention.

　　　　c. The fluid removal plan during dialysis should take into account the 0.2 L that the patient will receive at the end of dialysis in the form of saline to rinse the dialyzer and any other fluid ingested or administered during the hemodialysis session.

　　　　d. As noted above, if it is the initial dialysis, the length of the dialysis session should be limited to 2 hours. However, if a large amount of fluid (e.g., 4.0 L) must be removed, it is impractical and dangerous to remove such an amount over a 2-hour period. In such instances, the dialysis solution flow can initially be shut off and isolated ultrafiltration (see Chapter 13) can be performed for 1–2 hours, removing 2–3 kg of fluid. Immediately thereafter, dialysis can be performed for 2 hours, removing the remainder of the desired fluid volume. (If severe electrolyte abnormalities, such as hyperkalemia, are present, dialysis may have to be performed prior to isolated ultrafiltration.)

　　　　An alternative approach is to dialyze such a patient for 4–5 hours at a reduced blood flow rate and remove the fluid at 1 L per hour. Blood flow rates lower than 200 mL per minute through adult-size dialyzers may increase the risk of dialyzer clotting. One approach that might reduce clotting risk is to use a small-surface-area dialyzer.

　　　　e. In general, it is best to remove fluid at a constant rate throughout the dialysis treatment. This is best done by a dialysis machine that incorporates an ultrafiltration controller. If the dialysis solution sodium level has been set lower than the plasma value (e.g., in the treatment of hypernatremia), the ultrafiltration rate should initially be reduced to compensate for the osmotic contraction of blood volume that will occur as the plasma sodium concentration is being lowered.

　　　　In patients with acute renal failure, it is extremely important to avoid hypotension at all times, including during dialysis. In a rat model of acute renal failure, Kelleher et al. (1987) showed that the renal autoregulatory response to systemic hypotension is greatly impaired. They found that transient episodes of hypotension caused by blood withdrawal caused further renal damage and delay of functional renal recovery.

2. **Impact of dialysis frequency on ultrafiltration needs.** It is difficult in an acute setting to limit a patient's fluid gain to <2 L per day. Often 3 L per day is absorbed in patients receiving parenteral nutrition. Use of a daily (six or seven times per week) dialysis schedule reduces the amount of fluid that needs to be removed with each dialysis, thereby lowering the risk of intradialytic hypotension and further ischemic damage to an already impaired set of kidneys.

II. Hemodialysis procedure

A. Rinsing and priming the dialyzer (single-use setting). Thorough rinsing of the dialyzer is important because it may reduce the incidence or severity of anaphylactic dialyzer reactions by virtue of removal of leachable allergens (e.g., ethylene oxide in ethylene oxide–sterilized dialyzers).

B. Obtaining vascular access

1. **Percutaneous venous cannula.** Clot or residual heparin is first aspirated from each catheter lumen. Patency of the catheter lumina is checked by irrigating with a saline-filled syringe. For acute dialysis, heparin-free dialysis is becoming more popular and is routinely used in some centers. If heparin is to be used, the heparin loading dose is administered into the venous catheter port and is flushed in with saline. After 3 minutes (to allow heparin to mix with the blood), blood flow is initiated. (Some nephrologists administer the heparin into the arterial line leading to the dialyzer and start blood flow immediately thereafter.)

2. **Arteriovenous (AV) fistula** (see also Chapter 7). Both needles are placed in the vein downstream to the anastomosis. Flow through the venous limb is distal to proximal; hence, the arterial needle is placed distally. Some tips regarding needle placement are as follows:

   a. In a patient with a poorly distended venous limb, brief application of a tourniquet may be helpful in defining its location. This tourniquet should be removed during dialysis, as its presence will encourage recirculation.

   b. A 16-gauge (or 15-gauge) needle should be used.

   c. Prepare the needle insertion sites with povidone–iodine for a full 10 minutes.

   d. Arterial needle. Insert it first, at least 3 cm away from the site of the AV anastomosis. The needle should be inserted bevel up, at a 45-degree angle, pointing either upstream or downstream.

   e. Venous needle. Insert bevel up, at a 45-degree angle, pointing downstream (usually this will be toward the heart). The insertion point should be at least 3–5 cm downstream to the arterial needle to minimize entry of dialyzed blood into the arterial needle (recirculation).

3. **AV graft.** The anatomy of the graft should be known and preferably diagrammed in the patient's chart. The guidelines for placing needles are the same as for the AV fistula. Use of a tourniquet is never necessary.

After the needles have been placed, if heparin is to be used, the heparin loading dose is given into the venous

needle and flushed in with saline. After 3 minutes, flow
through the blood circuit is initiated.
C. Initiating dialysis. The blood flow rate is initially set
at 50 mL per minute, then 100 mL per minute, until the entire blood circuit fills with blood. As the blood circuit fills, the
priming fluid in the dialyzer and tubing can either be given
to the patient or disposed of to drain. In the latter instance,
the venous blood line is kept to drain until the blood column
passes through the dialyzer and reaches the venous air trap.
In unstable patients, the priming fluid is usually administered
to the patient to help maintain the blood volume.

After the circuit is filled with blood and proper blood levels in the venous drip chamber are ensured, the blood flow
rate should be increased promptly to the desired level (usually about 350 mL per minute for acute dialysis). The pressure
levels at the inflow (arterial) monitor, between the access site
and blood pump, and of the outflow (venous) monitor, between
the dialyzer and venous air trap, are noted, and the pressure
limits are set, slightly above and below the operating pressure
to ensure that the blood pump will stop and alarms will sound
in the event of a line separation. If a line separation does occur,
the pressure in the blood line will rapidly approach zero. As
it does, it should trigger a properly set pressure limit switch.
The lower pressure limit on the venous pressure gauge should
be set within 10–20 mm Hg of the operating pressure; a
larger gap can cause failure of the alarms to trigger with line separation. Unfortunately, properly set venous pressure limits may
not stop the pump if the venous needle dislodges; most of the
flow resistance to blood return is in the needle, and the venous blood line return pressure may not change much after the
needle becomes dislodged. (See Sandroni, 2005 reference cited
in Chapter 4.I.D. for more information.) The dialysis solution
flow can now be initiated, and the transmembrane pressure
(TMP), calculated as described in Chapter 3, is set by adjusting the pressure level at the dialysis solution outflow line. In
machines with an ultrafiltration controller, the desired fluid
removal rate is simply dialed in.
D. Beeps, buzzers, and alarms. As introduced in Chapter
4, the monitors on the dialysis solution machine include the
following:

Blood circuit	Dialysis solution circuit
Inflow pressure	Conductivity
Outflow pressure	Temperature
Air detector	Hemoglobin

  1. Blood circuit (see Fig. 4-1)
    a. Inflow (prepump) pressure monitor. Usually, the
    inflow pressure (proximal to the blood pump) is −80 to −
    200 mm Hg, with −250 mm Hg being considered the usual
    limit beyond which one does not go.
      If the access is not providing sufficient blood to the
    pump, the suction proximal to the blood pump will in-
    crease, and the alarm will sound, shutting off the blood
    pump. Once the blood pump is shut off, the suction will
    be relieved; the alarm will then deactivate, and the pump

will resume operation until suction again builds up, repeating the cycle.

(1) Causes of excessive inflow suction

(a) Venous catheter access. Usually improper tip position or ball-valve thrombus or fibrin plug at the catheter tip.

(b) AV access

(i) Improperly positioned arterial needle (needle not in vessel or up against vessel wall)

(ii) Decrease in the patient's blood pressure (and hence flow through the access)

(iii) Spasm of the access vessel (AV fistula only)

(iv) Stenosis of the arterial anastomosis of an AV graft

(v) Clotting of the arterial needle or of the access

(vi) Kinking of the arterial line

(vii) Collapse of the access due to elevation of the arm (if this is suspected, sit the patient up, blood pressure permitting, until the access site is below heart level)

(viii) Use of too small a needle for the blood flow rate being used. In general, 15-gauge needles should be used whenever a blood flow rate >350 mL per minute is desired.

(2) Management

(a) Venous catheter. Check lines for kinking. Sometimes changing arm or neck position or moving the catheter slightly makes the catheter work. Reversing the catheter ports is another maneuver that sometimes works. If these initial steps do not work, subsequent steps include urokinase or tissue plasminogen activator infusion, checking catheter position in the radiology suite, or fibrin sleeve stripping as described in Chapter 6.

(b) AV access

(i) Reduce blood flow rate to the point that inflow suction decreases and the alarm stays off.

(ii) Verify that the patient's blood pressure is not unusually low. If the pressure is low, correct it by administering fluid or reducing the ultrafiltration rate.

(iii) If a patient's pressure is not unusually low, untape the arterial needle, move it up or down slightly, or rotate it.

(iv) Turn up blood flow rate to previous level. If inflow suction remains excessive, repeat (iii).

(v) If improvement is not obtained, continue dialysis for a longer time at a lower blood flow rate or place a second arterial needle (leaving the original, flushed with heparinized saline, in place until the end of dialysis), and dialyze through the second needle.

(vi) If excessive inflow suction persists despite needle change, the inflow to the vascular access may be stenosed. Occlude the access between the arterial and venous needles by transient pressure with two fingers. If the negative pressure at the prepump monitor increases markedly when the intraneedle segment is occluded, this is a sign that some of the inflow was coming from the downstream access limb and that blood flow through the upstream limb of the access is inadequate.

b. Outflow (venous) pressure monitor. Usually, the pressure here is $+50 - +250$ mm Hg, depending on needle size, blood flow rate, and hematocrit.

(1) Causes of high venous pressure

(a) The pressure may be as high as 200 mm Hg when using an AV graft because the high arterial pressure in the graft is often transmitted to the venous line.

(b) High blood flow rate when using a relatively small (16-gauge) venous needle

(c) Clotting in the venous blood line filter if one is being used. Clotting of the filter may be the first sign of inadequate heparinization and of incipient clotting of the entire dialyzer.

(d) Stenosis (or spasm) at the venous limb of the vascular access

(e) Improperly positioned venous needle or kinked venous line

(f) Clotting of the venous needle or venous limb of the vascular access

(2) Management of high venous pressure

(a) If clotting of the venous blood line filter is at fault, the dialyzer should be rinsed with saline (by opening up the saline infusion line and briefly clamping the blood inlet line proximal to the saline infusion port). If the dialyzer is not clotted (fibers appear clear on saline rinse), then a new venous line can be rapidly primed with saline and substituted for the partially clotted line, and dialysis can be resumed after adjusting the heparin dose.

(b) The presence or absence of obstruction at the venous needle or in the venous limb of the access can be assessed by shutting off the blood pump, quickly clamping the venous blood line, disconnecting the venous blood line from the venous needle, and irrigating through the venous needle with saline and noting the amount of resistance.

(c) Occlude the access between the arterial and venous needles by pressing down gently with two fingers. If stenosis downstream is causing outflow obstruction through the vascular access, the positive pressure measured at the venous monitor will increase further when the upstream access is occluded.

(3) Effects of high venous pressure on ultrafiltration rate (older machines only). When an ultrafiltration controller is not used, high pressure in the blood compartment can result in excessive ultrafiltration. This is especially a problem when a dialyzer with a high permeability to water (high K_U) is used. To limit the amount of ultrafiltration, the pressure in the dialysate compartment should be increased to approach (but not exceed) the pressure in the blood compartment (in some older machines the pressure in the dialysate compartment cannot be increased above zero). The patient's weight and blood pressure should be carefully monitored, and intravenous fluids given as necessary.

c.   Air detector. The danger of inadvertent air entry is greatest between the vascular access site and the blood pump, where the pressure is negative. Common sites of air entry include the region around the arterial needle (especially if the inflow suction is very high), via leaky tubing connections, via broken blood tubing as it passes through the roller pump, or via the saline infusion set. Air can also enter the patient if air return is improperly performed at the end of dialysis. Many air emboli occur after the air detector has been turned off because of false alarms. This practice should be avoided. Air embolism can be fatal.

d.   Blood line kinking and hemolysis. Severe hemolysis may occur due to kinking of the blood line between the pump and dialyzer. *This is a relatively common cause of dialysis machine/blood line malfunction causing patient injury.* Blood lines configured for prepump pressure will not alarm if high pressures are encountered in the segment between pump and dialyzer. Even if a blood line with a postpump pressure monitor is being used, if the kink is upstream to the monitoring line, high pressure due to the kink will not be detected.

2.   Dialysis solution circuit monitors. The dangers of dialyzing against an excessively concentrated, dilute, or hot dialysis solution have been discussed in Chapter 4.

a.   Conductivity. The most common cause of increased dialysis solution conductivity is either a kink in the tubing routing purified water to the dialysis machine, or low water pressure, resulting in insufficient water delivery to the machine. The most common cause of a reduced conductivity is an empty concentrate bottle. Otherwise, the cause is usually in the proportioning pump. The dialysis solution bypass valve is activated as soon as conductivity deviates from the specified limits, diverting the abnormal dialysis solution away from the dialyzer to the drain.

b.   Temperature. Abnormal temperature is usually caused by some malfunction in the heating circuit. Again, a properly functioning bypass valve protects the patient.

c.   Hemoglobin (blood leak). False alarms may be due to the presence of air bubbles in the dialysis solution, to dialysate bilirubin in jaundiced patients, or to a dirty sensor. The dialysate may not appear to be discolored to the naked eye. A blood leak alarm should be confirmed by testing the effluent dialysate with a test strip of the sort used for detecting hemoglobin in the urine.

If a leak is confirmed, the dialysate compartment pressure should be set to −50 mm Hg or lower to minimize entry of bacteria or their products from the dialysis solution into the blood side of the extracorporeal circuit. The blood should be returned and dialysis discontinued, although small leaks in hollow-fiber dialyzers may seal themselves off with continued dialysis.

E. Patient monitoring and complications. The patient's blood pressure should be monitored as often as necessary, but at least every 15 minutes for an acute dialysis in an unstable patient. The manifestations and treatment of hypotension and other complications during dialysis are discussed in Chapter 10.

F. Termination of dialysis. The blood in the extracorporeal circuit can be returned using either saline or air. If saline is used, the patient usually receives 100–200 mL of this fluid during the rinse-back procedure, nullifying the corresponding amount of fluid removed by ultrafiltration. However, if the patient's blood pressure is low at the end of dialysis, the saline bolus will help to raise the blood pressure quickly. When air is used, the blood pump is first shut off, and the arterial blood line is clamped close to the patient. The arterial blood line is then disconnected just distal to the clamp, opening it to air. The blood pump is restarted at a reduced rate (20–50 mL per minute), and the air is allowed to displace the blood in the dialyzer. When the air reaches the venous air trap, or when air bubbles are first seen in the venous blood line, the venous line is clamped, the blood pump shut off, and the return procedure terminated. Use of air to return the blood increases the risk of air embolism, and the termination procedure should be extremely carefully supervised when air return is employed.

G. Postdialysis evaluation

    1. Weight loss. The patient should be weighed after dialysis whenever possible, and the postdialysis weight compared with the predialysis weight. It is not uncommon for the weight loss to be greater or less than that anticipated based on the calculated ultrafiltration rate. Sources of error include the following:

        a. With an ultrafiltration controller: Use of a dialyzer with low water permeability in a patient where a high rate of ultrafiltration was needed

        b. When an ultrafiltration controller has not been used (older machines only): Overestimation of dialyzer water permeability due to coating of the membrane with protein or clot, or dialyzer lot variation; difficulty in maintaining the desired TMP during dialysis due to changes in venous resistance; use of a dialyzer that is highly permeable to water, with small errors in the TMP translating into larger errors in fluid removal

        c. Additional errors: Failure to take into account fluid administered to the patient during dialysis in the form of saline, medications, hyperalimentation, or oral fluid ingestion

    2. Postdialysis blood values. Blood can be sampled promptly after dialysis to confirm the adequacy of urea nitrogen removal and correction of acidosis. For urea nitrogen, sodium, and calcium, the postdialysis specimen can be drawn 10 seconds to 2 minutes after dialysis, although a postdialysis increase in the plasma urea level of 10%–20% usually occurs within 30 minutes due to re-equilibration of urea between various body compartments. The method of obtaining the postdialysis blood sample is quite important; if access recirculation is present, contamination of the inlet blood sample with dialyzed outlet blood can occur, yielding erroneously low plasma urea nitrogen values. Reliable methods of obtaining the postdialysis sample are described in Chapter 3 and also summarized in Chapter 9.

  a.   Urea nitrogen. The methods described in Chapters 3 and 9 can be used to estimate a predicted Kt/V and urea reduction ratio. If the plasma urea nitrogen value has fallen to a lesser extent, possible causes include partial clotting of the dialyzer, an error in setting of the blood flow rate, and recirculation at the vascular access site.

  b.   Potassium. The change in the plasma potassium level as a result of dialysis is difficult to predict because of concomitant shifting of potassium into cells due to correction of acidosis or to cellular uptake of glucose. In acute patients, it is best to sample blood for potassium at least 1 hour after the end of dialysis.

SELECTED READINGS

Casino FG, Marshall MR. Simple and accurate quantification of dialysis in acute renal failure patients during either urea non-steady state or treatment with irregular or continuous schedules *Nephrol Dial Transplant* 2004;19:1454–1466.

Emmett M, et al. Effect of three laxatives and a cation exchange resin on fecal sodium and potassium excretion. *Gastroenterology* 1995;108:752–760.

Evanson JA, et al. Measurement of the delivery of dialysis in acute renal failure. *Kidney Int* 1999;55:1501–1508.

Gardiner GW. Kayexalate (sodium polystyrene sulphonate) in sorbitol associated with intestinal necrosis in uremic patients. *Can J Gastroenterol* 1997;11:573–577.

Herrero JA, et al. Pulmonary diffusion capacity in chronic dialysis patients. *Respir Med* 2002;96:487–492.

Hussain S, et al. Phosphorus-enriched hemodialysis during pregnancy: two case reports. *Hemodial Int* 2005;9:147–150.

Kanagasundaram NS, et al. for the Project for the Improvement of the Care of Acute Renal Dysfunction (PICARD) Study Group. Prescribing an equilibrated intermittent hemodialysis dose in intensive care unit acute renal failure. *Kidney Int* 2003;64(6):2298–2310.

Kelleher SP, et al. Effect of hemorrhagic reduction in blood pressure on recovery from acute renal failure. *Kidney Int* 1987;31:725.

Ketchersid TL, Van Stone JC. Dialysate potassium. *Semin Dial* 1991;4:46.

Kyriazis J, et al. Dialysate magnesium level and blood pressure. *Kidney Int* 2004;66(3):1221–1231.

MacLeod AM, et al. Cellulose, modified cellulose and synthetic membranes in the haemodialysis of patients with end-stage renal disease. *Cochrane Database Syst Rev* 2006;1.

Madias NE, Levey AS. Metabolic alkalosis due to absorption of "nonabsorbable" antacids. *Am J Med* 1983;74:155–158.

Nappi SE, et al. QTc dispersion increases during hemodialysis with low-calcium dialysate. *Kidney Int* 2000;57:2117–2122.

Palevsky PM, et al. VA/NIH acute renal failure trial network: study design [Abstract]. *J Am Soc Nephrol* 2003;14:512A.

Roy PS, Danziger RS. Dialysate magnesium concentration predicts the occurrence of intradialytic hypotension [Abstract]. *J Am Soc Nephrol* 1996;7:1496.

Schiffl H, Lang SM, Fischer R. Daily hemodialysis and the outcome of acute renal failure. *N Engl J Med* 2002;346(5):305–310.

Subramanian S, Venkataraman R, Kellum JA. Related articles, links influence of dialysis membranes on outcomes in acute renal failure: a meta-analysis. *Kidney Int* 2002;62(5):1819–1823.

Sweet SJ, et al. Hemolytic reactions mechanically induced by kinked hemodialysis lines. *Am J Kidney Dis* 1996;27:262–266.

van der Sande FM, et al. Effect of dialysate calcium concentrations in intradialytic blood pressure course in cardiac-compromised patients. *Am J Kidney Dis* 1998;32:125–131.

Ward RA, et al. Hemodialysate composition and intradialytic metabolic, acid–base and potassium changes. *Kidney Int* 1987;32:129.

Yu AW, et al. Raising plasma phosphorus levels by phosphorus-enriched, bicarbonate-containing dialysate in hemodialysis patients. *Artif Organs* 1992;16:414.

WEB REFERENCES

Acute dialysis—recent articles and abstracts: http://www.hdcn.com/ddacut.htm

9

Chronic Hemodialysis Prescription: A Urea Kinetic Approach

John T. Daugirdas

Please review Chapter 3 at this time. Many concepts developed in Chapter 3 will be only briefly touched on here.

I.   Introduction: Urea as a marker solute. Although uremic toxicity is due to both small and large molecular weight solutes, small toxins appear to be of greater importance. For this reason (and there are practical, laboratory measurement issues as well), the amount of dialysis prescribed is based on removal of urea, which has a molecular weight of 60 daltons. Urea is only slightly toxic per se, and so its plasma level is only reflecting concentrations of other, presumably more harmful, uremic toxins.

A.   Removal versus serum level. Both removal and serum level should be monitored when checking dialysis adequacy. Monitoring of urea removal is more important. If removal is inadequate, then dialysis is inadequate, regardless of the serum level. On the other hand, a low serum urea level does not necessarily reflect adequate dialysis. Serum level depends not only on the rate of removal but also on the rate of urea generation. The generation rate is linked to the protein nitrogen appearance rate because most protein nitrogen is excreted as urea. A low serum urea level may be found in patients in whom removal is poor but in whom the generation rate is also low (e.g., due to poor protein intake).

B.   Measures of urea removal. These are the urea reduction ratio (URR), the single-pool Kt/V (spKt/V), the equilibrated Kt/V (eKt/V), and the weekly standard Kt/V (std-Kt/V) (see Chapter 3).

C.   Thrice-weekly dialysis

  1.   National Kidney Foundation's (NKF) Kidney Disease Outcome Quality Initiative (KDOQI) 2006 adequacy guidelines. In large cross-sectional studies, mortality increases when spKt/V falls below 1.2. Accordingly, the current dialysis adequacy standard in the United States, the set of KDOQI guidelines, recommends keeping spKt/V above 1.2, or the URR above 65% when three treatments per week are being given. These are the minimum values and not the target values. Dose targets are 1.4 for spKt/V and 70% for URR. Whether or not larger amounts of dialysis might be beneficial is controversial. In the National Institutes of Health (NIH)–sponsored HEMO study, in which patients were randomized to receive spKt/V levels of about 1.3 versus 1.7, patients assigned to the higher dose of dialysis did not live longer, were not hospitalized less frequently, and were not found to manifest nutritional or other benefits.

2. Effect of gender. Observational studies have suggested that women may benefit more from higher doses of dialysis than men. In the randomized analysis of the HEMO trial, the women assigned to the higher dose of dialysis survived longer than women assigned to the standard dose. Survival in the men assigned to the higher dialysis dose was slightly worse, so the overall effect of dose in the HEMO trial was negative, and it is not clear if this dose-gender interaction was real or just a statistical fluke. If women need more dialysis, the reason is unclear. As detailed in Chapter 3, an alternative method of scaling dialysis dose might be to go by body surface area (BSA) instead of by urea distribution volume (V). Because the ratio of V:BSA is about 15% different in men than in women, under current dosing guidelines, if a man and a woman have the same level of V, they will get the same dose of dialysis; however, BSA in the woman will be 15% higher, so her dialysis dose as scaled to BSA will be 15% lower. Recognizing this theoretical issue plus the trends in the HEMO trial as well as evidence from observational data sets, the 2006 KDOQI adequacy work group issued a "clinical practice recommendation" that dialysis dose targets be increased in women.

3. Smaller patients. Similarly, another 2006 KDOQI clinical practice recommendation is to give more dialysis to smaller patients. There are two main reasons: (a) small patients (those with small values for V) would get a slightly larger amount of dialysis if dose were scaled to body surface area, and (b) the KDOQI dose targets are in the form of spKt/V and not eKt/V. It is well known that postdialysis urea rebound tends to be larger in smaller patients (see Chapter 3).

4. Malnourished patients. Yet another KDOQI 2006 clinical practice recommendation was a suggestion to give more dialysis to patients whose weights are substantially below the weights of their peers, or to patients who have lost substantial weight without other explanation. The idea is that one would like to scale dialysis for patients by their weights as they were before weight loss occurred to assist them to return to their healthier, premorbid condition.

5. Dialysis session length. Urea is only one measure of dialysis adequacy. To ensure minimum removal of sodium and water as well as other, less–well-dialyzable substances, the KDOQI 2006 adequacy work group also recommended a minimum session length of 3 hours for patients dialyzed three times per week with little residual renal function. The effect of dialysis treatment time on outcome in a three times per week setting has been debated for a long time. Clearly there are outcomes benefits when session length is increased to 6–8 hours per treatment, as is done in Tassin, France, with one main benefit being better control of fluid status and blood pressure. In the DOPPS database (Saran et al., 2006), treatment times longer than 4 hours have been associated with increased survival. The KDOQI 2006 minimum treatment time recommendation of 3 hours serves as another layer of protection for small patients, in whom an adequate spKt/V might otherwise be delivered over a shorter time interval.

6. Equilibrated *Kt/V*. This generally is about 0.15–0.2 Kt/V units lower than spKt/V (see Chapter 3); hence, by inference, KDOQI minimum and target spKt/V values of 1.2 and 1.4 would translate roughly into minimum and target eKt/V values of 1.05 and 1.25. The European guidelines recommend dose targets using eKt/V and suggest a target eKt/V value of 1.4, so the European guidelines recommend a higher amount of dialysis than KDOQI 2006.

7. KDOQI guidelines regarding residual renal urea clearance (K_{ru}). The 2006 KDOQI and European Best Practice committees took different approaches in terms of incorporating residual renal clearance into dose targets for dialysis. The European approach was to include residual renal function in the target dialysis dose for virtually all patients. The KDOQI group took a more conservative "stop" and "cap" approach, being concerned that residual renal function may dwindle fairly quickly, and that its measurement may not always be reliable. The "stop" was set at a residual renal urea clearance (K_{ru}) of 2.0 mL per minute per 1.73 m^2. This is equivalent to a residual glomerular filtration rate (GFR; as estimated from the average of urea and creatinine clearance) of about 4.0. The "stop" approach means that for patients with K_{ru} <2.0, the minimum and target dialysis doses are set as if K_{ru} were equal to zero. For patients with K_{ru} values >2.0, the minimum and target spKt/V doses were reduced by about 20%–25%. The amount of dose reduction was derived from a kinetic analysis (Table 9–1).

The KDQOI work group decided to "cap" the dose reduction at this amount, and therefore patients with residual renal urea clearances of 3, 4, or 5 mL per minute per 1.73 m^2 would still be required to achieve the same spKt/V as

Table 9-1. Minimum^a sp*Kt/V* values for various frequency schedules of dialysis (achieving an estimated standard *Kt/V* = 2.0)

Schedule^b	K_r <2 mL per min per 1.73 m^2	K_r >2 mL per min per 1.73 m^2
Two times per week	Not recommended	2.0
Three times per week	1.2	0.9
Four times per week	0.8	0.6

Assumes session lengths of 3.5–4 hours.
^{a}Target spKt/V values should be about 15% higher than the minimum values shown.
^{b}Values for five and six times per week are given in Chapter 14.

a patient with 2 mL per minute K_{ru}. This was done for reasons of safety as well as simplicity. The KDOQI recommendations for minimum dialysis dose using a three times per week schedule are easy to remember: 1.2 for patients with K_{ru} <2.0 mL per minute per 1.73 m^2, and 0.9 for those patients in whom K_{ru} >2.0 can be documented. The recommended target spKt/V values were set at 15% above the minimum values, so target three times per week spKt/V values would be 1.4 and 1.15 in patients without and with the threshold amount of residual renal function, respectively.

D. Session spKt/V values for schedules other than 3x/week. The 2006 KDOQI adequacy work group also made recommendations for dialysis adequacy for patients being dialyzed other than three times per week. They issued only clinical practice "recommendations," because there are so few outcome data for such schedules. The approach taken was to choose minimum doses that would result in a standard weekly Kt/V of 2.0 with each schedule for an average-sized patient. The standard Kt/V value of 2.0 was chosen because this is the value that would be achieved with an spKt/V of 1.2 when given three times per week. The resulting minimum recommended spKt/V values are given in Table 9-1.

The same type of "stop" and "cap" approach was used to incorporate residual renal function into these other treatment schedules. When residual renal urea clearance was <2.0 mL per minute per 1.73 m^2, K_{ru} was ignored when calculating the required standard weekly Kt/V of 2.0. When residual clearance was >2.0 mL per minute per 1.73 m^2, the amount of dose reduction was capped at the level calculated for $K_{ru} = 2.0$ in an average-sized patient.

A **twice-weekly dialysis schedule** was not recommended for patients without a qualifying amount of residual urea clearance (2.0); it was allowed for patients with K_{ru} >2.0, and for them the minimum spKt/V was set at 2.0, assuming a session length of 4 hours.

For **four times per week schedules,** in patients without residual urea clearance, the minimum spKt/V per session was 0.8, and with K_{ru} >2.0, the minimum spKt/V was 0.6. Similar values were also computed for five and six times per week schedules, and these are detailed in Chapter 14.

1. Calculating standard Kt/V (std-Kt/V) in patients with and without K_{ru}. One can use Table A-7 in the Appendix to compute the standard Kt/V for any schedule based on the spKt/V. The results depend on session length, and a more detailed web calculator for this is available on hdcn.com. The minimum std-Kt/V should be at least 2.0. It may be prudent to set this minimum target a bit higher in women and small patients (Table A-6). For patients with K_{ru} >2, the minimum std-Kt/V target (excluding renal clearance) can be set to 1.7 for twice-a-week schedules, and 1.6 for 3 to 7 treatments per week schedules. This gives results that are consistent with 2006 KDOQI guidelines across all dialysis schedules.

II.   Writing the initial prescription
A.   The dialysis dose: $K \times t$.
A dialysis prescription involves only two main components: K, the dialyzer clearance, and t, the dialysis session length. K, in turn, depends on the dialyzer size used, the blood flow rate, and the dialysate flow rate, as discussed in detail in Chapter 3.

1.   **K usually ranges from 200 to 260 mL per minute.** For adult patients, given that dialyzer K_0A values, blood flow rate, and dialysate flow rate are usually within fairly narrow ranges, K (corrected for blood water and flow reduction due to prepump pressure as per Table A-1) will usually be about 230 ± 30 mL per minute. As a rule of thumb, if one uses a high-efficiency (K_0A 800) dialyzer, rapid (450 mL per minute) blood flow rate, and a dialysate flow rate of 500 mL per minute, K will be about 260 mL per minute. Increase dialysate flow rate to 800 mL per minute, and K will go up to about 290 mL per minute. One needs to connect a second dialyzer in series or in parallel to get any clinically meaningful increase in clearance beyond this level. On the other hand, in a patient with a venous catheter access, a lower blood flow of 300–350 mL per minute, and a smaller (K_0A = 600) dialyzer, with Q_D of 500 mL per minute, K will be about 200 mL per minute.

If we assume that K will be 250 mL per minute, for dialysis session lengths of 3 and 4 hours, $K \times t$ will be $250 \times 180 = 45,000$, and $250 \times 240 = 60,000$ mL, respectively, or 45 and 60 L. These represent the total volumes of plasma cleared of urea during the dialysis session.

2.   **Adjusting $K \times t$ for patient size: The Kt/V.** This is done by dividing $K \times t$ by the patient's urea distribution volume, which is approximately 55% of body weight, but which can be more accurately estimated from a nomogram (Figs. A-5 and A-6) or from an anthropometric equation (e.g., Watson equations, Table A-2).

Assume that we have a clearance of 250 mL per minute and session lengths of 3 and 4 hours. How large a patient could we dialyze and still meet KDOQI guidelines? Remember that the guidelines suggest using a prescribed ($K \times t$)/V of 1.4 to ensure that the delivered dose stays above 1.2.

For the 3-hour session, we are predicting 45 L of $K \times t$. If ($K \times t$) = 45, and ($K \times t$)/V is 1.4, then V must be $45/1.4 = 32$ L. A patient who has a V of 32 L would have a weight of about $32/0.55$ (assuming $V = 55\%$ of body weight), or 58 kg. This means that if we can reliably deliver a K of 250 mL per minute, most patients up to 58 kg could be dialyzed for 3 hours and still meet KDOQI guidelines. For the 4-hour session, we are delivering 60 L of $K \times t$, and if we want a Kt/V of 1.4 prescribed, V must be $60/1.4 = 43$ L, corresponding to a weight of about 78 kg. From this analysis, it is clear that as long as a blood flow rate of 450 mL per minute and a dialyzer with a K_0A of about 800 mL per minute are used, patients weighing about 60–80 kg can be dialyzed for 3–4 hours and usually still meet KDOQI guidelines.

B. The initial prescription for a specific patient to achieve a desired spKt/V. The general strategy is as follows:

Step 1: Estimate the patient's V.

Step 2: Multiply V by the desired Kt/V to get the required $K \times t$.

Step 3: Compute required K for a given t, or the required t for a given K.

1. Estimate V. This is best done from anthropometric equations incorporating height, weight, age, and gender as devised by Watson (Table A-2). If the patient is African American, add 2 kg to the Watson value for V_{ant}. Alternatively, one can use the Hume-Weyers equations or the nomogram derived from them (Table A-2, Figs. A-5 and A-6). Assume that, in this case, the estimated V is 40 L.

2. Compute the required $K \times t$. If the desired Kt/V is 1.5 and estimated V is 40 L, then the required $K \times t$ is 1.5 times V, or $1.5 \times 40 = 60$ L.

3. Compute the required t or K. The required $K \times t$ can be achieved with a variety of different combinations of K (which depends on K_0A, Q_B, and Q_D) and t. A variety of urea modeling programs are available that will do a computer simulation of various scenarios and come up with many possible combinations of K and t. Internet-based calculators can be accessed via the Web References cited at the end of this chapter.

C. Given a desired session length t, how to compute required K. One approach is to input a session length t and then ask: What kind of dialyzer, blood flow rate, and dialysate flow rate would I then need to achieve the required $K \times t$? Again, simple algebra is sufficient. From the previous example:

Desired sp$Kt/V = 1.5$; $V_{ant} = 40$ L, K $\times$ t $= 60$ L

First, convert $K \times t$ to milliliters to get 60,000 mL. If the desired session length is 4 hours, or 240 minutes:

Desired $t = 240$ minute

Desired $K = (K \times t)/t = 60{,}000/240 = 250$ mL per minute

Now we know that the patient needs a combination of K_0A, Q_B, and Q_D that will result in a dialyzer clearance of 250 mL per minute. How does one now choose K_0A, Q_B, and Q_D? A simple way is to select the most rapid value of Q_B that can be reliably and consistently delivered. Assume in this patient that a blood pump speed of 400 mL per minute will be possible. One can then go to the K-K_0A-Q_B nomogram (Fig. A-1a) to find the approximate dialyzer K_0A value that will be required to achieve a K of 250 mL per minute at a blood flow rate of 400 mL per minute.

To find the required dialyzer K_0A, find 400 (which is Q_B) on the horizontal axis, then go up until you find 250 (desired K) on the vertical axis. At this point, you are on a K_0A line of about 900, so a dialyzer with a K_0A value of at least 900 mL per minute will be needed. If such a high-efficiency dialyzer is not available, one will need to dialyze longer than 4 hours. One way of avoiding the need to go to a longer session length might be to use a dialysate flow rate of 800 mL per minute. Fig. A-1a is set up for $Q_D = 500$ mL per minute. One would need a separate nomogram for $Q_D = 800$, and all of the K_0A lines would be moved upward a bit. At blood flow rates over 400 mL per minute, use of an 800 mL per minute dialysate flow rate will result in an increase in clearance of about 10% over what is reported in Figure A-1a. One can do detailed computation of expected clearance using the equations in Table A-1.

D.   Given an actual blood flow rate (Q_B), how to compute required session length given two possible choices of dialyzers. A common situation occurs when the maximum blood flow rate that can be reliably delivered is known. Often one has a choice between using a larger (more expensive) or a smaller (slightly cheaper) dialyzer. Let us assume that one is constrained to using a dialysate flow rate of 500 mL per minute. What would the dialysis session length then need to be to achieve a target spKt/V of 1.5? Let us assume that we are prescribing for the same patient, with an estimated V of 40 L, which means that $K \times t$ again must be 60 L, or 60,000 mL. Assume that the projected blood flow rate is 450 mL per minute. Of the two dialyzers available, we look up their K_0A (maximum clearance) values and find they are 800 mL per minute for the big one and 600 mL per minute for the smaller one. So how long do we need to dialyze this patient with each of the two dialyzers?

Step 1: From Figure A-1a (which we can use because $Q_D = 500$ mL per minute), find the K corresponding to Q_B of 450 mL per minute (x-axis value) for each of the two dialyzers. K will be the value on the vertical axis that corresponds to the intersection of the 800- and 600-K_0A lines with a perpendicular rising from the horizontal axis (Q_B) at a point representing 450 mL per minute. We find that the K values are about 250 mL per minute for the big ($K_0A = 800$) dialyzer and 220 mL per minute for the smaller ($K_0A = 600$) dialyzer.

Step 2: We know that sp$Kt/V = 1.5$ and $V_{ant} = 40$ L, forcing $K \times t$ to be 60 L, or 60,000 mL. By algebra:

$$600\text{-}K_0A \text{ dialyzer, } K = 220: \text{t} = \frac{(K \times t)}{K} = \frac{60,000}{220} = 273 \min$$

$$800\text{-}K_0A \text{ dialyzer, } K = 250: \text{t} = \frac{(K \times t)}{K} = \frac{60,000}{250} = 240 \min$$

Our calculations, thus, suggest that we will need to dialyze for one-half hour longer using the smaller ($K_0A = 600$) dialyzer.

E.   How weight change during dialysis affects the dialysis prescription. In patients who have large weight gains, one will need a higher Kt/V to get a given URR than in patients with minimal weight gain (see Fig. A-2). For example, to get a URR of 70%, one needs to prescribe a Kt/V of only 1.3

if no fluid is removed, but that one needs a Kt/V of 1.5 if the weight loss during dialysis (UF/W) is usually about 6% (0.06 UF/W line in Fig. A-2).

III. Checking the delivered dose of dialysis. What was discussed above was how to prescribe an initial dose of dialysis. Now one must monitor the delivered dose of dialysis, on a monthly basis, according to KDOQI guidelines, by drawing a predialysis and postdialysis blood urea nitrogen (SUN). The pre- and post-SUN values are used to compute the URR, which then is combined with information concerning UF/W and with some other adjustments to compute the delivered spKt/V. One caveat: When checking the URR, one must be sure to use a properly drawn postdialysis blood specimen. In the presence of access recirculation, the postdialysis blood may be low due to admixture with dialyzer outlet blood unless a slow-blood-flow or a stop-dialysate-flow technique is used. Two KDOQI-suggested techniques for blood drawing are given in Table 9-2, and the reasons behind them are explained in detail in Chapter 3.

A. Methods of computing spKt/V from the pre- and post-SUN

1. Nomogram method. One uses Figure A-2 as described before. Assume that a URR of 0.70 or 70% is measured. Depending on whether 0%, 3%, or 6% of the body weight was removed during the dialysis treatment, the delivered spKt/V for that treatment was 1.3, 1.4, or 1.5, respectively.

2. More exact methods. The standard method recommended by the KDOQI guidelines is a urea kinetic modeling

Table 9-2. Guidelines for obtaining the postdialysis plasma urea nitrogen sample

Principles
The effect of access recirculation will reverse quickly. When blood flow is slowed to 100 mL per minute, the inflow urea concentration will rise in about 10–20 seconds (depending on the amount of dead space in the arterial line; usually about 10 mL).

Method
1. Set ultrafiltration (UF) rate to zero.
2. Slow the blood pump to 100 mL per minute for 10–20 seconds.
3. Stop the pump.
4. Draw a sample, either from the arterial blood line sampling port or from the tubing attached to the arterial needle.

Alternate Method
1. Set UF rate to zero.
2. Put dialysate into bypass.
3. Keep blood flow going at usual rate; wait 3 minutes.
4. Draw the sample.

program. The basic principles of how such programs work are described in Chapter 3. These programs are available commercially, and one is available on the Internet (see Web References). An alternative method that is approved by KDOQI is to use the following equation (Daugirdas, 1993):

$$\text{sp}Kt/V = -\ln(R - 0.008 \times t) + (4 - 3.5 \times R) \times 0.55 \times \text{UF}/V_{\text{ant}}$$

where R is $(1 - \text{URR})$, or simply post-SUN/pre-SUN, t is the session length in hours, $-\ln$ is the negative natural logarithm, UF is the weight loss in kilograms, and V_{ant} is the anthropometric urea distribution volume in liters. V_{ant} can be computed using the Watson equations as discussed above or the Hume-Weyers nomogram in Appendix A, or simply estimated as $0.55 \times$ postdialysis weight W. In the last instance, $0.55 \times \text{UF}/V$ simplifies to UF/W. (See Chapter 3 for a more complete discussion of this formula.)

IV. Adjusting the initial dialysis prescription. When patients are put on a particular dialysis prescription, even when there are no apparent changes in therapy, the delivered spKt/V derived from the measured URR often will vary considerably from month to month. The reasons are not completely clear, but laboratory error in measuring the SUN values in the samples, possible variations in how the postdialysis blood is drawn and variations in actual session length, time-averaged blood flow rate, and dialyzer clearance may all have a role. It may be useful to average the spKt/V value from three monthly treatments to determine whether or not the standard minimum spKt/V of 1.2 is being delivered.

Example: For the above patient, with a target Kt/V of 1.5, one might get URR values that, based on Figure A-2, convert to the following spKt/V values:

Month	spKt/V
Jan	1.40
Feb	1.35
Mar	1.54
Apr	1.30

The average of these values is 1.40. Although this is well within KDOQI targets for dialysis adequacy, if one wishes to achieve the original spKt/V goal of 1.5, one needs to increase the numerator $(K \times t)$ in Kt/V by a factor of 1.5/1.4, or 1.07 (7%).

One now has a choice in that either the K or the t term can be increased by 7% (or each one can be increased so that their product increases by 7%). A simple way is to increase dialysis session length (the t term in $K \times t$) by 7%. This would mean adding 17 minutes to a 4-hour treatment $(1.07 \times 240 = 257$ minutes). Another option is to try to increase the K term by going to a higher blood flow rate, going to a larger dialyzer, or increasing the dialysate flow rate. However, it is often difficult to increase the blood flow rate further or to change to a dialyzer large enough to increase K by 7%. The easiest maneuver is to increase dialysate flow rate to 800 mL per minute, which typically results in about a 10% increase in clearance as long as the blood flow rate is >400 mL per minute. So in this particular patient, appropriate changes in prescription would be to add 17 minutes to the dialysis session length or to increase the dialysate flow rate to 800 mL per minute.

A.   The concept of modeled V. In this patient, with an anthropometric estimate for V of 40 L, the Kt/V target undershot by 7%. One of the advantages of using spKt/V over the URR is that one can take the value of spKt/V computed from the URR, UF, and W, and then use it to compute a kinetically modeled patient urea distribution volume V. How is this done?

Step 1: Compute spKt/V from the URR, session length (t), and UF/W.

Step 2: Input values for K and t.

Step 3: Using algebra, if Kt/V is known, and if K and t are known, one can compute V.

In this patient, the delivered spKt/V now averages 1.40. Since the $(K \times t)$ term is 60 L, modeled V is 60/1.40 = 43 L.

If we are using a urea kinetics program, the program reasons as follows: It was told that V was 40 L, and it computed a value of K from the entered values for dialyzer K_0A, Q_B, and Q_D. It also assumes that the value of t is correct. Based on what it was told, the computer continues to assume that $K \times t$ is 60 L. But now the computer finds that $K \times t/V$ (which it computes from the monthly URR and UF/W and other adjustments) is 1.4 instead of the prescribed 1.5. The only way that the computer can maintain its sanity is to reason that the patient's urea volume is actually somewhat larger than it was told, that is, 43 L instead of 40 L. With a 43 L value for V, the computer takes $K \times t = 60$ L, divides by 43 L instead of 40 L, and finds that $K \times t/V$ is now 60/43 = 1.4, which is equal to the spKt/V being computed from the URR. The computer then reports this volume as a modeled (single pool) urea volume, or V_{sp}.

After all, our initial estimate of a 40 L V in this patient (V_{ant}) was based only on our patient's height, weight, age, and sex. We do know that V_{ant} often deviates from the modeled urea distribution volume. V_{sp} will vary from treatment to treatment, but an average modeled V is more accurate than an anthropometric estimate (V_{ant}) and is best used for any further prescription changes.

B.   Changing the prescription based on V. Above, we discussed changing the prescription based on spKt/V. spKt/V was 1.4 instead of 1.5, so the conclusion was that $K \times t$ needed to be increased by a ratio of 1.5:1.4, or by 7%. Another way is to now use the modeled V. The initial prescribed $K \times t$ was computed using a V_{ant} of 40 L. Now we know that the mean V is probably closer to 43 L. So if we write a new prescription, to keep spKt/V at 1.5, we find we need to increase $K \times t$ a ratio of 43 to 40 L, or by a factor of 1.07 or 7%. It is plain that the two methods of making prescription changes are identical. Ideally, every month one should not only compute a spKt/V, but also sequentially follow the V.

C. V is a fictitious quantity. It is important to recognize that V is a tool that is used to assess dialysis adequacy. It does not always reflect the true urea distribution volume. Computers are not very smart in the sense that they use only the information given to them. For example, if the URR and hence spKt/V suddenly decrease due to a batch of bad dialyzers, all the computer knows is that the spKt/V has suddenly fallen, but it is not told that the dialyzer clearance (K) has changed. Also, the session length (t) has not changed. How, then, can the computer explain the sudden decrease in spKt/V? All it knows is that ($K \times t$)/V is down and that ($K \times t$) is unchanged. The only way the computer can explain this scenario is to assert that the patient's urea distribution volume (V) must have increased. Actually, the true urea distribution volume changes only rarely. This point is amplified in some of the examples discussed below.

D.   An equilibrated postdialysis SUN sample should not be used to compute V. As discussed in Chapter 3, eKt/V will be about 0.2 unit lower than spKt/V. If one takes a pre-SUN sample in the usual fashion followed by a 30-minute post-SUN sample, one can use these two numbers to compute eKt/V directly (Chapter 3). However, now you have a Kt/V value that is lower by about 15%–20%. If you now ask the computer to compute a V, it will tell you that the only way this 15%–20% reduction in Kt/V could have occurred is if the patient has somehow increased in size. Accordingly, the use of a 30-minute postdialysis SUN sample will result in a 15%–20% overestimation of V.

E.   Monitoring modeled V in individual patients. After the initial 3–6 months of dialysis, one can take the average value for V and use it as a quality assurance tool. However, to do this, one needs to first understand that the value for V can vary markedly from session to session.

Example 1. In our original patient, the prescription ($K \times t$) is now increased by 7% based on the new value for V of 43 L. The spKt/V and V values (computed from the URR and from the UF/W) for the ensuing 5 months are as follows:

Month	spKt/V	V
May	1.5	43
Jun	1.43	45
Jul	1.7	38
Aug	1.8	36
Sep	1.1	58

What should be done at this point? The usual coefficient of variation for V (standard error as a percentage of the mean) is about 10%. This means that the 95% confidence limits for V extend out by 20% from either side of the mean. In the example above, a transient increase in the value for V was found in September due to an unexpectedly low value for the spKt/V. Twenty percent (2 standard deviations [SD]) of 43 is about 9, so the V of 58 L is more than 2 SD away from the previous mean value of 43 L.

Step 1: Review the dialysis run sheet for the September treatment. The low spKt/V and the apparent rise in V most probably reflect an unrecorded decrease in K or t. Was the treatment shortened? Was the blood flow rate reduced during all or part of the treatment? Did the dialysate concentrate run out? Were there problems with access during the treatment? If the answer to these questions is no, it can be assumed that the aberrant result was most likely due to measurement error.

Step 2: The prescription should not be changed at this point. One approach is to obtain one or more additional pre-/post-SUN measurements to determine if the low spKt/V value was a fluke or something about which to be concerned. In this case, as the September spKt/V measure is still 1.1, which is close to the minimum KDOQI guideline of 1.2, one could justify waiting for the next regular monthly blood draw.

Caveat: If, on the other hand, the spKt/V value for September was 0.7 instead of 1.1, and if no obvious shortening of the session length or problems with the treatment were found, a repeat post-/pre-SUN should be drawn during a subsequent dialysis. A repeat spKt/V is then calculated, and if the repeat value is still low, some major problem exists in delivering either the prescribed K or t. The most likely explanation that would cause a decrease of spKt/V of this magnitude would be the development of severe access recirculation or upstream placement of the venous dialysis needle (needle reversal).

Example 2 (sustained rise in V, associated with a fall in spKt/V). Suppose that in the same patient the following results were obtained (prescribed sp$Kt/V = 1.5$, average $V = 43$ L) for October and November:

Month	spKt/V	V
May	1.5	43
Jun	1.43	45
Jul	1.7	38
Aug	1.8	36
Sep	1.1	58
Oct	1.2	54
Nov	1.15	56

In this case, it appears in retrospect that the September increase in V was a sustained event. The mean V for September, October, and November is now 55 L, a 28% increase over the previous value of 43 L. What could account for such a phenomenon? It is highly unlikely that the patient's true V increased, and this possibility can be quickly excluded by checking the patient's serial weights.

So something happened in September that caused $K \times t$ to decrease by about 28%. This is where the sleuthing begins (Table 9-3) and the initial evaluation should start at the dialysis run sheet.

Step 1: Check the dialysis run sheet:
  a. Was the full session length delivered?

Table 9-3.   Reasons why the urea reduction ratio–based delivered single-pool Kt/V (spKt/V) may be different than prescribed Kt/V

Reasons why delivered Kt/V may be less than prescribed (in this case modeled V will be increased)

Patient's V greater than initial estimate (initial R_x only)

Actual blood flow less than that marked on the blood pump (very common when prepump negative pressure is high)

Blood flow temporarily lowered (symptoms or other reasons)

Actual dialysis session length shorter than prescribed

Dialyzer K_0A less than expected (manufacturer specifications incorrect, decreased due to reuse, etc.)

Access recirculation or inadvertent needle reversal (when postdialysis SUN is drawn properly using a slow-flow period prior to the draw)

Rebound (use of delayed postdialysis SUN to compute spKt/V and V)

Reasons why delivered Kt/V may be greater than prescribed (in this case, modeled V will be decreased)

Patient's V less than initial estimate (initial R_x only) or recent, severe weight loss

Postdialysis SUN specimen artifactually low

Access recirculation or inadvertent needle reversal, and postdialysis blood contaminated with dialyzer outlet blood (slow-flow period not used)

Specimen drawn from dialyzer outlet blood line

Session length longer than the time recorded

Recent correction of access recirculation or inadvertent needle reversal

SUN, serum urea nitrogen.

    b. Was the prescribed blood flow rate delivered for the entire treatment?

Step 2: Check for access recirculation or needle placement. Again, if explanations a and/or b above are accepted, they must together account for an almost 30% reduction in therapy from the prescribed values. A key potential culprit whenever V increases is access recirculation due either to access flow problems or to upstream venous needle placement. If there is no obvious major decrease in t or K, then the presence of access recirculation should be evaluated using methods described in Chapter 3, and flow direction in the access (to check for reversal of needle placement) should be evaluated.

Step 3: Make sure that there has been no change in how the pre- and post-SUN blood samples are being drawn. For example, a delay in drawing the pre-SUN sample will lower URR and spKt/V. If there is marked delay in drawing the post-SUN sample, some rebound will occur. Then one will be measuring eKt/V instead of spKt/V. eKt/V on average is about 0.2 unit lower than Kt/V, so this may be a potential explanation.

Step 4: See if there might be problems with delivered blood flow rate. The dialysis machine blood pump might be mis-calibrated. The roller pump may not be completely occluding the blood line, reducing stroke volume. If one is using a small (e.g., 16-gauge) needle with a high blood flow rate, there might be a high negative prepump pressure causing collapse of the blood tubing segment and reduced stroke volume leading to reduced blood flow rate during dialysis.

Step 5: Ensure that the machine is delivering the proper dialysate flow rate.

Step 6: Check dialyzer clearance and reuse procedure. These are discussed in Chapter 11. Briefly, if the fill volume of the dialyzer falls by more than 20%, the dialyzer should be discarded. Also, one may simply have a bad batch of dialyzers (unlikely in this age of quality control).

Example 3 (sustained fall in V). Suppose that in another patient we have a sustained increase in spKt/V, causing a decrease in apparent V:

Month	spKt/V	V
Jul	1.2	54
Aug	1.15	56
Sep	1.35	48
Oct	1.18	55
Nov	1.5	43
Dec	1.43	45
Jan	1.5	43
Feb	1.43	45
Mar	1.7	38
Apr	1.47	43

Here we have a patient whose V was initially about 54 L, and then, sometime around November, the V appeared to decrease suddenly by about 11–44 L. What could cause this (Table 9-3)?

Step 1: The first possibility to rule out is a true decrease in V, which can occur either because of better removal of chronic overhydration or because of loss of lean body mass due to intercurrent illness. The first step, then, is to check the patient's weight to exclude this possibility.

Step 2: Review the dialysis run sheets. Again, if the patient's weight is unchanged, the true V probably has not decreased. Rather, the $K \times t$ must have increased in some manner somewhere around October. The goal is to explain how this could have occurred. One needs to compare the run sheets before and after October. It is possible that a pre-existing problem in delivering the entire session length or prescribed blood flow rate that was active prior to October was corrected in October and the months that followed.

Step 3: Access recirculation/needle placement. If there was a change in access in October, then this might have resulted in cessation of access recirculation, or perhaps prior to October the needles were reversed, and in October the problem was found and corrected.

Step 4: Check to see if there was a systematic change in how the blood samples were collected. This is unlikely, of course. One pernicious problem occurs when a slow-flow technique is not used. Consider the following scenario: This patient always had access recirculation (or upstream venous needle placement). However, prior to October, the postdialysis sample was drawn using a proper slow-flow method. Then, in October a new technician arrived, who drew the post-samples after simply stopping the blood pump, without any antecedent slow-flow period to clear the blood line of recirculated blood. This would result in a sudden, unexplained drop in the postdialysis SUN, which would translate to an apparent, factitious rise in the URR and spKt/V, with a concomitant fall in V.

Step 5: A previously existing delivered blood flow or dialysate flow problem may have been corrected; perhaps, prior to October, a problem with blood pump calibration, occlusion, or reduced stroke volume secondary to use of a small needle were corrected, or perhaps a malfunctioning dialysate pump was fixed.

F.   Monitoring changes in V for the entire unit as a quality assurance tool. Whereas large fluctuations in V can occur in individual patients, averaging the modeled V for the entire unit is useful as a quality assurance tool and can identify several problems associated with dialysis delivery. Here a small change in V for the unit over time can often be detected. It is useful to compute both an anthropometric V (V_{ant}) and the modeled V for each patient, and to follow the ratio of the two. Unit wide, V/V_{ant} should average close to 0.90–1.0. A ratio >1 suggests that one or both components of $K \times t$ are being overestimated.

G.   Inability to reach the desired spKt/V. Patients in whom it is difficult to reach an spKt/V of at least 1.2 fall into three categories: (a) patients with poor access, resulting in either limitation of blood flow and/or access recirculation; (b) very large patients; and (c) patients with frequent hypotension, angina, or other side effects, resulting in frequent reductions in blood flow during dialysis.

   1.   Simultaneous use of two dialyzers. Although not yet supported officially by dialyzer manufacturers or machines, in such a patient, one can add a second dialyzer downstream to the first, connecting them both in series. Parallel connection of two dialyzers also has been described. In the case of a serial connection, the K_0A values of the two dialyzers are additive, giving a K_0A value for the combination of about 1,600 mL per minute. Use of a second dialyzer will result in an additional 20%–40% increase in K, allowing a proportional shortening of the treatment time. Great care must be taken to ensure that a proper rinsing procedure is used when two dialyzers are used, as it may be more difficult to remove residual processing material from the dialyzer fibers. Use of two dialyzers in series or in parallel is not specifically approved by the U.S. Food and Drug Administration, although to the best of our knowledge it is not forbidden, and the method is being done routinely in some dialysis units.

It should be pointed out that the benefits of using a second dialyzer depend on the extraction percentage in the first dialyzer. At slow blood flow rates, a large dialyzer easily removes 90% of urea. A second dialyzer will then remove 90% of what is left, but the overall increase is only 9%. At more rapid blood flow rates, the extraction ratio (see Chapter 3) is only 60%. The second dialyzer then removes 60% of the remaining 40%, or an additional 24%, and the increase in clearance is 84/60, or 1.4, or 40%. Therefore, for patients in whom maximum achievable blood flow rate is severely curtailed due to access problems, the use of a second dialyzer to increase clearance is not very effective.

2. Therapy four times per week. Four sessions per week schedules are becoming increasingly popular for treating larger patients as well as patients with hypertension and problems with removing excess fluid. The 2006 version of the KDOQI clinical practice recommendations suggest that with such schedules, when residual renal urea clearance is below 2.0 mL per minute per 1.73 m^2, the minimum spKt/V value can be reduced from 1.2 to about 0.8 (Table 9-1).

3. Patients with intradialytic symptoms. There is concern among some practitioners that use of a high blood flow rate might result in increased intradialytic symptoms. Many dialysis technicians will reduce the blood flow rate at the first occurrence of cramps, hypotension, angina, or other symptoms. Reduction of blood flow rate is not logical in a setting where bicarbonate dialysate is being used and where the ultrafiltration rate is being volumetrically controlled and therefore is independent of the blood flow rate. There is no documented proof that reduction of blood flow rate (assuming bicarbonate dialysis and volumetric ultrafiltration control) has any benefit. Because reduction of the blood flow rate can result in underdialysis, it should be avoided as much as possible. In such patients, symptoms are usually due to an excessively high ultrafiltration rate. The dialysis session length should be increased to the maximum extent possible, which will also help to ensure that adequate dialysis is taking place. When possible, conversion to a four sessions per week schedule should be considered for such patients.

H. Problems associated with a high blood flow rate
1. Need for special needles/blood tubing sets. Sixteen-gauge needles are adequate for blood flow rates of up to 350 mL per minute. With higher blood flow rates, one should use 15-gauge needles or, even better, 14-gauge needles with ultrathin walls. In addition, short blood tubing lines should be used. Many physicians prefer to use smaller needles in fistulas, either indefinitely or during the early maturation phase only.

    a. High negative prepump pressures. When high blood flow rates are used, especially when using a small arterial needle, a high negative pressure can develop in the blood tubing segment between the arterial needle and the roller pump. When this prepump pressure exceeds − 200 mm Hg, the tubing walls begin to flatten, causing the pump to deliver less blood flow than is indicated on the dial. The falloff in flow is usually about 5% at −200 mm Hg prepump pressure, and 12% at −300 mm Hg pressure, although it may be higher with certain tubing sets. −250 mm Hg is the usual limit for prepump vacuum set by dialysis unit policy.

Manufacturing companies have recently addressed the problem of blood line tubing segments flattening out under negative pressure, and use of such improved blood lines largely eliminates the problem of reduced pressure at higher prepump negative pressures. Whether hemolysis actually is a problem when prepump negative pressures are lower than −250 mm Hg has been questioned (Twardowski, 2000), so this is not an absolute limit below which safe dialysis cannot be performed.

2.   High venous pressure. The pressure in the venous blood lines is a function of blood flow rate. Normally, a high venous pressure will not reduce the ability of the blood pump to deliver the calibrated blood flow. In older machines without volumetric ultrafiltration control, the high pressure in the blood compartment of the dialyzer will drive a large amount of "spontaneous ultrafiltration," and this can result in patient dehydration.

3.   Increased access recirculation. Many peripheral accesses deliver extracorporeal blood flow rates of 600 mL per minute or greater. However, in a patient with poor vessels or a partially stenosed access, it may be difficult to obtain an extracorporeal blood flow rate of even 300 mL per minute. Some fistulas work for an extended period of time with low fistula flow rates. As the blood pump demands more flow than the access can deliver, a large amount of access recirculation may occur, reducing the expected amount of dialysis.

V.   Computing and monitoring the normalized protein nitrogen appearance rate (nPNA). This is described in Chapters 3 and 28.

VI.   Dialyzer

A.   Membrane material. Issues pertaining to biocompatibility and acute dialyzer reactions are discussed in Chapters 4, 8, and 10.

B.   Should a high-flux dialyzer be used? This question was partially answered by the NIH HEMO trial. Although randomization to high-flux membranes was associated with about a 10% increased survival, this did not attain statistical significance. Significant benefits in survival were measured in the predefined subgroup of patients who were on dialysis longer than 3.7 years (the median level for the HEMO patients). Also, cardiovascular mortality appeared to be reduced in all patients assigned to high-flux dialysis. These data, plus a number of observational studies that also suggested about a 10% improvement in mortality with high-flux dialysis and a number of studies showing improvement of β_2-microglobulin–associated amyloid disease with high-flux dialysis, led the 2006 KDOQI adequacy work group to recommend routine use of high-flux membranes whenever proper dialysate and water treatment systems are available. This was left as a strong clinical practice recommendation and not as a guideline, given that high-level evidence for an outcomes benefit was not quite attained in the HEMO trial. The European Best Practice guidelines also recommend use of high-flux membranes where proper water treatment is available.

VII.   Fluid removal orders

A.   Concept of "dry weight." The so-called dry weight is the postdialysis weight at which all or most excess body fluid has been removed. If the dry weight is set too high, the patient will remain in a fluid-overloaded state at the end of the dialysis session. Fluid ingestion during the interdialysis interval might then result in edema or pulmonary congestion. If the dry weight is set too low, the patient may suffer frequent hypotensive episodes during the latter part of the dialysis session. Patients who have been ultrafiltered to below their dry weight often experience malaise, a washed-out feeling, cramps, and dizziness after dialysis.

In practice, the dry weight of each patient must be determined on a trial-and-error basis. The dry weight often changes periodically (e.g., due to seasonal variations in the amount of body fat) and therefore should be re-evaluated at least every 2 weeks. A progressive decrease in the dry weight can be a clue to an underlying nutritional disturbance or disease process.

When setting the ultrafiltration rate, allow for the 0.2 L that the patient will receive at the end of dialysis during the blood return procedure. Also, compensate for any fluid ingestion or parenteral fluid administration during the treatment session.

1.   Frequent resetting of the dry weight. A common error in dialysis units is failure to re-evaluate the dry weight often enough. If a patient then loses flesh weight, the previously set dry weight become too high, and if maintained, can result in overhydration and hospitalization for fluid overload.

B.   Fluid removal rate. Usually fluid is removed at a constant rate during dialysis. There is some interest in using a nonconstant fluid removal rate during a dialysis session. In one approach, the fluid removal rate is increased during the initial 1–2 hours of dialysis and reduced toward the end of dialysis. The dialysis solution sodium level also may be increased during the initial phase of dialysis to help maintain the blood volume osmotically. The benefits of this approach remain controversial.

VIII.   Dialysis solutions (Table 9-4)

A.   Flow rate. The standard dialysis solution flow rate is 500 mL per minute. When the blood flow rate is high (e.g., >400 mL per minute) and when a high-K_0A dialyzer is used, increasing the dialysis solution flow rate to 800 mL per minute will increase dialyzer clearance (K) by about 10%.

Table 9-4. Dialysis solution orders

Flow rate:
  500 mL per minute
Base:
  Bicarbonate (35 mM)/plus acetate (4 mM)
Electrolytes and dextrose
Potassium = 2.0 mM (3.0 mM for patients taking digitalis, or
  patients with a low-normal potassium predialysis)
Sodium = 135–145 mM
Dextrose = 200 mg/dL (11 mmol/L)
Calcium = 1.25–1.75 mM (2.5–3.5 mEq/L; depends on type of
  phosphate binder used)
Magnesium = 0.25–0.50 mM (0.5–1.0 mEq/L)

B. **Composition**
    1. **Bicarbonate concentration.** Bicarbonate dialysis so-
    lution is the fluid of choice, and use of acetate-based
    dialysate is now considered obsolete in most countries.
        The concentration of base should be adjusted to achieve
    a predialysis plasma bicarbonate concentration of 20–23
    mmol/L. There has been some interest in increasing dialysis
    solution bicarbonate level, or giving supplementary oral bi-
    carbonate to increase the predialysis HCO_3 level. A definite
    clinical benefit of raising predialysis HCO_3 beyond 20–23
    has not been shown. Metabolic alkalosis may result post-
    dialysis in such patients, with theoretical increased risk of
    calcium–phosphorus precipitation, and of cardiac arrhyth-
    mia should alkalemia due to sudden hyperventilation su-
    pervene.
    2. **Potassium.** The usual dialysis solution potassium level
    is 2.0 mM unless the patient's usual predialysis plasma
    potassium concentration is <4.5 or unless the patient is re-
    ceiving digitalis. In the latter two instances, the dialysis so-
    lution potassium level should usually be 3.0 mM. Should the
    interdialytic serum potassium levels be high because of the
    use of this 3 mM dialysis solution, chronic administration of
    sodium polystyrene sulfonate resin may be required. Mal-
    nourished patients may have low predialysis serum potas-
    sium levels, and in these patients the dialysate potassium
    level can and should be increased to avoid hypokalemia. Use
    of 1.0 mM potassium dialysate on a chronic basis to control
    hyperkalemia has been associated with increased incidence
    of cardiac arrest (Lafrance et al., 2006).
    3. **Sodium.** The usual dialysis solution sodium level is be-
    tween 135 and 145 mM. Levels above 140 mM are associ-
    ated with increased thirst and weight gain between dialyses,
    although the extra fluid often can be removed during dialy-
    sis with fewer symptoms. The blood pressure may increase.
    Dialysis solution sodium levels lower than 135 mM predis-
    pose to hypotension and cramps.
        One study suggests that patients may have individual
    "set points" for sodium (Keen et al., 1997). In patients with
    a low sodium set point, a lower dialysis sodium level can

logically be used, which should minimize postdialysis thirst and weight gain.

4. Dextrose. It is routine to add dextrose (200 mg/dL or 11 mmol/L) to dialysis solutions for all patients. The presence of dextrose may reduce the incidence of hypoglycemia during dialysis.

5. Calcium. Dialysis solution calcium levels normally range from 1.25 to 1.75 mM (2.5–3.5 mEq/L). The usual level in patients taking calcium-containing phosphorus binders is 1.25 mM (2.5 mEq/L), but the level may have to be adjusted upward or downward depending on clinical response and parathyroid hormone status. In patients taking the newer resin-based phosphate binders, which do not contain calcium, the dialysis solution calcium level may need to be increased to avoid negative calcium balance.

6. Magnesium. The usual dialysis solution magnesium level is 0.25–0.5 mM (0.5–1.0 mEq/L).

C. Temperature. The dialysate temperature should be set as low as possible without engendering patient discomfort, generally in the range of 34.5–36.5°C.

IX. Anticoagulation orders. See Chapter 12.

X. Standing orders for complications. Complications are discussed in depth in Chapter 10. Frequently occurring complications, such as hypotension, cramps, restlessness, nausea, vomiting, itching, and chest pain, can be managed with a set of standing orders. However, symptoms during dialysis may be the result of a more serious disease process that can require immediate diagnosis and specific treatment.

XI. Patient monitoring

A. Prior to and during the treatment session

1. Prior to dialysis

a. Weight. The predialysis weight should be compared with the patient's last postdialysis weight and with the target dry weight to obtain some idea of interdialysis weight gain. A large interdialysis weight gain, especially when coupled with symptoms of orthopnea or dyspnea, should prompt a complete cardiovascular examination and reassessment of the target dry weight (it may be too high). Patients should strive to keep their interdialysis weight gain below 1.0 kg per day. They also need to be counseled about limiting sodium rather than fluid intake, as the water intake generally follows that of salt. Excessive thirst may be due to a high dialysis solution sodium level or to high plasma renin activity, and may be mitigated by use of an angiotensin-converting enzyme inhibitor, although evidence for this is controversial. Complaints of a washed-out feeling or of persistent muscle cramps after dialysis suggest that the target dry weight is too low.

b. Blood pressure. Predialysis hypertension is often volume related. However, in many patients, hypertension appears to be renin mediated or due to some other unknown factor(s). In these patients, blood pressure can increase during dialysis despite fluid removal. In one report, even volume-resistant hypertensive patients benefited from further fluid removal (Fishbane et al., 1996).

Patients with hypertension are routinely counseled to withhold their blood pressure medication on the day of dialysis to limit the incidence of dialysis hypotension. This is not absolutely necessary, especially for patients who will be dialyzed in the afternoon. Management of high blood pressure is described in Chapter 31, but basically focuses on sodium restriction, lengthening the dialysis session, and, if available, moving to a more frequent dialysis schedule.

    c.   Temperature. The patient's temperature should be measured. The presence of a fever prior to dialysis is a serious finding and should be investigated diligently. The manifestations of infection in a dialysis patient may be subtle. On the other hand, a rise in body temperature of about $0.5°C$ during dialysis is normal and not necessarily a sign of infection or pyrogen reaction.

    d.   Access site. Whether or not fever is present, the vascular access site should always be examined for signs of infection before each dialysis.

  2.   During the dialysis session. Blood pressure and pulse rate are usually measured every 30–60 minutes. Any complaints of dizziness or of a washed-out feeling are suggestive of hypotension and should prompt immediate measurement of the blood pressure. Symptoms of hypotension may be quite subtle, and patients sometimes remain asymptomatic until the blood pressure has fallen to dangerously low levels.

B.   Laboratory tests (predialysis values)

  1.   Serum urea nitrogen. This should be measured monthly as part of the URR.

The predialysis urea nitrogen can be measured prior to the first treatment of the week or prior to the midweek session. A urea kinetic modeling program can then be used, along with determination of residual renal urea clearance, to compute spKt/V, V, and nPNA. The clinical significance of a low or high serum UN is difficult to interpret, as this depends on both spKT/V and urea nitrogen generation rate. Very low or decreasing serum UN values are associated with poor outcome, as they often reflect a poor nutritional state. It is best to compute the nPNA from a modeling program to verify that a low SUN is due to a low nPNA.

  2.   Serum albumin. The predialysis serum albumin level should be measured every 3 months. The serum albumin concentration is an important indicator of nutritional state. A low serum albumin level is a very strong predictor of subsequent illness or death in dialysis patients. The increased mortality risk begins at serum albumin levels <4.0 g/dL (40 g/L). Patients with serum albumin levels <3.0 g/dL (30 g/L) are at high risk of morbid events, and every effort should be made to find the cause of the low albumin value and correct it. The optimum serum albumin level is >4.0 g/dL (40 g/L), but setting a single target is difficult because the range of normal values depends on the assay method used. Specifically, two methods commonly used, involving bromcresol purple or bromcresol green, give levels that differ by about 0.4 g/dL (4.0 g/L).

3. Serum creatinine. The predialysis serum creatinine level is measured monthly. The usual mean value in hemodialysis patients is 12–15 mg/dL (1,060—1,330 mcmol/L), with a common range of 8–20 mg/dL (700–1,770 mcmol/L). Paradoxically, in dialysis patients, high serum creatinine levels are associated with a low risk of mortality, probably because the serum creatinine value is an indicator of muscle mass and nutritional status.

The serum creatinine and urea nitrogen levels should be examined in tandem. If parallel changes in both occur, then alteration in the dialysis prescription or degree of residual renal function should be suspected. If the serum creatinine level remains constant but a marked change occurs in the serum urea nitrogen value, the change in the latter is most likely due to altered dietary protein intake or altered catabolic rate of endogenous body proteins.

4. Serum total cholesterol. The serum total cholesterol level is an indicator of nutritional status. A predialysis value of 200–250 mg/dL (5.2–6.5 mmol/L) is associated with the lowest mortality risk in dialysis patients. Low serum total cholesterol values, especially <150 mg/dL (3.9 mmol/L), are associated with an elevated mortality risk in dialysis patients, probably because they reflect poor nutritional status.

5. Serum potassium. Dialysis patients with a predialysis serum potassium level of 5.0–5.5 mmol/L have the lowest mortality risk. The mortality risk increases greatly for values over 6.5 and under 4.0 mmol/L.

6. Serum phosphorus. Measure monthly. The predialysis value associated with the lowest mortality is below 5.5 mg/dL (1.8 mmol/L). Mortality rates increase sharply for values over 9.0 mg/dL (2.9 mmol/L) and under 3.0 mg/dL (1.0 mmol/L) . Current KDOQI targets are 3.5–5.5 mg/dL (1.1–1.8 mmol/L). Serum phosphorus values tend to be substantially higher on Monday/Tuesday, that is, after the two-day interdialytic interval.

7. Serum calcium. Measure monthly (more often when changing the dose of vitamin D). The lowest mortality is associated with values of 9–12 mg/dL (2.25–3.0 mmol/L). Mortality rates increase markedly at values over 12 mg/dL (3.0 mmol/L) and under 7 mg/dL (1.75 mmol/L). The target value should be a calcium within the normal range. Targeting the upper range of normal serum calcium is no longer recommended, for fear of precipitating vascular calcification.

8. Serum alkaline phosphatase. Measure every 3 months. High values are a sign of hyperparathyroidism or liver disease. Lowest mortality is for values <100 units/L (normal being 30–115 units/L). Mortality doubles for values >150 units/L.

9. Serum bicarbonate. Measure monthly. Lowest mortality is for values between 20 and 22.5 mmol/L. Mortality increases for both lower and higher values. Marked increases in mortality are noted when the predialysis value is under 15 mmol/L. Predialysis acidosis can be corrected by administration of alkali between dialyses.

10. Hemoglobin. The optimal predialysis hemoglobin level is not known but is at least 110 g/L, according to KDOQI guidelines, and 11–13 g/dL is the current target range. Spontaneously high hemoglobin levels (without erythropoietin therapy) may be a sign of polycystic kidney disease, acquired renal cystic disease, hydronephrosis, or renal carcinoma.

Serum ferritin levels, iron levels, and iron binding capacity, as well as erythrocyte indexes, should be checked every 3 months (see Chapter 32).

11. Serum aminotransferase values are usually checked monthly. High values may unmask silent liver disease, especially hepatitis or hemosiderosis. The blood should be screened for the presence of hepatitis B surface antigen and for hepatitis C (see Chapter 33).

12. Serum parathyroid hormone levels and serum aluminum concentrations should be measured as needed, whenever the possibility of hyperparathyroidism or aluminum intoxication is suspected.

SELECTED READINGS

Cheung AK, et al. Effects of high-flux hemodialysis on clinical outcomes: results of the HEMO study. *J Am Soc Nephrol* 2003;14(12): 3251–3263.

Fishbane S, et al. Role volume overload in dialysis-refractory hypertension. *Am J Kidney Dis* 1996;28:257–261.

Daugirdas JT. Second generation logarithmic estimates of single-pool variable volume *Kt/V*: an analysis of error. *J Am Soc Nephrol* 1993;4:1205–1213.

Daugirdas JT, et al. Relationship between apparent (single-pool) and true (double-pool) urea distribution volume. *Kidney Int* 1999;56(5):1928–1933.

Depner T, et al. Dialysis dose and the effect of gender and body size on outcome in the HEMO Study. *Kidney Int* 2004;65(4): 1386–1394.

Eknoyan G, et al. Effect of dialysis dose and membrane flux in maintenance hemodialysis. *N Engl J Med* 2002;347(25):2010–2019.

Hanson JA, et al. Prescription of twice-weekly hemodialysis in the USA. *Am J Nephrol* 1999;19:625–633.

Karnik JA, et al. Cardiac arrest and sudden death in dialysis units. *Kidney Int* 2001;60(1):350–357.

KDOQI Adequacy Guidelines, 2006 update. *Am J Kidney Dis* 2006; in press.

Keen M, et al. Plasma sodium (CpNa) "set point": relationship to interdialytic weight gain (IWG) and mean arterial pressure (MAP) in hemodialysis patients (HDP) [Abstract]. *J Am Soc Nephrol* 1997;8:241A.

Lafrance J, et al. Predictors and outcome of cardiopulmonary resuscitation (CPR) calls in a large haemodialysis unit over a seven-year period. *Nephrol Dial Transplant* 2006;21:1006–1012.

Saran R, et al. Longer treatment time and slower ultrafiltration in hemodialysis: associations with reduced mortality in the DOPPS. *Kidney Int* 2006;69:1222–1228.

Twardowski ZJ. Safety of high venous and arterial line pressures during hemodialysis. *Semin Dial* 2000;13(5):336–337.

WEB REFERENCES

HDCN adequacy channel: http://www.hdcn.com/ch/adeq/

NKF KDOQI guidelines for hemodialysis adequacy: http://www.kidney.org

NKF KDOQI guidelines for peritoneal dialysis adequacy: http://www.kidney.org

Urea kinetics calculators: http://www.hdcn.com/calc.htm

Complications During Hemodialysis

Richard A. Sherman, John T. Daugirdas, and Todd S. Ing

I. Common complications. The most common complications during hemodialysis are, in descending order of frequency, hypotension (20%–30% of dialyses), cramps (5%–20%), nausea and vomiting (5%–15%), headache (5%), chest pain (2%–5%), back pain (2%–5%), itching (5%), and fever and chills (<1%).

A. Hypotension (Table 10-1)

  1. Common causes

    a. Hypotension related to excessive or rapid decreases in blood volume. Hypotension during dialysis results primarily from a reduction in blood volume from fluid removal (ultrafiltration) during treatment that is accompanied by insufficient hemodynamic compensation. Maintenance of blood volume during dialysis depends on refilling of the blood compartment from surrounding tissue spaces, a process that varies in rapidity among patients. A decrease in blood volume results in decreased cardiac filling, which, in turn, causes reduced cardiac output and, ultimately, hypotension.

      (1) Therapeutic implications

        (a) Use an ultrafiltration controller. Ideally, the rate of fluid removal should be closely controlled throughout the dialysis session. When an ultrafiltration control device is not used, the fluid removal rate as well as the total volume of fluid removed can fluctuate considerably as the pressure across the dialyzer membrane varies. Transiently rapid rates of fluid removal can then occur, causing acute contraction of the blood volume and hypotension. Dialysis machines now routinely have an ultrafiltration control device. If such a machine is not available, then one should use a dialyzer membrane with a relatively low permeability to water, so that the unavoidable fluctuations in the transmembrane pressure during dialysis will translate to small changes in the fluid removal rate.

        (b) Avoid large interdialytic weight gain or short treatment. To avoid the necessity for rapid ultrafiltration rates, patients should be counseled to limit their salt intake and hence their interdialytic weight gain (IDWG; e.g., to <1 kg per day). An emphasis on salt restriction is far more effective in decreasing IDWG than an emphasis on fluid restriction (Tomson, 2001). An increase in treatment

Table 10-1.   Causes of intradialytic hypotension

1. **Volume related**
   a. Large weight gain (high ultrafiltration rate)
   b. Short dialysis (high ultrafiltration rate)
   c. Low target ("dry") weight
   d. Nonvolumetric dialysis (inaccurate or erratic ultrafiltration)
   e. Low dialysis solution Na (intracellular fluid shift)
2. **Inadequate vasoconstriction**
   a. High dialysis solution temperature
   b. Autonomic neuropathy
   c. Antihypertensive medications
   d. Eating during treatment
   e. Anemia
   f. Acetate buffer
3. **Cardiac factors**
   a. Diastolic dysfunction
   b. Arrhythmia (atrial fibrillation)
   c. Ischemia
4. **Uncommon causes**
   a. Pericardial tamponade
   b. Myocardial infarction
   c. Occult hemorrhage
   d. Septicemia
   e. Dialyzer reaction
   f. Hemolysis
   g. Air embolism

time is also an effective way of decreasing ultrafiltration rate (same weight loss, longer time) and the frequency of intradialytic hypotension (IDH). Using a four times per week schedule, configured so as to avoid a two-day interdialytic interval, is also quite effective. The new KDOQI 2006 adequacy guidelines recommend that treatment time not be reduced below 3 hours (for thrice-weekly dialysis) in patients with little or no residual urine output regardless of how high their Kt/V may be.

(c)   Choose a patient's "dry weight" carefully. A patient's true dry weight can be reliably found only with testing that is not routinely available in the clinic (e.g., bioimpedance devices, inferior vena cava diameter ultrasonography, serum atrial natriuretic factor levels). Instead, the decision is made on a clinical basis taking into account a patient's blood pressure, presence of edema, and tolerance of ultrafiltration to the chosen weight. As the patient's dry weight is approached, the rate at which the blood compartment refills from surrounding tissue spaces is diminished. As a result, patients with large IDWG and ultrafiltration rate requirements may have diffi-culty reaching their true dry weight because the re-fill rate is too slow at the end of treatment to prevent transient hypovolemia and IDH. Such patients are commonly maintained at weights higher than their optimal euvolemic target weights. Attempts to ultra-filter these patients to their true dry weight or other patients to an incorrectly chosen dry weight (too low) will result in IDH and, often, postdialysis hypoten-sion with cramps, dizziness, malaise, and a washed-out feeling.

When intradialytic hematocrit monitors are available, they may be helpful in recognizing a dry weight that is (or has become, due to tissue weight loss) too high. A "flat-line" hematocrit response (e.g., lack of an increase during dialysis) despite fluid removal indicates rapid blood compartment refilling and suggests fluid overload. Identification of a specific level of hemoconcentration ("crash-crit") using these devices has been suggested as useful in avoiding IDH. Investigations in this area are ongo-ing. However, a recent randomized trial in which "flat-line" hematocrit responses were responded to paradoxically resulted in an increased, rather than a decreased, hospitalization rate (Reddan et al., 2005).

(d) Use an appropriate dialysis solution sodium level. When the dialysis solution sodium level is less than that of plasma, the blood return-ing from the dialyzer is hypotonic with respect to the fluid in the surrounding tissue spaces. To main-tain osmotic equilibrium, water leaves the blood com-partment, causing an acute reduction in the blood volume. This effect is most pronounced during the early part of dialysis, when the plasma sodium level is falling most abruptly. The higher the dialysis solu-tion sodium, the smaller will be the reduction in blood volume for any given amount of ultrafiltration. Un-fortunately, higher dialysis solution sodium levels in-crease IDWG, blood pressure, and postdialysis thirst.

So-called "sodium modeling" (or sodium gradient dialysis) is widely practiced. It generally involves use of a high dialysis solution sodium early in treatment (145–155 mM) with a progressive fall (linear, step, or logarithmic) to lower levels (135–140 mM) at the end of treatment. The objective is to obtain the benefits of high-sodium dialysis solution without its compli-cations. Review of the large literature on this subject shows that sodium modeling is of uncertain benefit (Stiller et al., 2001). It should also be noted that a patient's postdialysis serum sodium is a function of a treatment's time-averaged concentration of dialy-sis solution sodium, not the terminal level of dialysis solution sodium.

Instead of a "one size fits all" level of dialysis so-lution sodium, using a fixed level set close to the

patient's predialysis serum value—an **"individualized" dialysis solution sodium**—may reduce
symptoms as well as intradialytic thirst according
to a preliminary report (Santos et al., 2003).

(e) **Blood-volume control devices with feedback loop.** For a number of years now, software
has been allowing improved feedback control of ultrafiltration rate based on monitoring of blood volume during dialysis. Some randomized trials suggest
that such feedback devices can reduce the incidence
of dialysis-induced hypotension while avoiding a positive sodium balance (Santoro et al., 2002).

b. **Hypotension related to lack of vasoconstriction.** The hypovolemic state is one in which cardiac output is limited by cardiac filling; a reduction in peripheral
vascular resistance or cardiac filling in this setting can
precipitate hypotension. Under conditions of decreased
cardiac filling, increases in heart rate have little effect
on cardiac output. With more than 80% of the total blood
volume in veins, changes in venous capacity can have important effects on a patient's effective circulating blood
volume and cardiac output. Decreased arteriolar resistance increases transmission of arterial pressure to veins.
This causes passive stretching and distension, resulting
in increased sequestration of blood. While not important
in euvolemic patients given a vasodilator (because cardiac filling is more than adequate), with hypovolemia this
mechanism can result in hypotension (Daugirdas, 1991).
The degree of arteriolar constriction, or total peripheral
resistance (TPR), is also important because TPR will
determine the blood pressure for any level of cardiac
output.

(1) **Therapeutic implications**

(a) **Lower dialysis solution temperature.** Ideally, the dialysis solution temperature should be one
that maintains a patient's arterial blood temperature
at its initial level throughout dialysis. When the dialysis solution temperature is higher than this ideal
level, cutaneous vasodilation occurs to allow heat to
be dissipated. This vasodilation reduces vascular resistance and predisposes the patient to hypotension.
Blood temperature modules are available for dialysis
machines, which can provide patients with a euthermic treatment. Without such a device the choice
of dialysis solution temperature is problematic,
with even small (1.1°C) differences in temperature
having a notable impact on blood pressure (Sherman
et al., 1984). The widely used dialysis solution
temperature of 37°C is almost always in excess of
euthermic values. Levels of 35.5–36.0°C are better
initial choices with adjustment made up or down depending on tolerance (chills) and effectiveness (blood
pressure). The hemodynamic benefits of cool dialysis
solution are associated with a significant incidence of
patient discomfort only because of an inability to

deliver dialysate of the optimal (usually unknown) temperature; euthermic dialysis is not associated with shivering and only rarely with chills (Maggiore et al., 2002).

(b) Avoid intradialytic food ingestion in hypotension-prone patients. Eating during hemodialysis can precipitate or accentuate a fall in blood pressure (Sherman et al., 1988; Strong et al., 2001). The effect is probably a result of dilation of resistance vessels in the splanchnic bed, which reduces TPR and increases splanchnic venous capacity (Barakat et al., 1993). The "food effect" on blood pressure probably lasts at least 2 hours. Patients who are prone to hypotension during dialysis should avoid eating just before or during a dialysis session.

(c) Minimize tissue ischemia during dialysis. During any type of hypotensive stress, the resulting tissue ischemia causes release of adenosine. Adenosine blocks release of norepinephrine from sympathetic nerve terminals and also has intrinsic vasodilator properties. Severe hypotension can therefore amplify itself: Hypotension → ischemia→ adenosine release → impaired norepinephrine release → vasodilation → hypotension. This may be one reason for the clinical observation that patients with low hematocrit levels (e.g., <20%–25%) are very susceptible to dialysis hypotension (Sherman et al., 1986).

Since the advent of erythropoietin, few patients have levels of anemia severe enough to cause hypotension. However, in an acute dialysis setting, severely anemic patients with refractory IDH are seen; transfusion sufficient to raise the predialysis hemoglobin level to 11–12 g/dL may be beneficial.

(2) Midodrine in refractory cases. Midodrine, an orally acting α-adrenergic agonist, has been shown to limit intradialytic hypotension in several studies. A dose of 10 mg orally one-half to 2 hours before a dialysis session is typical, though use of as much as 40 mg has been reported. Supine hypertension is the major dose-limiting factor. Active cardiac ischemia (but not simply coronary artery disease) is a contraindication. Concomitant use of α-adrenergic blockers renders midodrine ineffective. No data exist as to whether the drug is especially useful in patients with autonomic insufficiency (half of the dialysis population) as might theoretically be the case.

(3) Antihypertensive medication (see Chapter 31)

(4) Consider a trial of sertraline. At least three reports indicated that 4 to 6 weeks of therapy with the selective serotonin reuptake inhibitor sertraline reduces the frequency of intradialytic hypotension. Some evidence suggests that the drug improves autonomic function (Yalcin et al., 2003).

c. Hypotension related to cardiac factors

(1) Diastolic dysfunction. A stiff, hypertrophied heart is especially prone to a reduction in output in response to minor reductions in filling pressure. So-called diastolic dysfunction is common in dialysis patients due to the effects of hypertension, coronary artery disease, and, probably, uremia itself.

(2) Heart rate and contractility. Most, but not all, dialysis hypotension is associated with decreased cardiac filling, a setting in which cardiac compensatory mechanisms can do little to increase output. In some patients, TPR may fall (due to temperature effects, food ingestion, or tissue ischemia) without a fall in cardiac filling. In this setting, impairment of cardiac compensatory mechanisms can play a direct role in the development of hypotension.

(a) Therapeutic implications. A dialysis solution calcium concentration of 1.75 mM helps maintain intradialytic blood pressure better than a level of 1.25 mM, especially in patients with cardiac disease (van der Sande et al., 1998). The mechanism is increased cardiac contractility. However, in the chronic outpatient (as opposed to an intensive care unit) setting, the frequency of symptomatic IDH does not improve with a higher dialysis solution calcium (Sherman et al., 1986). A positive calcium balance with potential vascular calcification risk may be a consequence of using a calcium of 1.75 mM in conjunction with calcium-containing phosphate binders long term. Dialysis solution magnesium levels may impact dialysis hypotension, but whether a higher or a lower level should be used is controversial (see discussion in Chapter 8).

2. Unusual causes of hypotension during dialysis. Rarely, hypotension during dialysis may be a sign of an underlying, serious event (Table 10-1).

3. Dialyzer membranes and hypotension. There has been much speculation that cellulosic membranes, by activating complement and a number of cytokine systems, might be associated with more dialysis hypotension than synthetic membranes. There is no evidence to support these contentions. Several good studies, several of them double blinded, have found no differences among membranes with regard to intradialytic hypotension.

4. Detection of hypotension. Most patients complain of feeling dizzy, light-headed, or nauseated when hypotension occurs. Some experience muscle cramps. Others may experience very subtle symptoms, which may be recognizable only to dialysis staff familiar with the patient (e.g., lack of alertness, darkening of vision). In some patients, there are no symptoms whatsoever until the blood pressure falls to extremely low (and dangerous) levels. For this reason, blood pressure must be monitored on a regular basis throughout the hemodialysis session. Whether this is done hourly, or half-hourly, or on a more frequent basis depends on the individual case.

5.   Management. Management of the acute hypotensive episode is straightforward. The patient should be placed in the Trendelenburg position (if respiratory status allows this) and a bolus of 0.9% saline (100 mL or more, as necessary) should be rapidly administered through the blood line. The ultrafiltration rate should be reduced to as near zero as possible. The patient should then be observed carefully. Ultrafiltration can be resumed (at a slower rate, initially) once vital signs have stabilized. As an alternative to saline, glucose, mannitol, or albumin solutions can be used to treat the hypotensive episode; albumin is costly and offers little benefit over other approaches (Knoll et al., 2004). Unless cramps are also present, use of hypertonic saline appears to offer no benefit over 0.9% saline for equivalent sodium loads. It is best avoided if a high dialysis solution sodium is being used. Nasal oxygen administration is not generally of benefit during hypotensive episodes, though it may have value in selected patients.

a.   Slowing the blood flow rate. In the past, part of the initial therapy for dialysis hypotension was to slow the blood flow rate, a practice developed at a time when plate dialyzers and acetate dialysis solution were in use and ultrafiltration control systems were not. The practice was believed beneficial at the time because reducing blood flow rates resulted in reductions in (a) dialyzer blood volume, (b) acetate (a vasodilator) transfer to the patient, (c) ultrafiltration rate, and (d) fistula "steal." The latter refers to the belief that lowering blood flow reduces access flow and allows systemic flow to increase, a concept that is very likely incorrect (Trivedi et al., 2005). With current dialysis practice, reduction of the blood flow rate to manage hypotension during dialysis should not routinely be done. If, however, the hypotension is severe or the patient is not responding to other treatment measures (stopping ultrafiltration and/or infusion of volume expanders), blood pump rates may be transiently reduced. One common cause of underdialysis is a reduction in solute removal due to repeated slowing of the blood flow rate to manage recurring hypotensive episodes.

6.   Prevention. A useful strategy to help prevent hypotension during dialysis is given in Table 10-2.

B.   Muscle cramps

1.   Etiology. The pathogenesis of muscle cramps during dialysis is unknown. The four most important predisposing factors are hypotension, hypovolemia (patient below dry weight), high ultrafiltration rate (large weight gain), and use of low-sodium dialysis solution. These factors all tend to favor vasoconstriction resulting in muscle hypoperfusion leading to secondary impairment of muscle relaxation. Muscle cramps most commonly occur in association with hypotension, although cramps often persist after seemingly adequate blood pressure has been restored. The frequency of cramping increases logarithmically with the weight loss

Table 10-2. Strategy to help prevent hypotension during dialysis

1. Use a dialysis machine with an ultrafiltration controller.
2. Counsel patient to limit salt intake, which will result in a lower interdialytic weight gain (ideally <1 kg per day).
3. Reassess the patient's dry weight.
4. Use a dialysis solution with a time-averaged concentration of sodium of 140–145 mM, as tolerated.
5. Give daily dose of antihypertensive medications after, not before, dialysis.
6. Use bicarbonate-containing dialysis solution.
7. Use a dialysis solution temperature of 35.5°C with adjustment downward (or upward) as needed and tolerated.
8. Ensure a predialysis hemoglobin level of ≥11 g/dL (110 g/L).
9. Do not give food or glucose orally during dialysis to hypotension-prone patients.
10. Consider use of a blood volume monitor.
11. Consider use of α-adrenergic agonist (midodrine) prior to dialysis.
12. Consider a 6-week trial of sertraline.
13. Extend the length of dialysis by 30 minutes.

requirements; weight losses of 2%, 4%, and 6% have, respectively, been associated with cramping frequencies of 2%, 26%, and 49%.

Cramping is also more common during the first month of dialysis than in subsequent periods. Diagnostically obscure elevations in serum creatinine phosphokinase levels on routine monthly laboratory tests may result from intradialytic muscle cramping. Hypomagnesemia may cause treatment-resistant muscle cramping during dialysis. Hypocalcemia should also be considered as a potential cause, especially in patients treated with relatively low-calcium dialysis solution (1.5 mM) and calcium-free phosphate binders and/or cinacalcet. Predialysis hypokalemia will be exacerbated by the usual level of dialysis solution potassium (2 mM) and may precipitate cramping as well.

2. Management. When hypotension and muscle cramps occur concomitantly, both may respond to treatment with 0.9% saline; however, it is not unusual for muscle cramps to persist. Hypertonic solutions (saline, glucose, mannitol) may be more effective in dilating muscle-bed blood vessels. These solutions are more effective in the acute management of muscle cramps. Since the concentrated sodium load associated with hypertonic saline administration can be problematic, hypertonic glucose administration is preferred for treatment of cramps in nondiabetic patients (Sherman et al., 1982). Mannitol may accumulate in dialysis patients particularly when administered late in treatment—the usual time for the occurrence of cramps. Nifedipine (10 mg) has also been found to reverse cramping. Though reportedly not causing a notable fall in blood pressure, nifedipine should be reserved for cramping in hemodynamically stable patients. Forced stretching of the muscle involved (e.g., ankle flexion for calf cramping) may provide relief. Massage varies in its utility on an individual basis.

3. Prevention. Prevention of hypotensive episodes will eliminate most cramping. The frequency of cramping is also inversely related to the dialysis solution sodium level. Raising sodium levels to just below the threshold for induction of postdialysis thirst will be beneficial. Avoiding low predialysis levels of magnesium, calcium, and potassium may also be helpful.

a. Quinine. Quinine sulfate before dialysis is quite effective in preventing intradialytic cramps; it is ineffective as an acute therapy for cramping. One or two doses (250–325 mg each) can be used. With the higher dose symptomatic (tinnitus) accumulation may occur, requiring a dose reduction. Quinine therapy may also be associated with thrombocytopenia.

b. Carnitine, oxazepam, and prazosin. Carnitine supplementation of dialysis patients may reduce intradialytic muscle cramps (Ahmad et al., 1990) as may oxazepam (5–10 mg, given 2 hours prior to dialysis) and prazosin, though hypotension may complicate therapy with the latter agent.

c. Stretching exercises. A program of stretching exercises targeted at the affected muscle groups may also be useful.

d. Compression devices. A type of sequential compression device may be of benefit (Ahsan et al., 2004).

C. Nausea and vomiting

1. Etiology. Nausea or vomiting occurs in up to 10% of routine dialysis treatments. The cause is multifactorial. Most episodes in stable patients are probably related to hypotension. Nausea or vomiting also can be an early manifestation of the so-called disequilibrium syndrome described below in section II A. Both type A and type B varieties of dialyzer reactions can cause nausea and vomiting. Gastroparesis, very common in diabetes but also seen in nondiabetic patients, is exacerbated by hemodialysis and may play a role in some patients. Contaminated or incorrectly formulated dialysis solution (high sodium, calcium) may cause nausea and vomiting as part of a constellation of symptoms. Dialysis patients appear to develop nausea and vomiting more readily than other patients (e.g., with an upper respiratory infection, narcotic usage, hypercalcemia); dialysis may precipitate these symptoms in such a predisposing setting.

2. Management. The first step is to treat any associated hypotension. Vomiting may be particularly problematic when associated with a hypotension-induced reduction in the level of consciousness due to the risk of aspiration. Antiemetics can be administered for other causes of vomiting as needed.

3. Prevention. Avoidance of hypotension during dialysis is of prime importance. Persistent symptoms unrelated to hemodynamics may benefit from metoclopramide. Sometimes a single predialysis dose of 5–10 mg is sufficient.

D. Headache

1. Etiology. Headache is common during dialysis; its cause is largely unknown. It may be a subtle manifestation of the disequilibrium syndrome (see II A). In patients who are coffee drinkers, headache may be a manifestation of caffeine withdrawal as the blood caffeine concentration is acutely reduced during the dialysis treatment. With atypical or particularly severe headache, a neurologic cause (particularly a bleeding event precipitated by anticoagulation) should be considered.

2. Management. Acetaminophen can be given during dialysis.

3. Prevention. Decreasing dialysis solution sodium also may be helpful in patients being treated with high sodium levels. A cup of strong coffee may help prevent (or treat) caffeine withdrawal symptoms. Patients suffering from headache during dialysis may be magnesium deficient (Goksel et al., 2006). A cautious trial of magnesium supplementation may be indicated, keeping in mind the risks of giving magnesium to patients with renal failure.

E. Chest pain and back pain. Mild chest pain or discomfort (often associated with some back pain) occurs in 1%–4% of dialysis treatments. The cause is unknown. There is no specific management or prevention strategy, though switching to a different variety of dialyzer membrane may be of benefit. The occurrence of angina during dialysis is common and must be considered in the differential diagnosis, along with numerous other potential causes of chest pain (e.g., hemolysis, air embolism, pericarditis). The management and prevention of angina is discussed in Chapter 37.

F. Itching. Itching, a common problem in dialysis patients, is sometimes precipitated or exacerbated by dialysis. Itching appearing only during the treatment, especially if accompanied by other minor allergic symptoms, may be a manifestation of low-grade hypersensitivity to dialyzer or blood circuit components. More often than not, however, itching is simply present chronically, and is noticed in the course of the treatment while the patient is forced to sit still for a prolonged period of time. Viral (or drug-induced) hepatitis should not be overlooked as a potential cause of such itching.

Standard symptomatic treatment using antihistamines is useful. Odansetron and naltrexone have failed to help in randomized trials; acupuncture has helped (Che-yi et al., 2005).

Chronically, general moisturizing and lubrication of the skin using emollients is recommended. Ultraviolet light therapy, especially UVB light, may be of help (Blachley et al., 1985). Pruritus often is found in patients with elevated serum calcium × phosphorus product and/or substantially elevated parathyroid hormone (PTH) level; reductions in phosphorus, calcium (to the lower end of the normal range), and PTH levels are indicated. Whether uremic pruritus is helped by an increased dose of dialysis, use of a high flux or polymethylmethacrylate (PMMA) membrane, capsaicin cream, oral activated charcoal, tacrolimus ointment, evening primrose oil, or erythropoietin (all reported to be of benefit) remain questions for further investigation. Recent small, randomized studies have suggested beneficial effects for gabapentin (Gunal et al., 2004) and for nalfurafine (a κ-opioid agonist) (Wikström et al., 2005).

G. Fever and chills. See Chapter 33.

II. Less common but serious complications. These include disequilibrium syndrome, hypersensitivity reactions, arrhythmia, cardiac tamponade, intracranial bleeding, seizures, hemolysis, and air embolism.

A. Disequilibrium syndrome

  1. Definition. The disequilibrium syndrome is a set of systemic and neurologic symptoms often associated with characteristic electroencephalographic findings that can occur either during or following dialysis. Early manifestations include nausea, vomiting, restlessness, and headache. More serious manifestations include seizures, obtundation, and coma.

  2. Etiology. The cause of the disequilibrium syndrome is controversial. Most believe it to be related to an acute increase in brain water content. When the plasma solute level is rapidly lowered during dialysis, the plasma becomes hypotonic with respect to the brain cells and water shifts from the plasma into brain tissue. Others incriminate acute changes in the pH of the cerebrospinal fluid during dialysis as the cause of this disorder.

    The disequilibrium syndrome was a much larger problem two or more decades ago, when acutely uremic patients with very high serum urea nitrogen values were commonly subjected to prolonged dialysis. However, milder forms of the syndrome may still occur in long-term dialysis patients, manifesting as nausea, vomiting, or headache. The full-blown disequilibrium syndrome, including coma and/or seizures, can still be precipitated when an acutely uremic patient is dialyzed too energetically.

  3. Management

    a. Mild disequilibrium. Symptoms of nausea, vomiting, restlessness, and headache are nonspecific; when they occur, it is difficult to be certain that they are due to disequilibrium. Treatment is symptomatic. If mild symptoms of disequilibrium develop in an acutely uremic patient during dialysis, the blood flow rate should be reduced to decrease the efficiency of solute removal and pH change, and consideration should be given to terminating the dialysis session earlier than planned. Hypertonic sodium chloride or glucose solutions can be administered as for treatment of muscle cramps.

    b. Severe disequilibrium. If seizures, obtundation, or coma occur in the course of a dialysis session, dialysis should be stopped. The differential diagnosis of severe disequilibrium syndrome should be considered (see Chapter 42). Treatment of seizures is discussed in Chapter 42. The management of coma is supportive. The airway should be controlled and the patient ventilated if necessary. Intravenous mannitol may be of benefit. If coma is due to disequilibrium, then the patient should improve within 24 hours.

4. **Prevention**

   a. **In an acute dialysis setting.** When planning dialysis for an acutely uremic patient, one should not prescribe an overly aggressive treatment session (see Chapter 8). The target reduction in the plasma urea nitrogen level should initially be limited to about 40%. Use of a low-sodium dialysis solution dialysis solution (more than 2–3 mM less than the plasma sodium level) may exacerbate cerebral edema and should be avoided. In hypernatremic patients, one should not attempt to correct the plasma sodium concentration and the uremia at the same time. It is safest to dialyze a hypernatremic patient initially with a dialysis solution sodium value close to the plasma level and then to correct the hypernatremia slowly post-dialysis by administering 5% dextrose.

   b. **In a chronic dialysis setting.** The incidence of disequilibrium syndrome can be minimized by use of a dialysis solution with a sodium concentration of at least 140 mM and a glucose concentration of at least 200 mg/dL (11 mmol/L). Using a high dialysis solution sodium concentration (145–150 mM) that declines over the course of treatment for patients has been advocated in this setting. The initially high dialysis solution sodium results in a rising plasma sodium that may counteract the osmotic effects of the initially rapid removal of urea and other solutes from plasma. There is evidence that use of this approach reduces the incidence of disequilibrium-type intradialytic symptoms.

B. **Dialyzer reactions.** This is a broad group of events that includes both anaphylactic and less well-defined adverse reactions of unknown cause (Jaber and Pereira, 1997). In the past, many of these reactions were grouped under the term "first-use" syndrome because they presented much more often when new (as opposed to reused) dialyzers were employed. However, similar reactions occur with reused dialyzers, and we now discuss them under the more general category used here. There appear to be two varieties: An anaphylactic type (type A) and a nonspecific type (type B). The occurrence of type B reactions appears to have diminished considerably during the past several years.

   1. **Type A (anaphylactic type)**

      a. **Manifestations.** When a full-blown, severe reaction occurs, the manifestations are those of anaphylaxis. Dyspnea, a sense of impending doom, and a feeling of warmth at the fistula site or throughout the body are common presenting symptoms. Cardiac arrest and even death may supervene. Milder cases may present only with itching, urticaria, cough, sneezing, coryza, or watery eyes. Gastrointestinal manifestations, such as abdominal cramping or diarrhea, may also occur. Patients with a history of atopy and/or with eosinophilia are prone to develop these reactions. Symptoms usually begin during the first few minutes of dialysis, but onset may occasionally be delayed for up to 30 minutes or more.

b.   Etiology

(1)   Ethylene oxide. Initially, about two thirds of patients with type A (anaphylactic) reactions were found to have elevated serum titers of immunoglobulin E (IgE) antibodies to ethylene oxide–altered protein. Ethylene oxide was used to sterilize almost all hollow-fiber dialyzers in the late 1980s, and it tended to accumulate in the potting compound used to anchor the hollow fibers, hampering efforts to remove it by degassing prior to sale. Ethylene oxide hypersensitivity reactions were observed exclusively during first use of dialyzers, often after less than adequate rinsing. Most of the initial reactions were reported in dialyzers made of unsubstituted cellulose. Current thinking is that the membrane itself plays no role in ethylene oxide hypersensitivity reactions. Recently, manufacturers have taken great pains to remove most residual ethylene oxide from dialyzers, and some have changed the composition of the potting compounds to reduce absorption of ethylene oxide during sterilization. Today ethylene oxide reactions are uncommon.

(2)   AN69-associated reactions. These were initially reported in patients dialyzed with the AN69 membrane who were also taking angiotensin-converting enzyme (ACE) inhibitors. The reactions are thought to be mediated by the bradykinin system. The negatively charged AN69 membrane activates the bradykinin system with the effects magnified because ACE inhibitors block bradykinin inactivation. Plasma bradykinin levels, higher at baseline in patients treated with AN69 dialyzers, rise substantially during reactions. The bradykinin effect should be less pronounced with angiotensin receptor blockers (Ball et al., 2003).

(a)   AN69 versus other polyacrylonitrile (PAN) membranes. The AN69 membrane is a copolymer of PAN and sodium methallyl sulfonate. Dialyzer membranes made of PAN with other copolymers also are available. It is unclear to what extent ACE inhibitor–associated reactions occur with other PAN-based membranes or with other non–PAN-based membranes.

(3)   Contaminated dialysis solution. Type A dialyzer reactions may be accounted for in some instances by dialysis solution contamination with high levels of bacteria and endotoxin. Such reactions are likely to occur promptly (within 2 minutes) of initiating dialysis; complement-mediated reactions are more delayed (15–30 minutes) in onset. Fever and chills are particularly common symptoms with these reactions. It should be noted that use of even grossly contaminated dialysis solution usually has no acute clinical consequences;

however, the higher the bacterial and endotoxin levels are, the greater the risk is of a reaction.

(4) Reuse. Clusters of anaphylactic-type dialyzer reactions have occurred in a reuse setting. The problem has often been linked to inadequate dialyzer disinfection during the reuse procedure, but in many cases the cause is unknown. Half of Centers for Disease Control and Prevention (CDC) investigations of outbreaks of bacteremia or pyrogenic reactions in dialysis patients over a 20-year period were ascribed to dialyzer reuse problems (Roth and Jarvis, 2000).

(5) Heparin. Heparin has occasionally been associated with allergic reactions, including urticaria, nasal congestion, wheezing, and even anaphylaxis. When a patient seems to be allergic to a variety of different dialyzers regardless of the sterilization mode, and dialysis solution contamination also has been reasonably excluded, a trial of heparin-free dialysis or citrate anticoagulation should be considered. Low molecular weight heparins are not a safe substitute in such patients due to cross-reactivity with heparin, which may result in anaphylactic reactions.

(6) Complement fragment release. Acute increases in pulmonary artery pressure have been documented in both animals and humans during dialysis with unsubstituted cellulose membranes. However, there is no good evidence that complement activation causes type A dialyzer reactions. Several studies have found no difference in reaction rates between membranes that readily activate complement (cuprophane) and those that don't (polysulfone, AN69).

(7) Eosinophilia. Type A reactions tend to occur more readily in patients with mild to moderate eosinophilia. Very severe reactions to dialysis or plasmapheresis were reported in patients with very high eosinophil counts; these were thought to be due to sudden eosinophil degranulation with release of bronchoconstrictive and other mediators.

c. Management. Identifying the actual cause of a dialyzer reaction is frequently not possible. It is safest to stop dialysis immediately, clamp the blood lines, and discard the dialyzer and blood lines *without returning the contained blood.* Immediate cardiorespiratory support may be required. According to the severity of the reaction, treatment with intravenous antihistamines, steroids, and epinephrine can be given.

d. Prevention. For all patients, proper rinsing of dialyzers prior to use is important to eliminate residual ethylene oxide and other putative allergens. In a patient with a history of type A reaction to an ethylene oxide–sterilized dialyzer, γ-irradiated or steam-sterilized dialyzers should be used (see Table 4-1). The necessity of using non–ethylene oxide–sterilized blood lines when switching to a γ-irradiated dialyzer has not been established. For patients whose mild type A symptoms persist following a switch to equipment free of ethylene oxide, predialysis administration of antihistamines may be of benefit. Placing the patient on a reuse program and subjecting even new dialyzers to the reuse procedure prior to first use may be of benefit due to enhanced washout of potential noxious substances or allergens. Changing or stopping heparin, trying a less complement–activating membrane, and substituting an angiotensin receptor blocking agent for an ACE inhibitor may also be tried. Latex exposure in a sensitive dialysis patient during dialysis initiation should be considered as well.

 2. **Nonspecific type B dialyzer reactions**

   a. **Symptoms.** The principal manifestations of a type B reaction are chest pain, sometimes accompanied by back pain. Symptom onset is usually 20–40 minutes after starting dialysis. Typically type B reactions are much less severe than type A reactions.

   b. **Etiology.** The cause is unknown. Complement activation has been suggested to be a culprit, but its etiologic role in the development of these symptoms is uncertain. Chest and back pain may occur less frequently with reused dialyzers than with new dialyzers, though this is controversial (see Chapter 11). Any beneficial effects may be due to increased biocompatibility from protein coating of the membrane (not seen with bleach reprocessing) or to washout of potentially toxic substances from the dialyzer. The incidence of type B reactions has declined in the United States. Other causes of chest and back pain must be excluded, and the diagnosis of a type B dialyzer reaction is one of exclusion. In particular, subclinical hemolysis must be ruled out. A syndrome of acute respiratory distress associated with heparin-induced thrombocytopenia has been described (Popov et al., 1997), which may superficially resemble a type B dialyzer reaction.

   c. **Management.** Management is supportive. Nasal oxygen should be given. Myocardial ischemia should be considered, and angina pectoris, if suspected, can be treated as discussed in Chapter 37. Dialysis can usually be continued, as symptoms invariably abate after the first hour.

   d. **Prevention.** Initiating dialyzer reuse or trying a different dialyzer membrane may be of value.

 C. **Arrhythmia.** Arrhythmias during dialysis are especially common in patients receiving digitalis and those with coronary artery disease (Kitano et al., 2004). Prevention and management are discussed in Chapter 37.

 D. **Cardiac tamponade.** Unexpected or recurrent hypotension during dialysis can be a sign of pericardial effusion or impending cardiac tamponade (see Chapter 37).

 E. **Intracranial bleeding.** Underlying vascular disease and hypertension combined with heparin administration can sometimes result in the occurrence of intracranial, subarachnoid, or subdural bleeding during the dialysis session (see Chapter 42).

F. Seizures. Children, patients with high predialysis plasma urea nitrogen levels, and patients with severe hypertension are the most susceptible to seizures during dialysis. Seizure activity can be one manifestation of the disequilibrium syndrome. Seizures are more fully discussed in Chapter 42.

G. Hemolysis. Acute hemolysis during dialysis may be a medical emergency.

  1. Manifestations

    a. Symptoms. The symptoms of hemolysis are back pain, tightness in the chest, and shortness of breath.

    b. Signs. A dramatic deepening of skin pigmentation may occur (Seukeran et al., 1997). Common are a port-wine appearance of blood in the venous blood line, a pink discoloration of the plasma in centrifuged blood samples, and a marked fall in the hematocrit.

    c. Consequences of hemolysis. If massive hemolysis is not detected early, then hyperkalemia can result due to release of potassium from the hemolyzed erythrocytes, leading to muscle weakness, electrocardiographic abnormalities, and, ultimately, cardiac arrest.

  2. Etiology. Acute hemolysis has been reported in two primary settings: (a) an obstruction or narrowing in the blood line, catheter, or needle; and (b) a problem with the dialysis solution. The possibility of hemolysis induced by the combination of G6PD deficiency and predialysis quinine sulfate therapy should be considered.

    a. Blood line obstruction/narrowing. Kinks may develop in the arterial blood line (Sweet et al., 1996). An epidemic of hemolysis also has been reported due to manufacturing defects in the link between the dialyzer outlet blood line and the venous air trap chamber (CDC, 1998). Hemolysis (usually subclinical) may also appear when blood flow rate is high and relatively small needle sizes are used (De Wachter et al., 1997). Routine blood line pressure monitoring will call attention to many, but not all, such problems.

    b. Problems with dialysis solution. These are:

      (1) Overheated dialysis solution

      (2) Hypotonic dialysis solution (insufficient concentrate-to-water ratio)

      (3) Dialysis solution contaminated with formaldehyde, bleach, chloramine (from city water supply), copper (from copper piping), fluoride, nitrates (from water supply), zinc, and hydrogen peroxide (see Chapter 5)

  3. Management. The blood pump should be stopped immediately and the blood lines clamped. The hemolyzed blood has a very high potassium content and should not be reinfused. One should be prepared to treat the resultant hyperkalemia and possible drop in hematocrit. The patient should be observed carefully and hospitalization should be considered. Delayed hemolysis of injured erythrocytes may continue for some time after the dialysis session. Severe hyperkalemia may occur, and this may require additional dialysis or other measures (e.g., administration of an Na/K ion exchange resin by mouth or rectum) to control. A complete blood count, reticulocyte count, and levels of haptoglobin, lactate dehydrogenase (LDH), and methemoglobin should be obtained. Dialysis solution water (chloramine, nitrates, metals) and, if reprocessed, the dialyzer (residual sterilant) need to be assessed as well.

4.   Prevention. Unless the problem is an obstruction in the blood path or faulty roller pump causing excessive blood trauma, the cause of the hemolysis must be assumed to be in the dialysis solution, and samples of dialysis solution must be investigated to determine the cause.

H.   Air embolism. Air embolism is a potential catastrophe that can lead to death unless detected and treated quickly.

1.   Manifestations

a.   Symptoms. These depend to an extent on the position of the patient. In seated patients, infused air tends to migrate into the cerebral venous system without entering the heart, causing obstruction to cerebral venous return, with loss of consciousness, convulsions, and even death. In recumbent patients, the air tends to enter the heart, generate foam in the right ventricle, and pass into the lungs producing dyspnea, cough, and chest tightness and arrhythmias. Further passage of air across the pulmonary capillary bed into the left ventricle can result in air embolization to the arteries of the brain and heart, with acute neurologic and cardiac dysfunction.

b.   Signs. Foam is often seen in the venous blood line of the dialyzer. If air has gone into the heart, a peculiar churning sound may be heard on auscultation.

2.   Etiology. The predisposing factors and possible sites of air entry have been discussed in Chapters 4 and 5. The most common sites of air entry are the arterial needle, the pre-pump arterial tubing segment, and an inadvertently opened end of a central venous catheter.

3.   Management. The first step is to clamp the venous blood line and stop the blood pump. The patient is immediately placed in a recumbent position on the left side with the chest and head tilted downward. Further treatment includes cardiorespiratory support, including administration of 100% oxygen by mask or endotracheal tube. Aspiration of air from the atrium or ventricle with a percutaneously inserted needle or cardiac catheterization may be needed if the volume of air warrants it.

4.   Prevention. See Chapters 4 and 8.

III.   Visual and hearing loss. The osmolar gradients that develop in dialysis between the blood and the intraocular fluid and vestibular system may alter sensory function. Transient blindness in patients with glaucoma and hearing loss due to endolymphatic hydrops have been reported to occur during dialysis (Evans et al., 2005). Complications of heparin administration (inner ear, vitreous or retinal hemorrhage) may result in similar clinical findings. Intradialytic hypotension or unrelated vascular events can also alter visual and auditory function.

IV. Dialysis-associated neutropenia and complement activation. As discussed in Chapter 8, dialyzer membranes made of unsubstituted cellulose have on their surface many exposed hydroxyl groups. The latter can activate the complement cascade in blood flowing through the dialyzer. The liberated complement fragments cause circulating blood neutrophils to migrate to the lungs, where they localize next to blood vessel walls, resulting in neutropenia. After 30– 60 minutes of dialysis, the circulating neutrophil count again rises to normal or even supranormal levels.

Cellulose membranes in which the hydroxyl groups have been chemically "covered" by either acetate (to form cellulose acetate) or a tertiary amino group (Hemophan) activate complement to a much lesser extent and cause less neutropenia. Most synthetic membranes (polysulfone, polycarbonate, polymethylmethacrylate) cause little complement activation or neutropenia. PAN activates complement but then adsorbs the complement fragments, obviating most of their secondary effects.

A. Clinical importance

   1. Symptoms. Whether complement activation and neutropenia during dialysis play an etiologic role in intradialytic symptoms (i.e., hypotension, nausea, chest pain, back pain) remains a matter of controversy. Most patients can be asymptomatically dialyzed using membranes of unsubstituted cellulose.

   2. Renal injury. Complement activation causes activation of leukocytes with increased generation of superoxide. In a rat model of ischemic renal failure, complement infusion or exposure to a complement-activating membrane causes sequestration of neutrophils in glomeruli and delay of recovery of renal function. The trials concerning use of complement-activating membranes for acute dialysis are discussed in Chapter 4.

   3. Chronic effects of complement-activating membranes on the immune system. Membranes of unsubstituted cellulose have deleterious effects on the immune system that persist over the subsequent interdialytic interval. However, there are no definitive studies linking use of unsubstituted cellulose membranes to an adverse outcome. One randomized trial (Parker et al., 1996) suggesting an adverse effect of complement-activating membrane use on patient dry weight and serum albumin value was not confirmed by a larger, multicenter randomized trial (Locatelli et al., 1996).

   4. Hypoxemia. See Section IV.

   5. Interference with complete blood count determination. Because the white blood cell count may be transiently reduced by 50%–80% during dialysis with a cellulose membrane, all blood counts done for diagnostic purposes should be drawn predialysis.

V. Dialysis-associated hypoxemia

A. Definition and clinical importance. During hemodialysis, the arterial blood P_{O_2} drops by 5–30 mm Hg. The fall in P_{O_2} is of no clinical significance in the typical patient but may be deleterious in a patient with severe pre-existing pulmonary or cardiac disease.

B.   Etiology. There are several possible reasons for the drop in PO_2 during dialysis.

   1.   Hypoventilation. Studies have shown that hypoventilation can almost always be implicated. Two mechanisms may contribute to hypoventilation during dialysis:

   a.   Acetate-containing dialysis solution. During dialysis against an acetate-containing dialysis solution, blood passing through the dialyzer loses carbon dioxide to the dialysis solution. The patient hypoventilates slightly, which maintains blood PCO_2 close to the baseline value but also causes hypoxemia. Bicarbonate-containing dialysis solution has an elevated Pco_2. For this reason, dialysis against a bicarbonate bath does not result in hypocapnia.

   b.   Bicarbonate-containing dialysis solution: Alkalosis. When a bicarbonate-containing dialysis solution is used, especially when bicarbonate levels are high (>35 mM), bicarbonate diffusion from the dialysis solution to the blood raises blood pH. This tends to suppress ventilation, causing hypoxemia.

   2.   Intrapulmonary diffusion block. As noted above, dialysis using unsubstituted cellulose membranes causes sequestration of neutrophils in the lung. Some studies have suggested that the alveolar-to-arterial oxygen gradient is increased very early during dialysis, presumably due to neutrophil embolization into the pulmonary capillaries. This concept is controversial; the absence of hypoxemia during dialysis when the patient is on mechanical ventilation (Huang et al., 1998) suggests that such a diffusion block is of little importance. Of some concern is a report suggesting that dialysis using unsubstituted cellulosic membranes may adversely (and apparently permanently) reduce pulmonary diffusing capability (Herrero et al., 2002).

C.   Management. Intervention is usually not required. With active cardiac ischemia or severe chronic obstructive pulmonary disease, nasal oxygen administration may be beneficial. In patients with carbon dioxide retention, delivery of oxygen by Venturi mask may be more appropriate.

D.   Prevention. Oxygen administration will prevent (as well as treat) hypoxemia. In high-risk patients, one might consider avoiding dialyzer membranes made of unsubstituted cellulose (uncertain benefit) and using a bicarbonate-containing dialysis solution with a bicarbonate concentration low enough to avoid alkalemia.

SELECTED READINGS

Ahmad S, et al. Multicenter trial of L-carnitine in maintenance hemodialysis patients. II. Clinical and biochemical effects. *Kidney Int* 1990;38:912–918.

Ahsan M, et al. Prevention of hemodialysis-related muscle cramps by intradialytic use of sequential compression devices: a report of four cases. *Hemodial Int* 2004;8:283–286.

Ball AM, et al. Bradykinin (BK) metabolism in hemodialysis (HD): comparison of angiotensin converting enzyme inhibitors (ACEi) and angiotensin II receptor blockers (ARB). ASN Annual Meeting—San Diego. *J Am Soc Nephrol* 2003;14:712A.

Barakat MM, et al. Hemodynamic effects of intradialytic food ingestion and the effects of caffeine. *J Am Soc Nephrol* 1993;3:1813–1818.

Blachley JD, et al. Uremic pruritus: skin divalent ion content and response to ultraviolet phototherapy. *Am J Kidney Dis* 1985;5:237–241.

Brunet P, et al. Tolerance of haemodialysis: a randomized cross-over trial of 5-h versus 4-h treatment time. *Nephrol Dial Transplant* 1996;11(Suppl 8):46–51.

Centers for Disease Control and Prevention (CDC). Multistate outbreak of hemolysis in hemodialysis patients. *JAMA* 1998;280:1299.

Che-yi C, et al. Acupuncture in haemodialysis patients at the Quchi acupoint for refractory uremic pruritus. *Nephrol Dial Transplant* 2005;20:1912–1915.

Cruz DN, et al. Midodrine and cool dialysis solution are effective therapies for symptomatic intradialytic hypotension. *Am J Kidney Dis* 1999;33:920–926.

Daugirdas JT. Dialysis hypotension: a hemodynamic analysis. *Kidney Int* 1991;39:233.

Daugirdas JT, Ing TS. First-use reactions during hemodialysis: a definition of subtypes. *Kidney Int* 1988;24:S37.

De Wachter DS, et al. Blood trauma in plastic haemodialysis cannula. *Int J Artif Organs* 1997;20:366–370.

Evans RD, Rosner M. Ocular abnormalities associated with advanced kidney disease and hemodialysis. *Semin Dial* 2005;18:252–257.

Franssen CFM. Adenosine and dialysis hypotension. *Kidney Int* 2006;69:789–791.

Goksel BK, et al. Is low blood magnesium level associated with hemodialysis headache? *Headache* 2006;46(1):40–45.

Gunal AL, et al. Gabapentin therapy for pruritus in hemodialysis patients: a randomized placebo-controlled, double-blind trial. *Nephrol Dial Transplant* 2004;19:3137–3139.

Gwinner W, et al. Life-threatening complications of extracorporeal treatment in patients with severe eosinophilia. *Int J Artif Organs* 2005;28(12):1224–1227.

Herrero JA, et al. Pulmonary diffusing capacity in chronic dialysis patients. *Respir Med* 2002;96(7):487–492.

Huang CC, et al. Oxygen, arterial blood gases and ventilation are unchanged during dialysis in patients receiving pressure support ventilation. *Respir Med* 1998;92:534.

Jaber BL, Pereira JBG. Dialysis reactions. *Semin Dial* 1997;10:158–165.

Jansen PH, et al. Randomised controlled trial of hydroquinine in muscle cramps. *Lancet* 1997;349:528.

Kitano Y, et al. Severe coronary stenosis is an important factor for induction and lengthy persistence of ventricular arrhythmias during and after hemodialysis. *Am J Kidney Dis* 2004;44:328–336.

Knoll GA, et al. A randomized, controlled trial of albumin versus saline for the treatment of intradialytic hypotension. *J Am Soc Nephrol* 2004;15:487–492.

Krieter DH, et al. Anaphylactoid reactions during hemodialysis in sheep are ACE inhibitor dose-dependent and mediated by bradykinin. *Kidney Int* 1998;53:1026–1035.

Lemke H-D, et al. Hypersensitivity reactions during haemodialysis: role of complement fragments and ethylene oxide antibodies. *Nephrol Dial Transplant* 1990;5:264.

Locatelli F, et al. Effects of different membranes and dialysis technologies on patient treatment tolerance and nutritional parameters. The Italian Cooperative Dialysis Study Group. *Kidney Int* 1996;50:1293–1302.

Maggiore Q, et al. The effects of control of thermal balance on vascular stability in hemodialysis patients: results of the European randomized clinical trial. *Am J Kidney Dis* 2002;40:280–290.

Parker TF 3rd, et al. Effect of the membrane biocompatibility on nutritional parameters in chronic hemodialysis patients. *Kidney Int* 1996;49:551–556.

Parnes EL, Shapiro WB. Anaphylactoid reactions in hemodialysis patients treated with the AN69 dialyzer. *Kidney Int* 1991;40:1148.

Pegues DA, et al. Anaphylactoid reactions associated with reuse of hollow-fiber hemodialyzers and ACE inhibitors. *Kidney Int* 1992;42:1232.

Poldermans D, et al. Cardiac evaluation in hypotension-prone and hypotension-resistant dialysis patients. *Kidney Int* 1999;56:1905–1911.

Popov D, et al. Pseudopulmonary embolism: acute respiratory distress in the syndrome of heparin-induced thrombocytopenia. *Am J Kidney Dis* 1997;29:449–452.

Reddan DN, et al. Intradialytic blood volume monitoring in ambulatory hemodialysis patients: a randomized trial. *J Am Soc Nephrol* 2005;16:2162–2169.

Ritz E, et al. Cardiac changes in uraemia and their possible relationship to cardiovascular instability on dialysis. *Nephrol Dial Transpl* 1990;5:93–97.

Robertson KE, Mueller BA. Uremic pruritus. *Am J Health Syst Pharm* 1996;53:2159—2170; quiz 2215—2216.

Roca AO, et al. Dialysis leg cramps. Efficacy of quinine versus vitamin E. *ASAIO J* 1992;38:M481.

Roth VR, Jarvis WR. Outbreaks of infection and/or pyrogenic reactions in dialysis patients. *Semin Dial* 2000;13:92–96.

Santoro A, et al. Blood volume controlled hemodialysis in hypotension-prone patients: a randomized, multicenter controlled trial. *Kidney Int* 2002;62:1034–1045.

Santos SFF, et al. The consequences of an individualized dialysate Na+ prescription on hemodialysis (HD) parameters. A short-term study. ASN Annual Meeting—San Diego. *J Am Soc Nephrol* 2003;14:55A.

Selby NM, McIntyre CW. A systematic review of the clinical effects of reducing dialysate fluid temperature. *Nephrol Dial Transplant* 2006;21:1883–1898.

Seukeran D, et al. Sudden deepening of pigmentation during haemodialysis due to severe haemolysis. *Br J Dermatol* 1997;137:997–999.

Sherman RA, et al. Effect of variations in dialysis solution temperature on blood pressure during hemodialysis. *Am J Kidney Dis* 1984;4:66–68.

Sherman RA, et al. Postprandial blood pressure changes during hemodialysis. *Am J Kidney Dis* 1988;12:37–39.

Sherman RA, et al. The effect of dialysis solution calcium levels on blood pressure during hemodialysis. *Am J Kidney Dis* 1986;8:244–227.

Sherman RA, et al. The effect of red cell transfusion on hemodialysis-related hypotension. *Am J Kidney Dis* 1988;11:33–35.

Sherman RA, et al. Acute therapy of hemodialysis-related muscle cramps. *Am J Kidney Dis* 1982;2:287–288.

Silver SM, et al. Dialysis disequilibrium syndrome (DDS) in the rat: role of the "reverse urea effect." *Kidney Int* 1992;42:161.

Steuer RR, et al. Reducing symptoms during hemodialysis by continuously monitoring the hematocrit. *Am J Kidney Dis* 1996;27:525.

Stiller S, et al. A critical review of sodium profiling for hemodialysis. *Semin Dial* 2001;14:337–347.

Straumann E, et al. Symmetric and asymmetric left ventricular hypertrophy in patients with end-stage renal failure on long-term hemodialysis. *Clin Cardiol* 1998;21:672–678.

Strong J, et al. Effects of calorie and fluid intake on adverse events during hemodialysis. *J Ren Nutr* 2001;11(2):97–100.

Sweet SJ. Hemolytic reactions mechanically induced by kinked hemodialysis lines. *Am J Kidney Dis* 1996;27:262.

Tomson CRV. Advising dialysis patients to restrict fluid intake without restricting sodium intake is not based on evidence and is a waste of time. *Nephrol Dial Transplant* 2001;16:1538–1542.

Trivedi H, et al. Effect of variation of blood flow rate on blood pressure during hemodialysis. ASN Annual Meeting—Philadelphia. *J Am Soc Nephrol* 2005;16:39A.

Van der Sande FM, et al. Effect of dialysis solution calcium concentration on intradialytic blood pressure course in cardiac-compromised patients. *Am J Kidney Dis* 1998;32:125.

Wikström B, et al. Kappa-opioid system in uremic pruritus: multicenter, randomized, double-blind, placebo-controlled clinical studies. *J Am Soc Nephrol* 2005;16:3742–3747.

Yalcin AU, et al. Effect of sertraline hydrochloride on cardiac autonomic dysfunction in patients with hemodialysis-induced hypotension. *Nephron Physiol* 2003;93:P21–P28.

Dialyzer Reuse

Allen M. Kaufman, Robert Levin,
Ravi Jayakaran, and Nathan W. Levin

After a dialyzer is used, it can be rinsed free of blood, chemically cleaned, disinfected, and reused. Dialyzer reuse is a safe and effective practice in the United States. In the late 1990s, dialyzer reuse was applied in the treatment of 80% of U.S. hemodialysis patients. Largely as a result of the decision of Fresenius Medical Care to phase out dialyzer reuse, reuse is currently utilized in the treatment of fewer U.S. hemodialysis patients. Although 78% of clinics continued to practice reuse in 2001 (U.S. Renal Data System, USRDS Annual Data Report, Bethesda MD, 2004), in 2005 this number dropped to <50%. Almost all reuse is performed utilizing hollow-fiber dialyzers. The average number of times that a dialyzer is reused varies from unit to unit, although many programs average >10 reuses per dialyzer.

I.   Reprocessing technique. The major steps in dialyzer reprocessing are rinsing, cleaning, measuring dialyzer performance, disinfecting/sterilizing, and removing germicides.

A.   Rinsing and reverse ultrafiltration. To maintain the patency of fibers and to minimize clotting after dialysis, blood should be returned with heparinized saline. After the patient has been disconnected, removal of residual blood can be accomplished by reverse ultrafiltration with dialysate while still at the dialysis station. Once the dialyzer has been removed from the machine, a pressurized rinse of both the blood and dialysate compartments should begin with minimal delay. If a delay is unavoidable, the dialyzers should be refrigerated within 2 hours (American Association of Medical Instrumentation Renal Disease Committee [AAMI RD] standard 47-2002 11.1). Facility practice should set limits for how long the dialyzers can be refrigerated before being reprocessed or discarded. Typically this maximum time varies between 36 and 48 hours from the end of treatment.

B.   Cleaning

1.   Water. Water used for reprocessing must, at a minimum, meet the specification of the current version of AAMI RD62, *Water treatment equipment for hemodialysis applications*.

A prolonged rinse with reverse-osmosis water followed by reverse ultrafiltration has been shown to be an effective means of cleaning dialyzers without the addition of chemicals.

2.   Bleach. Sodium hypochlorite (bleach), diluted to 0.6% or less, dissolves proteinaceous deposits that may occlude fibers. Bleach increases albumin losses in high-flux cellulose triacetate (CT 190) and polysulfone–polyvinylpyrrolidone (F80B) dialyzers. Albumin losses are generally not clinically significant unless bleach is used on high-flux membranes with exceptionally high water permeability (see III B, Clinical concerns). However, bleach can result in an increase in the ultrafiltration coefficient and overt membrane damage in cellulosic membranes, especially when used in high concentrations, at an elevated temperature, or for prolonged exposure times (Pizziconi, 1990).

3. Other cleaning agents. Hydrogen peroxide (3% or less) and peracetic acid/hydrogen peroxide/acetic acid mixtures (available in the United States as Renalin or Puresteril) are commonly used. These agents may not completely remove proteins deposited on the dialyzer membrane. For this reason, the ultrafiltration coefficient may become reduced in dialyzers cleaned with peroxide/acetic acid mixtures.

C. Tests of dialyzer performance. These check the integrity of the membrane and its clearance and ultrafiltration properties. The tests may be done manually or using automated techniques.

1. Pressure test for leaks. A blood path integrity test works by generating a transmembrane pressure gradient across the membrane and observing for a pressure fall in either the blood or the dialysate compartment. The gradient may be produced by instilling pressurized air or nitrogen into the blood side of the dialyzer or by producing a vacuum in the dialysate side. Only minimal amounts of air can leak through an intact wetted membrane; damaged fibers usually rupture when a transmembrane pressure gradient is applied. Leak tests also screen for defects in the dialyzer O-rings, potting compound, and end-caps.

2. Blood compartment volume. This test indirectly measures changes in membrane clearance for small molecules, such as urea. The blood compartment volume (total cell volume, TCV) is measured by purging the filled blood compartment (header volume and fiber volume) with air and measuring the volume of obtained fluid. Every dialyzer should be processed before the first use in order to obtain a dialyzer-specific baseline TCV. The change in TCV is then followed after each reuse. A reduction in TCV of 20% corresponds to 10% reduction in urea clearance, the maximum decrease acceptable for continued use. Meaningful tests of TCV cannot be done in plate dialyzers because their blood compartment volume changes with the amount of transmembrane pressure applied. In a given patient, repeated failure to reach a target number of reuses because of TCV test failures suggests excessive clot formation during dialysis and should prompt a review of the heparin prescription.

3. In vitro K_{Uf}. The dialyzer ultrafiltration coefficient (K_{Uf}; described in Chapter 3) is another indirect measure of membrane mass transfer properties because a change in the K_{Uf} reflects changes in membrane resistance, as well as surface area. The in vitro K_{Uf} can be measured by determining the volume of water passing through the membrane at a given pressure and temperature. However, changes in this parameter do not have a clinical impact when dialysis is being done using machines with ultrafiltration control.

   4.   Conductivity-based clearance. On-line determination of sodium or ionic clearance, which is comparable to urea clearance, is another acceptable method of monitoring dialyzer performance. See AAMI Renal Disease Committee (AAMI-RD) standard RD47-202.

D.   Disinfection/sterilization. Once cleaned, the dialyzer must undergo a physical or chemical process that renders all living organisms inactive. High-level disinfection differs from sterilization in that the former may not destroy spores. High-level disinfection is all that current standards require. Sterilization as defined legally is not easily accomplished in a dialysis facility.

   1.   Germicides. Germicides are generally instilled in both blood and dialysate compartments for 24 hours. Peracetic acid/hydrogen peroxide/acetic acid mixtures, formaldehyde, and glutaraldehyde (Diacide) are the most common germicides used. Formaldehyde vapor is effective in disinfecting fibers that do not come in direct contact with the liquid formaldehyde. Renalin or Puresteril offers the advantage of qualifying as a sterilant with the limitations mentioned above. Heated 1.5% citric acid at 95°C (Levin et al., 1995) or the original method with heated water at 105°C (Kaufman, 1992) are nonnoxious chemical alternatives to disinfection. Laboratory studies have shown that with this method of disinfection spores are destroyed.

   2.   Documenting the presence of germicide. The presence of germicide must be ensured through procedural controls and, ideally, should be verified in every dialyzer prior to use. When formaldehyde is the germicide used, an indicator substance, such an FD&C blue dye no. 1, can be added to the concentrated stock solution. When dilute (batch) solutions are made and instilled in the dialyzer, their light blue color indicates that formaldehyde is present. This method avoids the need to test each dialyzer individually for presence of germicide on a routine basis. However, daily verification that the concentration of formaldehyde in the batch solution is adequate is still required, as are periodic spot checks of dialyzers for formaldehyde presence and concentration. The usual concentration of formaldehyde is 4% when disinfection is performed at room temperature for 24 hours. A 2% solution should not be used at room temperature because some types of mycobacteria have been shown to survive 2% formaldehyde exposure for 24 hours. However, even 1% solutions of formaldehyde may have excellent germicidal efficacy when dialyzers are incubated at 40°C for 24 hours (Hakim et al., 1985). When using peroxide/acetic acid mixtures (Renalin or Puresteril) as a sterilant, potassium iodide or starch testing strips should be used to test the presence of peracetic acid during reuse; a minimum contact time of 12 hours is needed for the dialyzer to be sterile when filled with peracetic acid. To ensure that the correct concentration of peroxide/acetic acid mixtures in the dialyzer is obtained, a four-dialyzer priming volume of the mixture must be introduced into the dialyzer.

3. Germicide removal. Germicide removal is accomplished by either automated or manual techniques. The basic maneuvers include initial flushing of the blood compartment, followed by flushing of the dialysate compartment. Removal (by diffusion) of formaldehyde and peroxide/acetic acid mixtures can be accomplished by circulating saline through the blood compartment while coursing dialysate at usual temperatures through the dialysate compartment in a single-pass fashion for 15 minutes.

Air must be removed from the arterial line before flushing in order to avoid introduction of air into the blood compartment. Trapped air in the fibers or dialysate compartment may retard the effectiveness of germicide removal techniques. In addition, the dialyzer should be rotated at intervals during flushing to release trapped air in the dialysate compartment.

The blood circuit should be checked for residual germicide immediately prior to use by two individuals. Residual formaldehyde can be checked with modified Schiff reagent and should be within the currently acceptable levels of 5 ppm. Residual levels of other germicides can be checked with specific manufacturer-recommended test kits.

4. Heat sterilization. Germicide-free reprocessing utilizing high temperature to achieve sterilization obviates many of the concerns related to the use of chemicals to process dialyzers. In the original technique, the dialyzers are cleaned and tested in the usual manner, reverse-osmosis water is instilled, and the dialyzers are heated in a 105°C convection oven for 20 hours (Kaufman, 1992). An additional integrity test at the bedside is required prior to use. In a subsequent technique, 1.5% citric acid solution allows for heating at 95°C for 20 hours to achieve identical disinfection and to limit structural damage to the dialyzer (Levin et al., 1995). At present, polysulfone is the only membrane material that has proved sufficiently heat resistant for clinical use. In addition, potting compounds must meet certain design specifications for use under these conditions. In the case of heat methodology that utilizes a convection oven, appropriate temperature is ensured by a continuous temperature recorder and by heat-sensitive labels.

5. Final inspection. Dialyzers should not be used if they have an abnormal or unaesthetic appearance (e.g., if there is an overall brownish or blackish discoloration, if there are clots in the header, or if bands of clotted fibers are present).

II. Automated versus manual systems. Several types of automated machines are now manufactured; some provide the ability to process multiple dialyzers simultaneously. With automated methods, the cleansing cycles are highly reproducible and a variety of quality control tests measuring fiber bundle volume, ultrafiltration coefficient, and pressure holding are built in. Dialyzer labels can also be automatically printed. Computerized analysis of records and results are available with some of the systems. Although the use of automated

Table 11-1. Advantages and disadvantages of dialyzer reuse

Advantages

Allows more widespread use of costlier dialyzes (e.g., high-K_0A, high-flux, synthetic membranes with their attendant benefits)

Reduced exposure to residual industrial chemicals used in the manufacture of new dialyzers

Reduced incidence of intradialytic symptoms (controversial)

Enhanced dialyzer biocompatibility/reduced immune system activation (with unsubstituted cellulose membranes and when bleach is not used)

Reduction in treatment cost

Disadvantages

Potential for exposure of patient and personnel to chemicals

Potential for bacterial/endotoxin contamination of dialyzer

Potential for loss of dialyzer mass transfer (clearance) and ultrafiltration capacity

Potential for transmission of an infectious agent from one dialyzer to another during the reprocessing procedure

Potential loss of β_2-microglobulin clearance with certain reuse techniques

---

systems now predominates, manual reprocessing of dialyzers is still performed with success in some dialysis units.

III. Clinical issues. When reprocessing is performed in accordance with accepted standards and practices (ANSI/RD47:2002/A1:2003; AAMI, 2005), the risks of the procedure are negligible. The incidences of sepsis and hepatitis B infection are not different in patients treated with reused dialyzers from those treated with new dialyzers. There are no reports of transmission of HIV infection related to dialyzer reuse.

A. Clinical benefits (Table 11-1)

1. Wider use of costlier dialyzers. It is now well established that mortality in dialysis patients decreases as the amount of dialysis given is increased above substandard levels (Table 11-1). Large patients and patients who resist longer dialysis session lengths usually can be adequately dialyzed only when high-efficiency (high-K_0A) dialyzers are used (see Chapter 9). For a given dialysis session length and blood flow rate, use of a high-efficiency dialyzer results in more dialysis for every patient. Furthermore, evidence is accumulating that use of a high-flux synthetic membrane may confer an additional beneficial effect on survival (see Chapter 9). High-efficiency dialyzers, as well as high-flux synthetic dialyzers, can oftentimes be more widely offered by those units practicing reuse.

2. First-use reactions. In the past, anaphylactic reactions occurred less frequently with reprocessed dialyzers than with new dialyzers. Most likely, this was the result of removal of residual amounts of ethylene oxide or other substances used during manufacture. Milder, more common forms of "first-use syndrome" associated with cellulosic (Cuprophan) dialyzers may occur less frequently or are milder with reuse. It has been advocated that new dialyzers be reprocessed prior to clinical use. With this "preprocessing," the incidence of anaphylactic reactions during first use may be reduced, as may the incidence of symptoms during the first use (Charoenpanich et al., 1987).

3. Complement activation. With unsubstituted cellulose dialyzers, reuse lessens the degree of membrane-induced activation of complement and the resulting transient leukopenia. This may be the result of protein coating of the membrane during its first clinical use. The benefit disappears if bleach is used in the reprocessing method because bleach acts to remove or alter the protein coat from the membrane. Nonreused cellulosic dialyzers can cause chronic suppression of several aspects of the immune system. These adverse immune effects may occur to a lesser extent in a reuse situation.

B. **Clinical concerns**
1. **Formaldehyde**
   a. **Anti-N antibodies.** These can be produced when residual dialyzer formaldehyde levels are high and have been associated with hemolysis and with early transplant failure; one group has reported their development even when dialyzers were rinsed to the point that effluent formaldehyde levels were always below 2–3 ppm (Vanholder et al., 1988).
   b. **Acute formaldehyde reactions.** Immediate burning at the fistula site may indicate that formaldehyde has been improperly removed from the dialyzer. Under these circumstances, the dialysis should be stopped immediately, the venous blood line clamped, and the dialyzer contents checked for formaldehyde. Dialysis should continue with a new dialyzer.
   c. **Itching.** In some studies, itching during dialysis has improved after switching from formaldehyde to alternative disinfecting agents.
2. **Morbidity and mortality.** In an analysis of 49,273 incident Medicare patients from 1998 to 1999, Collins et al. (2004) reported that there were no significant differences in mortality among different reuse practices or no-reuse. However, Lowrie et al. (2004) reported that there is survival advantage when patients were switched from reuse to single use in a complicated study where the dialyzer type was also changed. Further studies on large population groups will need to be done to definitively analyze the impact of reuse on survival.
3. **Potential bacterial/pyrogen contamination.** Bacteremia and pyrogen reactions can result from improperly processed dialyzers. Clusters of pyrogen reactions occur slightly more often in centers that reuse dialyzers. In general, the source of such problems is generally the water used to rinse and clean the dialyzers and to prepare the germicides used for disinfection. Scrupulous attention to water treatment is required (Hoenich et al., 2003).
4. **Potential of anaphylactoid reactions with use of peracetic acid/hydrogen peroxide/acetic acid reuse**

agents and angiotensin-converting enzyme (ACE) inhibitors. An outbreak of anaphylactoid reactions to reused dialyzers occurred in patients dialyzed with cupram-monium cellulose, cellulose acetate, and polysulfone dialyzers reprocessed with peracetic acid/hydrogen peroxide/acetic acid. Most were being treated with ACE inhibitors (Pegues et al., 1992). Reuse of dialyzers with oxidizing agents, such as peracetic acid/hydrogen peroxide/acetic acid, can produce a strong negative charge on the protein-coated membrane and thereby activate factor XII, kininogen, kallikrein, and, subsequently, bradykinin. ACE inhibitor–induced inhibition of bradykinin degradation may poten-tiate the reaction. Similar reactions have been described with the use of polyacrylonitrile membrane and attributed to membrane-induced bradykinin generation. In another small case series, reactions in patients taking ACE in-hibitors began when bleach was added to the reuse pro-cedure and ceased when use of bleach was discontinued (Schmitter and Sweet, 1998).

5. Potential transmission of infectious agents. Of greatest concern are hepatitis B virus and HIV. The poten-tial inadvertent spillage of blood at the time that the dia-lyzer is reprocessed poses the theoretical risk of exposure of both staff and other patients to these viruses. However, bleach and germicides inactivate both the hepatitis B virus and HIV. For added safety, patients with sepsis or with acute hepatitis should not reuse dialyzers. Patients who are hep-atitis B surface antigen positive should not participate in a reuse program unless their dialyzers are reprocessed using a separate machine or manually in a separate area. Accord-ing to current Centers for Disease Control and Prevention (CDC) recommendations, patients with HIV may continue on a reuse program. The epidemiology of hepatitis C virus in the dialysis setting is under investigation. Currently, the CDC does not object to dialyzer reuse in patients infected with hepatitis C.

6. Potential for decreased dialyzer performance
   a.   Urea clearance. A reused hollow-fiber dialyzer ulti-mately becomes less efficient as a portion of its capillaries become plugged with protein or clot from previous uses. However, as long as the fiber bundle volume is at least 80% of the baseline value, urea clearance remains clini-cally acceptable. The HEMO study confirmed this data by reporting that the decrease in urea clearances in a large number of patients undergoing several different dialyz-ers and varying reuse methods (Cheung et al., 1999) is, at most, modest. The HEMO study found that, independent of the reuse method, urea clearance decreased 1.4%–2.9% over 20 uses.

   (1)   Heparin dosing. The reusability of dialyzers will deteriorate quickly unless adequate heparin anticoagu-lation is given. One group has reported increased num-bers of reuses with individual targeted heparin dosing (Ouseph et al., 2000). The use of low molecular weight heparin instead of unfractionated heparin may further increase the average number of reuses (Jayakaran, 2005, unpublished data).

(2) Bicarbonate dialysis solution containing citric acid. Bicarbonate dialysate containing a small amount of citrate (Citrasate) has been reported to result in increased urea clearance in a reuse setting (Ahmad et al., 2005). The mechanism of how this occurs is not known, but may be related to calcium chelation by citrate coming in from the dialysate at the membrane boundary layer, with perhaps reduced activation of clotting or protein deposition.

b. β_2-Microglobulin clearance. Protein deposits adsorbed by the membrane or convectively transported to the membrane surface and not removed by the reuse process may reduce the ultrafiltration rate and larger molecule clearance. The clearance of β_2-microglobulin (b2M, molecular weight 11,815) is negligible by low-flux dialyzers and does not change in a clinically significant way with reuse. High-flux dialyzer performance with respect to b2M clearance may be altered dramatically by reuse, depending on the type of membrane and type of reuse procedure (Cheung et al., 1999).

In the HEMO study, use of peracetic acid/hydrogen peroxide/acetic acid (which normally is used without a bleach cycle) reduced b2M clearance by 56% between the first use and the 15th–20th reuse in cellulose triacetate (CT 190) dialyzers. On the other hand, a minimal effect was observed on b2M clearance when polysulfone (F80A) dialyzers were reused in the same fashion. The use of bleach with formaldehyde in polysulfone dialyzers increased b2M clearance by 123% between the first use and the 15th–20th reuse. Glutaraldehyde with formaldehyde in polysulfone dialyzers increased b2M clearance by 11% through reuse 20. The effectiveness of bleach to increase b2M clearance was also noted with CT 190 dialyzers when peracetic acid/hydrogen peroxide/acetic acid was selected for reuse. Heated citric acid increased b2M clearance by 30% in polysulfone (F80B) dialyzers between the first use and the 10th–15th reuse, the maximum reuse utilized for this method. Thus, the effects of reuse on dialyzer flux are highly dependent on the dialyzer membrane property and the reuse method. Of most concern is the rapid falloff in b2M clearance when high-flux cellulose dialyzers are reused with peracetic acid/hydrogen peroxide/acetic acid without a bleach cycle.

7. Albumin loss. Some dialyzers exposed to bleach during reuse procedures may undergo an increase in permeability to albumin that correlates with the number of reuses. Non–high-flux membranes do not increase albumin losses in a clinically significant manner. However, when polysulfone dialyzers with very high water permeability (e.g., >60 mL per hour per mm Hg in vivo) are reused with methods that use bleach, losses of albumin can be substantial, particularly as the number of reuses increases to >20 (Kaplan et al., 1995). On the other hand, high-flux membranes of lesser water permeability (F80B, CT 190) exposed to bleach develop only limited albumin losses, with 1–2 g per dialysis reported over 20 reuses (Gotch et al., 1994). Albumin losses in high-flux polysulfone dialyzers reprocessed with peracetic acid or heat are negligible (Gotch et al., 1994). Thus, the effects of reuse on albumin losses, as noted for b2M, cannot be simply described. A full understanding requires knowledge of the type of dialyzer membrane and the reuse method.

IV.   Other issues

A.   Medico-legal aspects

1. **U.S. laws.** Federal regulations pertaining to dialyzer reprocessing follow, with some additions (*Reuse of hemodialyzers,* AAMI, 2005). Clinical practice guidelines are also discussed in the National Kidney Foundation's Kidney Dialysis Outcomes Quality Initiative (KDOQI).

2. **Manufacturer single-use recommendation.** Because of the widespread practice of reusing dialyzers labeled for single use only, the U.S. Food and Drug Administration (FDA) has developed guidelines that allow manufactures to label their dialyzers for multiple use, recommend an appropriate reuse method, and provide performance data of dialyzers over 15 reuses (FDA, October 6, 1995). Dialyzer manufacturers may choose to continue to label their dialyzers for single use only.

3. **Reuse of other dialysis disposables.** Health Care Finance Administration regulations do not allow reuse of transducer protectors. Guidelines for the reuse of blood tubing have been published (*Reuse of hemodialyzers,* AAMI, 2005). However, blood tubing reuse is permitted only when the manufacturer has developed a specific protocol that has been accepted by the FDA (via premarket notification, section 501[k] of the provision of the Food, Drug and Cosmetic Act).

4. **Informed consent.** Programs differ in the way that they define the patient's role in the decision to use reprocessed dialyzers. There are no federal requirements as to whether informed consent is needed, although commonly it is obtained. Patients should be fully apprised of the potential advantages and disadvantages of reuse. Given appropriate interaction with their physicians and the dialysis staff, most patients will cooperate with a recommendation for reuse. Once a patient has agreed to participate in a reuse program, it is recommended that he or she take an active role in the process. For example, federal guidelines recommend that the patient participate in the final checks for proper labeling of the reprocessed dialyzer just before its use.

B.   Cost. Although a reuse program requires increased staff and expenditure for supplies and equipment, reuse is cost effective. This is particularly true when high-efficiency or high-flux dialyzers (that are more expensive than conventional dialyzers) are prescribed. Even with the recent introduction of lower-priced high-flux single-use dialyzers, at current prices, the use of high-efficiency membranes with high ultrafiltration coefficients (high-flux membranes) are not economically feasible in some clinics under the current (U.S.) reimbursement schedules unless the dialyzers are reused.

C. Quality assurance. For safe and successful reuse of dialyzers, a quality assurance program must be in place that systematically ensures the implementation and effectiveness of the reuse policies and procedures. Audits of the program should be carried out on a regular basis by individuals not directly performing the reprocessing procedures.

   1. Record keeping. Records must be kept in a way that allows for identification of the individual completing each step in the reuse process. Documentation of all aspects of present and past reuse of a patient's individual dialyzers should be retrievable. Each patient's dialyzer is individually labeled with a unique identifier and with information related to the use number. A log is kept of all incoming materials used in the reuse process. A log is also kept of the weekly test results of the disinfectant stock for proper concentration. A percentage of the program's reused dialyzers are cultured weekly for bacteria and checked for proper disinfectant concentration. All equipment performance is monitored regularly. If dialyzers are incubated during disinfection, 24-hour temperature-recording devices are utilized to ensure consistent temperatures. A carefully monitored preventive maintenance program minimizes malfunction of equipment employed in the reuse process. Detailed files are kept for possible adverse clinical events related to reprocessed dialyzers.

D. Personnel and physical plant considerations. A comprehensive training course should be established for all personnel performing reprocessing. Competence should be verified for each item on the curriculum. The use of protective eyewear and clothing is stressed, as is proper handling of germicide spills. Where germicides are used, the work space should be designed with air turnover at least equivalent to the clinical area with forced inward air and additional ceiling exhaust ducts. Exposure to germicides is regulated by the U.S. Occupational Health and Safety Administration (OSHA). Current (1990) maximum allowable time-weighted average (TWA) exposure for formaldehyde is 1 ppm and for short-term exposure is 3 ppm. Maximum exposure limits for hydrogen peroxide is 1 ppm TWA and for glutaraldehyde is 0.2 ppm. There are no current OSHA exposure limits for peracetic acid.

E. Reuse water. Water purity is of crucial importance in the reuse process. It is preferable that reuse water be treated by reverse osmosis. Water used to prepare germicides should be tested weekly and have a bacterial colony count of <200 colony-forming units/mL and an endotoxin concentration (determined by limulus amebocyte lysate assay) of <2 endotoxin units/mL. Particularly with high-flux treatment, some authors believe that the currently accepted standards for water may be too liberal and perhaps ideally, sterile, pyrogen-free water should be used. For any system special attention should be paid to the occurrence of pyrogenic reactions, particularly in clusters. In general, this should prompt immediate checks of the water system for bacteria and endotoxins, as well as a

review of quality control procedures. The reverse osmosis system should be disinfected monthly to prevent biofilm growth.
V.   Patient monitoring. Measurements such as fiber bundle volume are only one aspect of the process of ensuring dialyzer performance. Careful evaluation of the patient's treatment and course is the primary validation of dialyzer performance. If conventional fluid removal systems are used, unexplained deviation from the ultrafiltration rate, as evidenced by unanticipated deviation of the postdialysis weight, may indicate altered dialyzer water permeability. However, this is not relevant in modern machines using ultrafiltration control. An unusual rise in predialysis plasma urea or creatinine concentration or a general deterioration of the patient's clinical condition may indicate reduced dialyzer solute permeability. Validation of the effectiveness of treatment by approaches such as urea kinetic modeling is also fundamental to the quality assurance process. Comparison of kinetically determined volume of total-body water with previous kinetically established values or demographically determined values serves as a useful screen for a number of technical problems including inadequate dialyzer clearance as a result of poor reprocessing technique. However, kinetic measurements are generally performed monthly and may not identify a problem in a timely manner. The recent practical development of online clearance provides immediate and direct information of dialyzer performance (Rahmati et al., 2003).

SELECTED READINGS

Ahmad S, et al. Increased dialyzer reuse with citrate dialysate. *Hemodial Int* 2005;9:264–267.

Association for the Advancement of Medical Instrumentation. *AAMI standards and recommended practices, vol. 3, Dialysis.* Arlington, VA: Association for the Advancement of Medical Instrumentation, 2005.

Charoenpanich R, et al. Effect of first and subsequent use of hemodialyzers on patient well being. *Artif Organs* 1987;11:123.

Cheung A, et al. Effects of hemodialyzer use on clearances of urea and beta-2 microglobulin. The Hemodialysis (HEMO) Study Group. *J Am Soc Nephrol* 1999;10:117–127.

Collins AJ, et al. Dialyzer reuse-associated mortality and hospitalization risk in incident Medicare haemodialysis patients, 1998–1999. *Nephrol Dial Transplant* 2004;19:1245–1251.

Fan Q, et al. Reuse-associated mortality in incident hemodialysis patients in the United States, 2000–2001. *Am J Kidney Dis* 2005;46:661–668.

Gotch FA, et al. Effects of reuse with peracetic acid, heat and bleach on polysulfone dialyzers [Abstract]. *J Am Soc Nephrol* 1994;5:415.

Hakim RM, Friedrich RA, Lowrie EG. Formaldehyde kinetics in reused dialyzers. *Kidney Int* 1985;28:936.

Hoenich NA, Levin R. The implications of water quality in hemodialysis. *Semin Dial* 2003;16:492–497.

Kaplan AA, et al. Dialysate protein losses with bleach processed polysulfone dialyzers. *Kidney Int* 1995;47:573–578.

Kaufman AM, et al. Clinical experience with heat sterilization for reprocessing dialyzers. *ASAIO J* 1992;38:M338–M340.

Kliger AS. Patient safety in the dialysis facility. *Blood Purif* 2006;24(1):19–21.

Levin NW, et al. The use of heated citric acid for dialyzer reprocessing. *J Am Soc Nephrol* 1995;6:1578–1585.

Lowrie EG, et al. Reprocessing dialysers for multiple uses; recent analysis of death risks for patients. *Nephrol Dial Transplant* 2004;19(11):2823–2830.

Ouseph R, et al. Improved dialyzer reuse after use of a population pharmacodynamic model to determine heparin doses. *Am J Kidney Dis* 2000;35:89–94.

Pegues DA, et al. Anaphylactoid reactions associated with reuse of hollow fiber hemodialyzers and ACE inhibitors. *Kidney Int* 1992;42:1232–1237.

Pizziconi VB. Performance and integrity testing in reprocessed dialyzers: a QC update. In: AAMI, ed. *AAMI standards and recommended practices. Vol 3. Dialysis.* Arlington, VA: 1990:176.

Rahmati MA, et al. On-line clearance: a useful tool for monitoring the effectiveness of the reuse procedure. *ASAIO J* 2003;49(5):543–546.

Schmitter L, Sweet S. Anaphylactic reactions with the additions of hypochlorite to reuse in patients maintained on reprocessed polysulfone hemodialyzers and ACE inhibitors. Paper presented at the annual meeting of the American Society for Artificial Internal Organs, New Orleans, April 1998.

Vanholder R, et al. Development of anti-N-like antibodies during formaldehyde reuse in spite of adequate predialysis rinsing. *Am J Kidney Dis* 1988;11:477–480.

Twardowski ZJ. Dialyzer reuse—part I: historical perspective. *Semin Dial* 2006;19(1):41–53.

Twardowski ZJ. Dialyzer reuse—part II: advantages and disadvantages. *Semin Dial* 2006;19(3):217–226.

US Renal Data System, USRDS Annual Report, Bethesda, MD, 2004.

Verresen L, et al. Bradykinin is a mediator of anaphylactoid reactions during hemodialysis with AN69 membranes. *Kidney Int* 1994;45:1497–1503.

Zaoui P, Green W, Hakim M. Hemodialysis with cuprophane membrane modulates interleukin-2 receptor expression. *Kidney Int* 1991;39:1020.

WEB REFERENCES

American Association for the Advancement of Medical Instrumentation (AAMI): http://www.aami.org/

Reuse: Recent literature and links: http://www.hdcn.com/hd/reuse

Anticoagulation

Andrew Davenport, Kar Neng Lai, Joachim Hertel, and Ralph J. Caruana

I. **Blood clotting in the extracorporeal circuit.** The patient's blood is exposed to intravenous cannulas, tubing, drip chambers, headers, potting compound, and dialysis membranes during the dialysis procedure. These surfaces exhibit a variable degree of thrombogenicity and may initiate clotting of blood, especially in conjunction with exposure of blood to air in drip chambers. The resulting thrombus formation may be significant enough to cause occlusion and malfunction of the extracorporeal circuit. Clot formation in the extracorporeal circuit begins with coating of the surfaces by plasma proteins, followed by platelet adherence and aggregation, thromboxane A_2 generation, and activation of the intrinsic coagulation cascade, leading to thrombin formation and fibrin deposition. Factors favoring clotting are listed in Table 12-1.
A. **Assessing coagulation during dialysis**
   1. **Visual inspection.** Signs of extracorporeal circuit clotting are listed in Table 12-2. Visualization of the circuit can be best accomplished by rinsing the system with saline solution while occluding the blood inlet temporarily.
   2. **Extracorporeal circuit pressures.** Arterial and venous pressure readings may change as a result of clotting in the extracorporeal circuit depending on the location of thrombus formation. An advantage of using blood lines with a postpump arterial pressure monitor is that the difference between the postpump and venous pressure readings can serve as an indicator of the location of the clotting. An increased pressure difference is seen when the clotting is confined to the dialyzer itself (increased postpump pressure, decreased venous pressure). If the clotting is occurring in or distal to the venous blood chamber, then the postpump and venous pressure readings are increased in tandem. If the clotting is extensive, then the rise in pressure readings will be precipitous. A clotted or malpositioned venous needle also results in increased pressure readings.
   3. **Dialyzer appearance after dialysis.** The presence of a few clotted fibers is not unusual, and the headers often collect small blood clots or whitish deposits (especially in patients with hyperlipidemia). More significant dialyzer clotting should be recorded by the dialysis staff to serve as a clinical parameter for adjustment of heparin dosing. It is useful to classify the amount of clotting based on the visually estimated percentage of clotted fibers in order to standardize documentation (e.g., <10% of fibers clotted, grade 1; <50% clotted, grade 2; >50% clotted, grade 3).
   4. **Measurement of residual dialyzer volume.** In units practicing dialyzer reuse, automated or manual methods are

Table 12-1. Factors favoring clotting of the extracorporeal circuit

Low blood flow
High hematocrit
High ultrafiltration rate
Dialysis access recirculation
Intradialytic blood and blood product transfusion
Intradialytic lipid infusion
Use of drip chambers (air exposure, foam formation, turbulence)

used to determine the clotting-associated fiber loss during each treatment. This is done by comparing the predialysis and postdialysis fiber bundle volumes. Dialyzers suitable for reuse characteristically have <1% fiber loss over each of the first 5–10 reuses.

II. Use of anticoagulants during dialysis. When no anticoagulant is used, dialyzer clotting rate during a 3- to 4-hour dialysis session is substantial (5%–10%), and when this occurs, it results in loss of the dialyzer and blood tubings, plus loss of approximately 100–150 mL of blood (the combined fill volume of the dialyzer and blood line in the extracorporeal circuit). This is an acceptable risk in many patients judged to be at moderate to high risk of anticoagulant-induced bleeding, since bleeding in such patients may often result in catastrophic consequences, and for such patients anticoagulation-free dialysis (described below) can be appropriately used. However, for the great majority of patients, who are judged not to be at a markedly increased bleeding risk, some form of anticoagulation must be employed. In programs reusing dialyzers, proper levels of anticoagulation during dialysis are key to obtaining reasonable reuse numbers.

There is considerable variability among regions of the world, countries, and even dialysis units about what type of anticoagulation is used during intermittent hemodialysis. Despite a number of promising alternatives, heparin is the most common anticoagulant used. In the United States unfractionated heparin is mostly used, whereas in the European Union, low molecular weight heparin is the anticoagulant of choice

Table 12-2. Signs of clotting in the extracorporeal circuit

Extremely dark blood
Shadows or black streaks in the dialyzer
Foaming with subsequent clot formation in drip chambers and venous trap
Rapid filling of transducer monitors with blood
"Teetering" (blood in the postdialyzer venous line segment that is unable to continue into the venous chamber but falls back into the line segment)
Presence of clots at the arterial-side header

recommended by the European Best Practice Guidelines (2002). A handful of dialysis units anticoagulate the blood circuit using trisodium citrate, and direct thrombin inhibitors such as argatroban are just beginning to be evaluated in clinical settings.

III. Measuring blood clotting during dialysis. While it is important to understand the principles of how clotting tests can be used to monitor heparin therapy, in the United States, because of economic constraints, the relatively low risk of bleeding complications from use of heparin during dialysis, and regulatory issues (the requirement for local laboratory certification), heparin therapy is ordinarily prescribed empirically, without monitoring of coagulation. In patients who are at an elevated risk of bleeding, the need to monitor anticoagulation is often circumvented by using heparin-free dialysis.

When clotting studies are done, blood for clotting studies should be drawn from the arterial blood line, proximal to any heparin infusion site, to reflect the clotting status of the patient rather than that of the extracorporeal circuit. It is very difficult to obtain baseline clotting studies from a venous catheter that has been locked with heparin, due to problems of residual heparin in the catheter, and this step is rarely attempted (Hemmelder, 2003).

A. Clotting tests used to monitor heparin therapy
   1. Activated partial thromboplastin time (APTT). This is for unfractionated heparin monitoring only. This is the most commonly used test in a hospital setting. Heparin resistance states can be falsely suggested due to elevated levels of factor VIII. Baseline levels may be prolonged because of lupus anticoagulant (see Olson, 1998).
   2. Whole-blood partial thromboplastin time (WBPTT). This is similar to above, but this is a bedside test. The WBPTT test accelerates the clotting process by addition of 0.2 mL of actin FS reagent (Thrombofax) to 0.4 mL of blood. The mixture is set in a heating block at 37°C for 30 seconds and then tilted every 5 seconds until a clot forms. The prolongation of the WBPTT is linearly related to the blood heparin concentration (in the range applicable to dialysis). It should not be used to monitor low molecular weight heparin therapy.
   3. Activated clotting time (ACT). The ACT test is similar to the WBPTT test but uses siliceous earth to accelerate the clotting process. ACT is less reproducible than WBPTT, especially at low blood heparin levels. Devices that automatically tilt the tube and detect clot formation facilitate standardization and reproducibility of both WBPTT and ACT. It is for unfractionated heparin monitoring only.
   4. Lee-White clotting time (LWCT). The Lee-White test is performed by adding 0.4 mL of blood to a glass tube and inverting the tube every 30 seconds until the blood clots. Usually, the blood is kept at room temperature. Disadvantages of the LWCT test include the long period of time required before clotting occurs, extensive use of technician time required, and the relatively poor standardization and reproducibility of the test. LWCT is the least desirable

method of monitoring clotting during hemodialysis. This test is now rarely used.

5. Factor Xa-activated ACT. This test has been proposed as a more sensitive test for monitoring anticoagulation during use of low molecular weight heparin (Frank, 2004).

IV. Anticoagulation techniques

A. Unfractionated heparin

1. Mechanisms of action. Heparin changes the conformation of antithrombin (AT), leading to rapid inactivation of coagulation factors, in particular factor Xa. Unfortunately, heparin does stimulate platelet aggregation and activation, but these undesirable effects are counterbalanced by interference with binding and activation of coagulation factors at the platelet membrane. Undesired side effects of heparin include pruritus, allergy, osteoporosis, hyperlipidemia, thrombocytopenia, and excessive bleeding.

2. Target clotting times. Heparin can usually be given liberally during dialysis without fear of precipitating a bleeding episode in patients who do not exhibit an abnormal bleeding risk. The effect of two routine heparin regimens on clotting time is shown in Figure 12-1. The goal is to maintain WBPTT or ACT at the baseline value plus 80% during most of the dialysis session (Table 12.3). However, at the end of the session, the clotting time should be shorter (baseline plus 40% for WBPTT or ACT) to minimize the risk of bleeding from the access site after withdrawal of the access needles.

The target clotting times using the Lee-White test are also listed in Table 12-3. With LWCT, in contrast to WBPTT or ACT, the target clotting times during dialysis are

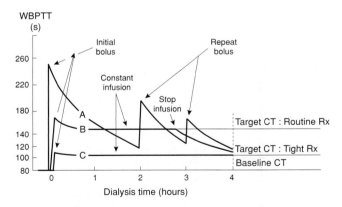

Figure 12-1. Effect of various heparin regimens on clotting time as reflected by the whole-blood partial thromboplastin time (WBPTT). CT, clotting time using the WBPTT test. A: routine regimen, repeated-bolus method; B: routine regimen, constant-infusion method; C: tight regimen, constant-infusion method.

Table 12-3. Target clotting times during dialysis

Test	Reagent	Baseline Value	Routine Heparin Desired Range During Dialysis	Routine Heparin Desired Range At End of Dialysis	Tight Heparin Desired Range During Dialysis	Tight Heparin Desired Range At End of Dialysis
WBPTT	Actin FS	60–85 sec	+80% (120–140)	+40% (85–105)	+40% (85–105)	+40% (85–105)
ACT[a]	Siliceous earth	120–150 sec	+80% (200–250)	+40% (170–190)	+40% (170–190)	+40% (170–190)
LWCT[b]	None	4–8 min	20–30	9–16	9–16	9–16

WBPTT, whole blood partial thromboplastin time; ACT, activated clotting time; LWCT, Lee-White clotting time.
[a]There are various methods of performing the ACT, and the baseline value with some methods is much lower (e.g., 90–120 seconds).
[b]Baseline values of the LWCT vary greatly depending on how the test is performed.

considerably greater than baseline plus 80%, and the target LWCT values at the end of the session are greater than baseline plus 40%.

3.   Routine heparin prescriptions. There are two basic techniques of administering routine heparin. In one method, a heparin bolus is followed by a constant heparin infusion. In the second, a heparin bolus is followed by repeated bolus doses as necessary. For the purpose of discussion, we present a typical prescription in each category.

R_x: **Routine heparin, constant-infusion method**

Administer the initial bolus dose (e.g., 2,000 units). The initial heparin dose is best administered to the patient via the venous access tubing and flushed in with saline (rather than being infused into the arterial blood line). Introducing heparin into the arterial blood line means that incoming nonheparinized blood will need to be pumped through the dialyzer until the loading dose has had time to pass through the extracorporeal circuit to anticoagulate blood in the body. Wait 3–5 minutes to allow heparin dispersion before initiating dialysis.

Start heparin infusion into the arterial blood line (e.g., at a rate of 1,200 units per hour).

R_x: **Routine heparin, single-dose-only or repeated-bolus method**

Administer the initial bolus dose (e.g., 4,000 units).

Then give an additional 1,000- to 2,000-unit bolus dose if necessary.

The prescriptions used in the United States, however, vary quite widely. Those centers that reuse dialyzers tend to use more heparin in order to maximize reuse number. Some centers give only a single initial dose (e.g., 2,000 units) of heparin, with no subsequent infusion or boluses. Some centers give a fairly large (75–100 units/kg) initial bolus dose followed by a 500- to 750-unit-per-hour infusion. At this point in time, there has been little research to convincingly demonstrate an optimal method of heparin dosing.

a.   Effect of body weight on the size of the heparin dose. Although in a population pharmacokinetic study the volume of distribution of heparin has been found to increase as body weight rises (Smith et al., 1998), many dialysis centers do not regularly adjust heparin dosage in accordance with body weights ranging between 50 and 90 kg. However, other centers do adjust both the loading and maintenance doses according to body weight.

b.   When to terminate the heparin infusion. The heparin half-life in dialysis patients averages 50 minutes but ranges from 30 minutes to 2 hours. For a patient with an average heparin half-life of 1 hour, if the heparin infusion during dialysis is prolonging WBPTT or ACT to the required baseline-plus-80% value, stopping heparin infusion approximately 1 hour prior to the end of dialysis will result in the desired WBPTT or ACT value of baseline plus 40% at termination of the session. With venous catheters, heparin infusions are commonly continued right up to the end of dialysis.

c. Posttherapy needle puncture site bleeding. When this occurs, in addition to re-evaluation of the heparin dose, the vascular access (graft or fistula) should be evaluated for the presence of outflow stenosis, as the increased intra-access pressure may be predisposing to posttreatment bleeding. There should also be an evaluation of needle insertion technique. Poor technique and failure to rotate puncture sites can lead to shredding of the wall of a graft so that it leaks following needle removal no matter how well anticoagulation is controlled.

4. Evaluation of clotting during routine heparinization. A small incidence of inadvertent clotting of the extracorporeal system is expected and generally does not necessitate a change in heparin prescription. When clotting occurs it is useful to evaluate the likely cause. Often the underlying cause may be correctable (e.g., access revision). Operator-induced errors, as listed in Table 12-4, must be considered and managed through education. Recurrent clotting warrants individual re-evaluation and adjustments in heparin dosing.

5. Bleeding complications of routine heparinization. The risk of increased bleeding due to systemic anticoagulation is 25%–50% in high-risk patients with bleeding gastrointestinal lesions (gastritis, peptic ulcer, angiodysplasia), recent surgery, or pericarditis. De novo bleeding can involve the central nervous system, retroperitoneum, and mediastinum. The tendency to bleed is potentiated by uremia-associated defects in platelet function and possibly by endothelial abnormalities.

Table 12-4.   Technical or operator-induced factors (resulting in clotting)

Dialyzer Priming
Retained air in dialyzer (due to inadequate priming or poor priming technique)
Lack of or inadequate priming of heparin infusion line

Heparin Administration
Incorrect heparin pump setting for constant infusion
Incorrect loading dose
Delayed starting of heparin pump
Failure to release heparin line clamp
Insufficient time lapse after loading dose for systemic heparinization to occur

Vascular Access
Inadequate blood flow due to needle/catheter positioning or clotting
Excessive access recirculation due to needle/tourniquet position
Frequent interruption of blood flow due to inadequate delivery or machine alarm situations

B. Tight heparin

   1. General comments. Tight heparinization schemes are recommended for patients who are at slight risk for bleeding, when the risk of bleeding is chronic and prolonged, and where use of heparin-free dialysis has been unsuccessful due to frequent clotting. When using WBPTT or ACT to monitor therapy, the target clotting time (see Table 12-3 and curve C in Fig. 12-1) is equal to the baseline value plus 40%. Target clotting times using the Lee-White method are given in Table 12-3. If the baseline WBPTT or ACT value is >140% of the average baseline value for patients in the dialysis unit, it is best not to use heparin and to proceed with a heparin-free or regional citrate technique.

   2. The tight heparin prescription. A bolus dose followed by a constant infusion of heparin is the best technique for administering a tight heparin prescription because constant infusion avoids the rising and falling clotting times that are inevitable with repeated-bolus therapy. A typical tight heparin prescription is as follows:

   R_x: Tight heparin, constant-infusion method

   Obtain baseline clotting time (WBPTT or ACT).
   Initial bolus dose = 750 units.
   Recheck WBPTT or ACT after 3 minutes.
   Administer a supplemental bolus dose if needed to prolong WBPTT or ACT to a value of baseline plus 40%.
   Start dialysis and heparin infusion at a rate of 600 units per hour.
   Monitor clotting times every 30 minutes.
   Adjust the heparin infusion rate to keep WBPTT or ACT at baseline plus 40%.
   Continue heparin infusion until the end of the dialysis session.

C. Heparin-associated complications. Apart from bleeding, complications of note are increase in blood lipids, thrombocytopenia, and the potential for hypoaldosteronism and exacerbation of hyperkalemia, especially in patients with substantial residual renal function.

   1. Lipids. Heparin activates lipoprotein lipase, and in this way can increase the serum triglyceride concentration. Lower levels of high-density lipoprotein (HDL) cholesterol also are associated with heparin use. Both lipid abnormalities are improved when using low molecular weight heparin (LMWH) (Elisaf et al., 1997).

   2. Heparin-associated thrombocytopenia. There are two types of heparin-associated thrombocytopenia (HIT). In type 1 HIT, the reduction in platelet count occurs in a time- and dose-dependent manner and responds to reduction in heparin dose. In type 2 HIT, there is agglutination of platelets and paradoxical arterial and/or venous thrombosis. Type 2 HIT, which is attributable to development of immunoglobulin G (IgG) or IgM antibodies against the heparin–platelet factor 4 complex, is more commonly induced with bovine versus porcine heparin. Given the frequency of HIT in the nondialysis population, it is surprising that it is not encountered more often in a dialysis setting. Diagnosis of type 2 HIT is by an abnormal platelet aggregation test or by an even more sensitive enzyme-linked immunosorbent assay (ELISA) using bound platelet factor 4 complexed with heparin.

LMWH should not be used to treat HIT, since there often is cross-reactivity of the heparin–platelet factor 4 antibodies with these drugs. Cross-reactivity is lower with the synthetic heparinoid danaparoid, and may be lower still with fondaparinux (Haase et al., 2005); however, regional citrate anticoagulation is a better alternative if heparin-free dialysis (without a heparin prerinse) cannot be performed (Davenport, 1998). Use of a direct thrombin inhibitor such as argatroban is also a tested alternative (Tang et al., 2005).

Warfarin should be used with caution or not at all in patients with HIT, as its use in such circumstances has been associated with skin necrosis and venous limb gangrene (Srinivasan et al., 2004).

3. Pruritus. Heparin can cause local itching when injected subcutaneously, and it has been speculated that heparin may be the cause of itching and other allergic reactions during dialysis. On the other hand, LMWH has been used to treat the itching associated with lichen planus, on the basis of inhibition of T-lymphocyte heparinase activity (Hodak et al., 1998). There is no evidence that removal of heparin from the extracorporeal circuit reliably improves uremic pruritus.

4. Anaphylactoid reactions. See Chapter 10.

5. Hyperkalemia. Heparin-associated hyperkalemia, attributable to heparin-induced suppression of aldosterone synthesis, has been well described. In oliguric dialysis patients, it has been speculated that aldosterone might still aid potassium excretion via a gastrointestinal mechanism. There is one report suggesting that changing from heparin to LMWH may improve the aldosterone/plasma renin activity ratio and result in slight improvement of hyperkalemia in dialysis patients (Hottelart et al., 1998).

6. Osteoporosis. Long-term administration of heparin can cause osteoporosis.

D. Heparin-free dialysis

1. General comments. Heparin-free dialysis is the method of choice in patients who are actively bleeding, who are at moderate to high risk of bleeding, or in whom the use of heparin is contraindicated (e.g., persons with HIT). The indications for heparin-free dialysis are listed in Table 12-5. Because of its simplicity and safety, many centers now use heparin-free dialysis routinely for most dialysis treatments being given in an intensive care unit setting.

2. The heparin-free prescription. There are a variety of techniques, but all are similar to the one given below:

R_x: Heparin-free dialysis

a. Heparin rinse. (This step is optional. Avoid if heparin-associated thrombocytopenia is present.) Rinse extracorporeal circuit with saline containing 3,000 units

Table 12-5. Anticoagulation strategy: indications for heparin-free dialysis

Pericarditis
Recent surgery, with bleeding complications or risk, especially:
  Vascular and cardiac surgery
  Eye surgery (retinal and cataract)
  Renal transplant
  Brain surgery
Coagulopathy
Thrombocytopenia
Intracerebral hemorrhage
Active bleeding
Routine use for dialysis of acutely ill patients by many centers

of heparin/L, so that heparin can coat extracorporeal surfaces and the dialyzer membrane to mitigate the thrombogenic response. To prevent systemic heparin administration to the patient, allow the heparin-containing priming fluid to drain by filling the extracorporeal circuit with either the patient's blood or unheparinized saline at the outset of dialysis.

b. High blood flow rate. Set the blood flow rate to 400 mL per minute if tolerated. If a high blood flow rate is contraindicated due to the risk of disequilibrium (e.g., small patient, very high predialysis plasma urea level), consider using a small-surface-area dialyzer and/or slowing the dialysate flow rate, or shortening the treatment sessions. Generally, double-lumen hemodialysis catheters deliver sufficiently high blood flows to be effective.

c. Periodic saline rinse. The utility of this step is controversial; one recent study suggested that use of a saline rinse may actually promote clotting (perhaps via introduction of microbubbles into the circuit) (Sagedal et al., 2006). The purpose of the periodic rinsing is to allow inspection of a hollow-fiber dialyzer for evidence of clotting and to allow for timely discontinuation of treatment or changing of the dialyzer. Also, periodic saline rinsing is believed by some to reduce the propensity for dialyzer clotting or interfere with clot formation.

Procedure: Rinse the dialyzer rapidly with 250 mL of saline while occluding the blood inlet line every 15 minutes. The frequency of the flushes can be increased or decreased as needed. The use of volumetric control is desirable for the accurate removal of volumes of ultrafiltrate equal to those of the administered saline rinses.

d. Different membrane materials and circuit design. There is no solid evidence to suggest that any one type of membrane material is better for heparin-free dialysis. Although heparin coatings and LMWH coatings are being tried, elimination of dead spaces in blood tubing and reducing the presence of air–blood interfaces in dialysis lines may be the most promising approaches to lower incidence of extracorporeal circuit clotting.

e.   Blood product transfusion or lipid administration. Administration via the inlet blood line has been reported to increase clotting risk during dialysis.

E.   Bicarbonate dialysis solution with low-concentration citrate (Citrasate). A small amount of citric acid is used instead of acetic acid as the acidifying agent. When the acid and base concentrates are mixed, the resulting dialysis solution commonly contains 0.8 mmol/L (2.4 mEq/L) citrate. This small amount of citrate, by complexing with calcium, has been suggested to inhibit blood coagulation and platelet activation locally at the dialyzer membrane surface, resulting in improved dialyzer clearance and increased dialyzer reusability (Ahmad et al., 2005). This type of dialysis solution can be used with a reduced dose of heparin, or as part of a heparin-free dialysis technique, with a reduced incidence of dialyzer clotting. The amount of citrate used is low enough such that monitoring of ionized calcium is not required. Unlike sodium citrate, citric acid does not increase the base load of a dialysate (since citric acid is metabolized to CO_2 and water only) and, therefore, has no alkalinizing influence.

V.   Other anticoagulation techniques

A.   LMWH. LMWH fractions (molecular weight = 4,000–6,000 daltons) are obtained by chemical degradation or sieving of crude heparin (molecular weight = 2,000–25,000 daltons). LMWH inhibits factor Xa, factor XIIa, and kallikrein, but causes so little inhibition of thrombin and factors IX and XI that partial thromboplastin time and thrombin time are only raised by 35% during the first hour and minimally prolonged thereafter, thus decreasing bleeding risk.

Hemodialysis using LMWH as the sole anticoagulant has been shown in some long-term studies to be safe and effective. LMWH's longer half-life permits anticoagulation with a single dose at the start of dialysis, though split dosing may be better.

LMWH is now commercially available in the United States but is not widely used there because it is more expensive and because it is not yet approved by the Food and Drug Administration for hemodialysis. The dose of LMWH is generally expressed in anti-factor Xa Institute Choay units (aXaICU). For a 4-hour dialysis treatment, a single loading dose of 10,000 or 15,000 aXaICU (125–250 aXaICU/kg) has been successful in providing adequate anticoagulation for hemodialysis with little or no prolongation of APTT. The lower dosage, 125 aXaICU/kg, should be used in patients who have a mildly increased risk of hemorrhage. (Lai et al., 1996). Coagulation tests are not routinely monitored during LMWH treatment, since the test to measure anti-Xa activity in blood is not yet widely available.

Potential benefits of LMWH, as discussed above, include an improved lipid profile and possibly some amelioration of hyperkalemia. Recent animal data revealed that LMWH does not inhibit osteoblast proliferation in vitro and may reduce the risk of heparin-induced osteoporosis associated with long-term heparin administration (Lai et al., 2001). The European

Best Practice Guidelines recommend LMWH over unfractionated heparin. One caveat: the lipid-related benefits of LMWH have been called into question (Nasstrom et al., 2005).

   1. Anaphylactic reactions to bolus low molecular weight heparin. As discussed in Chapter 10, so called "first-use" syndrome has been reported with both unfractionated heparin and also with low molecular weight heparin. When present, patients seem to react to all types of heparin. In one case report, apparently heparin-allergic patients could be dialyzed when the heparin was infused using a constant infusion method when a bolus dose was not given (De Vos et al., 2000).

   2. Bleeding complications. In chronic kidney disease patients being treated with LMWH who are also receiving clopidogrel and aspirin, bleeding complications have been reported (Farooq et al., 2004). Perhaps dialysis patients receiving clopidogrel and aspirin should be monitored more closely when LMWH is used as the anticoagulant for dialysis.

B. Heparinoids (danaparoid and fondaparinux). Danaparoid is a mixture of 84% heparin, 12% dermatan, and 4% chondroitin sulfates. Danaparoid affects predominantly factor Xa and therefore has to be monitored with anti-Xa assays. The half-life is prolonged in renal failure, such that monitoring is sometimes used to check anti-Xa activity prior to the succeeding dialysis session. In patients >55 kg, a 750-IU loading dose is recommended, and subsequent doses are titrated to achieve an anti-Xa activity of 0.25–0.35. Danaparoid may cross-react with HIT antibodies in up to 10% of cases. More recently a series of pentasaccharides, such as fondaparinux, have been developed, which do not cross-react with HIT antibodies.

C. Regional (high-concentration) citrate anticoagulation. An alternative to heparin-free dialysis is to anticoagulate the blood in the extracorporeal circuit by lowering its ionized calcium concentration (calcium is required for the coagulation process). The extracorporeal blood–ionized calcium level is lowered by infusing trisodium citrate (which complexes calcium) into the arterial blood line and by using a dialysis solution containing no calcium. To prevent the return of blood with a very low ionized calcium concentration to the patient, the process is reversed by infusion of calcium chloride into the dialyzer blood outlet line. About one third of the infused citrate is dialyzed away and the remaining two thirds are quickly metabolized by the patient. The advantages of regional citrate anticoagulation over heparin-free dialysis are (a) the blood flow rate does not have to be high and (b) clotting rarely occurs. The principal disadvantages are the requirement for two infusions (one of citrate and one of calcium) and the requirement for monitoring the plasma ionized calcium level. Because sodium citrate metabolism generates bicarbonate, use of this method results in a greater than usual increment in the plasma bicarbonate value. Hence, regional citrate anticoagulation should be used with caution in patients who are at risk for alkalemia. When citrate anticoagulation is to be used on a long-term basis, the dialysis solution bicarbonate level should be reduced (e.g., to 25 mM) if metabolic alkalosis is to be avoided (van der Meulen et al., 1992). Chronic citrate use may result in aluminum overload (aluminum contamination from glass container or from elsewhere). This technique is not widely used for intermittent hemodialysis but is more popular for the continuous forms of dialysis therapy. A theoretical advantage is the prevention of platelet activation/degranulation when using citrate anticoagulation (Gritters et al., 2006).

D.   Thrombin inhibitors. Argatroban, a synthetic peptide derived from arginine, acts as a direct thrombin inhibitor. It is primarily metabolized in the liver. Argatroban is licensed for treating patients with HIT. A typical loading dose for hemodialysis is 250 mcg/kg, followed by an infusion of 0.5–2.0 mcg/kg per minute, titrated to achieve an APTT of 1.5–2 times the normal ratio. A related drug, melagatran, has been used for anticoagulation when added to the dialysate, but this treatment remains experimental at this time (Flanigan, 2005).

SELECTED READINGS

Ahmad S, et al. Increased dialyzer reuse with citrate dialysate. *Hemodial Int* 2005;9:264.

Apsner R, et al. Citrate for long-term hemodialysis: prospective study of 1,009 consecutive high-flux treatments in 59 patients. *Am J Kidney Dis* 2005;45:557.

Caruana RJ, et al. Heparin-free dialysis: comparative data and results in high-risk patients. *Kidney Int* 1987;31:1351.

Davenport A. Management of heparin-induced thrombocytopenia during continuous renal replacement therapy. *Am J Kidney Dis* 1998;32:E3.

De Vos JY, Marzoughi H, Hombrouckx R. Heparinisation in chronic haemodialysis treatment: bolus injection or continuous homogeneous infusion? *EDTNA ERCA J* 2000;26(1):20–21.

Elisaf MS, et al. Effects of conventional vs. low-molecular-weight heparin on lipid profile in hemodialysis patients. *Am J Nephrol* 1997;17:153.

European Best Practice Guidelines. V.1–V.5 Hemodialysis and prevention of system clotting (V.1 and V.2); prevention of clotting in the HD patient with elevated bleeding risk (V.3); heparin-induced thrombocytopenia (V.4); and side effects of heparin (V.5). *Nephrol Dial Transplant* 2002;17[Suppl 7]:63.

Farooq V, et al. Serious adverse incidents with the usage of low molecular weight heparins in patients with chronic kidney disease. *Am J Kidney Dis* 2004;43:531.

Flanigan MJ. Melagatran anticoagulation during haemodialysis—'Primum non nocere.' *Nephrol Dial Transplant* 2005;20:1789.

Frank RD, et al. Factor Xa-activated whole blood clotting time (Xa-ACT) for bedside monitoring of dalteparin anticoagulation during haemodialysis. *Nephrol Dial Transplant* 2004;19:1552.

Gotch FA, et al. Care of the patient on hemodialysis. In: Cogan MG, Garovoy MR, eds. *Introduction to dialysis,* 2nd ed. New York, NY: Churchill Livingstone, 1991.

Gouin-Thibault I, et al. Safety profile of different low-molecular weight heparins used at therapeutic dose. *Drug Saf* 2005;28:333.

Gritters M, et al. Citrate anticoagulation abolishes degranulation of polymorphonuclear cells and platelets and reduces oxidative stress during haemodialysis. *Nephrol Dial Transplant* 2006;21: 153.

Haase M, et al. Use of fondaparinux (ARIXTRA) in a dialysis patient with symptomatic heparin-induced thrombocytopaenia type II. *Nephrol Dial Transplant* 2005;20:444.

Handschin AE, et al. Effect of low molecular weight heparin (dalteparin) and fondaparinux (Arixtra) on human osteoblasts in vitro. *Br J Surg* 2005;92:177.

Hemmelder MH, et al. Heparin lock in hemodialysis catheters adversely affects clotting times: a comparison of three catheter sampling methods [Abstract]. *J Am Soc Nephrol* 2003;14:729A.

Hodak E, et al. Low-dose low-molecular-weight heparin (enoxaparin) is beneficial in lichen planus: a preliminary report. *J Am Acad Dermatol* 1998;38:564.

Hottelart C, et al. Heparin-induced hyperkalemia in chronic hemodialysis patients: comparison of low molecular weight and unfractionated heparin. *Artif Organs* 1998;22:614.

Lai KN, et al. Use of low-dose low molecular weight heparin in hemodialysis. *Am J Kidney Dis* 1996;28:721.

Lai KN, et al. Effect of low molecular weight heparin on bone metabolism and hyperlipidemia in patients on maintenance hemodialysis. *Int J Artif Organs* 2001;24:447.

Lim W, et al. Safety and efficacy of low molecular weight heparins for hemodialysis in patients with end-stage renal failure: a meta-analysis of randomized trials. *J Am Soc Nephrol* 2004;15: 3192.

McGill RL, et al. Clinical consequences of heparin-free hemodialysis. *Hemodial Int* 2005;9:393.

Molino D, et al. In uremia, plasma levels of anti-protein C and anti-protein S antibodies are associated with thrombosis. *Kidney Int* 2005;68:1223.

Murray PT, et al. A prospective comparison of three argatroban treatment regimens during hemodialysis in end-stage renal disease. *Kidney Int* 2004;66:2446.

Nasstrom B, et al. A single bolus of a low molecular weight heparin to patients on haemodialysis depletes lipoprotein lipase stores and retards triglyceride clearing. *Nephrol Dial Transplant* 2005;20: 1172.

Olson JD, et al. College of American Pathologists Conference XXXI on laboratory monitoring of anticoagulant therapy: laboratory monitoring of unfractionated heparin therapy. *Arch Pathol Lab Med* 1998;122(9):782–798.

Ouseph R, et al. Improved dialyzer reuse after use of a population pharmacodynamic model to determine heparin doses. *Am J Kidney Dis* 2000;35:89.

Sagedal S, et al. Intermittent saline flushes during haemodialysis do not alleviate coagulation and clot formation in stable patients receiving reduced doses of dalteparin. *Nephrol Dial Transplant* 2006;21:444.

Schwab SJ, et al. Hemodialysis without anticoagulation. One year prospective trial in hospitalized patients at risk for bleeding. *Am J Med* 1987;83:405.

Smith BP, et al. Prediction of anticoagulation during hemodialysis by population kinetics in an artificial neural network. *Artif Organs* 1998;22:731.

Srinivasan AF, et al. Warfarin-induced skin necrosis and venous limb gangrene in the setting of heparin-induced thrombocytopenia. *Arch Int Med* 2004;164:66.

Tang IY, et al. Argatroban and renal replacement therapy in patients with heparin-induced thrombocytopenia. *Ann Pharmacother* 2005;39:231.

Van Der Meulen J, et al. Citrate anticoagulation and dialysate with reduced buffer content in chronic hemodialysis. *Clin Nephrol* 1992;37:36–41.

WEB REFERENCES

Anticoagulants during dialysis: Internet links: http://www.hdcn.com/hd/hepa

Slow Continuous Therapies

Boon Wee Teo, Jennifer S. Messer,
Emil P. Paganini, John T. Daugirdas,
and Todd S. Ing

The popularity of "slow continuous therapies" for the treatment of critically ill patients with renal failure is increasing. The techniques most commonly used are slow continuous hemodialysis and hemodiafiltration. Slow continuous hemofiltration and slow continuous ultrafiltration also are commonly used.

I. **Nomenclature.** In the *Handbook,* we abbreviate slow continuous hemodialysis as C-HD whether it is applied using an arteriovenous or venovenous access. Similarly, slow continuous hemofiltration is abbreviated as C-HF, and their combination, slow continuous hemodiafiltration, is C-HDF. Slow continuous ultrafiltration is abbreviated as SCUF. All these forms of extracorporeal therapies are popularly referred to as continuous renal replacement therapies (CRRTs). Others commonly insert "AV" or "VV" after the letter "C" to specify that the therapy is given using either an arteriovenous or a venovenous access, and these treatments are commonly named CAVHD or CVVHD (hemodialysis), CAVH or CVVH (hemofiltration), and CAVHDF or CVVHDF (hemodiafiltration).

A. **What are the differences among C-HD, C-HF, and C-HDF?** Each of these procedures involves slow, continuous passage of blood, taken from either an arterial or a venous source, through a filter. Table 13-1 shows a comparison of these techniques.

   1. **Continuous hemodialysis (C-HD).** In C-HD (Fig. 13-1), dialysis solution is passed through the dialysate compartment of the filter continuously and at a slow rate. In C-HD, diffusion is the primary method of solute removal. The amount of fluid that must be ultrafiltered across the membrane is low (3–6 L per day) and is limited to excess fluid removal.

   2. **Continuous hemofiltration (C-HF).** In C-HF (Fig. 13-2), dialysis solution is not used. Instead, a large volume (about 25–50 L per day) of replacement fluid is infused into either the inflow or the outflow blood line (predilution or postdilution mode, respectively). With C-HF the volume of fluid that needs to be ultrafiltered across the membrane includes both replacement fluid and excess fluid, and so is much higher than with C-HD.

   3. **Continuous hemodiafiltration (C-HDF).** This (Fig. 13-2) is simply a combination of C-HD and C-HF. Dialysis solution is used, and replacement fluid is also infused into either the inflow or the outflow blood line. The daily volume of fluid that is ultrafiltered across the membrane is high,

Table 13-1. Comparison of techniques

	IHD	SLED	SCUF	C-HF	C-HD	C-HDF
Membrane permeability	Variable	Variable	High	High	High	High
Anticoagulation	Short	Long	Continuous	Continuous	Continuous	Continuous
Blood flow rate (mL per minute)	250–400	100–200	100–200	200–300	100–300	200–300
Dialysate flow rate (mL per minute)	500–800	100	0	0	16–35	16–35
Filtrate (L per day)	0–4	0–4	0–5	24–96	0–4	24–48
Replacement fluid (L per day)	0	0	0	21.6–90	0	23–44
Effluent saturation %	15–40	60–70	100	100	85–100	85–100
Solute clearance mechanism	Diffusion	Diffusion	Convection (minimal)	Convection	Diffusion	Diffusion + convection
Urea clearance (mL per minute)	180–240	75–90	1.7	17–67	22	30–60
Duration (hours)	3–4	8–12	Variable	>24	>24	>24

IHD, intermittent hemodialysis; SLED, sustained, low-efficiency dialysis; SCUF, slow continuous ultrafiltration; C-HF, slow continuous hemofiltration; C-HD, slow continuous hemodialysis; C-HFD, slow continuous hemodiafiltration.
Modified from Metha RL. Continuous renal replacement therapy in the critically ill patient. *Kidney Int* 2005;67:781–795.

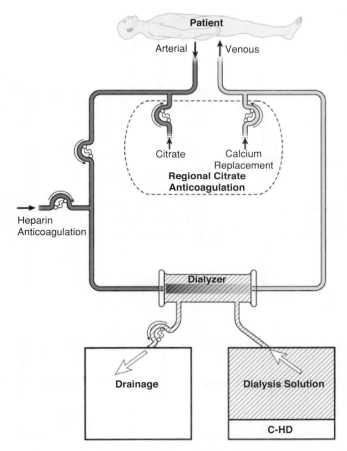

Figure 13-1. Typical circuit for slow continuous hemodialysis. Anticoagulation with either heparin or regional citrate is shown. For slow continuous ultrafiltration, the circuit is the same, except that dialysis solution inflow is not used.

but not as high as with C-HF, as the volume of replacement fluid used in C-HDF typically is much lower than with C-HF.

4. Slow continuous ultrafiltration (SCUF). Setup is similar to that for C-HD and C-HF, but neither dialysis solution nor replacement fluid is used. Daily ultrafiltered fluid volume across the membrane is low (3–6 L per day), similar to C-HD.

B. Sustained, low-efficiency dialysis (SLED). SLED is a form of intermittent hemodialysis using an extended (6- to 10-hour) session length and reduced blood and dialysate flow rates. Typically blood flow rates are about 200 mL per minute and dialysate flow rate is 100–300 mL per minute. Regular

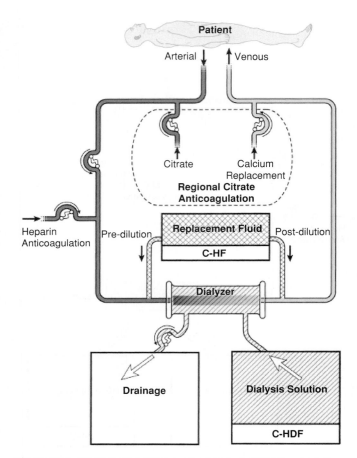

Figure 13-2.   Typical circuit for continuous hemofiltration and slow continuous hemodiafiltration. In slow continuous hemofiltration (C-HF), replacement fluid can be infused in the predilution mode, or postdilution mode, or both simultaneously. In slow continuous hemodiafiltration, hemodialysis is performed concurrently with C-HF. Anticoagulation with either heparin or regional citrate is shown.

hemodialysis equipment can be used, as long as low blood and dialysate flow rates are supported. The same machine used for intermittent hemodialysis (IHD) during the day often can be used for SLED during the night, and hemodialysis nurses can easily be trained to perform SLED, offering some economy of staff instruction. SLED allows units where CRRT equipment or personnel are unavailable to offer a treatment modality that should achieve similar benefits as CRRT.

    1.   SLED-F. Since increased middle molecule solute clearance may be beneficial to critically ill acute renal failure

Table 13-2. Potential advantages of slow continuous therapies

1. Hemodynamically well tolerated; smaller change in plasma osmolality
2. Better control of azotemia and electrolyte and acid–base balance; correct abnormalities as they evolve; steady-state chemistries
3. Highly effective in removing fluid (postsurgery, pulmonary edema, acute respiratory distress syndrome)
4. Facilitates administration of parenteral nutrition and obligatory intravenous medications (i.e., pressor, inotropic drugs) by creating unlimited "space" by virtue of continuous ultrafiltration
5. Less effect on intracranial pressure
6. New user-friendly machines available

patients on CRRT, SLED may not be able to achieve the much higher middle molecule clearance ascribed to truly continuous therapies. This has led to modification of the SLED technique to include infusion of replacement fluid, along with a higher ultrafiltration rate (hence SLED-F) and higher blood and dialysate flows.

II. Clinical indications. The potential advantages of the slow continuous procedures are listed in Table 13-2 and include a lower rate of fluid removal as well as enhanced control of azotemia when compared to standard IHD.

A. Comparisons between CRRT and IHD

1. Despite the seemingly obvious advantages of slow continuous therapies, there has been no evidence from several randomized trials that use of CRRT offers a survival advantage in the acute renal failure setting. Also, with the increasing popularity of daily hemodialysis for intensive care unit (ICU) patients as well as use of SLED, either on a daily or every-other-day basis, some of the advantages of continuous therapies with regard to a reduced rate of fluid removal and amount of delivered clearance become diminished.

III. Training and equipment costs. The use of continuous procedures requires an effort on the part of nursing staff in the ICU to become familiar with the procedures. In units with high staff turnover rates, and in units where continuous therapies are done infrequently, use of intermittent hemodialysis or SLED may be a more practical option. However, in high-volume units where continuous therapies are a common part of the dialysis armamentarium, use of such therapies will greatly aid in the fluid, solute, and nutritional management of the most challenging patients.

IV. Differences among C-HD, C-HF, and C-HDF in clearance of small and large molecular weight solutes

A. Urea clearance with C-HD. In C-HD, where the blood flow rate is 100–150 mL per minute or more, clearance of urea and other small molecules is determined primarily by the dialysis solution flow rate. Outflow dialysate is 90% or more saturated with urea, except when filters begin to clot or when very high dialysate flow rates are used. So urea clearance can be estimated by the total daily filter outflow volume (which includes dialysis solution used, plus any excess fluid removed). The standard dialysis solution inflow rate is now about 25–50 L per day. Thus, taking into account an additional 5 L per day for excess fluid removal, it is easy to achieve urea clearances with C-HD on the order of 30–55 L per day.

Assuming a urea volume of distribution of 40 L for an average-size patient, the daily Kt/V with C-HD can be computed. Assume a clearance of 40 L per day. This is the $(K \times t)$ term of Kt/V. To compute Kt/V, we divide $(K \times t)$ by V (40 L in this case) to get 40/40, or a Kt/V of about 1.0 per day or 7.0 per week. This compares favorably with the Kt/V delivered by thrice-weekly intermittent hemodialysis (usually 3.6 per week). With all CRRT therapies, urea removal is further enhanced (relative to intermittent hemodialysis) because urea clearance is operating continuously while the plasma urea concentration is at a steady-state level.

B.   Urea clearance with C-HF. C-HF is a purely convection-based blood cleansing technique. As blood flows through the hemofilter, a transmembrane pressure gradient between the blood compartment and the ultrafiltrate compartment causes plasma water to be filtered across the highly permeable membrane. As the water crosses the membrane, it convects small and large molecules across the membrane and thus leads to their removal from the blood. The ultrafiltrate is replaced by a balanced electrolyte solution infused into either the inflow (predilution) or the outflow (postdilution) line of the hemofilter.

Typically about 25–50 L of replacement fluid is infused per day. The filter outflow or "drainage fluid" is nearly 100% saturated with urea when postdilution mode is used. At high replacement fluid infusion rates in postdilution mode, the blood flow rate needs to be increased from the usual 100–150 mL per minute to prevent excessive hemoconcentration (and resultant clotting) in the filter. When replacement fluid is given in predilution mode, the drainage fluid will not be 100% saturated, because levels of waste products in the blood entering the filter will be diluted. For example, a replacement fluid infusion rate of 35 L per day is equivalent to 24 mL per minute. If the blood flow rate is 140 mL per minute, the dilution or desaturation will be 24/164 = 15%. Assuming that 35 L per day of replacement fluid is used and that 5 L per day of excess fluid is removed, daily "drainage volume," to borrow a term from the peritoneal dialysis literature, will typically be about 40 L per day. In postdilution mode, Kt will be 40 L. In predilution mode, Kt will be perhaps 15% less, 34 L, and so, assuming $V = 40$ L, then daily Kt/V with C-HF will be about 40/40 = 1.0 (postdilution) or 34/40 = 0.85 (predilution).

C.   Urea clearance with C-HDF. With C-HDF, one can either leave the dialysis solution flow rate high, in which case the replacement fluid infusion will add to the urea clearance, or use a lower dialysis solution flow rate, and make up for this using replacement fluid to achieve similar overall urea clearance, but a higher clearance of middle molecules (see D, below). The clearance calculations are the same, and depend primarily on the daily outflow volume.

D. Small versus large molecular weight solute removal with C-HF versus C-HD. On a milliliter for milliliter basis (plasma ultrafiltrate out vs. dialysate out), C-HF is more efficient than C-HD as a means for solute removal. With both treatments, dialyzer effluent is almost completely saturated with urea, but with C-HD, the outflow dialysate is not completely saturated with higher molecular weight substances because these move slowly in solution and thus have a lower diffusive transfer across the dialyzer membrane. With C-HF, the plasma ultrafiltrate is almost completely saturated with both low and middle molecular weight solutes, because the convective removal rates of small and larger molecular weight solutes are similar. Hence, C-HF is more efficient than C-HD if one considers larger molecules, such as inulin and vitamin B_{12}. However, the theoretical advantage of C-HF is technically demanding to realize, as it can be challenging to ultrafilter >25 L from patients using C-HF techniques. In particular, fluid balancing becomes critical when the replacement fluid infusion rate is high. Furthermore, with high-volume C-HF, any slowing of the blood flow rate will result in transient hemoconcentration in the hemofilter, with attendant risk of clotting. On the other hand, it is easy to perform C-HD using dialysis solution flow rates of 50 L per day. For this reason, in daily practice, C-HD tends to be the more popular therapy, and if enhanced removal of middle molecules is desired, a replacement fluid component is added (C-HDF).

V. Vascular access

A. Venovenous blood access. Vascular access is obtained using a dual-lumen cannula inserted into a large (internal jugular or femoral) vein. Some prefer to use two single lumen catheters separately. The subclavian vein can be used but is not the site of first choice. See Chapter 6.

B. Arteriovenous (AV) blood access. One can cannulate a large artery, usually the femoral artery, and propel blood through the extracorporeal circuit by using the patient's own arterial pressure instead of a pump. Blood is returned via any large vein. Use of AV blood access for CRRT is no longer widely practiced. There is risk of damage to the femoral artery with possible distal limb ischemia, plus AV access will often not deliver high enough blood flows to be able to support the more intensive CRRT therapies in common use today. However, CRRT using AV access may be lifesaving in situations where a mass catastrophe has occurred (e.g., earthquake with renal injury due to rhabdomyolysis) and electrical power sources are unreliable, since blood flow is then driven by a patient's own blood pressure and ultrafiltration is adjusted by using gravity via the height of the effluent collection container. For a detailed description of CRRT using an AV access, please refer to the third edition of the *Handbook*.

C. Catheter changes: Scheduled changes versus changing only when clinically indicated. CRRT catheters should be changed only if clinically indicated, and not changed according to some predetermined schedule in the hopes of minimizing the rate of catheter sepsis. The practice of routine, scheduled catheter changes, once popular, is not recommended by the Centers for Disease Control and Prevention (CDC) and studies do not support this approach.

VI. CRRT filters

A. Nomenclature. The terms "hemofilter" and "dialyzer" are used interchangeably in this chapter. Hemofilters initially had only one outlet in the housing, making use of dialysis solution impossible. Subsequently, a second port was added.

B. Choosing a dialyzer or hemofilter. The choice of a hemofilter or hemodialyzer depends somewhat on whether C-HD, C-HDF, or C-HF is being contemplated.

 1. **A water permeability coefficient (K_{Uf}).** For C-HF, where all small-molecule clearance will need to come from fluid ultrafiltered across the membrane, a high ultrafiltration rate will be required, and a higher membrane water permeability is a must, particularly when using a non-pumped system. For example, K_{Uf} should be at least 12 mL per hour per mm Hg for such treatments.

 2. **Dialyzer diffusivity is important when C-HD, SLED, or C-HDF is used.** If a diffusive method of solute transport is to be used (C-HD or C-HDF), then the layout of the membrane– dialysate interface in the filter becomes important. Some of the early devices designed primarily for C-HF had excellent water permeability and convective solute clearance, but had poor diffusive clearance when used for C-HD; there was poor optimization of contact between dialysis solution and all parts of the membrane in these filters. Practically all currently used CRRT filters allow urea in the blood compartment of the filter to equilibrate promptly with dialysate.

 3. **Filter surface area and size.** Contrary to regular hemodialysis, because of the low blood flow rates used in C-HD, there is no advantage in terms of clearance to use a large, high-efficiency dialyzer. The risk of clotting in large dialyzers may be increased, as they have been designed for much higher blood flow rates than those used in C-HD, and flow velocity through each fiber will be relatively decreased. Larger dialyzers can be used if higher blood flow rates are to be used, such as in some higher-efficiency SLED protocols, in order to maximize middle molecule solute clearances.

VII. Dialysis and replacement solutions. Premixed dialysis and replacement solutions are available as commercially prepared, sterile fluids, typically packaged in 2.5-L or 5-L bags. For example, Prismasate (Gambro Renal Products, Lakewood, CO) comes in a variety of fluid compositions, differing in calcium, magnesium, potassium, and bicarbonate concentrations. A lactate-based preparation is also available. Normocarb (B. Braun Medical, Inc., Bethlehem, PA) is a bicarbonate concentrate in a 240-mL vial; when injected into a 3-L sterile water bag, it will produce a calcium-free, bicarbonate-based dialysis solution. Alternatively, customized solutions can be prepared in the pharmacy, or by the dialysis machine method (see Leblanc et al., 1995). Commercially produced and pharmacy-made solutions have an advantage in that they can be used for infusion into the blood line, thus permitting their use in C-HF and C-HDF. Ultrapure dialysis solution produced by dialysis machines can only be used for C-HDF in those countries where regulatory approval for online hemodiafiltration has been granted.

A. Composition. Table 13-3 lists the concentrations of solutes in some commercially available solutions used for C-HD.

    1. Sodium. The sodium concentration of some commercial solutions is only 130–132 mM. To these solutions, 2 mL of hypertonic (23.4%) sodium chloride (4 mmol/mL) should be added to each liter to raise the sodium concentration to approximately 140 mM. When hypertonic trisodium citrate is used for anticoagulation, one can offset its high sodium concentration by using an ultralow (117 mM) sodium replacement solution. This is made by starting with a 5-L bag containing 0.45% saline, and then adding sufficient 23% sodium chloride to adjust the sodium level to 117 mM.

    2. Alkali. The choice of alkali depends on the clinical situation and availability (bicarbonate solutions are harder to prepare and store). Both lactate and bicarbonate can correct metabolic acidosis as lactate is metabolized to bicarbonate.

        a. Bicarbonate solutions. Bicarbonate has become the buffer of choice. Bicarbonate concentrations are typically 22–35 mM. When a higher dialysis solution flow rate (2 L per hour or more) is prescribed, levels of 32 mM or less may be indicated to prevent metabolic alkalosis. Lower bicarbonate concentrations are also indicated when using regional citrate anticoagulation, since citrate is metabolized to bicarbonate by the liver.

        b. Lactate solutions. Available lactate concentrations range from 28 to 49 mM. Use of lactate solutions often requires either a higher concentration of lactate or intravenous bicarbonate supplementation to achieve the desired target serum bicarbonate level. Blood lactate levels are generally higher when lactate-based solutions are used, complicating their use as a monitoring tool in intensive care patients. Hyperlactatemia can become pronounced during high-volume treatments and in patients with liver dysfunction. "Lactate intolerance" during CRRT is defined arbitrarily as a >5 mmol/L rise in serum lactate levels. This may trigger a decision to switch to bicarbonate-based therapy. In any event, bicarbonate-based fluids are preferred in patients with lactic acidosis and/or liver failure. Whether bicarbonate-based fluids are associated with more hemodynamic stability is controversial, although some studies show a benefit in this regard (e.g., Barenbrock et al., 2000).

        c. Acetate solutions. For some people who cannot bring themselves to use lactate-based solutions, acetate-containing Ringer solution can be also used. In the C-HF

Table 13-3. Composition of some continuous renal replacement therapy solutions

Component (mM)	Dialysis Machine Generated[a]	Peritoneal Dialysis Fluid[b]	Lactated Ringer Solution	Accusol[b] (2.5-L bag)	Prismasate[c] (5-L bag)	Prisma-sate-L[c] (5-L bag)	Nxstage[d] (5-L bag)	Nxstage[d] (5-L bag)	Normo-carb[e]
Sodium	140	132	130	140	140	140	140	140	140
Potassium	Variable	—	4	0 or 2 or 4	0 or 2 or 4	0	0 or 2 or 4	1 or 3	0
Chloride	Variable	96	109	109.5–116.3	108–120.5	109	109–113	100–112	106
Bicarbonate	Variable	—	—	30 or 35	22 or 32	—	35	—	35
Calcium	Variable	1.75 (3.5 mEq/L)	1.35 (2.7 mEq/L)	1.4 or 1.75 (2.8 or 3.5 mEq/L)	0 or 1.25 or 1.75 (0 or 2.5 or 3.5 mEq/L)	1.25 (2.5 mEq/L)	1.5 (3.0 mEq/L)	1.5 (3.0 mEq/L)	0.75 (1.5 mEq/L)
Magnesium	0.75 (1.5 mEq/L)	0.25 (0.5 mEq/L)	—	0.5 or 0.75 (1.0 or 1.5 mEq/L)	0.5 or 0.75 (1.0 or 1.5 mEq/L)	0.75 (1.5 mEq/L)	0.5 (1.0 mEq/L)	0.5 (1.0 mEq/L)	0.75 (1.5 mEq/L)
Lactate	2	40	28	0	3	35	0	35, 40, 45	0

Glucose (mg per dL)	100	1,360	—	0 or 110	0 or 110	110	100	100
Glucose (mM)	5.5	75.5	—	0 or 6.1	0 or 6.1	6.1	5.5	5.5
Preparation method	6-L bag via membrane filtration	Premix	Premix	Two-compartment bag	Two-compartment bag	Premix	Two-compartment bag	Vial mix added to 3-L sterile water bag
Sterility	No	Yes	Yes	Yes	Yes	Yes	Yes	Yes

aFrom Leblanc M, et al. Bicarbonate dialysate for continuous renal replacement therapy in intensive care unit patients with acute renal failure. *Am J Kidney Dis* 1995;26:910–917.
bBaxter Healthcare Corp., McGaw Park, IL.
cGambro Renal Products, Lakewood, CO.
dNxstage Medical, Inc., Lawrence, MA.
eB. Braun Medical, Inc., Bethlehem, PA.

setting at least, acetate does not seem to have adverse hemodynamic effects, probably because the amount of acetate infused per unit time is much lower than that absorbed during conventional, acetate-based hemodialysis.

3. Glucose (MW 180 dalton). Different dialysis solution dextrose (glucose monohydrate, MW 198 dalton) concentrations are available, ranging from 0.10% dextrose in commercial hemodiafiltration fluid to 1.5%–4.25% dextrose in peritoneal dialysis fluids adapted for use with continuous extracorporeal therapies. Use of high glucose–containing fluids results in an uptake of 1,300–2,400 glucose-derived kilocalories per day from the dialysis solution. Because of the rapid dissipation of the dialysate–blood glucose concentration gradient, increasing the concentration of dextrose to 4.25% in the dialysis solution does not result in much increased osmotic removal of fluid from the blood compartment of the dialyzer. However, use of a high dialysis solution glucose concentration may result in hyperglycemia and necessitate use of an insulin drip to control blood glucose levels.

B. Methods of preparing bicarbonate-based CRRT solutions when prepackaged solutions are not available. One can prepare sterile dialysis/replacement fluid manually to achieve solutions containing 30–35 mM bicarbonate. Bicarbonate is in equilibrium with carbonic acid, which breaks down to CO_2 and H_2O; therefore, bicarbonate solutions are unstable. Bicarbonate also forms insoluble salts when in solution with calcium and magnesium. Therefore, bicarbonate-based dialysis/replacement solutions should be prepared just before use.

1. Single-bag method. Dialysis or replacement solution containing bicarbonate and no lactate is made by adding (usually this is done by the hospital pharmacy service) $NaHCO_3$ and some additional NaCl to 0.45% NaCl obtained commercially. A small amount of $CaCl_2.2H_2O$ is added as well, and magnesium is given parenterally as needed.

Formulation: 1.0 L of 0.45% NaCl + 35 mL of 8.4% $NaHCO_3$ (35 mol) + 10 mL of 23% NaCl (40 mmol) + 2.1 mL of 10% $CaCl_2.2H_2O$ (1.45 mmol or 2.9 mEq); total volume 1.047 L.

Final concentrations in mM: Na 145, Cl 114, HCO_3 33, and Ca 1.35 (2.7 mEq/L)

2. Two-bag method. Bags of 0.9% saline with added calcium are alternated with bags of 0.45% saline with added bicarbonate.

Formulation: *Solution A:* 1.0 L of 0.9% saline + 4.1 mL of 10% $CaCl_2.2H_2O$ (2.8 mmol or 5.6 mEq) *Solution B:* 1.0 L of 0.45% saline + 75 mL of 8.4% $NaHCO_3$ (75 mmol); total volume 2.079 L.

Final concentrations in mM (when considered together): Na 147, Cl 114, HCO_3 36, and Ca 1.35 (2.7 mEq/L).

3. Dialysis machine method (C-HD only). One can also prepare bicarbonate-containing dialysis solution for C-HD by ultrafiltering dialysis solution prepared by a standard dialysis machine across a dialyzer (to remove bacteria) and storing the solution in a 15-L sterile drainage bag from a peritoneal dialysis cycler. Such solutions should be used promptly after preparation. This technique has since been modified by storing solutions in more convenient 6-L sterile bags. The fluid preparation does not show growth of bacteria for at least 72 hours and for up to 1 month in tests. Routinely, however, the bags were discarded if not used within 72 hours of preparation by protocol. In 10 years of use, there have been no reported adverse events, and Limulus Amebocyte Lysate assays for endotoxin are reliably below the limit of detection. (Teo et al., 2006)

C. Sterility. Sterile dialysis solution is used for C-HD and C-HDF because the slow dialysate transit time plus the extended time of use of the same circuit and dialyzer could otherwise encourage bacterial growth in the dialysate circuit. All replacement fluid infusions, given directly into the blood lines, must be sterile.

D. Temperature of dialysis solution/replacement fluid. Up until recently, most CRRT was set up so that dialysis solution and replacement fluid were infused at room temperature. This is a departure from conventional dialysis, where dialysis solution is warmed and use of room temperature fluid results in heat subtraction from the patient. In fact, the hemodynamic benefits of CRRT appear to be due largely to such thermal cooling effects. When applied over long periods, CRRT-associated heat subtraction may mask the presence of fever, thus reducing the reliability of body temperature as a marker for infection or inflammation. Whether this heat subtraction has an effect on the body's ability to resist infection has not been studied. Recent CRRT delivery systems have heating systems. Heating sometimes is associated with an appearance of bubbles in the replacement or dialysis solutions, especially with bicarbonate formulations; the biochemical and clinical significance of this effect remains to be determined. One study done in a septic shock model using sheep suggested that warming of blood in the extracorporeal circuit increased survival rate (Rogiers et al., 2006).

VIII. Prescribing and delivering CRRT

A. Predilution versus postdilution mode of replacement fluid infusion (for C-HF and C-HDF). Replacement fluid can be infused either into the arterial blood line leading to the hemofilter (predilution) or into the venous blood line leaving the hemofilter (postdilution). The standard method is postdilution. However, when using postdilution at high fluid removal rates (more than 25 L per day), the blood in the hemofilter can become concentrated as its water is rapidly removed, leading to difficulty in obtaining adequate ultrafiltration and to increased resistance in the blood flow pathway (which can lead to poor blood flow and clotting). As a rule of thumb, in postdilution mode, the ultrafiltration rate should not exceed 20% of the plasma flow rate. The problem can be solved by increasing the blood flow rate to 150–200 mL per minute, or by using the predilution mode. With predilution there is slight lowering of the urea concentration of ultrafiltrate (usually 80%–90% of the corresponding plasma value), but this is outweighed by the ability to deliver an increased replacement solution infusion rate, enhancing overall middle molecule clearances.

We recommend using predilution whenever it is desirable to remove more than 25 L per day. Predilution is also performed if the baseline blood viscosity is relatively elevated (e.g., if the hematocrit is >35%). Combination pre- and postdilution has been advocated by some practitioners.

B.   Dose versus outcome. Adequacy or dose of dialysis for acutely ill patients in an ICU setting has not been defined. One large, prospective, randomized study using C-HF found that, for a 70-kg patient, increasing the daily ultrafiltrate volume from 36 L per day to about 60 L per day resulted in a substantial reduction in mortality (Ronco et al., 2000), but this result was not confirmed in a subsequent trial (Brause et al., 2003). The issue of dialysis and CRRT dosing in ICU patients is currently the subject of a large study, the Veterans Administration/National Institutes of Health (VA/NIH) Acute Renal Failure Trial Network (ATN) study. Among the comparisons being studied in a randomized, prospective fashion are C-HDF at 20 mL/kg per hour versus 35 mL/kg per hour (about 35 vs. 60 L per day in a 70-kg patient).

C.   Empiric dosing. A "standard" or starting C-HD prescription for an adult patient of usual size would be to use 1.5 L per hour of inflow dialysis solution (36 L per day). If one is a believer in the importance of removal of molecules larger than urea, one can use a C-HDF approach and divide up this 36 L into 24 L of dialysis solution and 12 L of replacement fluid.

After factoring in removal of 4 L per day excess fluid, either of these approaches should result in a daily urea clearance of about 40 L per day. In hypercatabolic patients, this amount of urea removal will be insufficient to maintain a serum urea nitrogen (SUN) in the 40–60 mg/dL (14–21 mmol/L) range, and the dialysis solution inflow rate can be increased further, to as high as 70 L per day, if desired. In patients with normal or reduced rates of urea generation, provision of 40 L per day of clearance by continuous therapy will result in steady-state SUN levels well below 40–60 mg/dL (14–21 mmol/L). Residual renal function, if present, will also result in relatively low SUN levels. Our approach, however, even in patients with relatively low SUN levels, is to maintain 40 L per day dialysate/replacement fluid inflow, under the assumption that not all uremic toxins are represented by urea, and that residual renal function will not be reliably present.

D.   Kinetic dosing. Despite the difficulties with estimating urea generation rate and distribution volume, urea kinetic approaches can be used to prescribe CRRT when a desired target level of SUN is desired. However, it should be kept in mind that such a strategy may not be ideal for all patients, the biggest risk being undertreatment of patients with a low urea generation rate.

1. **Six steps to estimating the prescription**
   a. Estimate or measure the patient's **urea generation rate.**
   b. Decide on the **desired level of SUN.**
   c. Calculate the **total urea clearance** necessary to keep the SUN at the desired level for the urea generation rate obtained from step 1.
   d. Measure **residual renal urea clearance.** If desired, subtract this from the total urea clearance to obtain the **extracorporeal urea clearance** that will be required.
   e. Calculate the **required drainage fluid volume.** Set this equal to the required extracorporeal urea clearance, assuming 100% saturation. Exception: With predilution C-HF or with C-HD when using a dialysis solution inflow rate >2 L per hour, the urea saturation of the drainage fluid will be <100%. In such cases, the required "drainage volume" should be increased appropriately (usually by 15%–20%), based on a measurement of percent saturation.
   f. Calculate the **required dialysis solution/replacement fluid inflow rate.** This is simply equal to the required drainage volume minus the **expected removal (L per day) of excess fluid.**

2. **Sample problem:** A **60-kg** male patient has an SUN of **40** mg/dL (14 mmol/L) on day 1 and **65** mg/dL (23 mmol/L) on day 2. A 24-hour urine collection from day 1 to day 2 contains **5 g** (178 mmol) of urea nitrogen. On day 2, weight has increased to **64 kg.** Estimated edema fluid is **8 L** on day 1 and is **12 L** on day 2. Calculate the clearance necessary to maintain the SUN at 40 mg/dL (14 mmol/L).

   Solution:
   a. Determine urea nitrogen generation rate.
   (1) Estimate initial and final total-body water.
   Initial total-body water: Initial weight is 60 kg with 8 kg estimated edema fluid. Edema-free weight is then 52 kg. Estimate total-body water as 55% of the "edema-free" weight.
   Total-body water therefore is 8 L + (0.55 × 52) = 8 L + 28.6 L = **36.6 L.**
   Final total-body water: Final weight is 64 kg, or 4 kg higher, all of which is water, so final total-body water is 36.6 + 4 = **40.6 L.**
   (2) Estimate initial and final total-body urea nitrogen.
   (i) Initial and final SUN levels are 40 mg/dL and 65 mg/dL, respectively (about 14 and 23 mmol/L).
   (ii) Total-body urea nitrogen at time 1 = 36.6 L × 0.40 g/L = 14.6 g.
   In SI units: Total-body urea at time 1 = 36.6 L × 14.3 mmol/L = 523 mmol.
   (iii) Total-body urea nitrogen at time 2 = 40.6 L × 0.65 g /L = 26.4 g.
   In SI units: Total-body nitrogen at time 2 = 40.6 × 23.2 mmol/L = 942 mmol.

(3) Calculate change in total body urea nitrogen.

(i) Change in total-body urea nitrogen content from time 1 to time 2 is 26.4 g – 14.6 g = 11.75 g urea nitrogen (or, in SI units, 942 – 523 mmol = 420 mmol).

(ii) This 11.75-g change in urea nitrogen now needs to be corrected to a daily basis. If time 1 and time 2 are 24 hours apart, then the change in body urea nitrogen content is ~11.75 g per day (420 mmol per day).

(4) Account for urinary losses. Urinary urea nitrogen loss during the 24-hour observation period was measured to be 5 g per day (178 mmol per day).

(5) Calculate urea nitrogen generation rate. This is equal to 11.75 + 5 = 16.75 g per day (or, in SI units, 420 + 178 = 598 mmol per day).

b.   Decide on a target SUN level. As discussed above, let's say it should be 40 mg/dL (14.3 mmol/L).

c.   Calculate desired total clearance. Assume target SUN = 40 mg/dL = 0.40 g/L.

Urea N removal = clearance (K_D) × serum level = K_D × 0.40 g/L

At steady state, urea generation = removal, $16.75 = K_D$ × 0.40

K_D = (16.75 g per day)/(0.40 g/L) = **42 L per day**

In SI units: Assume target serum urea = 14.3 mmol/L.

Urea N removal = clearance (K_D) × serum level = K_D × 14.3 mmol/L

At steady state, urea generation = removal, $598 = K_D$ × 14.3

K_D = (598 mmol per day)/(14.3 mmol/L) = **42 L per day**

d.   Adjust for residual renal function. This patient actually had a urea clearance of about 10 L per day (about 7 mL per minute), so we can subtract this from the required total clearance. So required extracorporeal clearance is 32 L per day.

e.   Determine dialysis solution inflow rate. This should be 32 L per day (assuming 100% saturation) minus the volume of excess fluid removal. For example, if we need to remove 3 L of fluid per day to offset hyperalimentation and fluid given with medications, subtract 3 L from 32 L in the example to obtain a required dialysate inflow rate of 29 L per day. We usually ignore residual renal function, since this may be ephemeral, and so we would add back the 10 L per day and use a dialysis solution inflow rate of 39 L per day.

3.   Nomogram method. There are graphical methods that simplify these calculations. Thus, if one knows the urea generation rate and sets a goal steady-state SUN, the required clearance can be read from a graph as created by Garred and shown in Figure 13-3. In the present example, 17 g per day = 17,000 mg per 1,440 minutes = 12 mg per minutes of urea nitrogen generation. To use the nomogram in Fig. 13-3, one starts with the desired SUN level on the vertical axis (40 mg/dL) and then one extends a horizontal

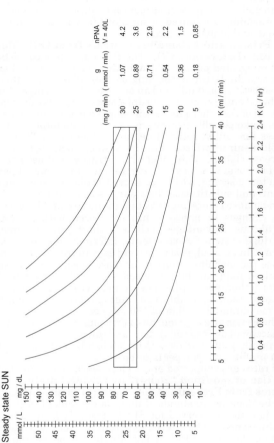

Figure 13-3.   Estimated total extracorporeal urea clearance required to attain various steady-state serum levels of urea nitrogen. Clearance, on the bottom, is read from the intersection of the urea nitrogen generation level (g) and the steady-state goal serum urea nitrogen. (From Garred LJ. Syllabus of the Second International Conference on CRRT, San Diego, CA, Feb 9, 1997, p. 7.)

line to the right until it intersects with the middle of the space between the curved lines representing g = 15 mg per minute and g = 10 mg per minute. Finally, one drops from this point to the horizontal axis to find the required drainage volume flow rate, in this case, about 1.8 L per hour, or 43 L per day.

IX. Equipment

A. Equipment. Considerations on the choice of CRRT equipment include the type of treatment modality chosen, whether blood warming is required, what blood flow rates need to be achieved, and dialyzer choices.

1. Prisma and Prismaflex systems from CGH Medical Inc. (Lakewood, CO). The Prisma system consists of four integrated pumps (blood, dialysate, effluent, and substitution fluid), three weighing devices (dialysate, effluent, and substitution fluid), and an anticoagulant syringe. When the blood pump stops (because of a pressure alarm, for example), all of the other pumps will stop. Four pressure-sensing pods make possible noninvasive pressure monitoring of the access line, filter, return line, and effluent line. There are no blood–air interfaces in the blood line, a feature that may decrease clotting. Control of ultrafiltration and net patient fluid removal is achieved using an integrated control panel with touch screen, which regulates the dialysis solution, effluent, and substitution fluid pump speeds. Filter clotting, fluid balance errors, air detection in the circuit, blood leaks, and changes in pressure are monitored with appropriate alarms. Advantages include a short priming time, a cartridge system for easy setup, informative screens, and alarms. In general, it is relatively easy to train ICU nurses to use the machine. Sources for dialysis solution and substitution fluid can be connected separately. One can also perform therapeutic plasma exchange with an optional cartridge system. A possible disadvantage of this system is the low maximum blood flow of 180 mL per minute.

The **Prismaflex** system has a fifth pump for prefilter fluid replacement or anticoagulation, and can perform simultaneous prefilter and postfilter C-HF up to 8 L per hour (4 L per hour prefilter and 4 L per hour postfilter). Also, higher blood flow rates are supported and a blood warmer is available.

2. Use of modified "2008H" or "2008K" dialysis machines from Fresenius USA (Walnut Creek, CA). C-HD can be done using standard dialysis equipment, although this is usually reserved for SLED. For C-HD, the dialysis machines need to be altered to permit delivery of a dialysis solution flow rate of 100 mL per minute, and potassium usually needs to be added to the dialysis solution. Blood lines and dialyzers are replaced every 24 hours. For SLED using this setup, blood flow rates of 200–300 mL per minute and dialysis solution flow rates of 300–400 mL per minute are used. SLED is done for 6–12 hours every day, with a rest period every night (see Kumar et al., 2000).

3. Use of upgraded "2008K" dialysis machines from Fresenius USA (Walnut Creek, CA). Further advancements have been introduced to allow C-HD to become an integrated treatment option without any machine alteration. Use is similar to that of the modified "2008H" machine, with dialysis solution flow rates between 100 and 300 mL per minute. Ultrafiltration or variable sodium profiles are not available and there is no ultrafiltrate time or target goal to set. The extracorporeal circuit, including dialyzer, should be replaced every 48 hours per manufacturer's recommendations.

4. **NxStage System One from NxStage Medical Inc. (Lawrence, MA).** This is a modular system that can be used as a portable home hemodialysis machine or as an ICU CRRT machine with enhancements including a touch-sensitive information screen, a fluid warmer, and a flash memory–based treatment history recorder. The key features include a drop-in cartridge design with or without a preattached filter, which minimizes machine contamination and disinfection. The cartridge has volume chambers for volumetric fluid balancing, thus eliminating the need for scales, and discharges effluent directly into the drain. By obviating the need to empty effluent collection bags, this design is considerably less labor intensive and offers a significant advantage over other CRRT machines.

5. **Braun Diapact from B. Braun Medical Inc. (Bethlehem, PA).** The Diapact CRRT system is a simple and compact dialysis unit originally designed for use in emergency situations where a purified water supply was not available. It operates on a three-pump system (blood, dialysis/infusion solution, and ultrafiltration) and an electronic single weighing cell. This machine also features a simplified user interface, an integrated fluid plate warmer, and choice of dialyzer capabilities. Flexible treatment options other than CRRT include intermittent hemodialysis and hemofiltration, as well as plasma exchange and plasma absorption/perfusion therapies.

6. **Accura from Baxter Heathcare (Deerfield, IL).** This system operates on four pumps incorporating three circuits—the extracorporeal (blood) circuit, filtrate circuit, and replacement fluid/dialysate circuit—and allows for a choice of dialyzers. It uses a weighing scale system, and is designed as a two-channel (control and protective) system for patient safety. Advantages of this machine include blood flow rates of up to 450 mL per minute, fluid exchange rates of up to 10 L per hour, an integrated fluid warmer and heparin pump, a preattached tubing set for easy priming, and a navigational information screen. Flexible treatment options include simultaneous pre- and postfilter replacement fluid infusion, therapeutic plasma exchange, and hemoperfusion therapies (although hemoperfusion using the Accura has not been approved in the United States). Hemodiafiltration can also be performed, but it requires a single source for both dialysis and replacement solutions due to tubing set design.

B. **Equipment for CRRT using an unpumped, AV access.** When a femoral circuit is used to obtain spontaneously driven blood flow, ultrafiltration is controlled simply by adjusting the height of the dialysate-side collection container. See the third edition of the *Handbook* for details.

C.   Setting the ultrafiltration rate

   1.   Automated modern systems. With most of the above equipment configurations, the ultrafiltration rate is simply "dialed in," and the machine achieves this as the difference between the drainage fluid outflow rate and the dialysis or replacement solution inflow rate. Scales or volumetric measurements reduce deviations from prescribed rates of ultrafiltration by automatically adjusting the pumps.

   2.   More primitive systems. For a detailed discussion, see the third edition of the *Handbook*. With some of the earlier equipment, one needs to manually adjust rates of the dialysate compartment outflow pump and the pump infusing either dialysis solution or replacement fluid. The two-pump method is limited to fluid infusion and/or ultrafiltration rates of about 20 L per day. Small errors in the dialysate inflow and outflow pumps can combine to generate a large error in the net amount of fluid removed from the patient. The output of many pumps is affected by the amount of negative or positive pressure present in the pump inflow and outflow lines. One should always monitor the patient's weight on a daily basis and compare the fluid removal rates as estimated from pump settings with actual weight loss. An alternative is to weigh the dialysis solution bags prior to infusion and compare this to the weight of the drainage bags.

D.   Anticoagulation. In most patients at low risk of bleeding, systemic heparin is routinely used as it is inexpensive and easy to implement. In immediate postoperative patients or patients at high risk of bleeding, heparin-free CRRT can be done, or else regional citrate anticoagulation (RCA) can be used. In patients with heparin-induced thrombocytopenia (HIT type I), RCA may also be employed. However, systemic anticoagulation therapy is often required in patients with HIT type II. These patients have venous or arterial thrombosis in addition to the thrombocytopenia. Systemic anticoagulation with lepirudin and argatroban have been described in these patients who also require CRRT.

   1.   Heparin. After attachment of the primed hemofilter or dialyzer, if baseline clotting times are not elevated, 2,000–5,000 units of heparin is injected into the patient using ideally the venous blood line. It is best to wait for 2–3 minutes to allow the heparin to mix with the patient's blood. Then, immediately, a constant infusion of heparin (at a rate of 500–1,000 units per hour) is begun via an intravenous infusion pump into the arterial line and blood flow through the extracorporeal circuit is begun. Heparin therapy is monitored as per Table 13-4.

   2.   Heparin-free method. In patients with liver disease, in postoperative patients, in patients with active or recent bleeding, or in patients with heparin-induced thrombocytopenia, CRRT can be performed without heparin, although the filter will clot periodically and need to be changed at more frequent intervals. If acute bleeding occurs while CRRT with heparin is being performed, the procedure can

Table 13-4. Heparin protocol for continuous therapies

1. *Initial therapy:* Heparin in priming and rinsing solution as described in text. At start of procedure, give 2,000–5,000 IU heparin to the patient via the venous line or other access. Wait 2–3 minutes for the heparin to mix with the circulation. Then start 500–1,000 IU per hour constant heparin infusion into the arterial (inlet) blood line.
2. *Monitoring:* PTT measured at the arterial and venous blood lines every 6 hours.
    Maintain arterial PTT 40–45 seconds.
    Maintain venous PTT >65 seconds.
    If arterial PTT >45 seconds, decrease heparin by 100 IU per hour.
    If venous PTT <65 seconds, increase heparin by 100 IU per hour, but only if arterial PTT <45 seconds.
    If arterial PTT <40 seconds, increase heparin by 200 IU per hour.

PTT, partial thromboplastin time.

be continued even after heparin administration has been stopped.

When heparin is not given, several steps may be taken to reduce the likelihood of clotting.

a. With C-HD, the dialysis solution inflow rate is increased by 20%–40%. The higher dialysate flow rate will compensate for the anticipated loss of clearance as the unheparinized dialyzer slowly clots. When using the heparin-free method for C-HD, we usually do not infuse saline into the arterial blood line on a periodic basis, in contrast to what is commonly practiced in the case of heparin-free intermittent hemodialysis.

b. In C-HF, predilution mode is preferred since prefilter fluid replacement reduces the hemoconcentration within the hemofilter when plasma water is removed. For C-HF done using an arterial access, using a larger-bore dialysis catheter (size 13.5 Fr) allows higher spontaneous blood flows of 200 mL per minute or more, and may also prevent early or excessive clotting.

When no heparin is used in patients without coagulation disturbances, the dialyzers will usually clot within 8 hours. A sign of early clotting is a reduction to <0.8 in the ratio of dialysate to serum urea nitrogen levels. When the ratio is <0.6, clotting is imminent.

3. Regional citrate anticoagulation (RCA). ACD-A solution (anticoagulant citrate dextrose form A) containing 3% trisodium citrate (2.2 g/mL 100 mL), citric acid (0.73 g/mL 100 mL), and dextrose (2.45 g/mL 100 mL) (Baxter-Fenwal Healthcare Corp., Deerfield, IL, USA) is preferred over trisodium citrate for routine RCA, as ACD-A is commercially prepared and is less hypertonic, thus potentially reducing mixing errors and dangers of overinfusion.

Many RCA protocols have been described for CRRT. The major complications of RCA are symptomatic reductions in serum ionized calcium levels and metabolic alkalosis from citrate metabolism.

We prefer RCA methods that minimize the amount of citrate infused, and these typically use calcium-free dialysis or replacement fluids, since the citrate infusion needs only to counteract the calcium in the patient's blood. Methods of RCA have been reported where calcium is maintained in the replacement fluid or the dialysis solution (Mitchell et al., 2003). These have an advantage of avoiding the return of a low-ionized calcium infusate close to the heart in the event that the calcium replacement solution pump fails.

   a. **Swartz protocol (Fig. 13-4).** As an example, here is a procedure for RCA in C-HD according to Swartz et al. (2004).

   (1) Attach the ACD-A 1,000-mL bag to an infusion pump infusing into the arterial line closest to the patient. A negative pressure valve is inserted into this line so that the infusion will occur in the direction of the blood pump and not directly into the patient should the blood pump stop. The rate of infusion in mL per hour is initially at 1.5 times the blood flow rate (BFR) in mL per minute. For example, when the BFR is set at 200 mL per minute, the citrate rate will then be 300 mL per hour.

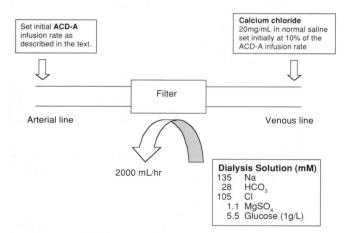

Figure 13-4. Circuit diagram for citrate slow continuous hemodialysis. The MgSO$_4$ level has been modified to 1.1 mM (versus 1.3 mM as originally depicted in the Swartz publication). (From Swartz R, et al. Improving the delivery of continuous renal replacement therapy using regional citrate anticoagulation. *Clin Nephrol* 2004;61:134–143.)

(2) A calcium chloride infusion (20 mg/mL in normal saline) is infused via a three-way stopcock valve placed at the venous port of the dialysis catheter. Initial calcium infusion rate should be set at 10% of the ACD-A infusion rate. For example, if the ACD-A rate is 300 mL per hour, then calcium infusion rate is 30 mL per hour. **(3)** Ionized calcium is sampled every 2 hours × 4, then every 4 hours × 4 for the first 24 hours, then every 6–8 hours thereafter. The ionized calcium should be checked within 1–2 hours whenever the site of the infusion or tubing is changed. The ionized calcium samples should be drawn from two sites and labeled carefully, one being "postfilter" from the postfilter venous sample port and the other from the patient via a systemic arterial or a venous line. Basic chemistries and total calcium should be checked every 6–8 hours. The titration of ACD-A citrate and calcium chloride infusions are done according to Table 13-5.

4. The dialysis solution is calcium free and contains sodium 135 mM, magnesium (in the form of magnesium sulfate) 1.1 mM (2.2 mEq/L), bicarbonate 28 mM, chloride 105 mM, sulfate 1.1 mM, and glucose 5.5 mM (1 g/L). The lower concentrations of sodium and bicarbonate help to counteract the tonicity and bicarbonate delivery from the infusion of ACD-A. Dialysis solution flow rate is 2.0 L per hour. Note:

Table 13-5. ACD-A citrate and calcium titration guidelines (for Swartz RCA protocol)

Postfilter Ionized Calcium (mM)	Adjustment of ACD-A Rate
<0.20	Reduce rate by 5 mL per hour
0.20–0.40	No adjustment
0.40–0.50	Increase rate by 5 mL per hour
>0.50	Increase rate by 10 mL per hour

Calcium chloride infusion is titrated to **systemic** ionized calcium level.

Systemic Ionized Calcium (mmol/L)	Adjustment of Calcium Infusion
>1.45	Reduce rate by 10 mL per hour
1.21–1.45	Reduce rate by 5 mL per hour
1.01–1.20	No adjustment
0.90–1.00	Increase rate by 5 mL per hour
<0.90	10 mg/kg calcium chloride bolus; increase rate by 10 mL per hour

ACD-A, Anticoagulant Citrate Dextrose Form A; RCA, regional citrate anticoagulation.

Table 13-6.   Dosing parameters for continuous renal replacement therapy with lepirudin or argatroban

	Lepirudin	Argatroban
Infusion rate	Initiate at 0.005–0.01 mg/kg per hour	Initiate at 0.5–1.0 mcg/kg per minute; start at lower does in patient with hepatic dysfunction
Monitoring test	aPTT	aPTT
Target	1.5–2.0 times normal	1.5–2.0 times normal

aPTT, activated partial thromboplastin time.

The dialysis solution magnesium concentration (1.1 mM) in the method shown is higher than that of most other available solutions (0.5–0.75 mM, Table 13-3).

5.   Anticoagulation with lepirudin and argatroban. See Table 13-6 for dosing parameters. Lepirudin (recombinant hirudin) and argatroban are direct thrombin inhibitors. Lepirudin is mainly eliminated by the kidneys. The dose has to be adjusted according to residual renal clearance and dialysis clearance. It can be administered as a continuous infusion or as repetitive boluses. Typical doses are 0.005–0.025 mg/kg body weight per hour. The anticoagulation effect is monitored by measuring the activated partial thromboplastin time (aPTT), aiming to keep it about 1.5–2.0 times normal, thereby ensuring anticoagulation without an excess of bleeding complications. After more than 5 days of lepirudin use, antilepirudin antibodies may develop. These antibodies enhance the anticoagulation effects of lepirudin, and a reduction of the infusion dose may be needed to minimize bleeding risk. It is recommended that with prolonged use of lepirudin, daily aPTT measurements be made. Argatroban is eliminated predominantly by liver metabolism and biliary secretion, and for this reason may be a preferred agent in renal failure patients. Argatroban is initiated at 0.5–1.0 mcg/kg per minute, using lower doses in patients with hepatic dysfunction. The anticoagulation effect is also monitored by measuring aPTT. The administration of fresh frozen plasma is required to reverse bleeding due to overdosage of lepirudin and argatroban. Hemofiltration with high-flux dialyzers can reduce the plasma concentration of hirudin.

6.   Other anticoagulants. Danaparoid has been described for use in CRRT but is currently unavailable in the United States. Fondaparinux, a synthetic pentasaccharide that inhibits factor Xa by binding to antithrombin, has been used in a HIT type II patient on intermittent hemodialysis. Monitoring anticoagulation requires measuring antifactor Xa activity, but its use in continuous therapies remains to be defined. Sagedal and Hartmann (2004) reviewed the use of low molecular weight heparins (LMWHs) in CRRT. Dalteparin probably can be used as a bolus of about 20 U/kg followed by an infusion of 10 U/kg per hour for adequate anticoagulation without an excess of bleeding in C-HDF. In a study with C-HD, a dalteparin dose of 35 U/kg bolus followed by 13 U/kg per hour had good filter patency rates but there were bleeding episodes. However, at a lower dose of 8 U/kg bolus and infusion of 5 U/kg per hour, circuit life was poor. Enoxaparin and nadroparin may also be used, but the experience is limited to two studies.

7. **Microbubbles.** Microbubbles can be introduced into the extracorporeal circuit during priming and any time a connection is made or reset upstream to the filter. These can get into the hollow fibers, and lead to clotting of the filter. Care should be taken to minimize this problem during priming and infusions.

8. **Signs of filter clotting.** Signs of markedly reduced blood flow include darkening of the blood in the extracorporeal circuit, coolness of blood in the venous blood line, and separation of erythrocytes and plasma in the extracorporeal circuit. A sustained reduction in the volume of ultrafiltrate to <150–200 mL per hour not attributable to blood pressure fall is suggestive of clotting in the filter or the line. Saline infusion can help diagnose a near-clotted system: This can make visible clots in transparent parts of the hemofilter.

One can check the filtrate urea nitrogen (FUN):SUN ratio. If it is <0.6, clotting is imminent. An ultrasound method has been used to measure filter fiber bundle volume (FBV) during use, but online FBV measurements have not been found to predict filter longevity. One problem is that the majority of clotting seems to occur in the venous air trap chamber rather than in the dialyzer (Liangos et al., 2002).

E. **Electrolyte imbalances.** With C-HD, as long as the dialysis solution used contains appropriate concentrations of electrolytes, electrolyte imbalances should be infrequent. With C-HF, monitoring and replacing sodium, calcium, and magnesium are important because of the large amount of ultrafiltrate removed. All intravenous fluids, including parenteral nutrition solutions and replacement fluids, should contain close to 140 mmol/L sodium (unless a low-sodium solution is being used with citrate anticoagulation). Adequate replacement of calcium, magnesium, potassium, and bicarbonate (given back as bicarbonate, lactate, or acetate) is also of key importance.

Phosphate clearance with CRRT is high, and intravenous phosphate replacement is usually required after several days of therapy. Two milliliters of a potassium phosphate solution (potassium 4.4 mmol and phosphorus 3.0 mmol/mL) can be added to 5-L bags of manufactured bicarbonate solutions (Hemosol), making a final phosphorus concentration of 1.2 mM (Troyanov et al., 2004). At this concentration, there was no evidence of precipitation. Furthermore, there were no adverse electrolyte changes in the solutions or in vivo during the course of therapy. Phosphate was added when the patients' serum phosphorus levels were <1.5 mmol/L. Alternatively, sodium phosphates may be used when potassium levels are high.

Table 13-7.   Approximate dosages of antibiotics in patients with acute renal failure while receiving slow continuous hemodialysis[a]

Cefuroxime	500–700 mg q12h
Ceftazidime	1 g q24h
Tobramycin	Loading dose followed by 60–80 mg per 24 hours
Gentamicin	Loading dose then 80–100 mg per 24 hours
Ciprofloxacin	200 mg q8h
Vancomycin	1 g q48h

[a]For a 70-kg patient. Blood levels should also be determined, if possible.
Modified from Davis SP, et al. Pharmacokinetic studies in patients with acute renal failure treated by continuous arteriovenous hemodialysis. In: Abstracts of the 1990 Interscience Conference on Antimicrobial Agents, 1990:213.

F.   Compensating for removal of therapeutic drugs during C-HD. Because of the high 24-hour cumulative clearances with C-HD, there is substantial incidental removal of therapeutic drugs and nutrient substances, such as crystalline amino acids in parenteral nutrition solutions. Table 13-7 lists the approximate dosages for antibiotics in renal failure patients being treated with C-HD. Antibiotic blood levels, if available, should be obtained because it is difficult to predict what the removal will be. The doses in Table 13-7 may need to be adjusted upward when the drainage volume is >30 L per day.

Total amino acids are removed in the amount of 12 g per 24 hours at dialysate flow rates of 1 L per hour and when standard parenteral nutrition solutions are infused at a rate of 60–100 mL per hour. The amount of pressor drugs removed during C-HD does not appear to be clinically important, and pressor infusion rates are usually adjusted to maintain a given hemodynamic response.

G.   Compensating for removal of therapeutic drugs by C-HF. The ultrafiltrate removed by C-HF also may contain any drugs present in the patient's plasma. Removal depends on the sieving coefficient, the degree of protein binding, and the ultrafiltration rate (Golper and Marx, 1998).

Table 13-8 gives some practical guidance regarding dosing of commonly used drugs when C-HF is being performed at ultrafiltration rates of 30–40 L per day. The C-HF procedure can be thought of as an extra kidney, the glomerular filtrate rate (GFR) of which will depend on the ultrafiltrate volume. Each 10 L per day of ultrafiltrate volume is equivalent to about 7 mL per minute of GFR (7.0 mL per minute × 1,440 minutes per day = 10.08 L per day). Thus, when prescribing drugs to otherwise anuric patients receiving C-HF, one should write the drug dose as for a patient with a GFR of 7 mL per minute for every 10 L of ultrafiltrate volume. For example, a 70-kg man being treated with CD at replacement fluid rates of 20 mL/kg per

Table 13-8. Estimated drug dosage during continuous hemofiltration ($Q_F = 30$–40 L per day)

Drug	(n)	Normal Dosage [mg per day]	Dosage from Kinetics [mg per day]	Dosage from Predictions [mg per day]	Practical Dosage [mg]
Amikacin	(4)	1,050[a]	280	273	250 q24h–bid
Netilmicin	(11)	420[b]	139	136	100–150 q24h
Tobramycin	(10)	350[b]	115	107	100 q24h
Vancomycin	(10)	2,000[b]	645	653	500 q24h–bid
Teicoplanin	(8)	400[b]	300	290	300 q24h
Ceftazidime	(11)	6,000[b]	1,675	1,622	1,000 bid
Cefotaxime	(13)	12,000[b]	3,235	3,380	2,000 bid
Ceftriaxone	(6)	4,000[b]	1,357	1,457	2,000 q24h
Ciprofloxacin	(9)	400[b]	98	167	200 q24h
Imipenem	(10)	4,000[b]	1,754	1,614	500 tid–qid
Metronidazole	(7)	2,100[b]	1,376	1,860	500 tid–qid
Piperacillin	(17)	24,000[b]	10,271	9,737	4,000 tid
Digitoxin	(9)	0.065	0.05	0.06	0.05 q24h
Digoxin	(9)	0.29[b]	0.07	0.10	0.10 q24h
Phenobarbital	(8)	233	330	480	100 bid–qid
Phenytoin	(2)	524	453	364	250 q24h–bid
Theophylline	(12)	720	889	745	600–900 q24h

[a]$p < 0.05$.
[b]$p < 0.01$; paired Wilcoxon-rank test.
From Kroh UF, et al. Management of drug dosing in continuous renal replacement therapy. *Semin Dial* 1996;9:161–165.

hour or 35 mL/kg per hour would have equivalent GFR values of 23 mL per minute and 40 mL per minute, respectively.

X.   Slow continuous ultrafiltration (SCUF) and isolated ultrafiltration (IU)

A.   Procedures. SCUF is achieved using the circuitry as for C-HD (Fig. 13-1) but omitting dialysis solution. IU is achieved using standard dialysis equipment by simply putting the dialysate in bypass, and can be performed prior to dialysis, after dialysis, or independently of dialysis. In patients with renal failure, IU is most often performed just prior to hemodialysis.

B.   Advantages and disadvantages

1.   IU. IU is usually carried out when IHD is being given. IU is useful to remove additional fluid while avoiding disequilibrium syndrome for the initial one or two dialysis treatments in acutely uremic patients. It also is used in some outpatient dialysis units in patients with difficulty in fluid removal. The principal advantage of IU is that fluid removal is better tolerated than with conventional hemodialysis. Today IU may no longer be a superior method of fluid removal. Historically, poor tolerance to fluid removal during intermittent hemodialysis was due partly to use of acetate-containing dialysis solution, excessively warmed dialysis solution, and solutions containing an inappropriately low sodium concentration (e.g., 5–10 mM below that of plasma). If these factors are avoided (i.e., if a bicarbonate-containing, high-sodium, slightly cooled dialysis solution is used), then the previous superiority of IU in terms of hemodynamic stability may no longer be apparent. Waste product removal is minimal during IU. For this reason, the subsequent hemodialysis session length should not be shortened, and thus the total treatment time for the separated IU–hemodialysis combination must be prolonged.

Despite the relatively good tolerance to fluid removal with IU, hypotension can still occur if the ultrafiltration rate is excessive. If overt edema is present, then hypotension is rare at ultrafiltration rates of 1.5–2.0 L per hour (for a 70-kg patient). It is best not to exceed an ultrafiltration rate of 30 mL/kg per hour. A rebound hyperkalemia has been reported after intensive IU, perhaps due to exit of intracellular potassium into the extracellular fluid. Although the existence of this complication is controversial, any possible hyperkalemia with IU can best be avoided by routinely following IU with a period of hemodialysis.

2.   SCUF. SCUF is used primarily in an ICU setting, to remove excess fluid from patients in whom residual renal function is substantial, and in whom electrolyte and acid–base imbalances are not an issue. It is also quite useful for inpatient treatment of patients with refractory heart failure and mildly impaired renal function as described below (section XII D). A disadvantage of SCUF is that acid–base disturbances and electrolyte imbalances need to be corrected indirectly by adjusting the composition of IV infusions given apart from the extracorporeal therapy.

XI.   Intermittent hemofiltration and hemodiafiltration. These are described in Chapter 15.

XII. CRRT pointers for certain groups of patients
A. Brain edema.
In critically ill patients with acute renal failure, CRRT has been shown to cause fewer changes in brain edema when compared to IHD. Furthermore, CRRT minimizes rapid and wide fluctuations to the cardiovascular system, particularly in blood volume and pressures, thereby reducing large variations in cerebral perfusion pressures and intracranial pressures. Patients with liver failure are one group at risk for developing cerebral edema, due to difficulty in maintaining cerebral autoregulation of blood flow. Davenport (1999) has used C-HF and C-HD to cope with the increased intracranial pressure and cerebral edema.

In patients at risk for cerebral edema, C-HF and C-HD systems using the new generation of continuous machines with tight volumetric control and biocompatible membranes should be used. If possible, anticoagulation should be avoided, as it may increase the risk of intracerebral hemorrhage either at the site of injury or around the intracranial pressure monitor.

Dialysis or replacement fluid should have a relatively higher sodium (>140 mM) and a lower bicarbonate (30 mM) concentration. A higher sodium concentration will reduce the blood–brain osmotic gradient and minimize water movement into the brain. A rapid rise in plasma bicarbonate increases CO_2 movement into brain cells. Since bicarbonate ions are charged, they enter cells less readily than CO_2, thus causing a paradoxical decrease in brain pH. A sudden decrease in brain pH results in the generation of idiogenic osmoles, which increase the osmotic gradient favoring water entry into the brain.

In severe cases of uncontrolled intracranial pressure, cooling of the dialysis or replacement solutions may be helpful, in addition to other measures used to cool the patient to 32°–33°C. At these temperatures, cranial oxygen demands are reduced (Davenport et al., 2001).
B. Sepsis and multiorgan failure
1. Multiple organ dysfunction syndrome occurs as a result of an outpouring of proinflammatory (tumor necrosis factor β, thromboxane B_2, platelet activating factor) and anti-inflammatory mediators (interleukin-10). This response is provoked by Gram-negative bacteria endotoxins, Gram-positive bacteria, viruses, splanchnic ischemia, and trauma. Many of these septic mediators are found in the filtrate of septic patients or adsorbed to the filter membrane, suggesting that C-HF has the ability to remove septic mediators from the circulation. Use of high-volume C-HF has been advocated for such patients. However, although septic mediator concentrations are reduced by such treatments, a clinical benefit has not been consistently seen, so the benefits of higher-volume (2 L per hour) C-HF for such patients remains controversial. Nevertheless, many centers will treat septic patients with C-HDF instead of C-HD to increase removal of potential sepsis-mediating molecules while retaining the efficiency associated with use of dialysis. Using a clearance dose of 35 mL/kg per hour and dividing equally between dialysis and hemofiltration is a common

strategy. Plasmapheresis for such patients has also been reported to be of benefit (see Chapter 16).

C.   Acute lung injury and acute respiratory distress syndrome (ARDS). Early institution of CRRT for volume removal may be helpful in improving oxygenation and ventilator parameters (PaO_2/FiO_2 ratio and oxygenation index) in patients with ARDS with concomitant acute renal failure. Respiratory improvement appears to be due more to the volume removal effect rather than to the removal of inflammatory mediators (Hoste et al., 2002).

D.   Congestive heart failure (C-HF). Patients with congestive heart failure may develop concomitant renal failure, resulting in fluid overload. They may have anuria, oliguria, or insufficient urine output (<1 L per day) despite optimal medical treatment with maximal doses of intravenous diuretics, inotropes, and natriuretic peptides. Ultrafiltration is a treatment option in such situations. While inpatient and outpatient intermittent isolated ultrafiltration for C-HF have been described, there are several advantages of SCUF that should be considered. Slow removal of fluid results in less hemodynamic issues, such as symptomatic hypotension. Also, many of these patients are volume overloaded substantially, sometimes 10–15 kg over their "feel good" weight; continuous therapy allows for larger volumes of fluid to be removed while minimizing the hemodynamic problems. Ultrafiltration techniques can be further enhanced by using a Swan-Ganz catheter for central volume monitoring, thereby guiding the endpoint of treatment, and by using an online blood volume monitoring instrument to protect against an excessive ultrafiltration rate. Recently a small, portable machine designed specifically for SCUF (C-HF Solutions, Aquadex Flex Flow, Brooklyn Park, MN) has become available in the United States.

E.   Prevention of radiocontrast-induced nephropathy. In patients with chronic renal failure (serum creatinine >2 mg/dL [180 mcmol/L]) undergoing coronary interventions requiring IV contrast administration, use of periprocedural C-HF was associated with a lower rate of acute renal failure requiring dialysis, compared to use of isotonic saline hydration. (Marenzi et al., 2003). Confirmatory studies are needed before CRRT can be recommended routinely for this purpose.

F.   Intoxication with dialyzable or filter-permeable drugs or toxins. Use of various modes of CRRT can be advantageous in treating various poisonings, especially when plasma levels are low. See Chapter 17.

G.   Extracorporeal membrane oxygenation (ECMO). SCUF or C-HD may be performed on patients receiving ECMO without the need for a separate CRRT system. The ECMO blood lines can be adapted to connect in parallel to a dialyzer. This allows C-HD or SCUF to be performed concurrently. Since these patients have ARDS or volume overload that requires ECMO in the first place, further volume removal may be helpful, especially in patients with chronic renal insufficiency. When C-HD is desired for the treatment of concomitant ARF in these patients, use of sterile dialysate solutions is preferred, as there may be high back-filtration due to high pressures in the ECMO circuit.

H. Infants and children. Use of CRRT in children is beyond the scope of this *Handbook*. See the review by Zobel et al. (1996).

SELECTED READINGS

Aronoff GR, et al. *Drug prescribing in renal failure dosing guidelines for adults,* 4th ed. American College of Physicians, Philadelphia, PA, 1998.

Augustine JJ, et al. A randomized controlled trial comparing intermittent with continuous dialysis in patients with ARF. *Am J Kidney Dis* 2004;44:1000–1007.

Barenbrock M, et al. Effects of bicarbonate- and lactate-buffered replacement fluids on cardiovascular outcome in CVVH patients. *Kidney Int* 2000;58:1751–1757.

Bouman CS, et al. Effects of early high-volume continuous venovenous hemofiltration on survival and recovery of renal function in intensive care patients with acute renal failure: a prospective, randomized trial. *Crit Care Med* 2002;30:2205–2211.

Brause M, et al. Effect of filtration volume of continuous venovenous hemofiltration in the treatment of patients with acute renal failure in intensive care units. *Crit Care Med* 2003;31:841–846.

Bunchman TE, Maxvold NJ, Brophy PD. Pediatric convective hemofiltration: Normocarb replacement fluid and citrate anticoagulation. *Am J Kidney Dis* 2003;42:1248–1252.

Cole L, et al. High-volume haemofiltration in human septic shock. *Intensive Care Med* 2001;27:978–986.

Dager WE, White RH. Argatroban for heparin-induced thrombocytopenia in hepato-renal failure and CVVHD. *Ann Pharmacother* 2003;37:1232–1236.

Davenport A. Is there a role for continuous renal replacement therapies in patients with liver and renal failure? *Kidney Int Suppl* 1999:S62–66.

Davenport A. Renal replacement therapy in the patient with acute brain injury. *Am J Kidney Dis* 2001;37:457–466.

Eichler P, et al. Antihirudin antibodies in patients with heparin-induced thrombocytopenia treated with lepirudin: incidence, effects on aPTT, and clinical relevance. *Blood* 2000;96:2373–2378.

Fischer KG, van de Loo A, Bohler J. Recombinant hirudin (lepirudin) as anticoagulant in intensive care patients treated with continuous hemodialysis. *Kidney Int Suppl* 1999;72:S46–50.

Golper TA. Update on drug sieving coefficients and dosing adjustments during continuous renal replacement therapies. *Contrib Nephrol* 2001;349–353.

Golper TA, Marx MA. Drug dosing adjustments during continuous renal replacement therapies. *Kidney Int Suppl* 1998;66:S165–168.

Henrich WL. *Principles and practice of dialysis,* 3rd ed. Philadelphia: Lippincott Williams & Wilkins, 2004.

Hoste EA, et al. No early respiratory benefit with CVVHDF in patients with acute renal failure and acute lung injury. *Nephrol Dial Transplant* 2002;17:2153–2158.

Jaski BE, et al. Peripherally inserted veno-venous ultrafiltration for rapid treatment of volume overloaded patients. *J Card Fail* 2003;9:227–231.

Kellum JA, et al. Continuous versus intermittent renal replacement therapy: a meta-analysis. *Intensive Care Med* 2002;28:29–37.

Kumar VA, et al. Extended daily dialysis: a new approach to renal replacement for acute renal failure in the intensive care unit. *Am J Kidney Dis* 2000;36:294–300.

Leblanc M, et al. Bicarbonate dialysate for continuous renal replacement therapy in intensive care unit patients with acute renal failure. *Am J Kidney Dis* 1995;26:910–917.

Liangos O, et al. Dialyzer fiber bundle volume and kinetics of solute removal in continuous venovenous hemodialysis. *Am J Kidney Dis* 2002;39:1047–1053.

Marenzi G, et al. Interrelation of humoral factors, hemodynamics, and fluid and salt metabolism in congestive heart failure: effects of extracorporeal ultrafiltration. *Am J Med* 1993;94:49–56.

Marenzi G, et al. The prevention of radiocontrast-agent-induced nephropathy by hemofiltration. *N Engl J Med* 2003;349:1333–1340.

Marshall MR, et al. Sustained low-efficiency daily diafiltration (SLEDD-f) for critically ill patients requiring renal replacement therapy: towards an adequate therapy. *Nephrol Dial Transplant* 2004;19:877–884.

McLean AG, et al. Effects of lactate-buffered and lactate-free dialysate in CAVHD patients with and without liver dysfunction. *Kidney Int* 2000;58:1765–1772.

Mehta RL. Indications for dialysis in the ICU: renal replacement vs. renal support. *Blood Purif* 2001;19:227–232.

Meier-Kriesche HU, et al. Unexpected severe hypocalcemia during continuous venovenous hemodialysis with regional citrate anticoagulation. *Am J Kidney Dis* 1999;33:e8.

Meier-Kriesche HU, et al. Increased total to ionized calcium ratio during continuous venovenous hemodialysis with regional citrate anticoagulation. *Crit Care Med* 2001;29:748–752.

Mitchell A, et al. A new system for regional citrate anticoagulation in continuous venovenous hemodialysis (CVVHD). *Clin Nephrol* 2003;59:106–114.

Morgera S, et al. Long-term outcomes in acute renal failure patients treated with continuous renal replacement therapies. *Am J Kidney Dis* 2002;40:275–279.

Rogiers P, et al. Blood warming during hemofiltration can improve hemodynamics and outcome in ovine septic shock. *Anesthesiology* 2006;104:1216–1222.

Rokyta R Jr, et al. Effects of continuous venovenous haemofiltration-induced cooling on global haemodynamics, splanchnic oxygen and energy balance in critically ill patients. *Nephrol Dial Transplant* 2004;19:623–630.

Ronco C, et al. Effects of different doses in continuous veno-venous haemofiltration on outcomes of acute renal failure: a prospective randomised trial. *Lancet* 2000;356:26–30.

Sagedal S, Hartmann A. Low molecular weight heparins as thromboprophylaxis in patients undergoing hemodialysis/hemofiltration or continuous renal replacement therapies. *Eur J Med Res* 2004;9:125–130.

Salvatori G, et al. First clinical trial for a new CRRT machine: the Prismaflex. *Int J Artif Organs* 2004;27:404–409.

Schindler R, et al. Removal of contrast media by different extracorporeal treatments. *Nephrol Dial Transplant* 2001;16:1471–1474.

Splendiani G, et al. Continuous renal replacement therapy and charcoal plasmaperfusion in treatment of amanita mushroom poisoning. *Artif Organs* 2000;24:305–308.

Swartz R, et al. Improving the delivery of continuous renal replacement therapy using regional citrate anticoagulation. *Clin Nephrol* 2004;61:134–143.

Teo BW, et al. Machine generated bicarbonate dialysate for continuous therapy: a 10-year experience. *Blood Purif* 2006;24:247–273.

Troyanov S, et al. Phosphate addition to hemodiafiltration solutions during continuous renal replacement therapy. *Intensive Care Med* 2004;30:1662–1665.

van der Sande FM, et al. Thermal effects and blood pressure response during postdilution hemodiafiltration and hemodialysis: the effect of amount of replacement fluid and dialysate temperature. *J Am Soc Nephrol* 2001;12:1916–1920.

Wang PL, et al. Bone resorption and "relative" immobilization hypercalcemia with prolonged continuous renal replacement therapy and citrate anticoagulation. *Am J Kidney Dis* 2004;44:1110–1114.

Wester JP, et al. Catheter replacement in continuous arteriovenous hemodiafiltration: the balance between infectious and mechanical complications. *Crit Care Med* 2002;30:1261–1266.

Yagi N, et al. Cooling effect of continuous renal replacement therapy in critically ill patients. *Am J Kidney Dis* 1998;32:1023–1030.

Zobel G, Ring E, Rodl S. Continuous renal replacement therapy in critically ill pediatric patients. *Am J Kidney Dis* 1996;28:S28–S34.

WEB REFERENCES

ADQI Initiative: http://www.adqi.org

HDCN CRRT Channel: http://www.hdcn.com/ch/cavh/

Intensive versus Conventional Renal Support in Acute Renal Failure Treatment Network (ATN) study: http://www.clinicaltrials.gov/show/NCT00076219

Frequent Hemodialysis

Gihad E. Nesrallah, Rita S. Suri,
Robert M. Lindsay, and Andreas Pierratos

Interest in providing dialysis more than the standard three times per week continues to garner interest worldwide. Two major variants have evolved: Short "daily" hemodialysis (SDHD) and long nocturnal (during sleep) hemodialysis (NHD). Prescriptions can range from five to seven treatments per week. SDHD is usually carried out for 1.5–3 hours per treatment, while NHD is done for 6–10 hours per session. These techniques lend themselves well to the home setting, although both are being performed in-center as well. Potential benefits include (a) better control of extracellular volume, with resulting improved blood pressure; (b) improved cardiac structure and function; (c) better nutritional status, with increased lean body weight, appetite, and albumin; (d) better control of phosphorus balance with reduced need for phosphorus binders; (e) reduced erythropoietin (EPO) requirements; (f) reduced intradialytic hypotensive episodes and intradialytic symptoms; (g) improved quality of life; and (h) reduced hospitalization.

I.   **Patient selection.** On average, it is estimated that approximately 20% of the dialysis patient population would be well suited to home hemodialysis. The proportion of these that would be willing to commit to a daily treatment regimen is unknown. There are few absolute contraindications. Inability to use heparin precludes NHD but not SDHD. High levels of comorbidity do not preclude use of either regimen. Patients with severe heart failure, malnutrition, hyperphosphatemia, or refractory hypertension, for example, have been shown to benefit greatly from more frequent dialysis therapy.

A.   **Home.** The primary prerequisite for SDHD or NHD in the home setting is a willing patient or partner who is able to learn to safely perform the dialysis procedure. The selection process should include a basic assessment of the patient's motor skills, strength, vision, hearing, reading ability, and motivation. Finally, the patient's home environment must be assessed to ensure adequate physical space for the HD machine and supplies, though patients have relocated in order to accommodate the necessary equipment.

B.   **In-center.** More frequent dialysis can also be delivered in-center. Reasons for choosing in-center over home-based SDHD or NHD include (a) patient safety concerns, (b) vascular access or cannulation problems, (c) patient or partner inability or unwillingness to perform the hemodialysis procedure at home, (d) unsuitable home environment (space, electrical, or plumbing limitations), and (e) patient preference. Transportation, proximity to the treatment center, patient lifestyle, and demands on the patient's family are important potential barriers to daily in-center therapy. In-center SDHD or NHD imposes increased demands on space, equipment, and nursing and technical support staff. Depending on the number of patients treated with SDHD or NHD, additional staff may need to be hired.

II.   Typical dialysis schedules

A.   SDHD versus NHD. The treatment schedule will depend on patient preference as well as clearance and ultrafiltration needs. Starting with one particular SDHD or NHD regimen does not preclude switching to another at any time, and many patients have used combinations of SDHD and NHD to accommodate work and other schedules.

Personal preference is the major arbiter of regimen selection. From a patient perspective, convenience and noninterference with work, sleep, and social schedules is of primary importance, and efforts should be made to accommodate these factors. Dietary factors including high phosphate and fluid intake may make NHD a preferable option. Patients with particularly large interdialytic weight gains may, for example, benefit from the longer time for ultrafiltration afforded by NHD where ultrafiltration rates of 0.5–0.8 L per hour are very well tolerated. Removing as much as 1.5 L per hour with SDHD, however, is generally well tolerated as well, since more fluid is close to the vascular compartment at the outset of a given dialysis session.

B.   Less frequent (three to four times per week) NHD. Nocturnal dialysis also has been provided on a three times per week, or every other night, schedule. The total weekly dialysis time with such schedules typically is in the range of 18–30 hours. Because patients may be more willing to come to a center three to four times per week, such regimens can be performed in existing dialysis units or in hospital inpatient dialysis rooms. In-center NHD improves overall utilization of these facilities, as it makes them functional during periods when they would not otherwise be in use.

III.   Technical considerations

A.   Training (home patients). The length of the training period depends on the patient's previous experience with HD. Patients recruited from self-care programs typically require less time than inexperienced patients; the latter typically need 6 weeks to become safe and proficient, although a prolonged training period in a self-care setting has facilitated the transition to fully independent treatment for some. Most training programs provide one-on-one instruction, though up to two patients have been successfully trained simultaneously. Educational materials in the form of manuals written at the appropriate reading and comprehension level are quite useful. Many programs require patients to "recertify" annually, by demonstrating in the training unit setting that they are able to accurately perform the dialysis procedure and troubleshoot effectively.

B.   Vascular access. With few exceptions, vascular access planning is the same as for regular dialysis patients. Native arteriovenous fistulas, synthetic grafts, and long-term central venous catheters are all acceptable options for use. Smaller needles providing a Q_B as low as 150 mL per minute are usually sufficient for NHD. In patients with arteriovenous (AV) fistulas, access longevity may be increased by using the "buttonhole" technique, which involves recannulation of precisely the same two or three sites (see Chapter 7). With synthetic grafts, needle sites are rotated in the usual fashion. Single-needle approaches are useful for NHD, where high dialysis efficiency is not required.

C. Patient safety and precautions (home patients). With an appropriately trained patient, and with appropriate supervision in place, both SDHD and NHD can be done safely at home. SDHD poses risks similar to home dialysis delivered on a standard schedule. NHD, in progress during sleep, requires additional precautions.

1. Hearing alarms. The patient must be able to hear the dialysis machine and its various alarms, and, if remote monitoring is to be used, the ringing of a telephone connected to the monitoring center.

2. Self-cannulation. Competence with the cannulation procedure and with securing the cannula are mandatory prerequisites for independent home treatment. Various products are available to help secure dialysis needles to the skin.

3. Accidental line disconnection. Plastic clamshell locking boxes have been used to prevent catheter-tubing separation, and have been available through the Humber program. A small patient connector clip (HemoSafe, Fresenius NA, Lexington, MA) is widely available. An enuresis alarm, such as the Drisleeper (Alpha Consultants Ltd., Nelson, New Zealand) can be attached to the cannula entry points to detect bleeding. Moisture sensors can be placed on the floor around the machine and near the water supply to detect blood, dialysate, and water leaks.

4. Prevention of air embolism. The InterLink System (Baxter Health Care, Deerfield, IL; Becton Dickinson, Franklin Lakes, NJ) is a catheter cap with a slit diaphragm that reduces the risk of air embolism. This can only be used for NHD, as it results in increased arterial and venous pressures at the higher pump speeds used in SDHD.

5. Using a two-pump single-needle system. This eliminates the risk of substantial blood loss due to accidental line disconnection. Single-needle dialysis does reduce clearance somewhat, but this is not much of an issue in NHD.

IV. Infrastructure requirements

A. Support staff. Specially trained support staff are required. Biomedical engineering personnel should be involved in the development of local policies governing practices, standards, and protocols for the installation and maintenance of equipment. The dialysis program's payment carrier should be informed of any changes to services provided. Dialysis programs offering home hemodialysis will already have much of this in place.

B. Home environment suitability. The home needs to be assessed by a renal technologist, focusing on (a) water quantity and quality, (b) electrical supply, (c) storage space, and (d) cleanliness. These rarely pose insurmountable barriers to home dialysis, though the patient must understand the nature and extent of the changes needed in order to accommodate the necessary equipment.

C. **Water supply.** Water quality must be assessed regardless of the source. Endotoxins, mineral content, and chloramines should be quantified. Rural water supplies must also be tested for coliform bacteria. Water pressure requirements are typically specified by the water purification system and hemodialysis equipment manufacturer.

    1. **Water purification.** Both reverse osmosis (RO) and deionization (DI) systems have been used successfully in home dialysis. Purification systems have become increasingly compact and quiet enough to install in a patient's bedroom, though more remote installation is also possible where desired. Patients should be instructed in maintenance procedures for their water systems, including filter changes and disinfection of lines and units. Ultrapure dialysate (generated by using an ultrafilter) has also been used by some programs and may be preferable for NHD, where the duration of dialysate exposure can compound the effects of inferior water quality. Disinfection and water sampling frequency (usually monthly) will depend on the system utilized and must follow national water standards.

D. **Dialysis membranes.** Currently there are no data to support the use of one kind of dialysis membrane over another in SDHD or NHD. Generally speaking, most centers have used high-flux dialyzers. Some have even used pediatric-sized dialyzers for NHD, given their suitability for the lower blood and dialysate flow rates commonly used. Dialyzer reuse has been described in SDHD or NHD, but has largely been abandoned with the fall in prices of dialysis membranes.

E. **Dialysis machines.** No existing data favor the use of any one type of hemodialysis machine over another; thus, any machine that can be used for in-center therapy can be used for home daily dialysis. For delivering NHD it is important that the machine be able to deliver a Q_B as low as 200 mL per minute; the ability to deliver a Q_D as low as 100–200 mL per minute can be helpful as well. Some machines are large, cumbersome, and difficult to use, though there appears to be a growing interest in producing machines that are more conducive to the home environment. Noise is a factor for machines used for NHD.

    1. **Equipment maintenance programs.** These are central to patient safety. Most manufacturers provide suggested maintenance schedules, and these should serve as a bare minimum requirement to minimize and prevent complications and equipment failure. In addition to a rigorous water purification maintenance schedule, microbiologic and endotoxin screening of product water and dialysis solution are critically important, particularly with high-flux membranes. Some advocate doing this monthly.

F. **Remote overnight monitoring.** A modem or high-speed connection to the hemodialysis machine and to specialized monitoring equipment can allow for software-based real-time monitoring to detect technical problems as they arise (e.g., air and blood leaks). Monitoring is also a useful means by which to track treatment adherence as well as physical parameters such as vital signs. It is typically only used in, but is not mandatory for, NHD delivery; such systems generally are not needed in SDHD. Available systems include the Cybernius DAX/DAXII (Cyberenius Medical Ltd., Edmonton, Alberta, Canada) and the iCare (Fresenius Medical Care, Lexington, MA); both have been used successfully. Although there are still no documented cases in which monitoring prevented a catastrophe, it is universally helpful in allaying patient anxiety during the first weeks at home alone. It is recommended that monitoring should be used for the first 3 months at home, and then monitoring can be continued thereafter if indicated. To offer patients optimum flexibility in treatment schedule, a monitoring center should be open 7 days a week, usually for at least 10 hours (e.g., 10 P.M. to 8 A.M). Monitoring staff should be present during the entire monitoring period and trained to respond to alarms; they should be available to call patients by telephone within a predetermined timeframe if an intervention is required. Automated telephone-response systems have been used with variable success. Most alarms result from minor and self-resolving problems such as venous or arterial line pressure changes (due to positional changes). In general, the frequency of alarms declines over time. Overnight monitoring can be costly, and use of regionalizing monitoring centers is a potential cost-saving strategy. Some centers abandon overnight monitoring as they gain experience with NHD.

V.   Adequacy and dose

A.   SDHD

    1.   Solute removal advantage of more frequent dialysis. Easily dialyzed solutes like urea are removed more efficiently using a six times per week schedule rather than a three times per week prescription. This is because the concentration of such solutes drops rapidly early in the course of dialysis. Once this happens, expending further time on dialysis gives relatively little additional solute removal, since the concentration of solute in the blood entering the dialyzer is no longer high. Thus, if total weekly dialysis time is held constant, time-averaged concentration of urea will be lower with a more frequent schedule. This advantage will be even larger for uremic solutes that may be sequestered in tissues during dialysis to a greater extent than urea.

    2.   Urea-based adequacy measures. Although there are no outcomes studies to support use of urea to quantify dialysis dose in SDHD, a conceptual framework of doing so is available using the standard Kt/V concept that has been described in Chapters 3 and 9.

        a.   Standard Kt/V (std-Kt/V). This concept is described in detail in Chapter 3 D 10 f and will only be summarized here. Std-Kt/V is a frequency-independent measure of dialysis dose. It is a weekly expression (normalized to V) of an equivalent urea clearance, which in turn is

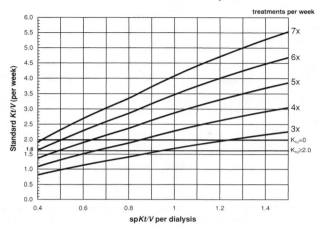

Standard *Kt/V*: a continuous clearance equivalent

Figure 14-1. The relationship between weekly std-*Kt/V* and per dialysis single pool *Kt/V* (sp*Kt/V*). (Data derived from Table A-7 in Appendix A).

defined as the urea generation rate divided by the mean peak predialysis serum urea nitrogen (SUN) level. The effect of dialysis frequency on the std-*Kt/V* can more easily be seen graphically, and is shown in Figure 14-1. It can be seen that, when three times per week dialysis sessions are given, each lasting about 3.5 hours and delivering an single-pool (sp) *Kt/V* of 1.2, the resulting std-*Kt/V* will be 2.0. Increasing the sp*Kt/V* using a three times per week schedule has only a marginal effect on increasing std-*Kt/V* (unless the session length is markedly lengthened). One also can see that, to achieve the same std-*Kt/V* of 2.0 using six times per week SDHD, an sp*Kt/V* of about 0.5 needs to be delivered during each session.

b. Equation for calculating std-*Kt/V*. An equation developed by Leypoldt can also be used to compute the approximate std-*Kt/V* of any dialysis prescription based on frequency and sp*Kt/V*. This is detailed in Appendix A, Table A-5.

3. Prescription recommendations. Patients following a six times per week SDHD schedule have been treated with session lengths ranging from 1.5–3 hours (Table 14-1) six times weekly, corresponding to weekly dialysis times of 9–18 hours. Blood flow rates are usually similar to those in conventional dialysis, but dialysate flows may be up to 800 mL per minute. What should the prescription be in a given individual? There are no hard outcomes studies. However, the majority of previous studies have achieved a weekly std-*Kt/V* of ~3.0. It is reasonable to start with 2-hour

Table 14-1. Typical SDHD and NHD prescriptions

	SDHD	NHD
Frequency (sessions per week)	6–7	5–7
Duration (hours)	1.5–3.0	6–10
Dialyzer (high flux preferred)	Any	Any (smaller)
Q_B (mL per minute)	400–500	200–300
Q_D (mL per minute)	500–800	100–300
Access	Any	Any
Remote monitoring	None	Optional
Dialyzer reuse	Optional	Optional

SDHD, short daily hemodialysis; NHD, nocturnal hemodialysis.

treatments, 12 hours per week. This schedule may then be adjusted depending on the measured delivered dose and patient satisfaction, remembering that every dialysis session need not be of the same length. In selected patients, further increases in dialysis session length (beyond 2 hours) should be considered, as this may be of help in removing more phosphate and also salt and water, as described below. On the other hand, SDHD sessions in the 1.5-hour range may also benefit many patients, especially those with substantial residual renal function.

a. The National Kidney Foundation's (NKF) Kidney Disease Outcome Quality Initiative (KDOQI) adequacy clinical practice recommendations for SDHD. In the absence of good outcomes data, the KDOQI adequacy workgroup, realizing that some sort of "logical" dose adequacy recommendations for SDHD may be helpful, took this std-Kt/V concept and came up with the data in Table 14-2. They took an average-size patient and computed the expected "session" spKt/V levels that would be required using different treatment schedules to achieve a

Table 14-2. Minimum spKt/V values for various frequency schedules of dialysis (achieving an estimated standard $Kt/V = 2.0$ for an average-size patient)

Schedule	K_r <2 mL per minute per 1.73 m^2	K_r >2 mL per minute per 1.73 m^2
Four times per week	0.87	0.62
Five times per week	0.64	0.46
Six times per week	0.51	0.37

Adapted from the National Kidney Foundation's (NKF) Kidney Disease Outcome Quality Initiative (KDOQI) 2006 adequacy guidelines, CPR #4. Based on a 120 minute treatment time.

std-Kt/V value of 2.0, and then set this as the "minimum" recommended amount of spKt/V for that given schedule. For a patient being dialyzed six times per week, the minimum spKt/V turned out to be about 0.5. They also considered the effect of residual renal function. With a urea clearance of around 2.0 mL per minute for an average-size patient, a target std-Kt/V of about 1.6 needs to be achieved by dialysis only. The calculations show that a session spKt/V of about 0.4 is required to deliver a weekly std-Kt/V of 1.6. A similar approach was taken to come up with the numbers in Table 14-2 for four times per week and five times per week dialysis schedules.

B. NHD. Once dialysis is given for 6- to 10-hour sessions three or more times per week, std-Kt/V values will typically be well above 2.0, assuming that an spKt/V of at least 1.0 is delivered per session. This is because the std-Kt/V is also affected by session length, and going from a 3.5- to a 6- to 10-hour session per se results in a marked increase in std-Kt/V, even for three times per week dialysis, even when spKt/V is unchanged. For the typical NHD prescriptions listed in Table 14-1, the std-Kt/V will be in the range of 4.0–5.0; for this reason, the KDOQI 2006 workgroup did not recommend routine monitoring of postdialysis SUN values with nocturnal therapies (assuming that total weekly time on dialysis is 18 hours or more). So here again, the optimal regimen has not been determined. Most experience has been obtained with a regimen of 6–10 hours 5–6 nights per week, using either single- or double-needle access and dialysate flows of 300–500 mL per minute. This is what we recommend as a starting point.

VI. Phosphorus. The basic ideas behind phosphorus balance are reviewed in Chapter 35. We consume about 1 g of phosphorus per day, mostly via protein. About 0.7 g of the element is absorbed per day. Total phosphorus absorption is therefore usually about 5 g per week. A single dialysis session removes about 0.8 g of phosphorus; so with three times per week dialysis, we are able to remove only $0.8 \times 3 = 2.4$ g. The shortfall in removal is the reason why phosphorus binders are universally required by almost all patients being dialyzed three times per week.

A. SDHD. The serum inorganic phosphorus level drops sharply during dialysis, and then remains at a very low plateau level during the session. For this reason, as for urea, there is some degree of increased phosphorus removal with SDHD relative to three times per week dialysis even when the weekly dialysis time of both therapies is the same. When SDHD is given six times per week with shorter (1.5- to 2.0-hour) session lengths, phosphorus control is not markedly improved, despite a moderately increased amount of phosphorus removal, probably because patients receiving SDHD sometimes feel better, have increased appetite, and increase their phosphorus intake. However, increasing total weekly dialysis time will substantially increase phosphorus removal, to the point that clinical benefits are observed. For example, when SDHD was given six times per week, 3 hours per session, control of serum phosphorus and Ca × P product was markedly improved, and the amount of phosphorus binders administered could be reduced (Ayus et al., 2005).

B.   NHD. About one third to one half of patients dialyzed 24–28 hours per week using NHD can go off phosphorus binders, and almost all patients being dialyzed six times per week can dispense with phosphorus binder therapy, provided that dialysate and blood flow rates are not reduced to very low levels. In fact, in many NHD patients, phosphorus needs to be added to the dialysis solution to prevent hypophosphatemia, as discussed below.

VII.   Other aspects pertaining to the dialysis treatment

A.   Dialysate composition. Dialysate composition for SDHD typically does not change when switching from conventional dialysis; occasional patients require a lower bicarbonate concentration. For NHD, dialysate composition must be individualized, particularly with respect to calcium and phosphorus content (see below). A typical dialysate contains Na^+ 135, K^+ 2, HCO_3^- 30–33, Ca^{++} 1.5–1.75 mM (3.0–3.5 mEq/L), Mg^{++} 0.5 mM (1 mEq/L), and usually phosphorus 0.32–0.65 mmol/L (1–2 mg/dL).

   1.   Phosphorus. Patients treated with NHD (or unusually, with longer SDHD sessions) may eventually have low predialysis serum inorganic phosphorus levels. If this persists after discontinuing phosphorus binders and liberalizing dietary phosphorus intake, then phosphorus must be added to the dialysate. Sodium phosphate preparations such as Fleet enema and Fleet phospho-soda laxative(C. B. Fleet Company, Lynchburg, VA) have been used, and can be added to the liquid form of either the acid or the bicarbonate concentrate by the patient. The Fleet enema preparation consisting of a mixture of $NaH_2PO_4.H_2O$ and $Na_2HPO_4.7H_2O$ and having a phosphorus (MW 31) content of 1.38 mmol/mL (43 mg/mL) is often used. The amount added can be adjusted to maintain normal pre- and postdialysis serum phosphorus levels. For example, should one select a three-stream, bicarbonate-based, dialysate delivery system having a dilution ratio of 1:1.83:34 (acid concentrate:bicarbonate concentrate:water) to generate 190.4 L of a final dialysate with a phosphorus level of 0.65 mM (2 mg/dL), one needs to add 124 mmol (3,837 mg) of phosphorus (i.e., 90 mL) of the above enema to either 5.17 L of the acid concentrate or 9.46 L of the bicarbonate concentrate.

   2.   Calcium. The ideal dialysate calcium concentration for an individual patient will vary with dietary calcium intake, ingestion of supplemental calcium (including calcium-based phosphorus binders), vitamin D analog use, and the level of parathyroid gland activity. Occasionally, measurement of pre- and postdialysis calcium levels can help identify an ideal bath calcium concentration. Since SDHD is not associated with marked changes in calcium levels, standard concentrations are typically used.

   In NHD, calcium depletion is a potential problem. Using a bath calcium concentration of 1.25 mM has been shown to result in hyperparathyroidism that is refractory to vitamin D analog therapy. This is particularly likely to happen when a patient is no longer taking calcium-based phosphorus binders because of normalization of serum phosphorus levels. Increasing the bath calcium concentration to 1.75 mM readily suppresses parathyroid hormone (PTH) release. Mass balance studies have shown that NHD results in a net calcium loss of approximately 2 mmol per hour when a 1.25 mM bath concentration is used, while a gain of 3.7 mmol per hour was observed with a 1.75 mM bath. Another series found that an average bath calcium concentration of 1.6 mM helped to maintain or improve bone mass as measured yearly using dual-energy x-ray absorptiometry (DEXA) densitometry. This level of dialysate calcium also suppressed PTH to the normal range, but was also associated with biopsy-proven low bone turnover in over half of patients. The ideal dialysate calcium is likely just under 1.6 mM, but individualization of therapy is essential and 1.6 mM appears to be a reasonable starting point. Dialysate calcium enrichment may be achieved through the addition of powdered calcium chloride in specifically prescribed amounts. The Humber program uses $CaCl_2.2H_2O$ USP.

B.   Anticoagulation. NHD generally cannot be performed without anticoagulation, while SDHD can be, if necessary. Standard heparin protocols may be used for either regimen. In the presence of heparin-induced thrombocytopenia, danaparoid has been used successfully.

VIII.   Monitoring and tailoring therapy

A.   Monitoring. Most patients should be seen within 2–4 weeks of starting home therapy, then monthly for 3 months, then every 2–3 months thereafter. This assumes that 24-hour on-call nursing support is always available. The use of dialysis "run sheets" allows for documentation of weights, blood pressures, and intradialytic complications. Patients should bring these to each clinic visit.

B.   Blood tests. Patients dialyzing at home can be provided with blood centrifuges and can be instructed in the handling of samples.

C.   Adjustment of antihypertensive medications. Improvement in blood pressure (BP) control may be noted as early as 1 week after changing to SDHD or NHD and is most marked within the first few months but may continue for up to 18 months later. Not uncommonly, the blood pressure may be so markedly improved by SDHD or NHD that a patient will no longer need antihypertensive drugs. Cardioprotective agents such as angiotensin-converting enzyme (ACE) inhibitors or beta-blockers may still be prescribed, if desired, but at lower doses as tolerated. If hypotension occurs, a slight increase in dry weight via liberalization of sodium intake may help raise blood pressure to an acceptable range.

IX.   Potential benefits

A.   Quality-of-life (QOL). Improvements in physical and social functioning have been documented, as well as reduced postdialysis fatigue, intradialytic symptoms, and Beck Depression Index scores. Most compelling of all is the ongoing patient willingness to commit to these regimens despite the increased treatment and setup time, inconvenience, and medicalization of their households.

B.   Cardiovascular. As noted above, BP control has been consistently improved with both NHD and SDHD, with less need for antihypertensive medication. NHD in particular appears to have potent antihypertensive effects that are independent of volume status. Total peripheral resistance falls as patients are switched from conventional therapy to NHD. Both SDHD (with increased weekly dialysis session time) and NHD appear to be associated with regression of left ventricular hypertrophy (LVH), and increases in ejection fraction have been documented. NHD also appears to restore a healthier type of heart rate variability, which is commonly impaired in uremia.

C.   Nutrition. Observational studies of both SDHD and NHD have shown improved nutritional status as measured by nPNA, serum albumin, and mean arm muscle area. NHD, and to a lesser extent SDHD patients enjoy unrestricted dietary and fluid intake. NHD patients treated five to six times per week generally do not require phosphorus or potassium restriction. Some studies have shown increases in high-density lipoprotein (HDL) cholesterol and reductions in both low-density lipoprotein (LDL) cholesterol and homocysteine. NHD tends to remove water-soluble vitamins; therefore, patients treated with NHD require supplements, which are typically given the morning after each dialysis session.

D.   Calcium and phosphorus balance. The management of hyperphosphatemia is made easier with NHD. Results with SDHD depend on the session length, with longer sessions (2.5–3 hours) consistently improving phosphorus control and calcium-phosphorus product (Ca $\times$ P). NHD can potentially result in phosphorus depletion unless phosphorus is added to the dialysis solution when needed, as described above. Symptomatic hypophosphatemia can have serious consequences. Long-term hypophosphatemia can also result in osteomalacia. Whether dialysis solution phosphorus supplementation will be needed depends primarily on the total weekly dialysis time, and, to a lesser degree, on the blood and dialysate flow rates. NHD given five to six times per week is the only extracorporeal therapy that can reverse the positive phosphorus balance of dialysis patients, and the potential benefits of this in terms of improving bone disease and vascular calcification are large but remain to be clarified. Of note, NHD also has caused dissolution of some fairly impressive soft tissue calcification deposits (extraosseous tumoral calcification).

E.   Anemia management. Studies have documented increases in hemoglobin with concomitant falls in EPO requirements with more frequent dialysis, but this has not been consistently found. Increasing the frequency of dialysis may theoretically increase blood loss in the circuit, so iron loss is an important issue. This remains an area for further study.

F.   Sleep. Conversion to NHD has been shown to normalize the frequency of apnea/hypopnea episodes and restore normal oxygen saturation during sleep in patients with obstructive sleep apnea. Another study, however, failed to show a reduction in daytime sleepiness. The effect of SDHD on sleep apnea is unknown.

G. Hospitalization. Some small observational studies have suggested that NHD and SDHD can reduce hospitalization rates. Various forms of bias and lack of randomization, however, limit the validity of these conclusions, and more rigorous and adequately powered studies are needed.

H. Survival. Improvements detailed above in Ca × P control and lower LVH may translate into improved survival using a more frequent dialysis approach. Such hard outcomes studies of SDHD or NHD documenting this supposition have not yet been done, however.

X. Economic aspects. Economic analyses in SDHD or NHD are complex and vary with practice environment and treatment setting. Expenditures must be weighed in the context of patient rehabilitation, clinical outcomes. and quality-of-life. Costs are approximately the same for NHD and SDHD done at home when the cost of overnight monitoring is excluded. Either regimen doubles the cost of consumables. Home dialysis entails further capital costs in the purchase and installation of dialysis machines and water treatment systems, though this equipment can be transferred from one patient's home to another in the event of a modality change or transplantation. Both SDHD and NHD may reduce costs due to decreased need for erythropoietin and lower hospitalization rates.

SELECTED READINGS

Al-Hejaili F, et al. Nocturnal but not short hours quotidian hemodialysis requires an elevated dialysate calcium concentration. *J Am Soc Nephrol* 2003;14(9):2322–2328.

Ayus JC, et al. Effects of short daily versus conventional hemodialysis on left ventricular hypertrophy and inflammatory markers: a prospective, controlled study. *J Am Soc Nephrol* 2005;16:2778–2788.

Blagg CR. A brief history of home hemodialysis. *Adv Ren Replace Ther* 1996;3(2):99–105.

Chan CT, et al. Short-term blood pressure, noradrenergic, and vascular effects of nocturnal home hemodialysis. *Hypertension* 2003;42(5):925–931.

Depner TA. Daily hemodialysis efficiency: an analysis of solute kinetics. *Adv Ren Replace Ther* 2001;8(4):227–235.

Diaz-Buxo JA, Schlaeper C, VanValkenburgh D. Evolution of home hemodialysis monitoring systems. *Hemodial Int* 2003;7(4):353–355.

Fagugli RM, et al. Short daily hemodialysis: blood pressure control and left ventricular mass reduction in hypertensive hemodialysis patients. *Am J Kidney Dis* 2001;38(2):371–376.

Gotch FA. The current place of urea kinetic modelling with respect to different dialysis modalities. *Nephrol Dial Transplant* 1998;13(Suppl 6):10–14.

Hanly PJ, Pierratos A. Improvement of sleep apnea in patients with chronic renal failure who undergo nocturnal hemodialysis. *N Engl J Med* 2001;344(2):102–107.

Ing TS, et al. Phosphorus-enriched hemodialysates: formulations and clinical use. *Hemodial Int* 2003;7:148–155.

Leitch R, et al. Nursing issues related to patient selection, vascular access, and education in quotidian hemodialysis. *Am J Kidney Dis* 2003;42(1 Suppl):56–60.

McFarlane PA. Reducing hemodialysis costs: conventional and quotidian home hemodialysis in Canada. *Semin Dial* 2004;17(2):118–124.

Mucsi I, et al. Control of serum phosphate without any phosphate binders in patients treated with nocturnal hemodialysis. *Kidney Int* 1998;53(5):1399–1404.

Nesrallah G, et al. Volume control and blood pressure management in patients undergoing quotidian hemodialysis. *Am J Kidney Dis* 2003;42(I Suppl):13–17.

Piccoli GB, et al. Vascular access survival and morbidity on daily dialysis: a comparative analysis of home and limited care haemodialysis. *Nephrol Dial Transplant* 2004;19:2084–2094.

Quotidian hemodialysis. In: Lindsay RM, Blagg C, eds. *Contributions in Nephrology.* 2004:145.

Suri RS, et al. Daily hemodialysis: a systematic review. *Clin J Am Soc Nephrol* 2006;1:33–42.

Walsh M, et al. A systematic review of the effect of nocturnal hemodialysis on blood pressure, left ventricular hypertrophy, anemia, mineral metabolism, and health-related quality-of-life. *Kidney Int* 2005;67:1501–1508.

Yuen D, et al. The natural history of coronary calcification progression in a cohort of nocturnal haemodialysis patients. *Nephrol Dial Transplant* 2006;21:1407–1412.

WEB REFERENCES

Home dialysis central: http://www.homedialysis.org

Home dialysis channel on HDCN: http://www.hdcn.com/ch/dailyhd

comparison—to high-flux hemodialysis—was not significantly different (Canaud, et al., 2006a).

B. Other potential benefits.

1. Intradialytic symptoms. Some have found a better tolerance to HDF than regular dialysis, particularly in cardiac-compromised patients and/or in hypotension-prone patients. This beneficial effect has been related to a vaso-modulation effect involving several factors including a negative thermal balance (due to replacement fluid infusion), a high sodium concentration of the substitution fluid, and removal of vasodilating mediators.

2. Residual renal function. Recent studies have suggested that high-flux therapy contributes to a longer and better preservation of residual renal function than conventional HD. This positive effect of high-flux therapy appears to be comparable to that observed in peritoneal dialysis patients. Although this phenomenon is not completely understood, it might be due in part to a reduction of microinflammation due to improvement in dialysis water quality in units performing HDF.

3. Lower levels of serum inflammatory markers. Based on sensitive markers of the acute-phase reaction (C-reactive protein, interleukin [IL]-1, IL-6, IL-1-RA, IL-6-RA, albumin), several prospective studies have shown that the behavior of these markers remains stable over time in HDF/HF modalities. This positive effect results from the combined use of synthetic biocompatible membrane and ultrapure dialysis fluid.

4. Anemia correction. This area is controversial, with both positive and negative attributes. A positive effect has been particularly noted when patients were switched from low-flux HD to high-flux HDF modalities or to HD with protein-leaking high-flux membranes, leading to the speculation that high-flux methods might remove some protein-bound erythropoietic inhibitor substance or lead to an overall reduced state of inflammation.

5. Malnutrition. Again, this is a controversial area. Some studies show that anthropometric parameters, such as dry weight and body mass index, tend to improve over time in patients treated with high-flux therapies. Serum albumin tends to increase when patients are treated with high-flux membranes. This is associated with an increase in dietary protein intake as evaluated by the urea generation rate. A positive effect of high-flux therapies might result from the combination of high-flux membranes with ultrapure dialysate and more speculatively with the removal of anorexia-inducing uremic toxins.

6. Dyslipidemia and oxidative stress. The regular use of high-flux membranes has been shown to improve lipid profile, to reduce serum markers of oxidative stress, and to lower serum AGE concentrations. Such beneficial effects may be partly due to the improved biocompatibility of the dialyzer and the ultrapurity of the dialysate.

a. Vitamin supplementation. The increased loss of natural antioxidant substances (vitamin C, vitamin E, selenium, etc.) may abolish part of the beneficial effect of high-flux therapies, particularly with high-flux convective modalities. To prevent the enhancement of oxidative stress by high-flux modalities, we advocate supplementing patients undergoing high-efficiency HDF with 300–500 mg per week of vitamin C.

7. β_2-**microglobulin amyloidosis.** β_2-microglobulin amyloidosis has become a major complication of long-term HD therapy. Using carpal tunnel syndrome as a crude and first manifestation of β_2-microglobulin amyloidosis in HD patients, it is commonly accepted that its incidence reaches 50% at 10 years and 100% at 20 years of conventional HD treatment. Several large studies indicate that the extended use of high-flux membranes has a beneficial impact on the development of β_2-microglobulin amyloidosis, reducing its incidence by 50%. Interestingly, it has been reported that the regular use of ultrapure water was also responsible for a significant reduction of carpal tunnel syndrome in HD patients. Indeed, almost all studies report a significant reduction of carpal tunnel incidence (by 50%) with the use of high-flux methods and ultrapure dialysis fluid.

IV. Potential risks and hazards

A. Related to dialysate/water contaminants. There is the potential risk of passage into the blood, either by direct infusion (cold sterilization failure) or dialysate back-transfer (massive dialysate contamination) of bacterial-derived products. Accordingly, two types of reactions might be encountered: An acute, clinical reaction or a chronic, subclinical reaction.

1. Acute reactions are usually observed when a large amount of pyrogenic substances enters the blood during the dialysis session. They can manifest as fever, hypotension, tachycardia, breathlessness, cyanosis, and general malaise. A comorbid condition of the patient may decompensate, and this can present as angina pectoris or abdominal pain. Fever usually abates within a few hours. Leukopenia is often observed, but blood cultures remain negative.

In HDF/HF, such acute reactions are rare, probably due to the ultrapurity of dialysis fluid used and the general level of safety of the online HDF/HF equipment used, including redundant ultrafilters.

2. Chronic reactions might be observed with low and/or repeated passage of bacterial-derived products into the patient's blood. Such passage is clinically asymptomatic, but the resulting chronic microinflammation might contribute to long-term, dialysis-related complications. However, patients regularly treated by online HDF/HF typically show a reduced, rather than enhanced, inflammatory profile when compared to patients treated by conventional hemodialysis.

B. Protein loss. The use of highly permeable membranes tends to facilitate albumin loss, although improvement of membrane fabrication is resulting in dialyzers in which albumin loss is very low, yet in which β_2-microglobulin clearance is substantial. For those membranes that do leak albumin, albumin loss is enhanced when used in an HDF/HF mode.

Albumin loss is also enhanced when postdilution modalities are employed. Clinical and biologic consequences of albumin loss must be evaluated with a focus on nutritional status.

C. Deficiency syndromes. Enhanced loss of nutrients is a theoretical risk of high-flux modalities. Soluble vitamins, trace elements, small peptides, and proteins may be lost during high-flux treatments. The total amount of nutrients lost per session is, however, sufficiently low to be easily compensated for by adequate oral intake.

V. Other techniques

A. Middilution HDF. Middilution HDF relies on a newly designed hemodiafilter with which very high β_2-microglobulin clearance values have been documented. Two high-flux fiber bundles are arranged in coaxial fashion in a single diafilter housing. The blood inlet and outlet are on the same header. Blood first enters the peripheral fiber bundle, flowing away from the blood header. It is subjected to hemodiafiltration, similar to what happens normally with postdilution HDF. Once the blood flow reaches the opposite header, it is diluted by replacement fluid infused at this header. Then the diluted blood reverses course and returns to the blood header through the central bundle of fibers. The returning blood is subjected to the equivalent of predilution HDF, but because the replacement is added in the middle of the blood pathway through the filter, the term "middilution" is used. Finally, the blood leaves the filter from the central fiber bundle via the blood header.

B. Additional methods. Other variants include push/pull hemodiafiltration, double high-flux hemodialysis, and paired hemodiafiltration. Their description is beyond the scope of the *Handbook.*

VI. Conclusions. HDF and HF are the most efficient methods for removing both small and middle molecule uremic toxins. Also, by virtue of their incorporation of ultrapure dialysis fluid and synthetic hemocompatible membranes, HDF/HF modalities also improve the global biocompatibility profile of the hemodialysis system. Preliminary clinical studies indicate that regular use of HDF/HF tends to reduce dialysis-related morbidity in long-term treated patients, although key "hard" outcome improvements will need to await the completion of ongoing large-scale, European prospective randomized studies (Canaud et al., 2006c). Combining an HDF approach with more frequent and/or longer treatment sessions may well have an additive beneficial effect on dialysis outcomes.

SELECTED READINGS

Altieri P, et al. Predilution haemofiltration—the Second Sardinian Multicentre Study: comparisons between haemofiltration and haemodialysis during identical *Kt/V* and session times in a long-term cross-over study. *Nephrol Dial Transplant* 2001;16(6):1207–1213.

Canaud B, et al. On-line haemodiafiltration. Safety and efficacy in long-term clinical practice. *Nephrol Dial Transplant* 2000;15(Suppl 1):60–67.

Canaud B, et al. Mortality risk for patients receiving hemodiafiltration versus hemodialysis: European results from the DOPPS. *Kidney Int* 2006a;69:2087–2093.

Canaud B, et al. Beta$_2$-microglobulin, a uremic toxin with a double meaning. *Kidney Int* 2006b;69:1297–1299.

Canaud B, et al. Overview of clinical studies in hemodiafiltration: what do we need now? *Hemodial Int* 2006c;10(Suppl 1):S5–S12.

Cheung AK, et al. Serum beta-2 microglobulin levels predict mortality in dialysis patients: results of the HEMO study. *J Am Soc Nephrol* 2006;17(2):546–555.

Chun-Liang L, et al. Reduction of advanced glycation end products levels by on-line hemodiafiltration in long-term hemodialysis patients. *Am J Kidney Dis* 2003;42:524.

Clark WR, Gao D. Low-molecular weight proteins in end-stage renal disease: potential toxicity and dialytic removal mechanisms. *J Am Soc Nephrol* 2002;13(1):S41–S47.

Eknoyan G, et al. Effect of dialysis dose and membrane flux in maintenance hemodialysis. *N Engl J Med* 2002;19:347.

European Best Practice Guidelines Expert Group on Hemodialysis, European Renal Association: Section II. Haemodialysis adequacy. *Nephrol Dial Transplant* 2002;17(Suppl 7):16.

Gupta BB, Jaffrin MY. In vitro study of combined convection-diffusion mass transfer in hemodialyzers. *Int J Artif Organs* 1984;7:263–268.

Hillion D, et al. Albumin loss with high-flux dialysers is underestimated. *J Am Soc Nephrol* 1999;10:283A.

Leypoldt JK, et al. Effect of dialysis membranes and middle molecule removal on chronic hemodialysis patient survival. *Am J Kidney Dis* 1999;33(2):349–355.

Locatelli F, et al. Comparison of mortality in ESRD patients on convective and diffusive extracorporeal treatments. The Registro Lombardo Dialisi E Trapianto. *Kidney Int* 1999;55(1):286–293.

Locatelli F, et al. Effects of different membranes and dialysis technologies on patient treatment tolerance and nutritional parameters. The Italian Cooperative Dialysis Study Group. *Kidney Int* 1996;50:1293.

Lonnemann G, Koch KM. Beta(2)-microglobulin amyloidosis: effects of ultrapure dialysate and type of dialyzer membrane. *J Am Soc Nephrol* 2002;13(Suppl 1):S72.

Lornoy W, et al. On-line haemodiafiltration. Remarkable removal of beta2-microglobulin. Long-term clinical observations. *Nephrol Dial Transplant* 2000;15(Suppl 1):49.

Lornoy W, et al. Impact of convective flow on phosphorus removal in maintenance hemodialysis patients. *J Ren Nutr* 2006;16(1):47–53.

McKane W, et al. Identical decline of residual renal function in high-flux biocompatible hemodialysis and CAPD. *Kidney Int* 2002; 61:256.

Morena M, et al. Convective and diffusive losses of vitamin C during haemodiafiltration session: a contributive factor to oxidative stress in haemodialysis patients. *Nephrol Dial Transplant* 2002;17:422.

Pedrini LA, De Cristofaro V. On-line mixed hemodiafiltration with a feedback for ultrafiltration control: effect on middle-molecule removal. *Kidney Int* 2003;64:1505.

Stein G, et al. Influence of dialysis modalities on serum AGE levels in end-stage renal disease patients. *Nephrol Dial Transplant* 2001;16:999.

Van der Sande FM, et al. Thermal effects and blood pressure response during postdilution hemodiafiltration and hemodialysis: the effect of amount of replacement fluid and dialysate temperature. *J Am Soc Nephrol* 2001;12:1916.

Vanholder R, Glorieux GL, De Smet R. Back to the future: middle molecules, high flux membranes, and optimal dialysis. *Hemodial Int* 2003;7:52.

Ward RA, et al. A comparison of on-line hemodiafiltration and high-flux hemodialysis: a prospective clinical study. *J Am Soc Nephrol* 2000;11:2344.

Zehnder C, Gutzwiller JP, Renggli K. Hemodiafiltration—a new treatment option for hyperphosphatemia in hemodialysis patients. *Clin Nephrol* 1999;52:152.

Plasmapheresis

Nuhad Ismail, Dobri D. Kiprov, and
Raymond M. Hakim

Therapeutic apheresis refers to an extracorporeal procedure in which blood separator technology is used to remove abnormal blood cells and plasma constituents. The terms **plasmapheresis, leukapheresis, erythrocytapheresis, and thrombocytapheresis** describe the specific blood element that is removed. In plasmapheresis, or therapeutic plasma exchange (TPE), large quantities of plasma are removed from a patient and replaced with fresh frozen plasma (FFP), albumin solution, and/or saline.

I.   Rationale. There are several mechanisms by which plasmapheresis exerts its beneficial effects (Table 16-1). Its major mode of action is rapid depletion of specific disease-associated factors. Another effect is its ability to remove other high molecular weight proteins that may participate in the inflammatory process (intact complement C3, C4, activated complement products, fibrinogen, and cytokines). Several other theoretical effects of TPE on immune function have been proposed, including immunomodulatory actions such as alterations in idiotypic/anti-idiotypic antibody balance, a shift in the antibody-to-antigen ratio to more soluble forms of immune complexes (facilitating their clearance), and stimulation of lymphocyte clones to enhance cytotoxic therapy. Therapeutic plasma exchange also allows the infusion of normal plasma, which may replace a deficient plasma component, perhaps the principal mechanism of action of TPE in thrombotic thrombocytopenic purpura (TTP).

A.   Principles of treatment

1.   Use of concomitant immunosuppression. Because of the immunologic nature of most diseases treated by plasmapheresis, therapy should almost always include concomitant immunosuppression (i.e., in most diseases, TPE should not be the sole modality of treatment). Adjunct drug protocols usually include high doses of corticosteroids and cytotoxic agents, such as cyclophosphamide. These agents would be expected to reduce the rate of resynthesis of pathologic antibodies and to further modulate cell-mediated immunity, which may contribute to many of these disorders.

2.   Treating early. Diseases that respond to plasmapheresis are best treated early to halt the inflammatory response that often contributes to disease progression. For example, plasmapheresis of anti–glomerular basement membrane (GBM) disease is most effective if therapy is initiated when serum creatinine is <5 mg/dL (440 mcmol/L).

Table 16-1. Possible mechanisms of action of therapeutic plasma exchange

Removal of abnormal circulating factor

Antibody (anti-GBM disease, myasthenia gravis, Guillain-Barré syndrome)
Monoclonal protein (Waldenström macroglobulinemia, myeloma protein)
Circulating immune complexes (cryoglobulinemia, SLE)
Alloantibody (Rh alloimmunization in pregnancy)
Toxic factor

Replenishment of specific plasma factor

TTP

Other effects on immune system

Improvement in function of reticuloendothelial system
Removal of inflammatory mediators (cytokines, complement)
Shift in antibody-to-antigen ratio, resulting in more soluble forms of immune complexes
Stimulation of lymphocyte clones to enhance cytotoxic therapy

GBM, glomerular basement membrane; SLE, systemic lupus erythematosus; TTP, thrombotic thrombocytopenic purpura.

II. Pharmacokinetics of immunoglobulin (Ig) removal
A. Plasma half-life. Immunoglobulins have relatively long half-lives, approaching 21 days for IgG and 5 days for IgM. Because of the relatively long plasma half-lives of the immunoglobulins, the use of immunosuppressive agents that decrease their production rate cannot be expected to lower the plasma levels of a pathogenic autoantibody for at least several weeks, even if production is completely blocked. This is the basic rationale for their removal by extracorporeal means.
B. Extravascular distribution and equilibration rate. Immunoglobulins have a substantial extravascular distribution (Table 16-2). The extent of intravascular versus

Table 16-2. Distribution volumes of immunoglobulins

Substance	Molecular Weight	% Intra-vascular	Half-Life (Days)	Normal Serum Conc. (mg/dL)
Albumin	69,000	40	19	3,500–4,500
IgG	180,000	50	21	640–1430
IgA	150,000	50	6	30–300
IgM	900,000	80	5	60–350
LDL-cholesterol (β-lipoprotein)	1,300,000	100	3–5	140–200

Ig, immunoglobulin; LDL, low-density lipoprotein.

extravascular distribution will determine *how effectively* they can be removed in the course of a single plasmapheresis session. Immunoglobulins exhibit an intravascular-to-extravascular equilibration that is approximately 1%–2% per hour, whereas extravascular-to-intravascular equilibration may be somewhat faster because it is governed by the rate of lymphatic flow. Still, since the extravascular-to-intravascular equilibration is relatively slow, the kinetics of immunoglobulin removal by plasma exchange can be calculated by using first-order kinetics governing removal rates from a single compartment (the intravascular space).

C. The macromolecule reduction ratio and V_e/V_p. In Chapter 3, the relationship between the urea reduction ratio (URR) and Kt/V was described, as depicted in Figure 3-6. A similar relationship holds for removal of immunoglobulins by TPE.

The kinetics of immunoglobulin removal by TPE follow an exponential relationship:

$$C_t = C_0 e^{-V_e/V_p},$$

where C_0 = the initial plasma concentration of the macromolecule in question, C_t = its concentration at time t, V_e = the volume of plasma exchanged at time t, and V_p = the estimated plasma volume, which, while smaller than the volume of distribution of many of these macromolecules, functions as the volume from which they are removed, given the slow rate of equilibration between the extravascular and intravascular compartments.

The macromolecule reduction ratio (MRR), expressed as a percentage, is $100 \times (1 - C_t/C_0)$, so MRR $= 100 \times (1 - e^{-V_e/V_p})$. If we plug in numbers for V_e from 1,400 mL to 8,400 mL (Table 16-3), and if we assume that a patient's V_p is 2,800 mL, we will get values of V_e/V_p from 0.5 to 3.0. TPE using these V_e/V_p ratios will result in values for the MRR (Table 16-3) ranging from 39% (when $V_e/V_p = 0.5$) to 95% (when $V_e/V_p = 3.0$). Note that for $V_e/V_p = 1.0$, the MRR is 63%. So

Table 16-3. Relationship between plasma volume removed and concentration of substance

Portion of Plasma Volume[a] Exchanged (V_e/V_p)	Volume Exchanged ($V_{e,mL}$)	Immunoglobulin or Other Substance Removed (MRR, %)
0.5	1,400	39
1.0	2,800	63
1.5	4,200	78
2.0	5,600	86
2.5	7,000	92
3.0	8,400	95

[a]Plasma volume = 2,800 mL in a 70-kg patient, assuming hematocrit = 45%.
V_e, volume of plasma exchanged; V_p, estimated plasma volume; MRR, macromolecule reduction ratio.

the largest decrease (MRR) occurs with removal of the first plasma volume; removal of subsequent plasma volumes during the same session becomes progressively less effective in decreasing the concentration of the macromolecule in question. For this reason, usually one, and at most two, plasma volume equivalents (V_e/V_p) are exchanged during a plasmapheresis session.

D. Reaccumulation. Subsequent to the removal of the macromolecule in question, there is a reaccumulation of its concentration in the vascular space from two sources: (a) lymphatic drainage into the vascular space, with a concentration of macromolecules that reflects its presence in the extravascular (primarily interstitial) space, as well as from diffusion of the macromolecule across capillaries from the interstitial to the intravascular space; and (b) endogenous synthesis. Endogenous synthesis has been documented in Goodpasture syndrome, in which the anti-GBM antibodies will be predictably lowered by a given plasma exchange treatment, but intertreatment increases in serum levels are too rapid to be compatible with simple re-equilibration from extravascular stores.

Thus, over the course of the 24–36 hours following a plasmapheresis treatment, the intravascular concentration of the macromolecule in question would rise from approximately 35% of basal levels to approximately 60%–65% of basal concentration. A second plasma exchange of one plasma volume would then reduce the plasma macromolecule concentration to 20%–25% of the original concentration, only to be followed by a gradual reaccumulation over the subsequent 24 hours to 38% of the original concentration as shown in Figure 16-1. At the time of the fourth or fifth TPE, the concentration of the macromolecule would be oscillating between 10% of basal

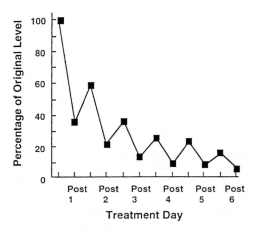

Figure 16-1. Plasma levels of immunoglobulin G before and after plasmapheresis.

levels at the end of the procedure to 20%–25% of basal levels before the next procedure. At this range of concentration, the efficiency of plasmapheresis is greatly reduced, and further plasma exchange is generally unwarranted.

E. Pharmacokinetic basis for TPE prescriptions. Based on these concepts, a rational approach to prescribing TPE is generally to recommend one plasma volume exchange daily for 5 consecutive days at intervals of 24 hours to allow for adequate lymphatic drainage into the vascular space. Clearly, the rate of accumulation and the frequency of TPE should also be targeted to the specific macromolecule that is pathogenic, if this is known. For example, whereas the half-life of IgG is approximately 21 days, that of IgM and IgA is much shorter (5–7 days). Therefore, if the macromolecule in question is IgM, there may be a role for a more extended period of TPE because the endogenous synthesis rate is expected to be higher for IgM than for IgG. If the substance to be removed is measurable by reliable quantitative means (such as with specific autoantibody), then the treatment schedule should be designed to achieve a significant reduction of that substance based on kinetic considerations. If treatments are performed without identification of the offending agent, then the physician remains dependent on empirical treatment regimens.

F. Estimation of plasma volume. An estimate of the plasma volume is required to arrive at an appropriate plasmapheresis prescription. For this purpose, there are several nomograms and equations using height, weight, and hematocrit (Hct). These have been incorporated into newer versions of the plasmapheresis equipment. A useful rule of thumb is to consider plasma volume to be approximately 35–40 mL/kg of body weight, with the lower number (35 mL/kg) applicable to patients with normal Hct values and 40 mL/kg applicable to patients with Hct values that are less than normal. For example, in a 70-kg patient with a normal Hct (45%), plasma volume (V_p) would be $70 \times 40 = 2,800$ mL.

Predicted blood volume equations have been derived by curve-fitting techniques using subjects' height (cm) and body weight (kg) compared with actual blood volumes measured by isotope (iodine-131 albumin) dilution techniques: $V_p = (1 - \text{Hct})(b + cW)$, where W = lean body weight, $b = 1,530$ for males, 864 for females, and $c = 41$ for males, 47.2 for females.

Kaplan (1992) uses a simplified method for predicting the estimated plasma volume:

$$V_p = [0.065 \times \text{weight (kg)}] \times (1 - \text{Hct})$$

III. Technical considerations. TPE can be performed using centrifugation blood cell separators or by membrane plasma separation (MPS). Centrifugation devices are commonly used for blood banking since they are capable of selective cell removal (cytapheresis) in addition to plasmapheresis. MPS utilizes highly permeable hollow-fiber filters, similar to dialyzers but with large pore sizes, and appropriately modified dialysis equipment. The advantages and disadvantages of each technique are summarized in Table 16-4.

Table 16-4. Comparison of membrane apheresis and centrifugal devices

	Advantages	Disadvantages
Membrane apheresis	Fast and efficient plasmapheresis No citrate requirements Can be adapted for cascade filtration	Removal of substances limited by sieving coefficient of membrane Unable to perform cytapheresis Requires high blood flows, central venous access Requires heparin anticoagulation, limiting use in bleeding disorders
Centrifugal devices	Capable of performing cytapheresis No heparin requirement More efficient removal of all plasma components	Expensive Requires citrate anticoagulation Loss of platelets

A. Centrifugal plasma separation. During centrifugation, blood cells are separated by gravity, based on the different densities of the blood components. There are two centrifugation methods used in blood cell separators: Intermittent-flow (or discontinuous-flow) devices and continuous-flow devices. Red blood cells (RBCs) move to the outside of the spinning container while plasma, the lightest component, remains on the inside. Platelets and white blood cells (WBCs) localize between the red cell and plasma layers. Any of these components can be collected, discarded, or reinfused.

In the intermittent-flow separation, multiple aliquots of blood are sequentially withdrawn in a bowl, processed, and reinfused. In the continuous method, blood is withdrawn, centrifuged, and separated, and the desired component removed or returned to the patient in a continuous mode using a hoop-shaped annulus that has sampling ports for the collection of plasma, RBCs, WBCs, and platelets. The intermittent-flow method requires a single-needle vascular access while the continuous-flow system requires two venous accesses (one for withdrawal and a second one for return). Discontinuous-flow blood cell separators (Haemonetics Corporation, Braintree, MA) are rarely used today for therapeutic apheresis. The continuous-flow devices are preferred for therapeutic procedures because of their smaller extracorporeal blood volume, significantly shorter procedure time, and lesser amount of anticoagulant requirement. The most widely used centrifugal blood cell separator in the United States is the Cobe Spectra (Gambro BCT, Lakewood, CO). It utilizes continuous-flow technology and helpful computerized automation. Another automated blood cell separator (available in the United States) is the Fresenius AS104 (Fresenius HemoCare, Redmond, WA).

B. Membrane plasma separators. Plasma separators use membranes with a molecular weight cutoff of about 3 million, generally sufficient to allow passage of immune complexes (MW $\approx$1 million). They can be manufactured in either a hollow-fiber or parallel-plate configuration. An example of a hollow-fiber plasma separator is the Plasma-Flo made by Asahi (Apheresis Technologies, Palm Harbor, FL). The membrane allows plasma only to pass, as the pores are small enough to hold back the formed elements of the blood. The membrane has a sieving coefficient (ratio of concentration in filtrate to blood) between 0.8 and 0.9 for albumin, IgG, IgA, IgM, C3, C4, fibrinogen, cholesterol, and triglycerides (at a blood flow rate of 100 mL per minute and a transmembrane pressure [TMP] of 40 mm Hg). The Asahi plasma flow filter can be used with ACCURA (Baxter, Deerfield, IL) or Diapact (B. Braun, Bethlehem, PA) continuous renal replacement therapy (CRRT) equipment. TPE is also provided as an option on Prisma (Gambro, Lakewood, CO), but this requires use of a dedicated disposable set with preconnected plasma filter and fluid circuitry.

MPS must be performed at low TMP ($<$500 mm Hg) to avoid hemolysis. With hollow-fiber devices, the blood flow rate should exceed 50 mL per minute to avoid clotting. The ideal blood flow rate (Q_B) is usually 100–150 mL per minute. When the blood flow rate is 100 mL per minute, a plasma removal rate of 30–50 mL per minute can be expected. Thus, the average time required to perform a typical membrane filtration (V_e = 2,800 mL) is $<$2 hours (40 mL per minute × 60 minutes = 2,400 mL per hour).

C. Comparison of MPS and centrifugation devices. Centrifugal blood cell separators are the preferred therapeutic apheresis devices in the United States. These are capable of performing cytapheresis (leukapheresis, erythrocytapheresis, and thrombocytapheresis) in addition to plasmapheresis. Centrifugal devices also operate at lower whole blood and plasma flow rates (Q_B in the range of 40–50 mL per minute). Such blood flows can be obtained from a large peripheral vein (antecubital vein), eliminating the risks associated with central vascular access in many cases.

MPS is more efficient and faster for performing plasmapheresis. However, it is unsuitable for treating patients with the hyperviscosity syndrome due to paraproteinemia (most commonly Waldenström macroglobulinemia) or patients with cryoglobulinemia, because the available devices are not efficient in removing very large macromolecules. MPS is normally performed using heparin as an anticoagulant; when treating bleeding disorders such as TTP, heparin should not be used, and a citrate-based method is indicated instead.

IV. Vascular access. For the centrifuge device systems, Q_B in the range of 40–50 mL per minute is required. This can sometimes be obtained from a large peripheral vein (antecubital vein). On the contrary, a central venous access is indicated when using MPS because a blood flow rate between 100 and 150 mL per minute is required for the successful and efficient operation of the filtration system. The best approach is the use of a large-bore, dual-lumen catheter similar to the ones used for dialysis and especially dedicated for apheresis. The majority of intravascular devices available for nondialysis use, such as Swan-Ganz catheters and triple-lumen catheters, almost never provide adequate blood flow for plasmapheresis, although they may be suitable for blood return.

Citrate infusion (see later) causes an acute reduction in the plasma ionized calcium level, which can have a local effect on the cardiac conduction system and can generate life-threatening arrhythmia, particularly when blood is returned centrally close to the atrioventricular node of the heart. Use of a femoral vein is preferable to the subclavian or internal jugular vein to decrease the risk of arrhythmias arising from return of low–ionized calcium blood so close to the heart. Although the presence of a catheter in the femoral vein limits the patient's mobility, it is a safer alternative to the subclavian or internal jugular vein, and in many patients treated with TPE, mobility may not be possible and treatment is of short duration. Cardiac rhythm should be monitored, and blood-warming devices should be used, especially if processed blood is returned centrally.

When the nature of the disease requires chronic TPE (e.g., hypercholesterolemia, cryoglobulinemia), the creation of a permanent access is preferred. Patients may undergo placement of a central catheter for long-term use, such as the Broviac Hickman catheter, or long-term access may be achieved using an arteriovenous fistula or polytetrafluoroethylene graft.

V. Anticoagulation. Anticoagulation is mandatory for plasmapheresis procedures whether by MPS devices or by centrifugal devices. Citrate solutions and heparin may be used in either type of device. In general, filtration devices use heparin, whereas centrifugal machines mostly operate with citrate.

A. Heparin. Heparin sensitivity and half-life vary greatly in patients, and individual adjustment of dosage is necessary. For most patients, heparin can be used at an initial loading dose of 50 units/kg, followed by an infusion rate of 1,000 units per hour. Frequent monitoring (half-hour) of the activated clotting time (ACT) to maintain an ACT of 180–220 seconds is desirable (1.5–2.0 times normal). Heparin doses may need to be increased in patients with low Hct (increased volume of distribution) and when the plasma filtration rate is high (a high plasma filtration rate results in increased net removal of heparin, which has a sieving coefficient of 1.0).

B. Citrate. Anticoagulant citrate dextrose (ACD) is used as the anticoagulation solution for most therapeutic plasma exchange procedures. Citrate chelates calcium, which is a necessary cofactor in the coagulation cascade, and this inhibits thrombus formation and platelet aggregation. ACD comes in two standard formulations. Formula A (ACD-A) contains 2.2 g/dL of sodium citrate and 0.73 g/dL of citric acid. Formula B (ACD-B) contains 1.32 g/dL of sodium citrate and 0.44 g/dL of citric acid. ACD-B is commonly used for the Haemonetics centrifugal system, and ACD-A is used for the Cobe centrifugal and membrane (TPE) systems. Citrate solutions (ACD-A) can be infused into the blood access at a ratio of citrate to blood of 1:15–1:25. The higher citrate flow ratios (1:10–1:15) tend to be used for the continuous centrifugal flow system (except when FFP, which contains citrate, is used as a replacement fluid). Lower citrate flow ratios (1:15–1:25) are recommended for membrane therapeutic plasma exchange.

Although bleeding is uncommon with citrate, low plasma ionized calcium levels commonly occur (60%–70% of the overall complications during TPE). Therefore, symptoms and signs of hypocalcemia must be carefully watched for (perioral and/or acral paresthesias; some patients may experience shivering, light-headedness, twitching, tremors, and, rarely, continuous muscular contractions that result in involuntary carpopedal spasm). If plasma ionized calcium levels fall more severely, symptoms can progress to frank tetany with spasm in other muscle groups, including life-threatening laryngospasm. Grand mal seizures have been reported. These symptoms and signs may be accentuated by alkalosis due to hyperventilation. Reductions of ionized calcium values also lengthen the plateau phase of myocardial depolarization, manifested electrocardiographically by prolongation of the QT interval. Very high citrate levels, with corresponding low ionized calcium, lead to depressed myocardial contractility, which, though very rare, can provoke fatal arrhythmias in apheresis patients.

1. Prevention of low ionized calcium levels during citrate anticoagulation. The following measures can be considered.

a. Limiting the rate of citrate delivery to the patient. The rate of citrate infusion must not exceed the capacity of the body to metabolize citrate rapidly. The ability to metabolize citrate varies from patient to patient. Because the amount of citrate infused will be proportional to the blood flow rate, very high blood flow rates should not be used in small patients. When ACD-A is being infused in a 1:10, 1:15, or 1:25 volumetric dilution with blood, the blood flow rates should not exceed 60, 100, or 150 mL per minute, respectively, for an average-size patient. In smaller patients, the maximum blood flow rate will be even less. The maximum recommended blood flow rate can be estimated in milliliters per minute as a proportion of body weight depending on the ACD-A:blood ratio being used:

ACD-A:blood ratio	Maximum blood flow rate (mL per minute)
1:10	1.2 × body weight (kg)
1:15	2.0 × body weight (kg)
1:25	3.0 × body weight (kg)

For example, when using an ACD-A:blood dilution ratio of 1:15 in a 30-kg patient, the maximum recommended blood flow rate would be 2 × 30 = 60 mL per minute. One of the systems, the Cobe Spectra (Gambro BCT Laboratories, Lakewood, CO), estimates the patient's blood volume by a nomogram. It then automatically sets the blood flow rate to limit the rate at which citrate is being infused.

Patients with liver disease may have an impaired ability to metabolize citrate, and in these patients, citrate infusion should be performed with great caution. FFP contains up to 14% citrate by volume. In cases where FFP, instead of albumin, is being used as the replacement fluid, the citrate reinfusion rate should be lowered even further.

b. Providing additional calcium to the patient during the plasmapheresis procedure. Calcium can be given either orally or intravenously. One can, for example, give orally 500-mg (5.0-mmol) tablets of calcium carbonate every 30 minutes. Another approach is to infuse calcium gluconate 10% continuously intravenously, in a proportion of 10 mL of the calcium gluconate solution per liter of return fluid (Weinstein, 1996). In addition to these measures, intravenous boluses of calcium (10 mL of 10% $CaCl_2$ infused over 15–30 minutes) can be given whenever symptoms of hypocalcemia become manifest.

2. Alkalosis during citrate infusion. There is the danger of developing metabolic alkalosis (although this is a very rare occurrence) because citrate is metabolized to bicarbonate. In patients with liver disease, who may have impaired ability for citrate metabolism, acid–base status during plasmapheresis using citrate anticoagulation should be monitored with special care.

VI. Replacement solution. The selection of the type and amount of replacement fluids is an important consideration in the prescription of plasmapheresis. The diversity of disease and patient conditions makes the elaboration of uniform suggestions for replacement fluid difficult. Nevertheless, certain guidelines are useful, and they can be modified by the specific conditions encountered.

In most plasmapheresis procedures, replacement by colloidal agents is essential to maintain hemodynamic stability. In practice, this is limited to albumin, generally in the form of an isonatric 5% solution, or to plasma in the form of FFP. The advantages and disadvantages of each are listed in Table 16-5.

A. FFP. FFP has the advantage of being similar in composition to the filtrate being removed from the patient but is

Table 16-5. Choice of replacement solution

Solution	Advantages	Disadvantages
Albumin	No risk of hepatitis Stored at room temperature Allergic reactions are rare No concern about ABO blood group Depletes inflammation mediators	Expensive No coagulation factors No immunoglobulins
Fresh frozen plasma	Coagulation factors Immunoglobulins "Beneficial" factors Complement	Risk of hepatitis, HIV transmission Allergic reactions Hemolytic reactions Must be thawed Must be ABO-compatible Citrate load

HIV, human immunodeficiency virus.

associated with side effects, such as allergic reactions. Urticaria and hives, which may be severe, are frequently present with the use of FFP. Rarely, anaphylactic reactions result in a form of noncardiogenic pulmonary edema caused by passive transfusion of leukoagglutinins. Another cause of anaphylaxis is infusion of IgA-containing FFP to a patient with selective IgA deficiency. Because FFP may contain appreciable amounts of anti-A and anti-B isoagglutinins, ABO compatibility between donor and recipient is necessary. As noted above, FFP contains citrate, and use of FFP increases the risk of citrate-mediated low ionized calcium reactions. Also, there is a small but measurable incidence of transmission via FFP of hepatitis B (0.0005% per unit), hepatitis C (0.03% per unit), and HIV (0.0004% per unit). Although these infectious risks are now much smaller with predonation and postdonation testing, it should be kept in mind that with each plasmapheresis treatment where 3 L of plasma is replaced with FFP, the 3 L of replacement FFP is made up of 10–15 units of plasma coming from an equal number of donors.

Use of FFP as the replacement fluid makes measurement of the efficacy of plasmapheresis more difficult in certain patients (e.g., one cannot simply follow serum levels of IgG and other immunoglobulins). Also, FFP may replenish some factors removed during plasmapheresis that could participate in the inflammatory process.

At present, the specific indications for replacing some or all of the removed plasma with FFP during plasma exchange are (a) thrombotic thrombocytopenic purpura–hemolytic uremic syndrome (TTP/HUS), (b) preexisting defect in hemostasis and/or low pretreatment serum fibrinogen level (<125 mg per dL), and (c) risk of cholinesterase depletion.

With regard to TTP/HUS, there is a rationale for using FFP as the sole replacement fluid because infusion of FFP by itself may be therapeutic and because in the presence of thrombocytopenia the risk of bleeding as a consequence of minor perturbations in the coagulation factors may be higher.

In general, because plasmapheresis also depletes coagulation factors, replacement by albumin and crystalloids alone may deplete these factors and place the patient at increased risk of bleeding. This is not likely to occur after one or two plasma exchanges, particularly if they are performed more than a day apart, because the half-life for most clotting factors is approximately 24–36 hours. Nevertheless, we recommend measurement of prothrombin time (PT) and partial thromboplastin time (PTT) before the third and subsequent procedures. If the PT and PTT are more than 1.5 times longer than control samples, we recommend infusion of at least 2 or 3 units of FFP as part of the replacement solution.

B. Albumin. Because of the above concerns with the use of FFP, we recommend albumin as the initial replacement solution. Albumin, at a concentration of 5 g/dL (50 g/L) in 0.9% saline, can be replaced in a volume equal to that of the removed filtrate. With modern equipment this can be done simultaneously and at the same rate as plasma removal. However, because a substantial proportion of the albumin that is infused early during the procedure is exchanged during the course of a plasmapheresis procedure, a more economical approach (when exchange volume is equal to one plasma volume and in the absence of hypoalbuminemia) is to replace the initial 20%–30% of the removed plasma volume with crystalloid, such as normal saline or Ringer's lactate, and then substitute the balance with 5% albumin. This method would result in a final concentration of albumin in the vascular space of approximately 3.5 g/dL (35 g/L), sufficient to maintain oncotic pressure and avoid hypotension.

Purified human serum albumin (HSA) solutions do not transmit viral diseases because of prolonged heat treatment during processing and have become a favored replacement fluid in TPE. They have an excellent overall safety record. The incidence of adverse reactions of any kind has been estimated to be 1 in 6,600 infusions. Severe, potentially life-threatening reactions occur in approximately 1 of every 30,000 infusions. When preparing 5% albumin solution from more concentrated solutions, 0.9% saline (with addition of supplementary electrolytes as needed) must be used as the diluent; use of water as a diluent has resulted in severe hyponatremia and hemolysis (Steinmuller et al., 1998).

The amount of fluid replacement given depends on the patient's volume status. The replacement volume can be adjusted, either manually or automatically, from 100% of the removed volume to less than 85%. Use of lower replacement volumes is generally not recommended, since this may contract the intravascular volume and result in hemodynamic instability.

Table 16-6.   Complications of plasmapheresis

Related to vascular access

Hematoma
Pneumothorax
Retroperitoneal bleed

Related to the procedure

Hypotension from externalization of blood in the extracorporeal
  circuit
Hypotension due to decreased intravascular oncotic pressure
Bleeding from reduction in plasma levels of coagulation factors
Edema formation due to decreased intravascular oncotic
  pressure
Loss of cellular elements (platelets)
Hypersensitivity reactions

Related to anticoagulation

Bleeding, especially with heparin
Hypocalcemic symptoms (with citrate)
Arrhythmias
Hypotension
Numbness and tingling of extremities
Metabolic alkalosis from citrate

VII.   **Complications.** The side effects observed in plasma
exchange are generally not severe and can be managed easily if they are anticipated. The main side effects are listed in
Table 16-6.

Complications range from 4% to 25%, with an average of
10%. Minimal reactions occur in about 5% of treatments and
are characterized by urticaria, paresthesias, nausea, dizziness, and leg cramps. Moderate reactions (5%–10% of treatments) include hypotension, chest pain, and ventricular ectopy. All are usually brief and without sequelae. Severe events
occur in <3% of treatments and are mainly related to anaphylactoid reactions associated with FFP administration. The estimated mortality rate associated with plasmapheresis is 3–6
per 10,000 procedures. The majority of deaths include anaphylaxis associated with FFP replacement, pulmonary embolism,
and vascular perforation. The most important complications
are summarized in Table 16-6. Strategies for avoidance and
management of these complications are summarized in Table
16-7.

A.   **Hemodynamic complications.** Hypotension (2% overall incidence) is due mainly to intravascular volume depletion, which may be exaggerated by the large (250–375 mL)
volume of blood externalized in the extracorporeal circuit of
centrifugal-type cell separators. Other causes include vasova-
gal episodes, use of hypo-oncotic fluid replacement, delayed
or inadequate volume replacement, anaphylaxis, cardiac arrhythmia, and cardiovascular collapse.

Table 16-7. Strategies to avoid complications during plasmapheresis

Complication	Management
Low ionized calcium	Prophylactic infusion of 10% $CaCl_2$ during treatment
Hemorrhage	Two units of fresh frozen plasma at the end of the session
Thrombocytopenia	Consider membrane plasma separation.
Volume-related hypotension	Adjust volume balance.
Infection postapheresis	Infusion of intravenous immunoglobulin (100–400 mg per kg)
Hypokalemia	Ensure a potassium concentration of 4 mM in the replacement solution.
Membrane biocompatibility	Change membrane or consider centrifugal method of plasma separation.
Hypothermia	Warm replacement fluids.
ACE inhibitors	Discontinue ACE inhibitor therapy 24–48 hours before treatments.
Sensitivity to replacement fluids	Consider diagnostic evaluation (anti–IgA antibody, anti–ethylene oxide antibody, anti–human serum albumin antibody, endotoxin assay, bacterial cultures of replacement fluid, etc.). Consider using starch-based fluids. Premedication regimen for sensitized individuals: (a) prednisone 50 mg orally 13 hours, 7 hours, and 1 hours before treatment; (b) diphenhydramine 50 mg orally 1 hour before treatment; and (c) ephedrine 25 mg orally 1 hour before treatment.

ACE, angiotensin-converting enzyme; Ig, immunoglobulin.
Modified from Mokrzycki MH, Kaplan, AA. Therapeutic plasma exchange: complications and management. *Am J Kidney Dis* 1994;23:817.

B. Hematologic complications. Hemorrhagic episodes are rare. Bleeding postinsertion of a femoral catheter, bleeding from a previous catheter site, hematemesis, and epistaxis have been described.

After a single plasma exchange, the serum fibrinogen level typically falls by 80%, and prothrombin and many other clotting factor levels also fall by about 50%–70%. The PTT usually increases by 100%. Recovery of plasma levels of coagulation factors is biphasic, characterized by a rapid initial increase up to 4 hours postapheresis and followed by a slower increase 4–24 hours postexchange. Twenty-four hours after treatment, fibrinogen levels are approximately 50% and antithrombin III levels are 85% of initial levels; both require 48–72 hours for complete recovery. One day following treatment, the prothrombin level is 75% and factor X is 30% of the original level; by this time, all other coagulation factors will have completely recovered to normal values. When multiple treatments are performed over a short period, the depletion in clotting factors is more pronounced and may require several days for spontaneous recovery. As stated before, when multiple closely spaced treatments are given, it is advisable to replace 2 units of FFP at the end of each treatment. Device-specific thrombocytopenia has been reported as a result of TPE, and this has caused confusion in assessing response during treatment of disorders such as TTP (Perdue et al., 2001).

C. Angiotensin-converting enzyme (ACE) inhibitors. Anaphylactic or atypical anaphylactoid reactions have been reported in patients taking ACE inhibitors during hemodialysis, low-density lipoprotein (LDL) affinity apheresis, and staphylococcal protein A affinity apheresis. These reactions have been related to negatively charged membranes or filters. Experimental evidence has shown that this reaction is not related to the extracorporeal circulation alone. It is speculated that the fragments of prekallikrein-activating factor present in human albumin lead to endogenous bradykinin release. The severity of the reactions depends on different variables, including drug type and lot of albumin (which may contain different concentrations of the prekallikrein-activating factor). Ideally, therefore, short-acting ACE inhibitors should be held for 24 hours, and long-acting ACE for 48 hours, prior to plasma exchange.

D. Infection. The true incidence of infection in TPE is controversial. Studies have not clearly shown a significantly higher occurrence of opportunistic infections among patients treated with immunosuppression and therapeutic plasma exchange than with immunosuppressive therapy alone. However, if a severe infection develops in the immediate post–plasma exchange period, a reasonable approach would be a single infusion of immunoglobulins (100–400 mg/kg intravenously).

E. Electrolyte, vitamin, and drug removal
   1. Hypokalemia. When the replacement solution is albumin in saline, there could be a 25% reduction in serum potassium levels in the immediate postapheresis period. The risk

of hypokalemia can be reduced by adding 4 mmol of potassium to each liter of replacement solution.

2. Metabolic alkalosis. This may result from infusion of large amounts of citrate.

3. Drugs. In general, drugs that are significantly cleared by plasma exchange are the ones that have small volumes of distribution and extensive protein binding. Evidence shows that supplemental dosing of prednisone, digoxin, cyclosporine, ceftriaxone, ceftazidime, valproic acid, and phenobarbital is not necessary after plasma exchange. In contrast, the dosages of salicylates, azathioprine, and tobramycin should be supplemented. The many reports of phenytoin clearance are conflicting; thus, it is necessary to carefully monitor unbound drug levels. Therefore, we generally recommend that all scheduled medications be given immediately after the procedure.

VIII. Indications for plasmapheresis. In this section, emphasis will be placed on a few diseases in which plasmapheresis has been shown to have a clear benefit, either as primary or adjunctive therapy (categories I and II). Category I indications are those for which TPE is standard and acceptable, but this does not imply that it is mandatory in all situations. Evidence is usually derived from controlled and well-designed clinical trials. Category II indications are those for which TPE is generally accepted; however, it is considered to be supplemental to other more definitive treatments rather than serving as primary therapy. Table 16-8 lists diseases for which plasmapheresis is definitely indicated as well as diseases in which plasmapheresis has been used as adjunctive treatment, although in some of the listings, use of plasmapheresis is still somewhat controversial (e.g., myeloma) as new studies continue to be reported.

A. Indications for emergency plasmapheresis. Life-threatening or organ-threatening situations that may require emergency plasmapheresis include:

1. Anti-GBM disease and/or pulmonary hemorrhage in Goodpasture syndrome

2. Hyperviscosity syndrome with signs and symptoms suggesting impending stroke or loss of vision

3. Microangiopathic thrombocytopenia (TTP/HUS)

4. Presence of very high factor VIII inhibitor levels in patients requiring urgent surgery (the purpose of plasmapheresis is to reduce the risk of intrasurgical and postsurgical bleeding complications)

5. Respiratory insufficiency in Guillain–Barré syndrome

6. Myasthenia gravis with respiratory distress not responding to medication

7. Acute poisoning with certain mushrooms or with other strongly protein-bound poisons, such as parathion or paraquat, depending on the severity of the intoxication

IX. Treatment strategies. General orders for plasmapheresis are listed in Table 16-9. The following sections describe plasmapheresis treatment prescriptions in selected diseases.

Table 16-8. Potential indications for plasmapheresis

Goodpasture syndrome (anti-GBM disease)
TTP/HUS
Cryoglobulinemia
Hyperviscosity syndrome
Myeloma cast nephropathy (controversial)
Acute demyelinating polyneuropathy (Guillain-Barré)
Homozygous familial hypercholesterolemia (selective
    adsorption)
Myasthenia gravis crisis
Chronic inflammatory demyelinating polyneuropathy
Eaton-Lambert myasthenic syndrome
Posttransfusion purpura
Refsum disease
Cutaneous lymphoma (photopheresis)
HIV-related syndromes (polyneuropathy, hyperviscosity, TTP)
Coagulation factor inhibitors
Rapidly progressive glomerulonephritis (without anti-GBM)
Paraproteinemic peripheral neuropathy
Systemic vasculitis associated with ANCA
ABO-incompatible marrow transplant
SLE (in particular SLE cerebritis)
Bullous pemphigoid
Pemphigus vulgaris
Immune thrombocytopenia (staphylococcal protein A
    adsorption)
Hemolytic disease of the newborn

GBM, glomerular basement membrane; TTP, thrombotic thrombocytopenic purpura; HUS, hemolytic uremic syndrome; HIV, human immunodeficiency virus; ANCA, antineutrophil cytoplasmic autoantibody; SLE, systemic lupus erythematosus.

A. Anti-GBM disease

1. Early use of plasmapheresis is strongly indicated, and the response rate is highest when serum creatinine is still low. In patients with severe disease (oliguria requiring dialysis), plasmapheresis should probably be reserved for treatment of pulmonary hemorrhage because renal function is unlikely to recover even with aggressive treatment.

2. The frequency of plasmapheresis should be high enough to rapidly decrease the circulating level of anti-GBM antibodies; exchange of two plasma volumes daily for 7 consecutive days is indicated in this disease. Because of the consequences of even small titers of circulating antibody, our practice is to continue plasmapheresis for a second week on an alternate-day basis to allow the cytotoxic effects of immunosuppressive medicines to become evident. Note that serial measurements of circulating anti-GBM antibody may be positive in only 65%–70% of cases. A renal biopsy is often indicated for definitive diagnosis of any rapidly progressive renal failure. However, if the index of suspicion for the presence of the anti-GBM disease is high and the clinical

Table 16-9. General orders for plasmapheresis

Calculate the plasma volume.

Measure the preplasmapheresis PT, PTT, and platelets.

When feasible, measure the plasma level of the substance targeted for removal (e.g., anti-GBM antibody titer, acetylcholine receptor antibody, cryoglobulin).

Space treatments approximately 24 hours apart (variable).

For heparin anticoagulation (low bleeding risk patient):
Heparin 50 units/kg initially, then 1,000 units per hour. Target ACT (when baseline mean control value = 145 seconds) during the procedure is about 180–220 seconds. If the ACT is <3 minutes, increase the infusion rate by 500 units per hour. If the ACT is >4 minutes, discontinue heparin infusion, continue to measure the ACT, and resume heparin infusion at a reduced rate when appropriate. Stop heparin infusion about 30 minutes prior to the end of the procedure.

For citrate anticoagulation, use ACD-A at 1:15 to 1:25 dilution with blood.

Use calcium infusion if necessary.

Cardiac monitor.

Administer scheduled medications only at the end of the session.[a]

Provide catheter care per routine.

---

[a]Especially cyclophosphamide and azathioprine. Prednisone and prednisolone are minimally removed by TPE and supplemental dosing after TPE has been found to be unnecessary.

PT, prothrombin time; PTT, partial thromboplastin time; GBM, glomerular basement membrane; ACT, activated clotting time; ACD-A, anticoagulant citrate dextrose formula A; TPE, therapeutic plasma exchange.

situation is suggestive (rapidly rising creatinine, lung hemorrhage), and because of the time needed for renal biopsy and the necessity for being cautious about plasmapheresis for 24 hours after biopsy to reduce the risk of bleeding, our recommendation is to initiate plasmapheresis of large plasma volumes (two plasma volumes each day) for 2 days before biopsy and defer biopsy to a time when the level of circulating antibodies is low. Citrate anticoagulation may be particularly indicated in this case to decrease the risk of pulmonary or renal bleeding. Plasmapheresis beyond a second week may be necessary, and both clinical course as well as anti-GBM antibody titers (if available) will dictate such a need.

3. Replace removed plasma (milliliter for milliliter) with isonatric 5% albumin. If the patient is in fluid overload, reduce the amount of albumin solution infused to 85% (but not less) of the removed plasma volume. In patients with pulmonary hemorrhage and patients who had a recent renal biopsy, replace the last liter with FFP.

B. TTP and HUS

1. TTP with central nervous system and renal complications can be a fulminant and rapidly fatal disorder, and it requires the institution of plasmapheresis as soon as possible. The recommended regimen is 1.5 plasma volumes for the first three treatments followed by one plasma volume exchange thereafter. The procedure is performed daily until the platelet count is normalized and hemolysis has largely ceased (as evidenced by lactate dehydrogenase level below 400 IU/L). Serum creatinine and urine output have a delayed recovery, generally improving after resolution of thrombocytopenia. Usually, 7–10 treatments are required to induce remission. Because relapse may occur in 50% of patients within a few days of stopping treatment, it is advised not to remove the vascular access catheter until the platelet count is at least 100,000/mm^3 for 5 days without treatment. If platelet count decreases to <100,000/mm^3, one can resume plasmapheresis on an every-other-day schedule until the platelet count and LDH normalize again.

In cases resistant to TPE alone, immunomodulating drugs (steroids, vincristine, cyclophosphamide, rituximab) and splenectomy should be considered.

2. Removed plasma is replaced milliliter for milliliter with FFP. It should be emphasized that the citrate present in FFP may exacerbate hypocalcemic symptoms. Cryopoor plasma has also been shown to be an effective replacement fluid in TTP.

3. In children, HUS is frequently a benign illness that often responds to supportive therapy. Although plasmapheresis is effective in shortening the duration of the illness, the difficulties of plasmapheresis in children outweigh the benefit in most cases. However, there may be a role of plasmapheresis in pediatric cases where supportive therapy does not reverse a rapidly deteriorating clinical condition.

4. Considering the severe prognosis (maternal and fetal) of TTP in pregnancy and the clear benefit in nonpregnant patients, TPE is also the treatment of choice for TTP during pregnancy despite the possibility of treatment-induced removal of pregnancy-maintaining hormones.

5. Except for mitomycin-induced TTP and cancer-associated HUS, in which plasma perfusion over a staphylococcal protein A immunoadsorbent column has been found to be more effective than the conventional exchange, the general recommendation is the use of standard plasma exchange for secondary causes of TTP/HUS.

C.   Cryoglobulinemia. Plasma exchange has been used for 20 years for the treatment of cryoglobulinemia. Although there are no randomized, controlled studies to document the efficacy of plasmapheresis in the disease, almost all of the published reports demonstrate the efficacy of plasmapheresis if the patient has overt symptoms or has progressive renal failure. Indications for TPE include (a) thrombocytopenia (platelet count <50,000/mm^3) or petechiae, or both; (b) hyperviscosity syndrome; (c) cryoglobulin titer >1%; (d) patient about to undergo surgery requiring hypothermia; and (e) renal insufficiency.

In general, patients are treated with immunosuppression and plasma exchange, but some investigators are concerned that this approach may have detrimental effects when cryoglobulinemia is associated with chronic hepatitis C infection.

A suggested prescription is to exchange one plasma volume three times weekly for 2–3 weeks. The replacement fluid can be isonatric 5% albumin, which must be warmed to prevent precipitation of circulating cryoglobulins. IgM antibodies may reaccumulate rapidly and may require chronic treatment once a week.

Selective removal techniques can be used to eliminate or minimize the need for replacement fluid. Double-cascade filtration, which allows separation of cryoglobulins (based on their high molecular weight), is a new technique that can substantially eliminate the need for replacement fluid, yet it is time consuming, relatively expensive, conducive to clotting, and increasingly difficult to obtain in the United States. Cryofiltration is another method that selectively removes cryoglobulins with a special filter by cooling plasma in an extracorporeal system. After removal of cryoglobulins, the remaining plasma is rewarmed and reinfused. Clinical trials are needed to determine the efficacy of these new approaches.

D. Pauci-immune rapidly progressive (necrotizing) glomerulonephritis (RPGN). Patients usually have Wegener granulomatosis, polyarteritis nodosa, or "renal-limited" disease. Many have antineutrophil cytoplasmic autoantibodies (ANCAs) in their circulation. ANCA titers often correlate with disease activity, and ANCAs seem to contribute to the pathophysiology of pauci-immune RPGN through reactivity with neutrophils, endothelial cells, and other inflammatory mechanisms. Available data indicate that 80% of these patients progress to end-stage renal disease without therapy with high-dose immunosuppression or cytotoxic drugs. The results of five randomized trials argue against a role for plasma exchange in mild forms of pauci-immune RPGN. However, Pusey et al. (1991) in a randomized trial on 48 patients showed a potential benefit when plasma exchange was used as an adjunct to conventional immunosuppressive therapy in patients who were originally dialysis dependent. These results probably reflect the efficacy of immunosuppression in controlling the inflammatory response and preservation of renal function.

Plasma exchange should be performed at least daily for 4 days for the first week, using 4-L exchanges with albumin and FFP to avoid coagulopathy. Response to therapy should be monitored with repeated assessments of urine output, serum creatinine values, and possibly ANCA titers. For those patients with positive ANCAs, there is a subpopulation with IgM ANCA who might be at a particular risk for pulmonary hemorrhage. If these antibodies are pathogenic, then a centrifugal method of plasma exchange may be required because standard MPS may be relatively inefficient in removing the large IgM-containing immune complexes.

E. Multiple myeloma and paraproteinemias. Renal failure complicates 3%–9% of cases of multiple myeloma and is associated with a poor prognosis. Renal impairment is caused by toxicity of myeloma light chains to renal tubules, although other factors can also contribute, including hypercalcemia, hyperuricemia, cryoglobulinemia, amyloidosis, light-chain deposition, hyperviscosity, infections, and chemotherapeutic agents. Serum levels of light chains and severity of renal damage are the main factors determining the recovery of renal function. Acute renal failure secondary to multiple myeloma or other paraproteinemia may respond to TPE. Randomized trials have reached conflicting conclusions. If chemotherapy is successful in limiting new light-chain synthesis, then a single prescription of five consecutive plasma exchanges may be sufficient to control the deleterious effects of light chains. Additional treatments may be necessary if there is continued light-chain production. Having identified a given abnormal "spike" as a light chain by immunofixation, regular monitoring by serum protein electrophoresis is an easy means to detect recurrent light-chain accumulation.

A recent randomized, controlled trial in patients with myeloma who presented with acute renal failure did not demonstrate conclusive evidence that TPE substantially reduces a composite outcome of death, dialysis dependence, or glomerular filtration rate <30 mL per minute per m^2. The authors admitted that a major limitation of this study was the lack of renal biopsy information, which would have helped in better patient selection for inclusion in the study (Clark et al., 2005).

F.   Lupus nephritis. Several prospective, randomized, controlled trials do not support a role for plasma exchange in the routine treatment of lupus nephritis. There is experimental and clinical evidence that rapid removal of circulating antibody by plasma exchange triggers a rebound B-cell clonal proliferation and enhanced antibody synthesis. Because proliferating cells have increased vulnerability to cytotoxic agents, it has been suggested that plasma exchange may be useful in patients with lupus nephritis if synchronized with pulse cyclophosphamide (with the latter administered shortly after plasma exchange).

An international trial has been designed to take advantage of this proposed mechanism. More than 170 patients enrolled from 35 centers in Europe, Canada, and the United States. Partial reporting from the study center in Germany has described a rapid beneficial response in all 14 patients undergoing the synchronized protocol, with eight remaining off all therapy for a mean of 5.6 years. Unfortunately, 4 of 14 patients developed irreversible amenorrhea, and one patient developed a squamous cell carcinoma of the oropharynx within 17 months of treatment initiation. The international trial was suspended because some participants developed severe infections. In a different approach, rescue therapy for refractory lupus using immunoadsorption onto protein A (see Section XI, below) has been tried with good results in a small number of patients.

G.   Recurrent focal segmental glomerulosclerosis (FSGS). Following renal transplantation, FSGS has an estimated recurrence of 15%–55%, with a rapid onset of proteinuria. A protein that has a molecular weight $<100,000$, which is capable of increasing glomerular permeability to albumin, has been characterized in these patients.

In one study of posttransplant recurrent FSGS, standard plasma exchange (1.5 plasma volumes with isonatric 5% albumin as replacement fluid for 3 consecutive days, then every other day up to a total of nine treatments) was performed in patients soon after the recurrence of proteinuria. Protein excretion was reduced from 11.5 to 0.8 g per day in six of nine patients. In another study in similar patients with rapid progression of native disease and those in whom urinary protein concentration remained >100 mg/dL, plasmapheresis appeared to have a poor result (Wolf, 2005).

H. Henoch-Schönlein purpura (HSP). Nine children with rapidly progressive HSP nephritis were treated with plasmapheresis as sole therapy. Four recovered, two had residual hematuria, and three progressed. Effectiveness remains to be proven in a randomized trial.

I. Hyperviscosity syndrome. This occurs most commonly with Waldenström macroglobulinemia (50% of the time) and occasionally with myeloma (2% of the time) and cryoglobulinemia. Rarely do other causes of elevated serum proteins, such as benign monoclonal gammopathy and rheumatoid arthritis, cause hyperviscosity. It is produced by very high plasma concentrations of monoclonal immunoglobulins, which increase red blood cell aggregation and impede overall blood flow, leading to ischemia and dysfunction of all organ systems. Usually, symptoms do not occur until plasma viscosity is three to four times that of water. The clinical syndrome includes neurologic symptoms, a bleeding diathesis due to effects of the protein on platelets and clotting factors, retinopathy with dilation and segmentation of retinal and conjunctival vessels, retinal hemorrhages, papilledema, hypervolemia, distention of peripheral blood vessels, increased vascular resistance, and congestive heart failure. The therapeutic goal is to reduce the plasma viscosity to normal and reverse the neurologic symptoms, stop the bleeding diathesis, reverse or stop the visual impairment, and reverse the cardiovascular effects, including hypervolemia and increased vascular resistance. Therapy includes plasma exchange as well as treatment of the primary disorder. The suggested TPE regimen includes daily one–plasma volume sessions for 2 days and continuation of daily one–plasma volume exchanges for 5 days if serum IgM levels remain above normal.

J. Multiorgan failure with disseminated intravascular coagulation (preliminary). One uncontrolled study of patients with multiorgan failure and sepsis with disseminated intravascular coagulation achieved a survival rate of 82% after treating with 1–14 plasmapheresis treatments. This interesting preliminary study (Stegmayr et al., 2003) needs to be confirmed.

X. New techniques

A. Extracorporeal immunoadsorption. Extracorporeal immunoadsorption is a treatment modality based on the use of special ligands to specifically remove blood components considered pathogenic for different diseases, mainly immune complexes and lipids. Separated plasma is passed through a column containing the specific ligand for the substance to be removed, and the depleted plasma is then returned to the patient. Different substances have been used as ligands, with staphylococcal protein A being most widely used, due to its ability to selectively bind IgG. The only Food and Drug Administration–approved protein A column is Prosorba (Fresenius HemoCare, Redmond, WA). These columns also cause transient production of beneficial antibodies. Prosorba columns also stimulate the activity of natural killer cells, granulocytes, and macrophages. The main disadvantages are cost and the requirement of trained personnel to set up and monitor the procedure. The Prosorba column is approved for the treatment of immune thrombocytopenic purpura and rheumatoid arthritis. Rescue therapy for patients with refractory lupus has also been tried in one small study with good results.

SELECTED READINGS

Braun N, et al. Immunoadsorption onto protein A induces remission in severe systemic lupus erythematosus. *Nephrol Dial Transplant* 2000;15(9):1367–1372.

Clark WF, et al. Plasma exchange when myeloma presents as acute renal failure a randomized, controlled trial. *Ann Intern Med* 2005;143:777–784.

Hakim RM. Plasmapheresis. In: Jacobson HR, et al., eds. *The principles and practice of nephrology*, 2nd ed. St. Louis: Mosby–Year Book, 1995:713–721.

Hakim RM, et al. Successful management of thrombocytopenia, microangiopathic anemia, and acute renal failure by plasmapheresis. *Am J Kidney Dis* 1995;5:170–176.

Hattori M, et al. Plasmapheresis as the sole therapy for rapidly progressive Henoch-Schonlein purpura nephritis in children. *Am J Kidney Dis* 1999;33(3):427–433.

Kale-Pradhan PB, Woo MH. A review of the effects of plasmapheresis on drug clearance. *Pharmacotherapy* 1997;17:684–695.

Kaplan AA. Toward the rational prescription of therapeutic plasma exchange: the kinetics of immunoglobulin removal. *Semin Dial* 1992;5:227–229.

Kaplan AA. Plasma exchange in renal disease. *Semin Dial* 1996;9:61–70.

Kaplan AA. Plasma exchange for non-renal indications. *Semin Dial* 1996;9:265–275.

Kiprov DD, et al. Adverse reactions associated with mobile therapeutic apheresis: analysis of 17,940 procedures. *J Clin Apheresis* 2001;16:130–133.

Kiprov DD, Hofmann J. Plasmapheresis in immunologically mediated polyneuropathies. *Ther Apheresis Dial* 2003;7(2):189–196.

Klemmer PJ, et al. Plasmapheresis therapy for diffuse alveolar hemorrhage in patients with small-vessel vasculitis. *Am J Kidney Dis* 2003;42:1149–1154.

Levy JB, et al. Long-term outcome of anti-glomerular basement membrane antibody disease treated with plasma exchange and immunosuppression. *Ann Intern Med* 2001;134:1033–1042.

Matsuzaki M, et al. Outcome of plasma exchange therapy in thrombotic microangiopathy after renal transplantation. *Am J Transplant* 2003;3(10):1289–1294.

McLeod B, et al. Special issue, clinical applications of therapeutic apheresis. *J Clin Apheresis* 2000;15(1/2):1–159.

Montagnino G, et al. Double recurrence of FSGS after two renal transplants with complete regression after plasmapheresis and ACE inhibitors. *Transpl Int* 2000;13(2):166–168.

Perdue JJ, et al. Unintentional platelet removal by plasmapheresis. *J Clin Apheresis* 2001;16:55–60.

Pusey CD, et al. Plasma exchange in focal necrotizing glomerulonephritis without anti-GBM antibodies. *Kidney Int* 1991;40:757–763.

Saddler JE, et al. Recent advances in thrombotic thrombocytopenic purpura. *Hematology* 2004:407–423.

Siami G, et al. Cryofiltration apheresis for treatment of cryoglobulinemia associated with hepatitis C. *ASAIO J* 1995;41:M315–M318.

Stegmayr B, et al. Plasma exchange as rescue therapy in multiple organ failure including acute renal failure. *Crit Care Med* 2003;31:1730–1736.

Steinmuller DR, et al. A dangerous error in the dilution of 25 percent albumin [letter]. *N Engl J Med* 1998;38:1226–1227.

Strauss RG. Mechanisms of adverse effects during hemapheresis. *J Clin Apheresis* 1996;11:160–164.

United States Centers for Disease Control. Renal insufficiency and failure associated with IGIV therapy. *Morb Mortal Weekly Rep* 1999;48:518–521.

Weinstein R. Basic principles of therapeutic blood exchange. In: McLeod BC, *Apheresis: principles and practice,* 2nd ed. Bethesda, MD: AABB Press, 2003:295–320.

Weinstein R. Prevention of citrate reactions during therapeutic plasma exchange by constant infusion of calcium gluconate with the return fluid. *J Clin Apheresis* 1996;11:204–210.

Wolf J, et al. Predictors for success of plasmapheresis on the long-term outcome of renal transplant patients with recurrent FSGS [Abstract]. *J Am Soc Nephrol* 2005;SA-FC026.

Zucchelli P, et al. Controlled plasma exchange trial in acute renal failure due to multiple myeloma. *Kidney Int* 1988;33:1175–1180.

Use of Dialysis and Hemoperfusion in Treatment of Poisoning

James F. Winchester, Adin Boldur, Chima Oleru, and Chagriya Kitiyakara

Hemodialysis, hemoperfusion, and peritoneal dialysis, particularly the first two procedures, can be useful adjuncts in the management of drug overdose and poisoning. However, these treatments should be applied selectively, in the context of a comprehensive management strategy that includes cardiorespiratory support, early gastric lavage (when indicated and safe), and administration of multiple-dose activated charcoal (MDAC) or specific antidotes (Kulig, 1992). Also, in patients with reasonably adequate renal function, forced diuresis along with alkalinization or acidification of the urine can accelerate removal of a number of drugs from the body. A review of data from the American Association of Poison Control Centers shows that MDAC and alkalinization treatments far outnumber treatments by hemodialysis, and these in turn far outnumber treatments using hemoperfusion.

I. Dialysis and hemoperfusion
A. Indications. Extracorporeal techniques should be considered when the conditions listed in Table 17-1 apply. Any procedure used in poisoning treatment should have a greater effect on drug elimination than that which occurs spontaneously. Early use of dialysis or hemoperfusion can also be considered if the serum levels of a drug or poison are found to be increased to values known to be associated with death or serious tissue damage. Critical serum concentrations for several drugs are listed in Table 17-2. The information given in Tables 17-1 and 17-2 represents a set of guidelines only; the decision to institute dialysis or hemoperfusion must be made on an individual basis.

B. Choice of therapy
  1. Peritoneal dialysis (PD) is not very effective in removing drugs from the blood, being one eighth to one fourth as efficient as hemodialysis. Nevertheless, when hemodialysis is difficult to institute quickly, such as in small children, a prolonged session of peritoneal dialysis can be a valuable adjunctive treatment for poisoning. Also, under certain conditions, such as in the hypothermic poisoned patient, PD maybe useful, as it also may be used to help in core rewarming.

  2. Hemodialysis is the therapy of choice for water-soluble drugs, especially those of low molecular weight along with a low level of protein binding, which will diffuse rapidly across the dialyzer membrane. Examples are ethanol, ethylene

Table 17-1. Criteria for consideration of dialysis or hemoperfusion in poisoning

1. Progressive deterioration despite intensive supportive therapy
2. Severe intoxication with depression of midbrain function leading to hypoventilation, hypothermia, and hypotension
3. Development of complications of coma, such as pneumonia or septicemia, and underlying conditions predisposing to such complications (e.g., obstructive airways disease)
4. Impairment of normal drug excretory function in the presence of hepatic, cardiac, or renal insufficiency
5. Intoxication with agents with metabolic and/or delayed effects (e.g., methanol, ethylene glycol, and paraquat)
6. Intoxication with an extractable drug or poison, which can be removed at a rate exceeding endogenous elimination by liver or kidney.

glycol, lithium, methanol, and salicylates. Water-soluble drugs that have high molecular weights (e.g., amphotericin B [MW 9,241] and vancomycin [MW 1,500]) diffuse across dialyzer membranes more slowly and are less well removed; removal rate is accelerated by use of high-flux membranes and hemodiafiltration. Hemodialysis is not very useful in removing lipid-soluble drugs (e.g., glutethimide) with large volumes of distribution or drugs with extensive protein binding.

3. Hemoperfusion is a process whereby blood is passed through a device containing adsorbent particles. Most commonly the adsorbent particles are activated charcoal or some sort of resin. Hemoperfusion is more effective than hemodialysis in clearing the blood of many protein-bound drugs because the charcoal or resin in the cartridge will compete with plasma proteins for the drug, adsorb the drug, and

Table 17-2. Serum concentrations of common poisons in excess of which hemodialysis (HD) or hemoperfusion (HP) should be considered

Drug	Serum Concentration[a]		Method of Choice
	(mg/L)	(mcmol/L)	
Phenobarbital	100	430	HP, HD
Glutethimide	40	180	HP
Methaqualone	40	160	HP
Salicylates	800	4.4 mmol/L	HD
Theophylline	40	220	HP, HD
Paraquat	0.1	0.4	HP > HD
Methanol	500	16 mmol/L	HD
Meprobamate	100	460	HP

[a]Suggested concentrations only: Clinical condition may warrant intervention at lower concentrations (e.g., in mixed intoxications).

thereby remove it from the circulation. Similarly, hemoperfusion will remove many lipid-soluble drugs from the blood much more efficiently than hemodialysis.

If a drug is equally well removed from the blood by hemoperfusion and hemodialysis, then hemodialysis is preferred as potential problems of cartridge saturation are avoided and any coexisting acid–base disturbances can be treated.

4. Continuous hemodiafiltration, hemoperfusion. Prolonged continuous treatment is potentially useful in drugs with moderately large volumes of distribution (V_D) and slow intercompartmental transfer times to prevent posttherapy rebound of plasma drug levels. Clear advantages of continuous treatment over repeated conventional treatment for drug rebound remain to be demonstrated. Continuous hemoperfusion has been used successfully in meprobamate, theophylline, and phenobarbital toxicity and continuous hemodiafiltration has been used in ethylene glycol and lithium toxicity (Leblanc et al., 1996).

C.   Importance of volume of distribution. The volume of distribution (V_D) is the theoretical volume into which a drug is distributed. Heparin, for example, a drug confined to the blood compartment, has a V_D of approximately 0.06 L/kg. Drugs distributed primarily in the extracellular water (e.g., cephalothin) will have a V_D of approximately 0.2 L/kg. Some drugs will have V_D values exceeding the volume of total body water (0.6 L/kg) because they are extensively bound to, or stored in, tissue sites.

With drugs that have a high V_D (e.g., digoxin, glutethimide, tricyclics), the amount of drug present in the blood represents only a small fraction of the total body load. Thus, even if a hemodialysis or hemoperfusion treatment extracts most of the drug present in the blood flowing through the extracorporeal circuit, the amount of drug removed during a single treatment session will represent only a small percentage of the total body drug burden. Subsequently, additional drug will enter the blood from tissue stores, sometimes causing a recurrence of the toxic manifestations. On the other hand, even transiently lowering the blood concentration of many drugs may mitigate certain important toxic effects of these agents. Hence, hemodialysis or hemoperfusion can sometimes effectively reduce drug toxicity even when the V_D is large.

D.   Technical points
  1. Vascular access for hemodialysis or hemoperfusion in poisoning. In patients without permanent vascular access in place, percutaneous cannulation of a large central vein using a dialysis catheter is required. See Chapter 6.
  2. Choice of hemodialyzer. High-flux, high-efficiency dialyzers with high urea clearances should generally be used. Biocompatible membranes may have theoretical advantages in unstable patients.
  3. Choice of a hemoperfusion cartridge. Some of the available cartridges are listed in Table 17-3. Typical sorbents are activated carbons (charcoals), ion exchange resins, or nonionic exchange macroporous resins. Sorbent

Table 17-3. Some available hemoperfusion devices (may vary by country)

Manufacturer	Device	Sorbent Type	Amount of Sorbent	Polymer Coating
Asahi	Hemosorba	Bead charcoal	170 g	Poly-HEMA
Clark	Biocompatible system	Charcoal	50, 100, 250 mL	Heparinized polymer
Gambro	Adsorba	Norit	100 or 300 g	Cellulose acetate
Organon-Teknika	Hemopur 260	Norit extruded charcoal	260 g	Cellulose acetate
Smith and Nephew	Hemocol or Haemocol	Sucliffe Speakman charcoal	100 or 300 g	Acrylic hydrogel
Braun	Haemoresin	XAD-4	350 g	None

N.B. Smaller devices for use in children.

particles have been rendered biocompatible by coating the surface with a polymer membrane. The cartridges contain various amounts of sorbent, the smaller ones being designed for pediatric use. No controlled comparative evaluation of in vivo performance of the various brands of cartridges has been published.

4. The hemoperfusion circuit. The hemoperfusion circuit is similar to the blood side of a hemodialysis circuit and includes an air detector and a venous air trap. Standard hemodialysis blood pumps and machines (without use of dialysis solution) are often used to drive the blood through the tubing and cartridge.

5. Priming the hemoperfusion circuit. Setup and priming procedures differ depending on the brand of cartridge used, and the manufacturer's literature should be consulted in all instances. The hemoperfusion cartridge must be primed in a vertical position with the arterial (blood inlet) side facing down. One manufacturer (Gambro) recommends that its cartridges be rinsed initially with 500 mL of 5% dextrose in water to load the charcoal with glucose. This maneuver is alleged to result in a lesser drop in the plasma glucose level during the hemoperfusion treatment. Not all manufacturers recommend a glucose rinse.

After the glucose rinse (if one is used), the cartridge is rinsed with 2 L of heparinized (2,500 units/L) 0.9% sodium chloride solution at a flow rate of 50–150 mL per minute. In rinsing Clark cartridges, the manufacturer recommends that the final liter of rinsing fluid be passed through the cartridge at a relatively rapid rate, that is, about 150% of the anticipated blood flow rate through the device (e.g., 300 mL per minute if the blood flow rate will be 200 mL per minute).

6. Heparinization during hemoperfusion. Once the cartridge has been primed, a bolus dose of heparin (usually 2,000–3,000 units) is administered into the arterial line, the cartridge is kept inlet side down, and blood flow through the cartridge is begun. As a rule, because of some adsorption on the sorbent, more heparin may be required for a hemoperfusion treatment (e.g., approximately 6,000 units or 10,000 units for charcoal and resin, respectively, per session) than for hemodialysis. Heparin should be given in amounts sufficient to maintain the patient's activated clotting time (ACT) or partial thromboplastin time at about twice the normal value.

7. Duration of hemoperfusion. A single 3-hour treatment will substantially lower the blood levels of most poisons for which hemoperfusion is effective. More prolonged use of a hemoperfusion cartridge is inefficient, because the charcoal tends to become saturated (especially when cartridges containing <150 g charcoal are used). Replacement of saturated devices with fresh ones is not usually required, and any rebound in blood drug concentrations consequent to tissue release can be treated with a second hemoperfusion session. On the other hand, a continuous hemoperfusion treatment may need to be prolonged for several days until clinical improvement or nontoxic blood level is achieved. Hemoperfusion devices may need to be changed every 4 hours in the course of continuous treatment.

E. Complications

　　1. Hemodialysis

　　　　a. Hypophosphatemia. In contrast to end-stage renal disease (ESRD) patients, patients being dialyzed for poisoning often do not have an elevated plasma phosphate value. Because phosphate is not present in standard dialysis solutions, intensive dialysis can severely lower the plasma phosphate level, resulting in respiratory insufficiency and other complications. Hypophosphatemia during dialysis can be avoided by supplementing the dialysis solution with phosphate (Chow et al., 1998).

　　　　b. Alkalemia. Standard hemodialysis solutions contain unphysiologically high concentrations of bicarbonate or bicarbonate-generating base and are designed to correct metabolic acidosis. Performing dialysis for poisoning in a patient with metabolic or respiratory alkalosis can provoke or worsen alkalemia unless the amount of base is appropriately reduced.

　　　　c. Disequilibrium syndrome in acutely uremic patients. In patients with both severe uremia and poisoning, it may be dangerous to carry out a prolonged high-clearance dialysis session initially. During a dialysis treatment for a Glucophage-induced lactic acidosis in a markedly uremic patient, enrichment of a dialysate with an appropriate amount of urea in an attempt to attenuate the manifestations of the disequilibrium syndrome has been successfully performed (Doorenboss et al., 2001). The disequilibrium syndrome is discussed in Chapter 10.

　　2. Hemoperfusion. Mild transient thrombocytopenia and leukopenia can occur but levels usually return to normal within 24 to 48 hours following a single hemoperfusion. Adsorption or activation of coagulation factors has also been observed rarely and may be clinically significant in patients with liver failure.

　　3. Continuous therapy. Fluid and electrolyte imbalances may be potential problems and require frequent monitoring. Prolonged anticoagulation may predispose to bleeding.

II. Management of poisoning with selected agents

A. Acetaminophen (MW 151). Activated charcoal should be given to those presenting within 4 hours after ingestion. Serum levels should be measured and plotted against the Rumack-Matthew nomogram to establish the risk for hepatotoxicity and requirement for N-acetyl cysteine (NAC) therapy. If serum acetaminophen levels are above 150 mg/L (1.0 mmol/L) at 4 hours, the likelihood of toxicity is high and NAC (PO or IV) should be given. Liver toxicity may be found at lower serum levels when acetaminophen ingestion is combined with even moderate amounts of ethanol. NAC, by increasing reduced glutathione stores, prevents the accumulation of the toxic byproducts. Its efficacy to prevent liver failure declines if started more than 10 hours after ingestion, although it may still be worth giving even after 24 hours. Although acetaminophen is moderately water soluble and is minimally protein bound and thus removed by dialysis or hemoperfusion, NAC remains the treatment of choice.

B.   Aspirin (acetylsalicylic acid, MW 180). In adults, severe aspirin poisoning is usually accompanied by metabolic acidosis with respiratory alkalosis, whereas in children isolated metabolic acidosis is often encountered. The appearance of central nervous system (CNS) symptoms is a sign of severe poisoning. The Done nomogram (Done and Temple, 1971), relating serum levels and time of ingestion to outcome, gives some idea of the seriousness of salicylate poisoning in an individual patient. MDAC should be initiated and alkaline diuresis carried out if substantial urine output is achievable, particularly when symptoms are present and serum salicylate levels are >50 mg/dL (2.8 mmol/L). Aspirin has a V_D of only 0.15 L/kg. Despite the fact that the drug is about 50% protein bound, aspirin is well removed by hemodialysis. Hemodialysis should be considered when the serum level exceeds 80 mg/dL (4.4 mmol/L) or the condition of the patient warrants aggressive management.

C.   Barbiturates. Toxic serum levels of phenobarbital (MW 232) are over 3 mg/dL (130 mcmol/L), and coma begins to appear at levels of 6 mg per dL (260 mcmol/L). MDAC should be considered as first-line therapy and alkalinization of the urine may also be useful in long-acting barbiturates such as phenobarbital. Phenobarbital is 50% protein bound, but its V_D is only 0.5 L/kg; the drug is well removed by either hemodialysis or hemoperfusion. Hemodialysis should be contemplated when coma is prolonged, especially when complications of coma, such as pneumonia, threaten. There is, however, no evidence that hemodialysis will improve overall survival.

D.   Digoxin (MW 781). The probabilities of digoxin-induced arrhythmias are 50% and 90% at serum levels of 2.5 and 3.3 ng/mL (3.2 and 4.2 nmol/L), respectively. Treatment includes correction of hypokalemia, hypomagnesemia, and alkalosis and administration of oral activated charcoal.

The V_D of digoxin is large (8 L/kg in normal patients, 4.2 L/kg in dialysis patients), and the drug is 25% protein bound. For these reasons, only 5% of the body load will be removed by a 4-hour hemodialysis treatment. Although hemoperfusion is more effective and has been shown to improve symptoms, it is not routinely recommended in the treatment of digoxin toxicity as the V_D of the drug is so large that total body clearance is limited. Digoxin-specific antibody fragments (Fab fragments) are indicated for massive ingestions, profound intoxication, or hyperkalemia in the presence of life-threatening arrhythmia. Although Fab has been used successfully in patients with coexisting renal failure, digoxin may be released from the Fab–digoxin complex, leading to a rebound in toxicity (Ujhelyi et al., 1993). Plasmapheresis performed soon after Fab fragment administration promotes removal of the Fab–digoxin complexes (Zdunek, 2000). In dialysis patients a judgment to employ hemoperfusion (made easier by the presence of an arteriovenous access) or digoxin antibody is required.

E. Toxic alcohols. Ethylene glycol and methanol are the commonest causes of fatal toxic alcohol poisoning. Ethylene glycol is found in antifreeze solutions, deicing solutions, hydraulic brake fluid, foam stabilizers, and chemical solvents. Methanol is found in windshield washing fluids, paints, solvents, copier fluids, and illegally manufactured (wood) alcohol. Methanol and ethylene glycol are relatively nontoxic, but both are metabolized via the enzyme alcohol dehydrogenase to produce the toxic metabolites formic acid and glycolic acid, respectively. In ethylene glycol poisoning, glycolate is further metabolized to oxalate, which can cause renal failure.

Coingestion of ethanol may delay formation of toxic metabolites and its associated clinical features. Poisonings with toxic alcohols should be suspected in patients with unexplained metabolic acidosis accompanied by increases in anion and osmolal gaps. However, an elevated anion gap and an elevated osmolal gap are rarely concomitantly present early or very late after ingestion of toxic alcohols. If a toxic alcohol has not been metabolized, the osmolal gap but not the anion gap will be increased. On the other hand, if a toxic alcohol has undergone metabolism, the anion gap but not the osmolal gap will be elevated. Therefore, a normal osmolal or anion gap does not eliminate the possibility of significant toxic alcohol ingestion.

Alcohols are rapidly absorbed and have the same V_D as water. MDAC or gastric lavage has a limited role in the management of alcohol poisoning. There is a competitive inhibition between either ethanol or fomepizole (4-methylpyrazole) on the one hand and a toxic alcohol on the other for the affinity of the enzyme alcohol dehydrogenase in the liver. Fomepizole has a greater affinity for alcohol dehydrogenase than ethanol. Either ethanol or fomepizole should be given as soon as possible after ingestion to delay the conversion to toxic metabolites and to allow time for the disposal of the parent drug and its toxic metabolites that might have been formed through the urinary, metabolic, and dialytic routes. Currently, there are insufficient data to define the relative roles of fomepizole and ethanol in the treatment of toxic alcohol poisoning. Ethanol can cause CNS depression, phlebitis, hypoglycemia, and respiratory depression, and requires close monitoring of serum ethanol levels. Fomepizole has advantages over ethanol in terms of validated efficacy, predictable pharmacokinetics, ease of administration, and fewer adverse effects. Ethanol has advantages over fomepizole in terms of clinical experience and lower drug cost (cost advantage upwards of 1:100). Fomepizole is probably safer in children and pregnant women. In mild intoxications prior to the toxic alcohols' metabolic breakdown (i.e., without metabolic acidosis) and in the face of adequate renal function, the toxic alcohols can be expected to be excreted in the urine in the course of treatment with ethanol or fomepizole. In the face of the toxic alcohols' breakdown with resultant metabolic acidosis and in the presence of poor renal function, however, removal of these toxic alcohols and their deleterious metabolites by hemodialysis or other extracorporeal measures is mandatory since neither ethanol nor fomepizole has the capacity to dispose of these substances from the body. For milder cases with adequate renal function, ethanol infusions alone (without extracorporeal treatment) over several days in the intensive care unit can be difficult to manage. In contrast, in the presence of adequate renal function, intensive care monitoring can be avoided in patients with mild toxic alcohol poisoning (without metabolic acidosis) and treated with fomepizole. Hemodialysis is highly effective in rapidly removing both toxic alcohols and their metabolites and in correcting metabolic abnormalities. Thus, the risks and costs of prolonged hospitalization and the cost of fomepizole must be weighed against those of hemodialysis. Since hemodialysis is so efficient in removing the toxic alcohols, the prolonged intensive care monitoring required for sole ethanol administration is less necessary if hemodialysis is added to the treatment regimen. On account of its lower cost, the use of ethanol may have an economic incentive in developing countries. Overall, prognosis correlates better with the severity of acidosis and toxic metabolite concentrations rather than the parent alcohol concentrations.

1.   Ethylene glycol (MW 62). The first phase of toxicity due to ethylene glycol occurs <1 hour after ingestion and is characterized by CNS depression similar to ethanol intoxication. In severe poisoning, this phase can result in coma and seizures and can last 12 hours. The second phase is due to the toxic effects of the metabolite, glycolic acid, on the cardiopulmonary system with the development of cardiac and respiratory failure 12 hours after ingestion. A severe metabolic acidosis commonly occurs. After 24–48 hours, renal failure often supervenes as a result of oxalate precipitation in the kidney, delaying the excretion of the poison. This is characterized by flank pain, hypocalcemia, and acute tubular necrosis accompanied by oxalate crystals in the urine.

Early aggressive management of acidosis with sodium bicarbonate is essential. Indications for the administration of an antidote (ethanol or fomepizole) are shown in Table 17-4. Indications for hemodialysis are shown in Table 17-5. Traditionally, an ethylene glycol level above 50 mg/dL (8.1 mmol/L) is an indication for dialysis. In the absence of **both** renal dysfunction and metabolic acidosis, the use of fomepizole may obviate the need for dialysis, even in patients with serum ethylene glycol levels above 50 mg/dL. However, if patients with serum levels of ethylene glycol above 50 mg/dL are not treated with hemodialysis but only with ethanol or fomepizole, the acid–base status should be monitored very closely and hemodialysis initiated promptly if acidosis develops. The dosing schedule for ethanol or fomepizole and the dose adjustments for hemodialysis are shown in Tables 17-6 and 17-7. Hemodialysis should be performed until acidosis has resolved and the ethylene glycol levels are <20 mg/dL (3.2 mmol/L). If ethylene glycol levels are unavailable, dialysis should be performed for at least

Table 17-4. Indications for treatment of ethylene glycol or methanol poisoning with ethanol or fomepizole

1. Documented plasma ethylene glycol or methanol concentrations >20 mg/dL
   or
2. Documented recent (hours) history of ingestion of toxic amounts of ethylene glycol or methanol and osmolal gap >10 mmol/kg
   or
3. History or strong clinical suspicion of ethylene glycol or methanol poisoning and at least two of the following criteria:
   (a) Arterial pH <7.3
   (b) Serum bicarbonate <20 mmol/L
   (c) Osmolal gap >10 mmol/kg[a]
   (d) Urinary oxalate crystals (in the case of ethylene glycol) or visual signs or symptoms (in the case of methanol) present

[a]Laboratory analysis by freezing point depression only.
Modified from Barceloux DG, et al. American Academy of Clinical Toxicology practice guidelines on the treatment of ethylene glycol poisoning. *J Toxicol Clin Toxicol* 1999;37:537; Barceloux DG, et al. American Academy of Clinical Toxicology practice guidelines on the treatment of methanol poisoning. *J Toxicol Clin Toxicol* 2002;40:415.

Table 17-5. Indications for hemodialysis in patients with severe ethylene glycol or methanol poisoning

1. Severe metabolic acidosis (pH <7.25–7.30)
2. Renal failure
3. Visual symptoms/signs
4. Deteriorating vital signs despite intensive supportive care
5. Ethylene glycol or methanol levels >50 mg/dL unless fomepizole is being administered and patient is asymptomatic with a normal pH[a]

[a]Such patients should be monitored very closely and hemodialysis should be initiated if acidosis develops. Withholding of dialysis in such patients may result in prolongation of hospitalization.
Modified from Barceloux DG, et al American Academy of Clinical Toxicology practice guidelines on the treatment of ethylene glycol poisoning. *J Toxicol Clin Toxicol* 1999;37:537; Barceloux DG, et al. American Academy of Clinical Toxicology practice guidelines on the treatment of methanol poisoning. *J Toxicol Clin Toxicol* 2002;40:415.

Table 17-6.   Guidelines for use of ethanol in toxic alcohol poisonings

1. Loading dose: 0.6 g/kg [intravenous 10% ethanol in D5W (7.6 mL/kg) or 43% oral solution or 86 proof undiluted liquor (34 g ethanol/dL) 1.8 mL/kg].
2. Maintenance dose:
   (a) In alcoholic patients 154 mg/kg per hour
   (b) In nonalcoholic patients 66 mg/kg per hour
   (c) Double dose during hemodialysis or enrich dialysate with 100 mg/dL ethanol[a]
   (d) Double dose if given orally with charcoal
3. Monitor serum ethanol concentrations every 1–2 hours and adjust infusion rate to maintain serum ethanol level of 100–150 mg/dL. Thereafter, monitor ethanol levels every 2–4 hours.
4. Continue until methanol or ethylene glycol concentrations are <20 mg/dL and patient is asymptomatic with normal arterial pH.

[a]From Wadgymar A, et al. Treatment of acute methanol intoxication with hemodialysis. *Am J Kidney Dis* 1998;31:897.

8 hours. Redistribution of ethylene glycol may result in rebound elevation of ethylene glycol levels within 12 hours after cessation of dialysis and repeat dialysis may be necessary. Thus, serum osmolality, electrolytes, and acid–base status should be monitored closely within 24 hours after dialysis. Pyridoxine (500 mg IM four times daily) and thiamine (100 mg IM four times daily) should be considered to increase the metabolism of glyoxylate. In addition, judicious intravenous fluids should be given to prevent calcium oxalate crystal deposition in the kidneys and acute renal

Table 17-7.   Guidelines for use of fomepizole in the treatment of ethylene glycol and methanol poisoning

1. Loading dose: 15 mg/kg IV in 100 mL 0.9% saline over 30 minutes to 1 hour.
2. Maintenance dose: 10 mg/kg every 12 hours for four doses, then 15 mg/kg every 12 hours.
3. Dose adjustments during hemodialysis: 15 mg/kg every 4 hours or 1–1.5 mg/kg per hour infusion during dialysis.
4. Continue until methanol or ethylene glycol concentrations are <20 mg/dL and patient is asymptomatic with normal arterial pH.

Modified from Barceloux DG, et al. American Academy of Clinical Toxicology practice guidelines on the treatment of ethylene glycol poisoning. *J Toxicol Clin Toxicol* 1999;37:537; Barceloux DG, et al. American Academy of Clinical Toxicology practice guidelines on the treatment of methanol poisoning. *J Toxicol Clin Toxicol* 2002;40:415.

failure. Hypocalcemia, the effects of which may be worsened by bicarbonate treatment, should be corrected if this is symptomatic or severe. It is uncertain if correction of hypocalcemia significantly increases calcium oxalate precipitation in tissues. Hypophosphatemia from intensive dialysis can be prevented by using a phosphate-enriched dialysis solution (Chow et al., 1998).

2. Methanol (MW 32). Methanol poisoning causes early temporary CNS depression followed by a latent period lasting 6–24 hours before the development of metabolic acidosis and visual symptoms. The latter include blurred vision, decreased visual acuity, photophobia, and visual field defects to complete blindness, due to formic acid accumulation. Early signs include optic disc hyperemia and decreased pupillary reflexes to light.

Initial management is similar to that for ethylene glycol toxicity, including the correction of acidosis with intravenous sodium bicarbonate to pH 7.35–7.4. Ethanol or fomepizole should be administered to prevent formation of formic acid according to indications (Table 17-4). Hemodialysis should be considered (Table 17-5) when there is significant metabolic acidosis (pH <7.25–7.3), abnormalities of vision, deteriorating vital signs, renal failure, or electrolyte abnormalities unresponsive to conventional therapy. Serum methanol concentration >50 mg/dL (15.6 mmol/L) is often used as an indication for hemodialysis. High serum methanol concentrations may require several days of treatment with ethanol or fomepizole. If a patient with high serum concentrations of methanol is not treated with hemodialysis, acid–base status should be monitored closely with hemodialysis initiated as soon as acidosis develops. Hemodialysis should be continued until acidosis is corrected and serum methanol levels are <20 mg/dL (6.3 mmol/L). When methanol concentrations are very high, dialysis of 18–21 hours may be required. In some patients with normal renal function receiving ethanol or fomepizole, dialysis may not be necessary once serum methanol falls below 50 mg/dL and anion gap acidosis is corrected. Ophthalmologic abnormalities may persist transiently or permanently and should not be considered an indication to continue dialysis. Redistribution of methanol may result in elevation of methanol concentrations after dialysis ceases, and repeat dialysis may be necessary. Consequently, serum osmolality and acid–base status should be monitored frequently for the first 24–36 hours after hemodialysis ceases. If dialysis is initiated, doses of ethanol or fomepizole should be increased (however, in the case of ethanol therapy, if ethanol is also used to enrich the dialysate, the systemic doses need not be increased) (Tables 17-6 and 17-7). Formic acid is converted by 10-formyl tetrahydrofolate synthetase to carbon dioxide and water. Folinic acid IV (1 mg/kg [up to 50 mg] in 5% dextrose over 30–60 minutes every 4 hours) should be given to enhance formic acid metabolism until methanol and formate have been cleared. If folinic acid is unavailable, folic acid can be used.

3. Isopropanol (MW 60). Isopropanol (isopropyl alcohol) is found in rubbing alcohol, antifreeze, and frost remover. Isopropanol is a common cause of poisoning but is only occasionally fatal. Isopropanol is oxidized by alcohol dehydrogenase to acetone. Unlike ethylene glycol and methanol, most of the clinical effects of isopropanol intoxication are due to the parent compound. Gastrointestinal and CNS symptoms, including confusion, ataxia, and coma, occur in 1 hour. Hypotension due to cardiac depression and vasodilation can occur in severe intoxication. Hypoglycemia can occur. Acidosis is rare in the absence of severe hypotension. Therefore, a high serum osmolal gap without acidosis in association with an increased urinary or serum acetone level is highly suggestive of isopropanol poisoning. Supportive treatment is usually all that is necessary. Inhibition of alcohol dehydrogenase is not warranted because acetone is less toxic than the parent compound. Hemodialysis might be considered if the isopropanol levels are >400 mg/dL (67 mmol/L) and significant CNS suppression, renal failure, or hypotension exists.

4. Other alcohols. Poisonings with other alcohols used in a variety of industrial and household products have also been reported with much less frequency. Metabolism of the parent compound may lead to the generation of toxic metabolites. Propylene glycol (MW 76) is an excipient often used in pharmaceuticals such as lorazepam and nitroglycerine to enhance solubility. Toxicity is associated with lactic acidosis and an elevated osmolal gap. 2-butoxyethanol (MW 118) is found in a number of resins, varnishes, and glass and leather cleaning solutions. Toxicity has been associated with metabolic acidosis, hepatic injury, and respiratory distress. Hemodialysis is effective in removing these alcohols and may be indicated in severe intoxications.

F. Lithium carbonate (MW for Li = 7). Most intoxications result from chronic accumulation, renal failure, diuretic use and dehydration, and interactions with angiotensin-converting enzyme (ACE) inhibitors and nonsteroidal anti-inflammatory drugs (NSAIDs). Mild (serum Li 1.5–2.5 mmol/L) and moderate (serum Li 2.5–3.5 mmol/L) lithium toxicity are characterized by neuromuscular irritability, nausea, and diarrhea. Severe toxicity (serum Li >3.5 mmol/L) can result in seizures, stupor, and permanent neurologic deficit. Initially diuretics should be stopped and half normal saline should be used to rehydrate the patient. As lithium is 0% protein bound with a V_D of 0.8 L/kg, it is removed very well by dialysis. Hemodialysis should be considered when (a) serum Li >3.5 mmol/L, (b) serum Li >2.5 mmol/L in patients with appreciable symptoms or in patients with renal insufficiency, or (c) when serum Li is between 2.5 and 3.5 mmol/L in asymptomatic patients but when levels are expected to rise (e.g., following recent massive ingestion) or are not expected to fall below 0.8 mmol/L in the next 36 hours, as predicted from a log/linear concentration versus time plot. As serum lithium may rebound following dialysis due to a shift from the intracellular compartment, dialysis should be performed using a high-clearance dialyzer for 8–12 hours. Repeated dialysis may be necessary until serum Li levels remain below 1.0 mmol/L for 6–8 hours after dialysis. Prolonged continuous hemodiafiltration may reduce the rebound of lithium levels post treatment (Leblanc et al., 1996), but further studies are necessary to confirm the utility of this method.

G. Mushroom poisoning. Ingestion of certain poisonous mushrooms is associated initially with severe gastrointestinal symptoms followed by hepatic insufficiency and cardiovascular collapse. The toxins of these mushrooms (α-amanitin and phalloidin, MW for both $\sim$900) are removed by hemodialysis and hemoperfusion in vitro, but the efficacy of hemodialysis or hemoperfusion in patients poisoned by mushrooms has been difficult to interpret because of lack of controls; some survival benefit has been alleged. Early referral to a liver transplantation unit is recommended. Plasmapheresis (see Chapter 16) is another experimental treatment option.

    1. Paraquat (MW 257). Delayed toxicity with pulmonary fibrosis and renal and multiorgan failure can occur following ingestion of more than 10 mL of paraquat concentrate. Survival is dependent on the amount ingested and the plasma levels with respect to time of ingestion (Proudfoot et al., 1979). Plasma levels of above 3 mg/L (12 mcmol/L) regardless of when they are measured are usually fatal. Initial management includes gastric lavage with administration of activated charcoal or Fuller Earth with cathartic. Hemoperfusion is effective in drug removal and should be considered when the plasma paraquat level is 0.1 mg/L (0.4 mcmol/L) or above. Repeated or continuous hemoperfusion may be needed for several days to maintain plasma levels below 0.1 mg/L as paraquat has a large V_D and a slow intercompartmental transfer rate. Although the evidence that hemoperfusion improves survival is controversial, the procedure should be considered since occasional patients have recovered despite massive ingestion and pulmonary involvement. Survival after treatment with plasmapheresis has been described (Dearaley et al., 1978).

H. Phenothiazines and tricyclic antidepressants. These agents are highly protein bound and have extremely large volumes of distribution (in the range of 14–21 L/kg). Hence, the total amount of these drugs removed by either hemodialysis or hemoperfusion is small. Hemoperfusion can be useful in temporarily lowering the plasma drug level and reducing acute toxicity, however. Treatment of intoxication with these agents is largely supportive, including correction of acidosis with bicarbonate.

I. Anticonvulsants

    1. Phenytoin (MW 252). Nystagmus and ataxia occur at serum values >20 and 30 mg/mL (79 and 119 mmol/L), respectively. Phenytoin is 90% protein bound (70% in uremic patients) and has a V_D of 0.64 L/kg. Phenytoin is removed poorly by hemodialysis, but is removed moderately well by hemoperfusion.

    2. Sodium valproate (MW 166). Valproate sodium has a small V_D, is metabolized by the liver, and has significant protein binding. In overdose, protein binding becomes saturated and free valproate can be subjected to extra-corporeal removal. High-flux hemodialysis with or without hemoperfusion should be considered when there is coma, severe liver dysfunction, or other organ failure.

J.   Sedatives and hypnotics. Older agents have greater toxicity and, fortunately, are less frequently used today. Since morbidity and mortality can be high, extracorporeal methods have been employed in overdose with these older drugs. Newer agents are associated with lower side effects, and supportive therapy is often sufficient to treat overdose.

1.   Diphenhydramine, an antihistamine commonly used as an over-the-counter sedative, is often taken in over-dose. Toxicity is usually limited to anticholinergic symptoms. Treatment is supportive and directed toward anti-cholinergic effects. Sodium bicarbonate may be beneficial if wide-complex tachycardia develops. Extracorporeal treatment has a limited role.

2.   Benzodiazepines (e.g., diazepam, clonazepam, flurazepam). Treatment is largely supportive for all of these drugs as the high degree of protein binding and the high V_D of some of these drugs limit drug removal by extra-corporeal therapy. Administration of flumazenil, a benzo-diazepine receptor antagonist, may be considered in severe benzodiazepine poisoning. Seizures may be precipitated and resedation may occur in patients who have awakened following flumazenil administration. The Multiple Adsorbent Recirculating System (MARS, Gambro Healthcare, Lund, Sweden) has been used experimentally to enhance drug removal. The benefit of this treatment modality is not clear in a clinical practice setting.

3.   Zolpidem and zaleplon are newer sedatives that act as selective benzodiazepine-1 receptor subtype agonists. These agents are increasingly used and are associated with fewer side effects even in overdose. Supportive treatment is usually sufficient.

4.   Meprobamate (MW 218) and chloral hydrate (MW 165). These older sedatives are lipid soluble and moderately protein bound, and have V_D values of 0.7 and 1.6 L/kg, respectively. Hemodialysis or hemoperfusion is indicated for patients who have been poisoned severely with these agents (Seyffart, 1997) and who have not responded to standard intensive care.

5.   Glutethimide (MW 217), methaqualone, methyprylon, ethchlorvynol. These older sedatives are highly lipid soluble and have a large V_D. They are poorly removed by hemodialysis and moderately well removed by hemoperfusion. After a hemoperfusion session, a rebound in plasma drug levels may occur and this may be sufficient to put the patient back into coma, necessitating a second or even a third hemoperfusion session. Continuous hemoperfusion may be useful to prevent rebound.

6.   Carbamazepine (MW 236). Hemoperfusion can be used for severe intoxications. High-flux hemodialysis has been reported to give good results, also (Kielstein et al., 2002; Koh et al., 2006).

Table 17-8. Drugs and chemicals removed with hemodialysis

Antimicrobials/ **Anticancer**	(Nafcillin)	(Miconazole)
Cefaclor	Penicillin	(Chloroquine)
Cefadroxil	Piperacillin	(Quinine)
Cefamandole	Temocillin	(Azathioprine)
Cefazolin	Ticarcillin	Bredinin
Cefixime	(Clindamycin)	Busulphan
Cefmenoxime	(Erythromycin)	Cyclophosphamide
Cefmetazole	(Azithromycin)	5-Fluorouracil
(Cefonicid)	(Clarithromycin)	(Methotrexate)
(Cefoperazone)	Metronidazole	
Ceforamide	Nitrofurantoin	**Barbiturates**
(Cefotaxime)	Ornidazole	Amobarbital
Cefotetan	Sulfisoxazole	Aprobarbital
Cefotiam	Sulfonamides	Barbital
Cefoxitin	Tetracycline	Butabarbital
Cefpirome	(Doxycycline)	Cyclobarbital
Cefroxadine	(Minocycline)	Pentobarbital
Cefsulodin	Tinidazole	Phenobarbital
Ceftazidime	Trimethoprim	Quinalbital
(Ceftriaxone)	Aztreonam	(Secobarbital)
Cefuroxime	Cilastatin	
Cephacetrile	Imipenem	**Nonbarbiturate**
Cephalexin	(Chloramphenicol)	**Hypnotics,**
Cephalothin	(Amphotericin)	**Sedatives,**
(Cephapirin)	Ciprofloxacin	**Tranquilizers,**
Cephradine	(Enoxacin)	**Anticonvulsants**
Moxalactam	Fluroxacin	Carbamazepine
Amikacin	(Norfloxacin)	Atenolol
Dibekacin	Ofloxacin	Betaxolol
Fosfomycin	Isoniazid	(Bretylium)
Gentamicin	(Vancomycin)	Clonidine
Kanamycin	Capreomycin	(Calcium Channel
Neomycin	PAS	Blockers)
Netilmicin	Pyrizinamide	Captopril
Sisomicin	(Rifampin)	(Diazoxide)
Streptomycin	(Cycloserine)	Carbromal
Tobramycin	Ethambutol	Chloral Hydrate
Bacitracin	5-Fluorocytosine	(Chlordiazepoxide)
Colistin	Acyclovir	(Diazepam)
Amoxicillin	(Amantadine)	(Diphenylhydantoin)
Ampicillin	Didanosine	(Diphenylhydramine)
Azlocillin	Foscarnet	Ethiamate
Carbenicillin	Ganciclovir	Ethchlorvynol
Clavulinic Acid	(Ribavirin)	Ethosuximide
(Cloxacillin)	Vidarabine	Gallamine
(Dicloxacillin)	Zidovudine	Glutethimide
(Floxacillin)	(Pentamidine)	(Heroin)
Mecillinam	(Praziquantel)	Meprobamate
(Mezlocillin)	(Fluconazole)	(Methaqualone)
(Methicillin)	(Itraconazole)	Methsuximide
	(Ketoconazole)	Methyprylon

Table 17-8. *Continued.*

Paraldehyde
Primidone
Valproic Acid

Cardiovascular Agents
Acebutolol
(Amiodarone)
Amrinone
(Digoxin)
Enalapril
Fosinopril
Lisinopril
Quinapril
Ramipril
(Encainide)
(Flecainide)
(Lidocaine)
Metoprolol
Methyldopa
(Ouabain)
N-Acetylpro-
  cainamide
Nadolol
(Pindolol)
Practolol
Procainamide
Propranolol
(Quinidine)
(Timolol)
Sotatol
Tocainide

Alcohols
Ethanol
Ethylene Glycol
Isopropanol
Methanol

**Analgesics, An-
  tirheumatics**
Acetaminophen
Acetophenetidin
Acetylsalicylic Acid

Colchicine
Methylsalicylate
(D-Propoxyphene)
Salicylic Acid

Antidepressants
(Amitriptyline)
Amphetamines
(Imipramine)
Isocarboxazid
Mao Inhibitors
Moclobemide
(Pargylline)
(Phenelzine)
Tranylcypromine
(Tricyclics)

Solvents, Gases
Acetone
Camphor
Carbon Monoxide
(Carbon
  Tetrachloride)
(Eucalyptus Oil)
Thiols
Toluene
Trichloroethylene

**Plants, Animals,
  Herbicides,
  Insecticides**
Alkyl Phosphate
Amanitin
Demeton
  Sulfoxide
Dimethoate
Diquat
Glufosinate
Methylmercury
Complex
(Organophosphates)
Paraquat
Snake Bite

Sodium Chlorate
Potassium Chlorate

Miscellaneous
Acipimox
Allopurinol
Aminophylline
Aniline
Borates
Boric Acid
(Chlorpropamide)
Chromic Acid
(Cimetidine)
Dinitro-O-Cresol
Folic Acid
Mannitol
Methylprednisolone
4-Methylpyrazole
Sodium Citrate
Theophylline
Thiocyanate
Ranitidine

Metals, Inorganics
(Aluminum)*
Arsenic
Barium
Bromide
(Copper)*
(Iron)*
(Lead)*
Lithium
(Magnesium)
(Mercury)*
Potassium
(Potassium
  Dichromate)*
Phosphate
Sodium
Strontium
(Thallium)*
(Tin)
(Zinc)

( ) implies poor removal.
( )*removed with chelating agent.

Table 17-9. Drugs and chemicals removed with hemoperfusion

Barbiturates
amobarbital
butabarbital
hexabarbital
pentobarbital
phenobarbital
quinalbital
secobarbital
thiopental
vinalbital

Nonbarbiturate hypnotics, sedatives and tranquilizers
carbamazepine
carbromal
chloral hydrate
chlorpromazine
(diazepam)
diphenhydramine
ethchlorvynol
glutethimide
meprobamate
methaqualone
methsuximide
methyprylon
phenytoin
promazine
promethazine
valproic acid

Analgesics, antirheumatic
acetaminophen
acetylsalicylic acid
colchicine
d-propoxyphyene
methylsalicylate
phenylbutazone
salicylic acid

Antimicrobials/ anticancer
(adriamycin)
ampicillin
carmustine
chloramphenicol
chloroq uine
clindamycin
dapsone
doxorubicin
gentamicin
ifosfamide
isoniazid
(methotrexate)
pentamidine
thiabendazole
(5-fluorouracil)
vancomycin

Antidepressants
(amitryptiline)
(imipramine)
(tricyclics)

Plant and animal toxins, herbicides, insecticides
amanitin
chlordane
demeton sulfoxide
dimethoate
diquat
endosulfan
glufosinate
methylparathion
nitrostigmine
(organophosphates)
phalloidin
polychlorinated biphenyls
paraquat
parathion

Cardiovascular
atenolol
cibenzoline succinate
clonidine
digoxin
(diltiazem)
(disopyramide)
flecainide
metoprolol
n-acetylprocainamide
procainamide
quinidine

Miscellaneous
aminophylline
cimetidine
(fluoroacetamide)
(phencyclidine)
phenols
(podophyllin)
theophylline

Solvents, gases
carbon tetrachloride
ethylene oxide
trichloroethane
xylene

Metals
(aluminum)*
(iron)*

( ) implies poor removal.
( )*removed with chelating agent.

317

K.   Theophylline (MW 180). Toxic reactions occur when theophylline levels exceed 25 mg/L (140 mcmol/L) (therapeutic levels being 10–20 mg/L [56–112 mcmol/L]). Chronic intoxication may have more pronounced symptoms at a given serum level. Seizures typically occur with levels >40 mg/L (224 mcmol/L) but may occur at levels as low as 25 mg/L (139 mcmol/L). Cardiovascular collapse is rare until levels are >50 mg/L (278 mcmol/L). Theophylline has V_D of 0.5 L/kg, poor intrinsic metabolism, and 56% protein binding, and is well adsorbed by charcoal, enabling efficacious removal by MDAC and hemoperfusion. MDAC should be used in significant poisonings even with intravenous theophylline overdose. Propranolol (1–3 mg IV) may be used to treat tachyarrhythmia, and hypokalemia should be corrected. Hemoperfusion or high-efficiency hemodialysis is indicated if vomiting prevents the use of MDAC, or it can be used in addition to MDAC in patients with seizures, hypotension, or arrhythmia. Hemoperfusion/hemodialysis should also be considered in patients with acute intoxication with levels above 100 mg/L (556 mcmol/L), in chronic toxicity with levels above 60 mg/L (333 mcmol/L), and in both the elderly or infants under 6 months of age above 40 mg/L (222 mcmol/L). Combining hemodialysis with hemoperfusion may further enhance clearance and prevent saturation of the hemoperfusion cartridge. Continuous hemoperfusion has also been used with success in severely toxic and hypotensive patients. Treatment should be continued until the plasma level is 25–40 mg/L (140–224 mcmol/L).

L.   Other drugs. Management of poisoning due to other agents is beyond the scope of this *Handbook*. The reader is referred to Haddad et al. (1998) and Tables 17-8 and 17-9.

SELECTED READINGS

Barceloux DG, et al. American Academy of Clinical Toxicology practice guidelines on the treatment of ethylene glycol poisoning. Ad Hoc Committee. *J Toxicol Clin Toxicol* 1999;37:537.

Barceloux DG, et al. American Academy of Clinical Toxicology practice guidelines on the treatment of methanol poisoning. *J Toxicol Clin Toxicol* 2002;40:415.

Chebrolu SB, et al. Extracorporeal methods in the treatment of poisoning. In: Henrich WL, ed. *Principles and practice of dialysis,* 3rd ed. Philadelphia: Lippincott Williams & Wilkins, 2004:570.

Chow MT, et al. Hemodialysis-induced hypophosphatemia in a normophosphatemic patient dialyzed for ethylene glycol poisoning: treatment with phosphorus-enriched hemodialysis. *Artif Organs* 1998;22:905.

Chyka PA. Multiple-dose activated charcoal and enhancement of systemic drug clearance: summary of studies in animals and human volunteers. *J Toxicol Clin Toxicol* 1995;33:399.

Dearaley DP, et al. Plasmapheresis for paraquat poisoning. *Lancet* 1978;1:162.

Done AK, Temple AR. Treatment of salicylate poisoning. *Modern Treat* 1971;8:528.

Doorenbos CJ, et al. Use of urea containing dialysate to avoid disequilibrium syndrome, enabling intensive dialysis treatment of a diabetic patient with renal failure and severe Glucophage induced lactic acidosis. *Nephrol Dial Transplant* 2001;16:1303.

Haddad LM, Shannon MW, Winchester JF, eds. *Clinical management of poisoning and drug overdose,* 3rd ed. Philadelphia: WB Saunders Co, 1998.

Jacobsen G, et al. Antidotes for methanol and ethylene glycol poisoning. *J Toxicol Clin Toxicol* 1997;35:127.

Kielstein JT, et al. High-flux hemodialysis—an effective alternative to hemoperfusion in the treatment of carbamazepine intoxication. *Clin Nephrol* 2002;57:484.

Koh KH, et al. High-flux haemodialysis treatment as treatment for carbamazepine intoxication. *Med J Malaysia* 2006;61:109.

Ku Y, et al. Clinical pilot study on high-dose intraarterial chemotherapy with direct hemoperfusion under hepatic venous isolation in patients with advanced hepatocellular carcinoma. *Surgery* 1995; 117:510.

Kulig K. Initial management of ingestions of toxic substances. *N Engl J Med* 1992;326:1677.

Leblanc M, et al. Lithium poisoning treated by high-performance arteriovenous and venovenous hemodialfiltration. *Am J Kidney Dis* 1996;27:365.

Litovitz TL, et al. 1998 annual report of the American of Poison Control Centers toxic exposure surveillance system. *Am J Emerg Med* 1999;17:435.

Martiny S, et al. Treatment of severe digoxin intoxication with digoxin-specific antibody fragments: a clinical review. *Crit Care Med* 1987;16:629.

Proudfoot AT, et al. Paraquat poisoning: significance of plasma paraquat concentrations. *Lancet* 1979;2:330.

Samtleben W, et al. Plasma exchange and hemoperfusion. In: Jacobs C, et al., eds. *Replacement of renal function by dialysis.* Dordrecht: Kluwer Academic Publishers, 1996:1260.

Seyffart G. *Poison index—the treatment of acute intoxication,* 4th ed. Scottsdale, AZ: Pabst Science Publishers, 1997.

Ujhelyi MR, et al. Disposition of digoxin immune Fab in patients with kidney failure. *Clin Pharmacol Ther* 1993;54:388.

Wadgymar A, et al. Treatment of acute methanol intoxication with hemodialysis. *Am J Kidney Dis* 1998;31:897.

Yip L, et al. Concepts and controversies in salicylate toxicity. *Emerg Med Clin North Am* 1994;12:351.

Zdunek M, et al. Plasma exchange for the removal of digoxin-specific antibody fragments in renal failure: timing is important for maximizing clearance. *Am J Kidney Dis* 2000;36:177.

Peritoneal Dialysis

Physiology of Peritoneal Dialysis

Peter G. Blake and John T. Daugirdas

Peritoneal dialysis is the method of renal replacement therapy used by approximately 120,000 patients worldwide. Since the introduction of continuous ambulatory peritoneal dialysis (CAPD) almost three decades ago, its popularity has increased greatly, mainly because of its simplicity, convenience, and relatively low cost.

I. What is peritoneal dialysis? In essence, peritoneal dialysis involves the transport of solutes and water across a "membrane" that separates two fluid-containing compartments. These two compartments are (a) the blood in the peritoneal capillaries, which in renal failure contains an excess of urea, creatinine, and other solutes, and (b) the dialysis solution in the peritoneal cavity, which typically contains sodium, chloride, and lactate or bicarbonate and which is rendered hyperosmolar by the inclusion of a high concentration of glucose. During the course of a peritoneal dialysis dwell, three transport processes occur simultaneously: Diffusion, ultrafiltration, and absorption. The amount of dialysis achieved and the extent of fluid removal depends on the volume of dialysis solution infused (called the dwell), how often this dialysis solution is exchanged, and the concentration of osmotic agent present.

As explained in detail in the next chapter (Chapter 19), chronic peritoneal dialysis is divided into CAPD and automated peritoneal dialysis (APD). CAPD typically involves four 2.0- to 2.5-L dwells daily, with each lasting 4–8 hours. In APD, from 3 to 10 dwells are instilled nightly using an automated cycler. In the daytime, the patient usually carries a dwell, which is drained each night before cycling recommences.

II. Functional anatomy

A. Anatomy of the peritoneal cavity. The peritoneum is the serosal membrane that lines the peritoneal cavity (Fig. 18-1). It has a surface area that is thought to be approximately equal to body surface area and so typically ranges from 1 to 2 m^2 in an adult. It is divided into two portions: (a) the visceral peritoneum, which lines the gut and other viscera, and (b) the parietal peritoneum, which lines the walls of the abdominal cavity.

The visceral peritoneum accounts for about 80% of the total peritoneal surface area and receives its blood supply from the superior mesenteric artery, whereas its venous drainage is via the portal system. In contrast, the parietal peritoneum, which may be more important in peritoneal dialysis, receives blood from the lumbar, intercostal, and epigastric arteries and drains into the inferior vena cava. Total peritoneal blood flow

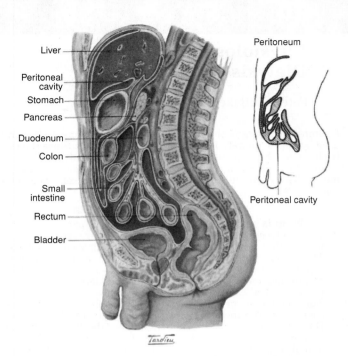

Figure 18-1. Simplified anatomy of the peritoneal cavity showing the visceral and parietal peritoneal membrane. (Adapted from Khanna R, et al., eds. *The essentials of peritoneal dialysis*. Dordrecht: Kluwer, 1993.)

cannot be directly measured but has been indirectly estimated at between 50 and 100 mL per minute. The main lymphatic drainage of the peritoneum and of the peritoneal cavity is via stomata in the diaphragmatic peritoneum, which ultimately drain via large collecting ducts into the right lymphatic duct. There is, however, additional drainage via lymphatics in both the visceral and parietal peritoneum.

B. Peritoneal membrane histology. The peritoneal membrane is lined by a monolayer of mesothelial cells that have microvilli and that produce a thin film of lubricating fluid. Under the mesothelium is the interstitium, which comprises a gel-like matrix containing collagenous and other fibers, and also the peritoneal capillaries and some lymphatics. The interstitium has been described as a two-phase system in which a colloid-rich, water-poor phase and a water-rich, colloid-poor phase are interspersed.

C. Models of peritoneal transport. Simplistically, the peritoneal membrane can be thought of as comprising six resistances to solute transport: (a) the stagnant capillary fluid film overlying the endothelium of the peritoneal capillaries,

(b) the capillary endothelium itself, (c) the endothelial basement membrane, (d) the interstitium, (e) the mesothelium, and (f) the stagnant fluid film that overlies the mesothelium.

Of these, a, e, and f (stagnant fluid films and the mesothelial layer) are thought to offer only trivial resistance to transport. Two concepts of peritoneal transport are popular; they are complementary and not mutually exclusive, and both emphasize the importance of peritoneal vasculature and interstitium. They are the three-pore model, which has helped explain how solutes of varying sizes, as well as water, are transported, and the distributed model, which has been used to develop the concept of effective peritoneal surface area.

1. The three-pore model. This model, which has been validated by clinical observations, tells us that the peritoneal capillary is the critical barrier to peritoneal transport, and that solute and water movement across it is mediated by pores of three different sizes (Fig. 18-2). These are:

a. Large pores with a radius of 20–40 nm. Macromolecules such as protein are transported by convection through these pores, which correspond to large clefts in the endothelium.

b. Small pores with a radius of 4.0–6.0 nm. There are a large number of these, which also likely represent interendothelial clefts; they are responsible for the

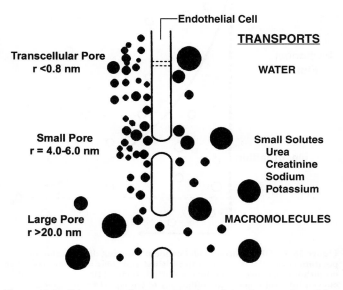

Figure 18-2. Diagrammatic representation of the three-pore model of peritoneal transport. (Adapted from Flessner MF. Peritoneal transport physiology: insights from basic research. *J Am Soc Nephrol* 1991;2:122.)

transport of small solutes, such as urea, creatinine, sodium, and potassium, in association with water.

   c. Ultrapores with a radius of <0.8 nm. These are responsible for the transport of water only and are thought to correspond to aquaporins, which are known to be present in the endothelial cell membranes of peritoneal capillaries. These ultrapores, or aquaporins, account for "sieving" by the peritoneal membrane (see below).

2. Distributed model and effective peritoneal surface area. The distributed model emphasizes the importance of the distribution of capillaries in the peritoneal membrane and of the distance water and solutes have to travel from the capillaries across the interstitium to the mesothelium (Fig. 18-3). Transport is dependent on the surface area of the peritoneal capillaries rather than on the total peritoneal surface area. Furthermore, the distance of each capillary from the mesothelium determines its relative contribution. The cumulative contribution of all of the peritoneal capillaries determines the effective surface area and the resistance properties of the membrane. From

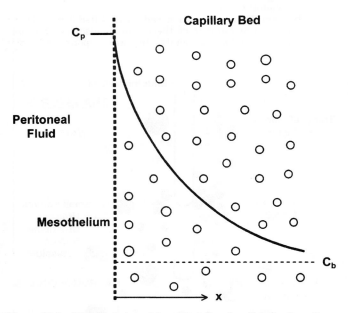

Figure 18-3. Distributed model concept showing distribution of peritoneal capillaries in the interstitium and their distances from the mesothelium, represented by the dotted, vertical line. Cp, the solid, curved line, represents the efficiency of transport from a given capillary to the peritoneal space, increasing for capillaries located closest to the mesothelial boundary. (Adapted from Flessner MF. Peritoneal transport physiology: insights from basic research. *J Am Soc Nephrol* 1991;2:122.)

the distributed model, the concept of "effective peritoneal surface area" has arisen. This is the area of the peritoneal surface that is sufficiently close to peritoneal capillaries to play a role in transport. Therefore, two patients with the same peritoneal surface area may have markedly different peritoneal vascularity and so also have very different effective peritoneal surface areas. In a given patient, effective peritoneal surface area may vary in different circumstances, increasing, for example, in peritonitis when inflammation increases vascularity.

III.   Physiology of peritoneal transport. As mentioned above, peritoneal transport comprises three processes that take place simultaneously: (a) diffusion, (b) ultrafiltration, and (c) fluid absorption.

A.   Diffusion. Uremic solutes and potassium diffuse from peritoneal capillary blood into the peritoneal dialysis solution, whereas glucose, lactate or bicarbonate, and, to a lesser extent, calcium diffuse in the opposite direction. Peritoneal diffusion depends on the following factors:

1.   The concentration gradient. For a substance such as urea, this is maximal at the start of a peritoneal dialysis dwell, when the concentration in the dialysis solution is zero. It gradually decreases during the course of the dwell. The diminishing concentration gradient effect can be counteracted partially by the performance of more frequent exchanges, as is typically done in APD, or by increasing dwell volumes, which allows the gradient to remain greater for a longer time.

2.   Effective peritoneal surface area. This can be increased by using larger fill volumes, which recruit more peritoneal membrane.

3.   Intrinsic peritoneal membrane resistance. This parameter is not well characterized but may reflect differences in the number of pores per unit surface area of capillary available for peritoneal transport and the distance across the interstitium of these capillaries from the mesothelium.

4.   Molecular weight of the solute concerned. Substances with lower molecular weight, such as urea (MW 60), are more quickly transported by diffusion than those with higher molecular weights, such as creatinine (MW 113) or albumin (MW 69,000).

a.   Mass transfer area coefficient. The combined effects of factors 2–4 are sometimes measured by an index called the mass transfer area coefficient (MTAC), which is analogous to the K_0A of a hemodialysis membrane. For a given solute, the MTAC is equivalent to the diffusive clearance of that solute per unit time in a theoretical situation in which dialysate flow is infinitely high, so that the solute gradient is always maximal. Typical MTAC values for urea and creatinine are 17 and 10 mL per minute, respectively. The MTAC is mainly a research tool and is generally not used in clinical practice.

b.   Peritoneal blood flow. It is important to note that diffusion does not generally depend on peritoneal blood flow, which, at 50–100 mL per minute, is already more than adequate relative to MTAC values for even the smallest solutes. Thus, in contrast to the situation in hemodialysis, diffusion in peritoneal dialysis is dependent on dialysate rather than blood flow. The ability of vasoactive agents to influence peritoneal transport is not related to their ability to increase peritoneal blood flow per se but rather to the associated recruitment of larger numbers of peritoneal capillaries that increase effective peritoneal surface area. The same effect is seen in peritonitis where inflammation increases peritoneal vascularity, and there is a consequent increase in peritoneal diffusion. It should be noted that the proportion of peritoneal blood flow involved in peritoneal dialysis is unknown, and it is possible that in some areas of the peritoneum blood flow may limit diffusion.

B.   Ultrafiltration. This occurs as a consequence of the osmotic gradient between the hypertonic dialysis solution and the relatively hypotonic peritoneal capillary blood. It is driven by the presence of high concentrations of glucose in dialysis solution and depends on the following:

1.   Concentration gradient for the osmotic agent (i.e., glucose). Again, this is typically maximal at the beginning of a peritoneal dialysis dwell and decreases with time due to dilution of the glucose by ultrafiltrate and due to diffusion of glucose from the dialysis solution into the blood (Fig. 18-4). The gradient will of course be less in the presence

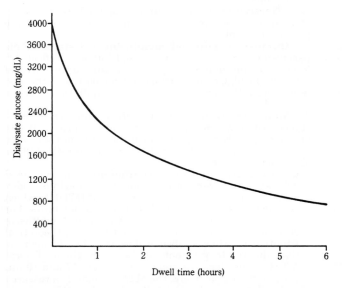

Figure 18-4.   Dialysate glucose level after instillation of a 4.25% dextrose (3.86% glucose) exchange into the peritoneal cavity. The initial level is close to 3,860 mg/dL (215 mmol/L).

of marked hyperglycemia. The gradient can be maximized by using more hypertonic solutions of dextrose or by doing more frequent exchanges, as is done with APD.

2. **Effective peritoneal surface area** (as described above)

3. **Hydraulic conductance of the peritoneal membrane.** This differs from patient to patient and perhaps reflects the density of small pores and ultrapores in the peritoneal capillaries, as well as the distribution of capillaries in the interstitium.

4. **Reflection coefficient for the osmotic agent (i.e., glucose).** This measures how effectively the osmotic agent diffuses out of the dialysis solution into the peritoneal capillaries. It is between 0 and 1; the lower the value, the faster the osmotic gradient is lost and the less sustained ultrafiltration is. For glucose the reflection coefficient is remarkably low (~ 0.03), indicating how imperfect an osmotic agent glucose is. The polyglucose preparation, icodextrin, has a reflection coefficient close to 1.0.

5. **Hydrostatic pressure gradient.** Normally, the capillary pressure (around 20 mm Hg) is higher than the intraperitoneal pressure (around 7 mm Hg), which should favor ultrafiltration. This effect is greater in an overhydrated and lower in a dehydrated patient. Rises in intraperitoneal pressure tend to oppose ultrafiltration, and this may occur when larger dwell volumes are used or when a patient is seated or standing.

6. **Oncotic pressure gradient.** Oncotic pressure acts to keep fluid in the blood, and so opposes ultrafiltration. In hypoalbuminemic patients, oncotic pressure is low, and ultrafiltration tends to be high.

7. **Sieving.** Sieving occurs when solute moves along with water across a semipermeable membrane by convection, but some of the solute is held back, or sieved. As a result, the solute concentration in the ultrafiltrate that has passed through the membrane is lower than that in the source solution. When sieving occurs, it renders ultrafiltration a less effective form of convective solute transport. Sieving coefficients for various solutes differ depending on solute molecular weight or charge, and also differ between patients. Values vary between 0 (complete sieving) and 1 (no sieving). In peritoneal dialysis, this sieving effect is due primarily to the presence of ultrapores, which are responsible for about half of total ultrafiltration and which transport only solute-free water (whereas ultrafiltrate moving through small pores, which are just clefts between the endothelial cells, probably is sieved to a much lesser extent if at all). See La Milia et al. (2005) for an experimental approach to quantify solute sieving.

8. **Alternative osmotic agents.** For many years, efforts have been made to develop osmotic agents that are more effective than glucose. The ideal osmotic agent would be safe and inexpensive, and would have a high reflection coefficient. Icodextrin is a large molecule with a high reflection coefficient, and so ultrafiltration using icodextrin is sustained

at a relatively steady level throughout even a long-duration dwell.

C.   Fluid absorption. This occurs via the lymphatics at a relatively constant rate. There is little or no sieving with fluid absorption, so that its net effect is to counteract both solute and fluid removal. Only a small proportion of fluid absorption occurs directly into the subdiaphragmatic lymphatics. The rest is absorbed across the parietal peritoneum into the tissues of the abdominal wall, from where it is subsequently taken up by local lymphatics and perhaps by peritoneal capillaries. Typical values for peritoneal fluid absorption are 1.0–2.0 mL per minute, of which 0.2–0.4 mL per minute go directly into the lymphatics. The determinants of this process are:

    1.   Intraperitoneal hydrostatic pressure. The higher this is, the greater the amount of fluid that is absorbed; intraperitoneal hydrostatic pressure is raised by increasing intraperitoneal volume as a result of more effective ultrafiltration or the use of larger infusion volumes. It is also higher when patients are sitting than when they are standing, and it is lower when they are supine (Fig. 18-5).

    2.   Effectiveness of lymphatics. The effectiveness of lymphatics absorbing fluid from the peritoneal cavity may differ markedly from person to person, for reasons that are not well understood.

IV.   Clinical assessment and implications of peritoneal transport

A.   Peritoneal equilibration test (PET). In clinical practice, indices such as the MTAC and hydraulic conductance of the peritoneal membrane are too complex for routine measurement and peritoneal transport is assessed using equilibration ratios between dialysate and plasma for urea (D/P urea), creatinine (D/P Cr), sodium (D/P Na), and so forth (Fig. 18-6). Equilibration ratios measure the combined effect of diffusion and ultrafiltration rather than either in isolation. However, they correlate well with MTAC values for the corresponding solutes. They are greatly influenced by the molecular weight of the solute concerned as well as by the membrane permeability and effective surface area. Interestingly, body size tends to have little relation to equilibration ratios despite its supposed equivalence to peritoneal surface area, suggesting that actual and effective peritoneal surface areas correlate poorly.

Conventionally, equilibration ratios are measured in a standardized PET that involves a 2-L 2.5% dextrose dwell with dialysate samples taken at 0, 2, and 4 hours and a plasma sample at 2 hours. A PET is also used to measure net fluid removal and the ratio of dialysate glucose at 4 hours to dialysate glucose at time zero (D/D$_0$ G). Patients are classified principally on the basis of their 4-hour D/P Cr into one of four categories: High, high-average, low-average, and low transporters (Fig. 18-7). The protocol for performing a PET and its use in the evaluation of ultrafiltration failure is further discussed in Chapter 23, whereas its role in peritoneal dialysis prescription is described in Chapter 22.

    1.   High transporters achieve the most rapid and complete equilibration for creatinine and urea, because they

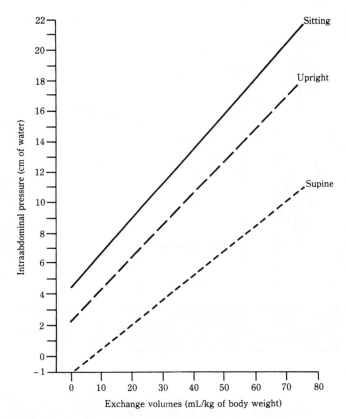

Figure 18-5.   Intra-abdominal pressure after infusing various volumes of dialysis solution. (Modified from Diaz-Buxo JA. Continuous cycling peritoneal dialysis. In: Nolph KD, ed. *Peritoneal dialysis*. Hingham: Martinus Nijhoff, 1985.)

have a relatively large effective peritoneal surface area or high intrinsic membrane permeability (i.e., low membrane resistance). However, high transporters rapidly lose their osmotic gradient for ultrafiltration because the dialysate glucose diffuses into the blood through the highly "permeable" membrane. Thus, high transporters have the highest D/P Cr, D/P Ur, and D/P Na values but have low net ultrafiltration and low D/D_0 G values. They also have higher dialysate protein losses and so tend to have lower serum albumin values.

2. Low transporters, in contrast, have slower and less complete equilibration for urea and creatinine, reflecting low membrane permeability or small effective peritoneal

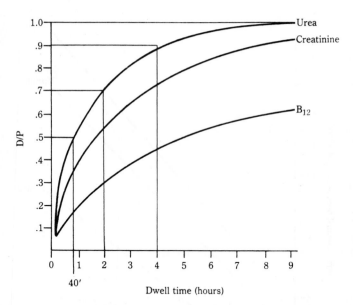

Figure 18-6.   Rate of entry of urea, creatinine, and vitamin B_{12} into peritoneal dialysis solution that has been left in the abdomen. Results are expressed as the ratio of the level in dialysate (D) to the level in plasma (P). Typical D/P ratios for urea at time points of 40 minutes, 2 hours, and 4 hours are indicated.

surface area. They thus have low D/P Ur, D/P Cr, and D/P Na and high D/D_0 G with good net ultrafiltration. Dialysate protein losses are lower, and serum albumin values tend to be higher.

3.   High-average and low-average transporters have intermediate values for these ratios and for ultrafiltration and protein losses.

4.   Clinical implications of transporter type. High transporters tend to dialyze relatively well but to ultrafiltrate poorly, whereas low transporters ultrafiltrate well but dialyze poorly, although these issues are often masked while residual renal function is still substantial. Theoretically, high transporters do best on peritoneal dialysis regimens that involve frequent short-duration dwells (e.g., APD), so that ultrafiltration is maximized. Conversely, low transporters should do best on regimens based on long-duration, high-volume dwells, so that diffusion is maximized. In practice, in most units, patient lifestyle and other nonmedical issues influence the peritoneal prescription more than transport status, and low transporters can be well managed on APD while high transporters can do CAPD provided the long nocturnal dwell is managed appropriately.

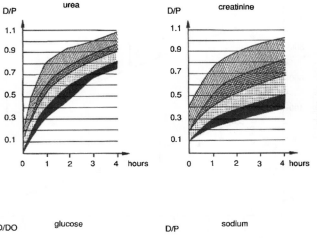

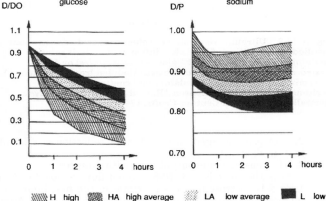

Figure 18-7.   **Standard peritoneal equilibration curves for urea, creatinine, and sodium, as well as glucose absorption showing ranges of values for high, high-average, low-average, and low transporters.** (Modified from Twardowski ZJ, et al. Peritoneal equilibration test. *Perit Dial Bull* 1987;7:138.)

B. Net fluid removal. Net fluid removal depends on the balance between peritoneal ultrafiltration and peritoneal absorption and thus on the determinants of these two processes. As lymphatic flow and the transport qualities of the membrane are not amenable to alteration, fluid removal in peritoneal dialysis can, in clinical practice, be enhanced by:

1. Maximizing the osmotic gradient
    a. Higher tonicity dwells (e.g., 4.25% dextrose)
    b. Shorter duration dwells (e.g., APD)
    c. Higher dwell volumes

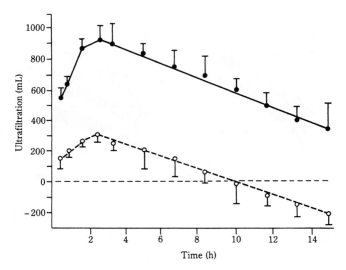

Figure 18-8. Ultrafiltration volume (volume drained minus volume instilled) as a function of time after infusion of dialysis solution containing 1.5% dextrose (1.35% glucose, *open circles*) or 4.25% dextrose (3.86% glucose, *closed circles*). (Modified from Diaz-Buxo JA. Intermittent, continuous ambulatory and continuous cycling peritoneal dialysis. In: Nissenson AR, et al., eds. *Clinical dialysis*. Norwalk, CT: Appleton-Century-Crofts, 1984.)

2. An osmotic agent with a higher reflection coefficient (e.g., icodextrin)
3. Increasing urine output (e.g., with diuretics)

As is shown in Figure 18-8, the net fluid removal with a 1.5% 2-L dextrose dwell is maximal in the first hour and intraperitoneal volume is greatest after 90 minutes. After this time, the volume being ultrafiltered is less than that being resorbed, and by 6–10 hours, the intraperitoneal volume falls below 2 L, and the patient is achieving net fluid gain. If the more hypertonic 4.25% dextrose dialysis solution is used, initial fluid removal is greater and more sustained, and intraperitoneal volume is greatest after about 3 hours and will not fall below 2 L until after many hours.

The effect of larger dwell volumes on net fluid removal is complex. On the one hand, fluid removal increases because the osmotic gradient persists longer due to the greater quantity of glucose in the peritoneal cavity and because the effective surface area over which water is transported is likely increased. On the other hand, fluid removal decreases because intraperitoneal pressure rises (Fig. 18-5), promoting peritoneal fluid absorption. The net effect of these forces varies and is difficult to predict.

C. Peritoneal clearance. Clearance for a given solute is defined as the volume of plasma cleared of that solute per unit time. Clearance is the net result of diffusion plus ultrafiltration minus absorption. It can be calculated as quantity of solute removed over a given period divided by plasma concentration. Clearance is maximal at the start of the dwell, when both diffusion and ultrafiltration are greatest, but becomes less as both urea concentration and glucose osmotic gradients diminish as the dwell remains in place. However, because peritoneal clearance is best expressed per day or per week rather than per minute or per hour, peritoneal dialysis is best modeled as a modality that delivers a low level of clearance continuously. Peritoneal clearance can be increased by (a) maximizing time on peritoneal dialysis (i.e., no "dry time"), (b) maximizing concentration gradient (i.e., more frequent exchanges as in APD and larger dwell volumes), (c) maximizing effective peritoneal surface area (i.e., larger dwell volumes), and (d) maximizing peritoneal fluid removal (as described above).

The mechanism by which increasing dwell volumes augment clearance is sometimes confusing. Larger dwell volumes enhance urea and creatinine diffusion from blood to dialysate because the greater volume makes the gradient stay higher for longer. Also, effective peritoneal surface area may increase because of recruitment of more membrane by the greater fluid volume, and consequently MTAC values may rise. This effect tends to be modest or absent once volumes exceed 2.5 L in adults, presumably because all of the available membrane has been recruited. These two effects increase diffusive clearance even though D/P ratios tend to be a little lower when larger dwell volumes are used. Another aspect of larger dwell volumes that tends to diminish clearance is the effect to diminish ultrafiltration slightly, which also lowers the amount of solute removed by convective transport. These last two factors conspire to limit the amount of increase in clearance with higher dwell volumes. For example, a switch from 2.0- to 2.5-L dwells represents a 25% increase in infused volume but might, for example, be associated with a decrease in D/P ratios of 3% and ultrafiltration of 5%, limiting the increase in clearance to 20%.

Urea versus creatinine: Changes in the peritoneal dialysis prescription alter urea and creatinine clearances to different degrees because the latter is more time dependent. Thus, a switch from CAPD to APD without a day dwell may lead to a much more marked decrease in creatinine than in urea clearance, whereas the introduction of a long day dwell in APD will cause a disproportionately greater enhancement in creatinine clearance. These effects are especially marked in low transporters whose creatinine clearance is particularly time dependent, as reflected by the flat shape of the creatinine equilibration curve.

1.   Measurement of clearance. Peritoneal clearance is easily measured and corresponds to the total daily dialysate drain volume multiplied by its solute concentration and divided by the plasma concentration measured during the dialysate collection period. Stated more simply, clearance equals the drain volume multiplied by the D/P ratio for the solute concerned.

In CAPD, the plasma urea does not alter significantly during the day because dialysis is continuous. Thus, the plasma sample can be taken at any convenient time during the day that dialysate is collected for analysis. In APD, there is significantly more intense dialysis at night than in the daytime; therefore, a constant plasma urea cannot be assumed, though variation is modest. Ideally, the plasma sample should be taken in the middle of the noncycling period (usually midafternoon) when the urea is about halfway between its lowest level (in the morning after cycling) and its highest level (at night before cycling).

Clearance is measured per day but expressed per week. It is conventional to normalize urea clearance to total-body water (V), which is typically estimated using the Watson nomogram (see Table 22-2). Creatinine clearance is normalized to 1.73 m^2 surface area, which is estimated using the formula of DuBois (see Table 22-2). For examples of peritoneal clearance calculations, see Table 22-3.

D.   Sodium removal. In peritoneal dialysis, it is helpful to consider sodium removal separately from water removal. As already mentioned, ultrafiltration in peritoneal dialysis involves sodium sieving, so that water losses are proportionately greater than sodium losses. At the end of a 4-hour dwell, dialysate sodium levels will have fallen from the initial 132 mM to about 122–125 mM (Fig. 18-7). In the early part of a dwell, dialysate sodium falls rapidly because it is diluted by ultrafiltrate containing only about 80 mM sodium. This effect is partly counteracted by diffusion, which becomes more significant as the concentration gradient for sodium widens. Thus, late in the dwell, when ultrafiltration is much lower, diffusion raises the dialysate sodium back up to about 125 mM. Overall, net sodium removal with a 4-hour, 1.5% dextrose, 2-L exchange is minimal, although with a 4-hour, 4.25% dextrose, 2-L dwell, it is typically in excess of 70 mmol. Thus, sodium removal requires the use of more hypertonic solutions. Lowering the sodium concentration in the dialysis solution would increase diffusive sodium removal but would require greater concentrations of glucose to achieve the same osmotic effect. Such solutions can be made up but are not commercially available.

E.   Protein losses. Obligatory dialysate protein losses are a feature of peritoneal dialysis and typically average 5–10 g daily, of which half is accounted for by albumin. These losses are probably the major cause of the lower serum albumin levels seen in peritoneal dialysis, as compared with hemodialysis, patients. Losses are greatest and serum albumin is lowest in high transporters. The losses or clearances of large molecular weight proteins such as albumin are relatively constant during the course of a dwell, but low molecular weight proteins such as lysozyme behave more like small solutes such as creatinine in that their clearance falls markedly as the dwell proceeds.

As already mentioned, protein losses are believed to occur via a relatively small number of large pores that correspond to interendothelial clefts. Peritoneal absorption of fluid is a form of "bulk flow" and so involves protein, as well as other solutes. It thus acts to decrease net peritoneal protein losses.

During peritonitis, protein losses increase markedly for a number of days, presumably due to an increase in effective peritoneal surface area consequent to increased vascularity. This effect is in part mediated by prostaglandins. Protein losses on intermittent peritoneal dialysis regimens appear to be somewhat less per day than on continuous regimens, presumably because the losses decrease during the "dry" interdialytic periods.

V.   Residual renal function. There is evidence that residual renal function persists longer and at a higher level in chronic peritoneal dialysis patients than in those on hemodialysis and that this plays an important part in the success of peritoneal dialysis. Residual function contributes to salt and water removal and to clearance of both small and medium-size molecular weight solutes. Creatinine clearance is disproportionately high with residual renal function as tubular secretion contributes to the overall clearance to a greater extent. The opposite is the case with urea clearances where tubular resorption is significant. The mean of urea and creatinine clearance is a reasonable estimate of true glomerular filtration rate in the failing kidney, and this estimate is customarily used when calculating the renal contribution to total creatinine clearance in patients on peritoneal dialysis. Residual renal function has been shown to be predictive of patient outcome in peritoneal dialysis, perhaps because it is associated with better preserved renal endocrine and metabolic function and superior volume homeostasis, as well as greater small- and large-molecule clearance.

SELECTED READINGS

Durand PY. Measurement of intraperitoneal pressure in peritoneal dialysis patients. *Perit Dial Int* 2005;25:333–237.

Flessner M. Water-only pores and peritoneal dialysis. *Kidney Int* 2006;69:1494–1495.

Flessner MF, et al. Blood flow does not limit peritoneal transport. *Perit Dial Int* 1999;19(Suppl 2):S208.

Flessner MF. The role of extracellular matrix in transperitoneal transport of water and solutes. *Perit Dial Int* 2001;21(Suppl 3):S24–S29.

Heimburger O, et al. A quantitative description of solute and fluid transport during peritoneal dialysis. *Kidney Int* 1992;41:1320–1332.

Krediet RT. The peritoneal membrane in chronic peritoneal dialysis. *Kidney Int* 1999;55:341–356.

Krediet RT, et al. Icodextrin's effect on peritoneal transport. *Perit Dial Int* 1997;17:35–41.

La Milia V, et al. Mini-peritoneal equilibration test: a simple and fast method to assess free water and small solute transport across the peritoneal membrane. *Kidney Int* 2005;68:840–846.

Ni J, et al. Aquaporin-1 plays an essential role in water permeability and ultrafiltration during peritoneal dialysis. *Kidney Int* 2006;69:1518–1525.

Parikova A, et al. The contribution of free water transport and small pore transport to the total fluid removal in peritoneal dialysis. *Kidney Int.* 2005;68:1849–1856.

Rippe B, et al. Fluid and electrolyte transport across the peritoneal membrane during CAPD according to the three-pore model. *Perit Dial Int* 2004;24:10–27.

Ronco C. The "nearest capillary" hypothesis: a novel approach to peritoneal transport physiology. *Perit Dial Int* 1996;16:121–125.

Twardowski ZJ, et al. Peritoneal equilibration test. *Perit Dial Bull* 1987;7:138.

WEB REFERENCES

HDCN peritoneal dialysis channel: http://www.hdcn.com/ch/perit/

Apparatus for Peritoneal Dialysis

Olof Heimbürger and Peter G. Blake

In this chapter, solutions and equipment for the various forms of peritoneal dialysis (PD) are described. Continuous ambulatory peritoneal dialysis (CAPD), automated peritoneal dialysis (APD), and hybrids of the two are discussed. Apparatus for acute PD is reviewed in Chapter 21.

I. CAPD. In CAPD, dialysis solution is constantly present in the abdomen. The solution is typically changed four times daily, with a range of three to five times depending on individual patient requirements. Drainage of "spent" dialysate and inflow of fresh dialysis solution are performed manually, using gravity to move fluid into and out of the peritoneal cavity. Technically, PD solution flows into the peritoneal cavity, and dialysate drains out (i.e., the solution does not become dialysate until dialysis has occurred, although the term "dialysate" is commonly used for fresh as well as for used or "spent" solution). In this chapter, the term dialysate is used correctly to refer only to PD solution after it has been instilled into the peritoneal space.

A. Dialysis solutions. CAPD solutions are packaged in clear, flexible plastic bags or, less commonly, in semirigid plastic containers. The bags are typically made from polyvinyl chloride though theoretical concern about phthalic acid leachates have led to bags of other composition being developed. Some new PD solutions are packaged with the different solution components in two- (or three-) chamber bags, which are mixed before infusion into the peritoneal cavity.

1. Dialysis solution volumes. For adult patients, CAPD solutions are available in volumes of 1.5, 2.0, 2.25, 2.5, or 3.0 L, depending on the manufacturer. The commonly used bags are routinely overfilled by about 100 mL to allow for flushing, as will be described in a subsequent section. The standard volume prescribed has been 2.0 L, but 2.5 L is also widely used. Generally, larger volumes are prescribed in order to increase solute clearance, but they may not always be tolerated by smaller patients because of symptoms induced by the consequent increase in intraperitoneal hydrostatic pressure.

2. Dialysis solution electrolyte concentrations. The electrolyte concentrations of CAPD solutions vary little by manufacturer. The standard formulations from the three large international manufacturers are shown in Table 19-1. Solutions contain no potassium and sodium levels are set at about 132–134 mM. Higher sodium concentrations would lead to less diffusive removal of sodium during dwells.

Table 19-1.   Commonly available peritoneal dialysis solutions

	Manufacturer	pH	Osmotic Agent	Na mM	Ca mM	Mg mM	Lactate mM	Bicarb mM	Pouches
Dianeal PD1	Baxter	5.5	Glucose	132	1.75	0.75	35	0	1
Dianeal PD4	Baxter	5.5	Glucose	132	1.25	0.25	40	0	1
Stay-safe 2/4/3	FMC	5.5	Glucose	134	1.75	0.5	35	0	1
Stay-safe 17/19/18	FMC	5.5	Glucose	134	1.25	0.5	35	0	1
Gambrosol Trio 10	Gambro	6.3	Glucose	132	1.75	0.25	40	0	3
Gambrosol Trio 40	Gambro	6.3	Glucose	132	1.35	0.25	40	0	3
Nutrineal	Baxter	6.5	Amino acids	132	1.25	0.25	40	0	1
Extraneal	Baxter	5.5	Icodextrin	132	1.75	0.25	40	0	1
Physioneal	Baxter	7.4	Glucose	132	1.75	0.25	10	25	2
Balance	FMC	7.4	Glucose	134	1.25 1.75	0.5	34	2	2
bicaVera	FMC	7.4	Glucose	134	1.75	0.5	0	34	2
bicaNova	FMC	7.4	Glucose	134	1.25	0.5	0	39	2

These may differ slightly in name and in formulation from region to region.
Note that all glucose-based solutions are available in three strengths (1.36, 2.27, and 3.86 g/dL equivalent to 1.5, 2.5, and 4.25 mg of dextrose/dL). However, some solutions in fact contain glucose 1.5, 2.5, 4.0, and 4.25 mg/dL.
To convert calcium from mM to mg/dL, multiply by 4.
To convert magnesium from mM to mg/dL, multiply by 2.43.
FMC, Fresenius Medical Care.

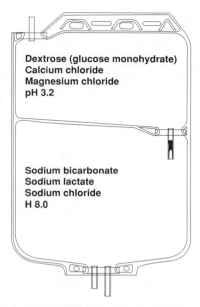

Dextrose (glucose monohydrate)
Calcium chloride
Magnesium chloride
pH 3.2

Sodium bicarbonate
Sodium lactate
Sodium chloride
H 8.0

Figure 19-1. Two-compartment continuous ambulatory peritoneal dialysis (CAPD) solution bag to allow delivery of a normal pH solution with low glucose degradation products (GDPs) and/or bicarbonate buffer.

Low-sodium solutions have been proposed as a means of augmenting sodium removal but would likely lead to hyponatremia, as well as a requirement for more glucose to maintain a given osmolarity.

Up until recently, all commonly marketed CAPD solutions contained lactate as the bicarbonate-generating base. Now bicarbonate-based PD solutions have become available in most countries, and are increasingly used. Both pure bicarbonate solutions and bicarbonate/lactate mixtures are available. A two-compartment bag system is used to keep the bicarbonate separate from the calcium and magnesium until just before use (Fig. 19-1). Bicarbonate solutions have a normal pH and so cause less discomfort on infusion than lactate-based solutions. They are theoretically more biocompatible, and it is hoped that they will enhance peritoneal host defenses and improve peritoneal membrane longevity and even patient survival. To date, however, there is little evidence that bicarbonate solutions improve long-term patient outcomes.

With the widespread use of calcium carbonate or calcium acetate as a phosphate binder, CAPD solutions containing

1.0–1.25 mM (2.0–2.5 mEq/L) rather than 1.75 mM (3.5 mEq/L) calcium are increasingly used with the goal of reducing the incidence of the hypercalcemia that is sometimes associated with oral calcium and vitamin D administration (see Chapter 35). However, the use of the lower calcium concentrations is sometimes associated with increasing parathyroid hormone (PTH) levels, and in these situations, vitamin D treatment may be indicated. Conversely, low turnover or adynamic bone disease is increasingly recognized in PD patients, and in this setting, low calcium solutions, as well as withdrawal of calcium carbonate and vitamin D, is typically required.

Solutions typically contain magnesium levels of 0.5 or 0.25 mM and this can occasionally result in magnesium depletion.

3. Dialysis solution dextrose concentrations. Dextrose (glucose monohydrate, MW 198) is the osmotic agent commonly used in CAPD solutions, and preparations containing 1.5%, 2.5%, and 4.25% dextrose are routinely available and are labeled as such in North America. The true anhydrous glucose (MW 180) concentrations in these solutions are 1.36%, 2.27%, and 3.86%, respectively, and this is how they are typically labeled in Europe. The approximate osmolarities of these solutions are 345, 395, and 484 mOsm/L, respectively.

An interesting preparation from Gambro is the tricompartmental Gambrosol Trio solution bag, which has one main compartment containing the solution and two other small compartments containing concentrated dextrose. This allows the osmolarity of the final infused solution to be varied. Opening the connection between one dextrose compartment and the rest of the bag gives a 1.5% solution. Opening the alternative dextrose compartment gives a 2.5% solution and opening both gives 3.9%. This avoids the need to store multiple different solution strengths but does increase complexity somewhat. This solution has the additional advantage of allowing the dextrose compartment solutions to be sterilized separately and at a lower pH than the usual 5.5 used for standard CAPD solutions. This minimizes caramelization of glucose and generation of toxic glucose degradation products (GDPs), which are increasingly believed to damage the peritoneal membrane. Strategies to minimize GDP generation are discussed below.

4. Nondextrose solutions. Dextrose as an osmotic agent in PD has the advantage of being familiar, relatively safe, and inexpensive, and also is a source of calories. There is concern, however, that it predisposes patients to hyperglycemia, dyslipidemia, obesity, and long-term peritoneal membrane damage, both directly and via GDPs and advanced glycosylation end products that result from their metabolism. In addition, it is not very effective in some patients, especially high transporters, and inadequate ultrafiltration may result. Alternative osmotic agents would be potentially helpful, and some are now available.

a. **Amino acid–based solutions** are used for nutritional supplementation as they are largely absorbed by the end of a 4- to 6-hour dwell. Studies have shown them to be modestly effective in nutritionally compromised patients. They are reasonably effective osmotically (comparable to the 1.5% dextrose solution) but can only be used once daily because in larger amounts they tend to cause acidosis, as well as a rise in the blood urea. These side effects may have to be addressed with oral alkali therapy and more dialysis, respectively.

b. **Icodextrin,** a polyglucose preparation, is now widely available. It is an iso-osmolar solution and induces ultrafiltration by its oncotic effect. Absorption of polyglucose to plasma is by the lymphatics and so is much slower compared to dextrose. The oncotic effect and the associated ultrafiltration are therefore more sustained than with dextrose. For this reason, the main indication is for the long nocturnal dwell in CAPD and for the long day dwell in APD, especially in patients with ultrafiltration failure (see Chapter 23). Icodextrin use is associated with unphysiologic blood levels of maltose and maltotriose, but no associated toxicity has been identified. However, the increased maltose levels will cause interference with the glucose dehydrogenase pyrroquinolone quinone assay (which reacts with both glucose and maltose) for blood glucose measurements. Therefore, blood glucose should be measured with other methods in patients using icodextrin solution. In addition, use of icodextrin solution is associated with low measured amylase levels, partly due to interaction between polyglucose metabolites and the assay. Icodextrin has been shown in randomized controlled trials to improve volume status in PD patients, though not convincingly to reduce blood pressure. Other potential advantages for icodextrin include a reduction in weight gain and in glucose-induced lipid abnormalities and better preservation of membrane function.

5. **Dialysis solution pH.** In the manufacturing process, the pH of traditional lactate-based PD solutions is lowered to about 5.5 to prevent caramelization of glucose and to minimize generation of GDPs during heat sterilization. Lowering pH further would decrease GDPs even more but would also cause infusion pain in patients. A pH of 5.5 on infusion is normally well tolerated, and rises rapidly as bicarbonate diffuses into the peritoneal cavity from the plasma. However, some patients complain of pain during inflow of dialysis solution. This pain can be relieved by neutralizing the dialysis solution pH with alkali prior to instillation.

The low pH of peritoneal dialysis has an adverse effect on leukocytes. Even brief exposure to such low pH solutions in vitro causes "stunning" of leukocytes, impairing their ability for phagocytosis, bacterial killing, and superoxide generation. It may also be harmful to the peritoneal membrane. As mentioned above, bicarbonate-based solutions with a physiologic pH are increasingly available. These solutions are supplied in dual-chamber bags that are mixed before infu-sion. Typically, the glucose chamber has a low pH to avoid formation of toxic GDPs during heat sterilization, whereas the bicarbonate compartment is alkalotic, resulting in a dialysis fluid with neutral pH after mixing (Fig. 19-1). Infu-sion pain resolves with use of neutral pH solutions.

6.   GDPs. As mentioned above, the heat sterilization pro-cess leads to generation of GDPs, which have toxic effects on the peritoneal membrane. The principal strategy to deal with this is the use of multicompartmental solution bags where the glucose, having been heat-sterilized at a very low pH that retards the formation of GDPs (e.g., pH 3.2), is kept separate from the rest of the solution, which can then be maintained at an alkaline pH. At the time of use, the glucose is allowed to mix with the rest of the solution, bringing the pH of the resultant mixture to close to normal. The higher pH and the reduced amount of GDPs are the main advan-tages of these solutions. It is important to note that these low GDP solutions in multicompartmental bags may or may not be bicarbonate based. For example, the Baxter Physioneal solution is a low GDP preparation with a mix of bicarbonate and lactate as the base. The Fresenius Balance and Gam-bro Unica solutions are completely lactate based, while the other Fresenius solution Bicavera is exclusively bicarbon-ate based. In other words, multicompartmental bags allow GDP generation to be reduced and also, if desired, bicarbon-ate buffer to be used.

7.   Sterility and trace metals. The preparation of PD so-lutions is carefully regulated to ensure that the final product is bacteriologically safe and has very low concentrations of trace metals.

8.   Dialysis solution temperature. PD solutions are usually warmed to body temperature prior to inflow. They can be instilled at room temperature, but uncomfortable lowering of the body temperature and shivering can result. The best warming method is to use a heating pad or special oven. Microwave ovens are frequently used, but this is not recommended by most manufacturers because "hot spots" may be produced during heating, in particular in the trans-fer sets. When using a microwave oven, great care must be taken to avoid overheating of the dialysis solution as this can chemically alter the dextrose and may cause discomfort on instillation. Also, accidental boiling of the solution in a con-fined space may cause an explosion. Heating methods that involve immersing the PD solution container completely in water are not recommended because contamination can result.

B.   Transfer sets. The CAPD solution bag is connected to the patient's peritoneal catheter by a length of plastic tubing called a "transfer set" (also sometimes called a "giving set"). There are three major types of transfer sets, each requiring a different method of performing the CAPD exchange. For the purpose of discussion, we will refer to them as the straight transfer set, the Y transfer set, and the double-bag system.

Note that some transfer sets are connected to the peritoneal catheter via a short extension tubing (see below).

1. Straight transfer set. This system is now rarely used because it is associated with high rates of peritonitis. However, a brief description is helpful in understanding how more modern systems have evolved.

  a. Design. The straight transfer set is a simple plastic tube. One end connects to the peritoneal catheter and the other end to the dialysis solution bag. All exchanges are performed by making and subsequently breaking the connection between the transfer set and the bag. This connection typically involves a spike or a Luer lock.

  b. Exchange procedure. Dialysis is performed as follows:

  (1) Dialysis solution is instilled by gravity.

  (2) The empty bag and transfer set are rolled up and stored in a pouch carried on the patient's body.

  (3) Dwell time is typically 4–8 hours.

  (4) The bag is unrolled and placed on the floor. The dialysate is drained into the bag. The bag is then disconnected from the transfer set and discarded.

  (5) A new bag is attached to the transfer set using a spike or Luer lock.

  (6) Fresh dialysis solution is instilled.

  Once every several months, the transfer set is changed. Extended-life transfer set tubing allows patients to dialyze for 6 months between transfer set changes.

2. The Y set (Fig. 19-2)

  a. Design. This is a Y-shaped piece of tubing that is attached by its stem to the patient's catheter or extension tubing at the time of each solution exchange. During the exchange, the afferent and efferent limbs of the Y are attached to a bag of fresh PD solution and to a drain bag, respectively. In some cases, the drain bag is the empty solution bag that was used in the previous exchange. Most Y sets are not connected directly to the catheter but rather to a short (15–24 cm) extension tubing inserted between the catheter and the stem of the Y set. This extension tubing is sometimes confusingly called a transfer set, but in this chapter that term is reserved for the tubing that connects the solution bag and drain bag to the extension tubing and catheter. The extension tubing avoids the need for, and the risk of damage associated with, repeated clamping of the catheter.

  b. Exchange procedure

  (1) Spike/lock: The fresh bag of PD solution is attached to the afferent limb of the Y set via a spike or Luer lock.

  (2) Connect: The stem of the Y set is connected to the extension tubing.

  (3) Drain: The stem and efferent limb of the Y are unclamped and the spent dialysate is drained from the peritoneal cavity into the drain bag.

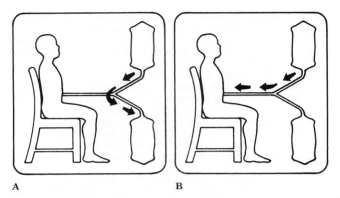

A   B

Figure 19-2.   Y-set system using flush-before-fill. A: A small volume of fresh dialysis solution is drained directly into the drainage bag (either before or just after drainage of the abdomen). This act washes away any bacteria that may have been introduced in the limb of the Y leading to the new bag at the time of connection. B: Fresh solution is introduced through the rinsed transfer set. The Y-set system illustrated is a double-bag one and differs only in that the fresh dialysis solution bag is incorporated into the Y tubing, and no connection to it is needed. In this situation the "flush-before-fill" step is solely to flush out any air in the tubing.

(4)   Flush: With the stem of the Y set clamped, approximately 100 mL of fresh solution is flushed from the new bag through the afferent limb of the Y into the efferent limb and so into the drain bag.

(5)   Fill: The efferent limb is clamped and the stem unclamped, and the peritoneal cavity is filled from the new bag of PD solution.

(6)   Disconnect: The Y set is then disconnected from the extension tubing. The Y set was developed to free patients from the requirement to remain attached to the transfer set and empty bag between exchanges. Early studies revealed a more important benefit—a peritonitis rate significantly lower than that with the straight set. This is thought to be due to the flush-before-fill procedure used to prime the tubing. Bacteria that may be introduced during the connection procedure are washed out of the Y set into the empty drainage bag rather than into the patient, as happens with the straight set. Also, because the tubing and bags are disconnected from the patient between exchanges, less mechanical stress may be placed on the catheter exit site and tunnel. This may result in fewer episodes of minor trauma to the catheter exit site and tunnel and therefore to fewer exit site and tunnel infections and associated peritonitis.

Because of this lower peritonitis rate and the convenience of allowing the patient to disconnect between exchanges, Y-set systems increasingly displaced the straight system as the transfer set of choice from the mid-1980s on. Nondisconnect Y sets, which are filled with sodium hypochlorite between exchanges, were initially popular but are now less so due to their complexity, lack of apparent additional benefit, and risk of painful accidental intraperitoneal hypochlorite infusion. Similarly, removable, reusable Y sets, called "O sets," in which the disconnected Y was filled with disinfectant between exchanges and stored with the two limbs connected to form an "O," are now of mainly historical interest.

3. Double-bag systems

a. Design. These systems are a variant of the Y set, in which the solution bag comes preattached to the afferent limb of the Y, so obviating the need for any spike or Luer lock connection. The drain bag is similarly preattached to the efferent limb, and the only connection the patient needs to make is thus between the transfer set and the extension tubing. A flush-before-fill step is still performed, but the purpose is only to flush out residual air and not to prevent peritoneal cavity contamination, as this is no longer relevant in the absence of a need to make a transfer set–to–solution bag connection.

These are now by far the most popular systems because of their ease of use and because of evidence that they are associated with even lower rates of peritonitis than the standard Y sets. Their only disadvantage is that their disposability results in increased use of materials as compared to older reusable systems.

b. Exchange procedure

(1) Connect: The patient connects the new transfer set to the extension tubing.

(2) Drain: The stem and efferent limb are unclamped and spent dialysate is drained from the peritoneal cavity into the drain bag.

(3) Flush: The stem is clamped, and the afferent limb of the Y is opened by breaking a "frangible" in the tubing. Then 100 mL of PD solution is flushed through from the fill bag to the drain bag to remove residual air from the tubing.

(4) Fill: The efferent limb is clamped, the stem is unclamped, and fresh PD solution is run into the peritoneal cavity.

(5) Disconnect: All limbs are clamped, and the transfer set is disconnected from the extension tubing.

C. Various connectors for PD. Over the years, a number of connectors and associated devices have been developed and marketed in an attempt to reduce the possibility of bacterial contamination while making either the catheter–to–transfer set or the transfer set–to–container connections.

1. Catheter–to–transfer set (or extension tubing–to–transfer set) connection

a. Catheter connector. Early in the history of CAPD, simple, plastic, plug-in connectors were used at the catheter–to–transfer set junction. Cracking of the plastic connector and accidental disconnection were frequent events that often led to peritonitis. A special Luer lock connector made of titanium was developed to prevent such problems. Titanium was chosen for its light weight and resistance to electrolyte-containing solutions. Designed for easier handling and a tighter connection, the new product functioned very well. Catheter–to–transfer set connectors constructed from more durable plastics are also available.

b. Quick connect–disconnect systems. With the advent of the disconnect Y sets and double bags, the need for an easy yet sterile connection at the catheter–to–transfer set joint (or adapter–to–transfer set joint) has arisen. A number of connector designs for this purpose are now available. Typically they include a "Luer lock"–type mechanism with a recessed orifice and an iodine-impregnated cap to minimize the risk of contamination. A more elaborate device is the "Stay Safe" device from Fresenius Medical Care, which regulates the fill and drain cycles as well as making the connection to the adapter tubing.

2. Transfer set–to–container connection. With the advent of double-bag systems, technologies to facilitate the connection between the transfer set and the peritoneal dialysis solution container are less relevant. However, some of them are still used, and brief mention will be made of them.

a. Spike-and-port design. The spike-and-port design is the oldest and simplest system used to connect the transfer set to the PD solution bag. It is operated by pushing a spike located at the end of the transfer set into a port on the solution bag.

b. Easy-lock connectors. Spiking the container is difficult for many patients because it requires reasonably good vision, depth and sensory perception, and strength. Mistakes can result in contamination and subsequent peritonitis. The spike has thus been replaced in many transfer sets by a Luer lock– or screw-type system, resulting in easier insertion. A modified form contains a recessed fluid pathway to prevent accidental contamination, a reservoir that can be filled with an antiseptic solution (e.g., povidone–iodine), and a silicon O-ring to provide a tight seal.

c. Specialized connection devices can reduce the risk of peritonitis associated with CAPD. However, most of the devices are bulky and cumbersome, and some require use of an electric power outlet or a somewhat heavy portable battery. These include:

(1) Mechanical devices to assist in spike–port insertion. Available devices make use of levers or gears to assist blind or arthritic patients in inserting the transfer set spike into the port on the dialysis solution container.

(2) Ultraviolet (UV) light sterilization device. This device combines a mechanical system that assists in spiking the port with UV light irradiation of the spike and port just before the connection is made.

II. Automated peritoneal dialysis. APD, using a cycler, is now the fastest-growing PD modality, and in some countries, including the United States, the majority of PD patients are treated this way. APD is traditionally divided into continuous cycling peritoneal dialysis (CCPD) and nocturnal intermittent peritoneal dialysis (NIPD), although the combination of cycler therapy at night with daytime exchanges is commonly used today (see Fig. 19-3). In CCPD (row 2 in Fig. 19-3), the patient carries PD solution in the abdominal cavity throughout the day but performs no exchanges and is not attached to a transfer set. At bedtime, the patient hooks up to the cycler, which drains and refills the abdomen with solution three or more times in the course of the night. In the morning, the patient, with the last dwell remaining in the abdomen, disconnects from the cycler and is free to go about daily activities. In NIPD (row 1 in Fig. 19-3), the patient drains out fully at the end of the cycling period, and so the abdomen is "dry" all day. Because of the absence of a long-duration day dwell, clearances are generally lower on NIPD than on CCPD, but its use may be indicated if there is good residual renal function or if there are mechanical contraindications to walking about with solution in the abdominal cavity (e.g., leaks, hernias, back pain).

A. Cyclers. These are machines that automatically cycle dialysis solution into and out of the abdominal cavity. Contemporary cyclers are not gravity dependent but instead use hydraulic pumps to deliver the solution from 3-, 5-, or 6-L bags to a "fill bag" and from there into the abdomen. The solution in the fill bag is warmed before inflow. With the aid of pressure alarms, clamps, and timers, inflow, dwell, and outflow of solution are regulated and overfilling prevented.

Recent cycler models are small and light enough to pack in a large suitcase and carry on trips. Advanced design and computer technology make them simple to set up and operate. The patient typically sets only the start time, volume of solution to be used, dwell volume, and length of dialysis or stop time desired. The cycler calculates the timing of the exchanges, measures volume of ultrafiltrate, and optimizes drain and inflow time by measuring flow rates and changing from drain to fill when flow slows down rather than waiting for a preset time. It also tests to determine whether flow has stopped because of obstruction. Some models incorporate "smart cards," which can be used to program the cycler prescription and to record the actual prescription delivered to the patient.

An extremely useful feature is the ability to draw dialysis solution from a separate solution container for the last instillation in the morning, called the "last bag option," because this last inflow, which will be in place throughout the day, may require a higher dextrose concentration than the other

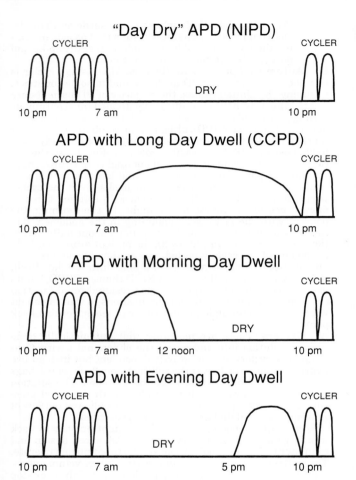

Figure 19-3. Visual representation of common APD prescriptions (see also Fig. 22-1 for additional PD prescription variants).

exchanges. More often, nowadays, the last bag option is used to deliver an alternative solution such as icodextrin or amino acids.

Typically, patients spend 8–10 hours a night cycling. Dwell volumes range from 1.5 to 3.0 L, and the number of cycles usually varies from 3 to 10 per night. The amount of fluid used is typically between 10 and 18 L but can range from 6 to 30 L.

B. Dialysis solution. Dialysis solution for APD is the same as that used for CAPD. Most cyclers are fed by a tube containing a multipronged manifold that can attach to as many as eight dialysis solution containers simultaneously to provide sufficient solution for the night. The total number of containers required, and thus the cost, can be reduced by using large containers holding 3, 5, or 6 L of dialysis solution, although lifting these can be a problem for older and frailer patients. Because the cycler can be fed from two or more containers simultaneously, with appropriate selection of the dextrose concentrations of the containers being hung, a number of intermediate dextrose concentrations (e.g., between those commercially available) can easily be delivered. New bicarbonate buffered solutions are generally not available in large-volume bags suitable for APD. Icodextrin and amino acid solutions are not appropriate for delivery by cycler, except as a "last bag option."

C. APD connections

    1. Transfer sets. One set of plastic tubing serves to interconnect several solution containers to the cycler and to connect the cycler to the patient. Shorter, simpler, and less expensive solution delivery sets are constantly being developed.

    2. Catheter–to–transfer set connection. The catheter–to–transfer set connection must be made every night and broken every morning. Previously, many patients had a standard Luer lock connector at the end of the peritoneal catheter. The procedure for connecting the catheter connector to the transfer set was tedious because it required sterile procedure and a lengthy antiseptic scrub. This older connector has largely been replaced by new, quick connect–disconnect systems that require no manual disinfection and therefore are much easier to use. Some of these systems also may fit CAPD transfer sets, allowing APD patients to use the CAPD method whenever desired (e.g., when traveling).

    3. Transfer set–to–container connections. The standard spike-and-port or, more often, Luer lock connections are used to connect the multipronged transfer set to the dialysis solution containers. It is ironic that this step, which has largely disappeared from CAPD with the dominance of double bags, is becoming commonplace again with the growth in APD. In order to minimize the risk of contamination, the newer cyclers allow for a flush option after this connection has been made. The same connection technologies used to assist CAPD patients with visual impairment, arthritis, or neuropathy (see above) can also assist APD patients in making the transfer set–to–container connections.

D. Tidal peritoneal dialysis (TPD). This variant of APD was designed to optimize solute clearance by leaving a large volume of dialysis solution in the peritoneal cavity throughout the dialysis session. It was thought that this would allow diffusive clearance to continue throughout the cycling period. Initially, the peritoneal cavity is filled with a volume of solution selected to be as large as possible without causing discomfort. The volume used depends on patient size and habitus but is typically 2 to 3 L. When TPD was introduced, a 50% tidal volume was common; for example, if 2 L is being used, the next fill volume (the tidal volume) is 1 L, the next drain volume is about 1 L, and so on. Clearances with TPD have been disappointing and, with usual solution volumes, are no better than those with similar amounts of solution, delivered by conventional cycling. Clearance benefits may be seen with high-volume TPD where solution volumes are >20 L, but these are not widely used because of high cost and inconvenience. Today, the commonest indications for TPD are to avoid low drain alarms in patients with poor catheter function or to avoid drain pain in patients who experience discomfort at the end of the drain phase. With this in mind, cyclers allow individualization of the tidal volume, and most commonly it is set to about 75%. TPD cycles are quite short, usually totaling <60 minutes, with dwell times for the replacement aliquot being only 10–40 minutes. The peritoneal cavity is drained completely only at the end of the dialysis session. At this stage, the peritoneal catheter can be capped and the peritoneal cavity left empty until the next treatment, as in NIPD. Alternatively, fluid can be left in the cavity, as in CCPD.

  1. **Technical problems.** Classical high-volume TPD has a number of technical problems, making it difficult to recommend for routine use. Therefore, mainly low-volume TPD is currently used.

   a. **Peritoneal catheter.** For classical high-volume TPD with 20–30 L of solution, the peritoneal catheter must have excellent inflow and drain characteristics, as flow must be 180–200 mL per minute during the drain phase. In contrast, low-volume TPD is often indicated to avoid alarms from low drain when the catheter function is poor.

   b. **Cost.** In adults, the advantages of TPD in terms of clearance are only seen with 20–30 L of solution per treatment and this is very expensive.

   c. **Ultrafiltration computations.** The ultrafiltration volume must be calculated and added to the drain volume with each exchange; otherwise, the intra-abdominal volume will become progressively larger. TPD is best performed with newer cyclers that have been modified, so that the outflow volume can be set to trigger a change to dialysate inflow mode. When the preset outflow volume is reached (e.g., 1.5 L), the machine changes immediately to inflow to infuse a fresh 1.5 L of dialysis solution. This system is quite different from that in most early cyclers, in which inflow/outflow cycles are regulated only by preset timers, not by volume.

III. Hybrid regimens. In an effort to improve the clearances and ultrafiltration associated with standard CAPD and APD without infringing unduly on patient lifestyle, a number of hybrid methodologies between CAPD and APD have evolved.

A. Night exchange device. This system was designed to provide a single extra exchange for CAPD patients, at a predetermined time, most often while the patient is asleep at night. In essence, it is a cycler that provides one exchange cycle. It was most often used to increase clearance by adding a fifth evenly spaced exchange at night, or to allow a fourth exchange for a patient who can only manage three during regular waking hours. Splitting the long nocturnal CAPD dwell in two also enhances ultrafiltration, and so the device is useful for patients, typically high transporters, who have net fluid resorption after long dwells. The night exchange device has become less popular as cyclers have decreased in cost and increased in flexibility and convenience.

B. APD with daytime exchanges. CCPD does not provide adequate clearances for some patients once residual renal function is lost. Additional day exchanges may be required (see rows 3 and 4 in Fig. 19-3). These exchanges improve clearance as the typical 14- to 16-hour, single day dwell in CCPD is unduly long and does not provide significant additional clearance after the first 4–6 hours. These additional day exchanges also improve ultrafiltration as the single day dwell is too long for effective net fluid removal. Indeed, in many patients, especially higher transporters, a single day exchange can result in significant net fluid resorption to a degree that is medically unacceptable. Additional day exchanges can be done manually using standard CAPD transfer sets, but this is relatively expensive in terms of solution and tubing costs and may be inconvenient for patients.

An alternative strategy, originally described as "PD Plus," involves using the cycler tubing to deliver the additional exchange(s). The patient returns to the cycler in the afternoon or evening, reattaches to the transfer set, drains the dialysate that has been in the peritoneal cavity since that morning, and then refills from the large-volume solution containers (3–5 L) that will be used to provide solution for cycling that night. The patient then detaches from the transfer set but is able to reattach to the same tubing later, either to do another exchange or to commence cycling that night. This is made possible by a modification of the transfer set that allows serial connections and disconnections to be performed or by simply using "caps" to protect the respective endings of the transfer set and adapter tubing while disconnected. This strategy, which has been described as using the cycler as a "docking station," can be easily performed with any of the newer-generation cyclers and is less costly because no additional transfer set is required and because the solution can be drawn from more economical, large-volume solution bags. It has the additional advantage that it can be set up for the patient in advance by a relative or a helper. However, for the working patient, the requirement to return to the cycler during the noncycling period may be a disadvantage, and in such cases, a manual CAPD-type exchange may be preferred.

In some patients, a second day dwell is not required for clearance reasons but a single long day dwell leads to net fluid resorption. In these cases, the cycler tubing can be used to drain the day dwell early without any subsequent fill (Fig. 19-3). Nowadays, a common alternative strategy in this setting is to use icodextrin solution, which generally maintains an adequate oncotic gradient, even during 16-hour cycles.

SELECTED READINGS

Brown EA, et al. Survival of functionally anuric patients on automated peritoneal dialysis: the European APD Outcome Study. *J Am Soc Nephrol* 2003;14:2948–2957.

Chagnac A, et al. Calcium balance during pulse alfacalcidol therapy for secondary hyperparathyroidism in CAPD patients treated with 1.0 and 1.25 mmol/L dialysate calcium. *Am J Kidney Dis* 1999;32:82–86.

Coles G, et al. A randomized controlled trial of a bicarbonate- and a bicarbonate/lactate-containing dialysis solution in CAPD. *Perit Dial Int* 1997;17:48–51.

Davies SJ, et al. Icodextrin improves the fluid status of peritoneal dialysis patients: results of a double-blind randomized controlled trial. *J Am Soc Nephrol* 2003;14:2338–2344.

Dombros N, et al., for the EBPG Expert Group on Peritoneal Dialysis. European best practice guidelines for peritoneal dialysis. 5 Peritoneal dialysis solutions. *Nephrol Dial Transplant* 2005;20 (Suppl 9):ix34–ix35.

Erixon M, et al. Take care in how you store your PD fluids: actual temperature determines the balance between reactive and non-reactive GDPs. *Perit Dial Int* 2005;25(6):583–590.

Feriani M, et al. Individualized bicarbonate concentrations in the peritoneal dialysis fluid to optimize acid-base status in CAPD patients. *Nephrol Dial Transplant* 2004;19:195–202.

Jones M, et al. Treatment of malnutrition with 1.1% amino acid peritoneal dialysis solution: results of a multicenter outpatient study. *Am J Kidney Dis* 1998;32:761–767.

Kiernan L, et al. Comparison of continuous ambulatory peritoneal dialysis–related infections with different "Y-tubing" exchange systems. *J Am Soc Nephrol* 1995;5:1835–1838.

Krishnan M, et al. Glucose degradation products (GDP's) and peritoneal changes in patients on chronic peritoneal dialysis: will new dialysis solutions prevent these changes [Review]? *Int Urol Nephrol* 2005;37(2):409–418.

Li PK, et al. Comparison of double-bag and Y-set disconnect systems in continuous ambulatory peritoneal dialysis: a randomized prospective multicenter study. *Am J Kidney Dis* 1999;33:535–540.

Lo WK, et al. A 3-year, prospective, randomized, controlled study on amino acid dialysate in patients on CAPD. *Am J Kidney Dis* 2003;42(1):173–183.

Mistry CD, et al. A randomized multicenter clinical trial comparing isosmolar icodextrin with hyperosmolar glucose solutions in CAPD. *Kidney Int* 1994;46:496–503.

Montenegro J, et al. Long-term clinical experience with pure bicarbonate peritoneal dialysis solutions. *Perit Dial Int* 2006;26(1): 89–94.

Ronco C, et al. Evolution of technology for automated peritoneal dialysis. *Contrib Nephrol* 2006;150:291–309.

Sitter T, Sauter M. Impact of glucose in peritoneal dialysis: saint or sinner [Review]? *Perit Dial Int* 2005;25(5):415–425.

Tranæus A, for the bicarbonate/Lactate Study Group. A long-term study of a bicarbonate/lactate-based peritoneal dialysis solution—clinical benefits. *Perit Dial Int* 2000;20:516–523.

Williams JD, et al. The Euro-Balance Trial: the effect of a new biocompatible peritoneal dialysis fluid (balance) on the peritoneal membrane. *Kidney Int* 2004;66:408–418.

Woodrow G. Can biocompatible dialysis fluids improve outcomes in dialysis patients? *Perit Dial Int* 2005;25:230–233.

Peritoneal Access Devices

Stephen R. Ash and John T. Daugirdas

The ideal peritoneal catheter allows adequate rates of dialysate inflow and outflow, drains the abdomen to less than a few hundred milliliters of residual fluid, minimizes infection at the skin exit site or in the peritoneum, avoids pericatheter leaks and hernias, and allows for successful resolution of peritonitis should it occur. Finally, it should be safely implantable without major surgery.

I. Acute versus chronic catheters. Peritoneal catheters may be categorized as acute or chronic.

A. Acute catheters. All acute catheters have the same basic design: A length of straight or slightly curved, relatively rigid tubing with numerous side holes at the distal end. A metal stylet or flexible wire over which the catheter slides is used to guide insertion. Acute catheters are designed to be placed "medically" at the bedside because even the short delays associated with surgical consultation and implantation may not be acceptable for patients in acute renal failure. Because acute catheters do not have cuffs to protect against bacterial migration from the skin site to the subcutaneous tract, the incidence of peritonitis increases prohibitively beyond 3 days of use. Also, risk of bowel perforation increases with duration of use. When it is anticipated that the need for peritoneal dialysis will be longer than a few days, a chronic catheter should be placed initially rather than an acute peritoneal dialysis catheter, whenever possible.

B. Chronic catheters. Chronic peritoneal catheters are constructed from silicone rubber or polyurethane and usually have two Dacron (polyester) cuffs. Like acute catheters, most chronic catheters have numerous side holes at the distal end. The Dacron cuffs provoke a local inflammatory response that progresses to form fibrous and granulation tissue within 1 month. This fibrous tissue serves to fix the catheter cuff in position and to prevent bacterial migration from the skin surface or from the peritoneal cavity (in cases of peritonitis) past the cuff into the subcutaneous tunnel.

Chronic peritoneal catheters, protected against migration of bacteria and fixed in position by the Dacron cuffs, are not restricted to a 3-day period of use as are the uncuffed acute catheters. Peritonitis usually can be treated successfully without catheter removal. Chronic catheters function successfully for 2 or more years, on average, before complications or modality changes necessitate their removal.

While chronic peritoneal dialysis catheters are typically implanted by surgical dissection in the operating room, effective and safe techniques for placement at the bedside or in an ambulatory surgical suite, utilizing guidewire and dilators or peritoneoscopy, also exist.

II. Types of chronic dialysis catheters

A. Tenckhoff catheter. A typical two-cuff straight Tenck-hoff catheter is shown in Figure 20-1, with the proper relationship of the various parts to the tissues of the abdominal wall. The proper location of the deep cuff is within the rectus muscle (lateral or medial border). Tissue ingrowth is faster in muscle than in subcutaneous tissue. The parietal peritoneum reflects along the catheter, forming a smooth tunnel, and stops at the deep cuff. The proper location of the subcutaneous cuff is 2–3 cm below the exit site. The stratified squamous epithelium reflects along the catheter and stops at the subcutaneous cuff. This epithelium has the capability to prevent bacterial penetration and limits seeping of fluid from the subcutaneous tissue. If the distance from the exit site to the subcutaneous cuff is >2 cm, for example, 4 cm, then the stratified squamous epithelium does not extend all the way to the cuff and instead granulation tissue is present, resulting in some exit site wetness and crusting. Exit site infection is then more likely.

The usual distance between the two cuffs in a two-cuff Tenckhoff is 5–6 cm. For obese patients with a large panniculus, the distance between the two cuffs of a standard Tenckhoff catheter may be too short to allow each cuff to be in proper position. Large adult catheters with more widely spaced cuffs are available. Single-cuff catheters are also available and can sometimes function as well as double-cuff catheters as long as the single cuff is properly placed within the rectus muscle and the distance from the cuff to the skin exit site is relatively short. Some physicians still advocate placing the single cuff in the superficial position, especially when using these catheters to perform acute peritoneal dialysis, in order to facilitate their subsequent removal.

B. Alternate chronic catheter designs. The standard Tenckhoff catheter almost always allows easy inflow of fluid.

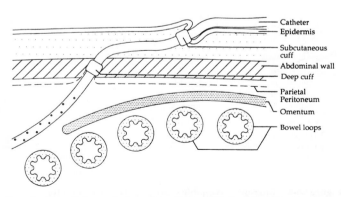

Figure 20-1. Schematic drawing of a straight Tenckhoff peritoneal catheter showing its proper relationship to adjacent tissues.

However, effective drainage of the abdomen may be variable and difficult. This is especially so in the later stages of the drain cycle when resistance to fluid outflow increases as the omentum and bowel loops are brought close to the catheter tip and sides and by the diminished volume of fluid in the abdomen. To minimize outflow obstruction, a number of alternative catheters have been devised (Fig. 20-2). These include designs where the tip of the catheter is curled—designs with a preformed or "swan neck" V-shaped arc (120 degrees) between the deep and superficial cuffs (Fig. 20-2, right). The bend allows the catheter to exit the skin facing downward yet enter the peritoneum facing toward the pelvis, as Tenckhoff originally suggested in 1968. Some versions also have a modified internal cuff to encourage the internal part of the catheter to point downward into the pelvic cavity. Another design, the Toronto-Western catheter, makes use of two perpendicular silicone disks to hold omentum and bowel away from the exit

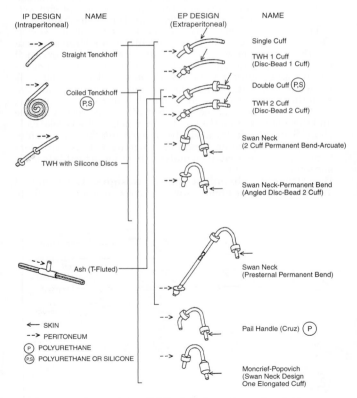

Figure 20-2. Currently available chronic peritoneal catheters showing their intraperitoneal (*left*) and extraperitoneal (*right*) portions.

holes. It also has a modified deep cuff to help ensure downward positioning of the intraperitoneal catheter end. The Advantage (T-fluted) catheter has grooves (flutes) on the outside of its two limbs to distribute flow widely; flow of fluid is through the middle "T" portion and then through the grooves or around the catheter. The T shape of the catheter places the limbs next to the parietal peritoneum so that external migration of the catheter is not possible (thus minimizing development of pericatheter leaks, pericatheter hernias, and exit site erosions of the cuff).

    1. Critical comparison of catheter designs. To what extent the new catheter designs are improvements over standard straight and curled Tenckhoff catheters has not been determined, despite a large number of retrospective studies and a few prospective trials. The standard curled and straight silicone Tenckhoff catheters still enjoy wide use and remain the standards against which the newer designs are judged. Some prospective studies have demonstrated small but significant advantages to two-cuff and to coiled catheters, but others have failed to demonstrate such advantages. Straight catheters remain somewhat less expensive than coiled catheters and other options. Table 20-1 gives a short list of catheter types, features, advantages, and disadvantages.

C. Presternal implantation. Presternal swan-neck catheters have an added subcutaneous extension to the swan-neck catheter (Fig. 20-2, right), allowing tunneling of the catheter under the skin to an exit site over the sternum. Such catheters are especially useful for obese patients, where the shifting of the abdominal wall would otherwise create excessive movement at the exit site and predispose to exit infection. Presternal catheters also are useful for patients wishing to bathe in a tub, allowing them to bathe without soaking the catheter exit site in the bath water.

III. Placement procedures

A. Acute catheters. The acute peritoneal catheter is designed to be placed blindly into an abdomen that has been prefilled with fluid. Insertion is guided by either a sharpened stylet or flexible guidewire. The potential complications of acute catheter placement should be understood. The incidence of complications is increased in patients with ileus, adhesions from previous abdominal surgery, or multiple prior acute catheter insertions. Placement is also difficult in comatose or uncooperative patients who cannot tense the abdominal wall during insertion of the catheter or prefilling needle. Surgical or peritoneoscopic placement of a chronic peritoneal catheter should be considered for such patients and for all patients for whom peritoneal dialysis is expected to be required for more than a few days.

    1. Procedure. Either a midline or a lateral abdominal entry site can be chosen (Fig. 20-3, solid black squares). The midline site is about 3 cm below the umbilicus. The lateral site is at the lateral border of the rectus muscle, on a line and halfway between the umbilicus and the anterior superior iliac spine (always above the anterior superior iliac

Table 20-1. Types of catheters

Type of Catheter	Placement Options	Removal Method for Internal Portion	Catheter Problems	Other Advantages/Disadvantages
Straight Tenckhoff	Dissection, blind, peritoneoscopy	Deep cuff dissection	Variable outflow volume, occasional omental attachment and outflow failure, deep and superficial cuff extrusion, pericatheter hernias	Easy to reposition by stylet or guidewire (though 50% failure rate)
Curled Tenckhoff	Dissection, blind, peritoneoscopy	Deep cuff dissection	Same but possibly less omental attachment	More difficult to reposition due to length of stylet or guidewire
Toronto-Western	Dissection only	Dissection to peritoneal level disk	Same but no deep and superficial cuff extrusion, fewer pericatheter hernias	Impossible to reposition
Missouri	Dissection only	Dissection to peritoneal level disk	Same but possibly less omental attachment and catheter migration, no deep and superficial cuff extrusion, fewer pericatheter hernias	Somewhat difficult to reposition
Advantage	Dissection, blind, peritoneoscopy	Deep cuff dissection	More uniform outflow volume, less omental attachment/outflow failure, no deep and superficial cuff extrusion, no pericatheter hernias	Small holes at junction of flutes with "T"; may clot, requiring irrigation; repositioning not possible but not required

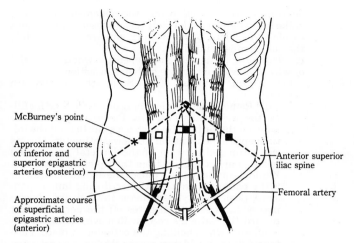

Figure 20-3. Deep-cuff locations for chronic peritoneal catheters. The solid squares show deep-cuff locations for catheters placed by peritoneoscopic or blind techniques. These are also the usual placement sites for "acute" catheters. The hollow squares locate alternative placement sites for chronic catheters placed by surgical dissection.

spine). The left lateral site is considered preferable because it avoids the cecum. When choosing an insertion site, avoid areas of previous catheter insertion or scars by at least 2–3 cm. The bladder must be empty, as a full bladder can inadvertently be penetrated by the stylet during insertion. The abdomen should be carefully examined to exclude the presence of massive enlargement of the liver, spleen, bladder, or other organs and to exclude other remarkable pathology (e.g., peritoneal carcinomatosis). A portable ultrasound unit is also of value in examination of the abdomen before placement of the catheter.

a. Carefully put on the mask, cap, gown, and sterile gloves. Wash, prep, and drape the skin overlying the desired insertion site. Anesthetize the full depth of the abdominal wall liberally at the desired site, using approximately 10 mL of local anesthetic agent, and the skin along the expected length of incision.

b. Make a 1- to 2-cm skin incision over the desired entry site. (Some prefer to make a smaller [e.g., 3-mm] incision.) Dissect down to the level of the fascia using a blunt hemostat. While asking the patient to tense the abdominal wall, insert a small needle or plastic tube into the abdomen (e.g., a 16-gauge Angiocath or a 14-gauge Verhees needle). The needle or tubing should be at least 6–8 cm long in order to reach the peritoneal space. If an Angiocath was used, remove the needle at this time, leaving the plastic tube in place. By gravity, infuse 1–2 L of 1.5%

dextrose dialysis solution into the abdomen, enough to make the abdomen moderately tense. Observe the patient carefully for signs of respiratory embarrassment while the abdomen is being filled.

c. The subsequent steps now depend on whether a stylet or wire will be used to guide catheter insertion.

    (1) Stylet method (for Stylocath or Trocath catheters)

        (a) Remove the plastic tubing or needle used for filling the peritoneum with fluid. Place the fingers of one hand on the catheter in such a way as to limit the initial depth of penetration to a few centimeters beyond the estimated location of the parietal peritoneum (usually about 6–8 cm from the tip of the catheter). While the patient again tenses the abdominal wall (or if the patient is on a ventilator, during lung expansion), push the stylet–catheter through the abdominal wall, aiming 20 degrees off the perpendicular toward the patient's coccyx. Remove the stylet immediately while holding the catheter in place. Peritoneal fluid should now escape through the catheter.

        (b) Reinsert the stylet partially, stopping 1 cm short of full insertion. Aim the stylet and catheter toward the left inguinal ligament, and angle the stylet to a plane as close as possible to that of the abdominal wall. Advance the catheter over the stylet down into the abdominal cavity without advancing the stylet itself until the catheter meets firm resistance, or until the "wings" or suture points descend to the skin surface. Redirect the catheter if it fails to advance at least 10 cm into the peritoneal space.

        (c) Remove the stylet, connect the catheter to the dialysis tubing, and immediately begin drainage of the peritoneal fluid. If no flow occurs, rotate or withdraw the catheter slightly.

        (d) Adjust the position of the catheter support wings so that they lie against the skin, and suture the catheter in place.

    (2) Guidewire method (for Cook peritoneal dialysis catheters)

        (a) Insert the guidewire through the plastic tubing or needle that was used to fill the abdomen with fluid. Remove the plastic tubing or needle.

        (b) Insert the catheter over the guidewire into the abdominal cavity in the same general direction as described for the stylet method. Some resistance is felt as the pointed end of the catheter passes through the rectus muscle and fascia. If it is necessary to reposition the catheter, reinsert the wire and readvance the catheter over the wire.

        (c) Suture the catheter in place.

2. Complications of acute catheter insertion

    a. Preperitoneal placement

        (1) Of the filling tubing or needle. Inflow of the fluid used to fill the abdomen will be slow, local swelling may be noted, and pain during filling may occur. It is important to recognize preperitoneal placement at this point and not proceed with catheter insertion at this site. As much fluid should be drained as possible and the plastic tubing or needle should be removed and reinserted at another site.

(2)   Of the catheter itself. Dialysis solution inflow will be slow and often painful. Outflow will be minimal and the return will quickly become blood tinged. Drain as much fluid as possible, then remove the catheter and insert at another site. The second catheter can be inserted at the same site if filling of the abdomen went well, or at a second site if there was any question about whether the filling tubing or needle was also placed preperitoneally.

b.   Blood-tinged dialysis solution return. In addition to preperitoneal placement of the catheter, blood-tinged outflow through the catheter can occur due to injury of a vessel in the abdominal wall or mesentery. The return will usually clear with continued dialysis. Use of room temperature dialysate may slow or stop capillary bleeding.

c.   Serious complications. These include grossly bloody effluent, a fall in the hematocrit, or a shock signal that a larger intra-abdominal blood vessel has been punctured; this usually requires urgent performance of a laparotomy. Unexplained **polyuria** and **glycosuria** can reflect inadvertent puncture of the urinary bladder. Feces or gas in the effluent or watery diarrhea having a high glucose concentration indicates bowel perforation. In case of bowel perforation, it is sometimes possible merely to remove the catheter and observe the patient carefully while treating with intravenous antibiotics. In the case of more significant peritoneal contamination, surgical repair may be necessary. If surgical repair is planned, leave the catheter in place so that the bowel entry site may be identified. Peritoneal dialysis should be delayed for several days after any bowel perforation, even if the bowel has been surgically repaired.

B.   Chronic catheters. There are four options for placement of chronic peritoneal catheters: (a) surgical placement by dissection, (b) surgical placement using laparoscopy, (c) blind placement using a guidewire, and (d) minitrocar placement using peritoneoscopy. Catheters with a disk-ball at the peritoneal surface such as the Toronto-Western and Missouri models must be placed surgically. Straight and curled Tenckhoff catheters (Fig. 20-2), with or without a swan-neck section, and the Advantage catheter may be placed by any technique.

1.   Chronic catheter implantation methods. These are beyond the scope of the *Handbook,* and the reader is referred to a special supplementary section on the Internet, available via the Hypertension, Dialysis, and Clinical Nephrology (HDCN) Web site, where these are described in detail. See the Internet references at the end of this chapter for the proper hyperlink.

2.   Relative advantages and disadvantages of various methods of chronic catheter placement. The advantage of surgical placement, with or without laparoscopy, is direct visualization; disadvantages include the requirement for general anesthesia in some patients (with subsequent risk of postoperative ileus), a larger incision relative to the other methods, more trauma near the catheter (resulting in slower healing or increased bleeding), inability to inspect the entire course of the catheter in the peritoneum, higher overall cost, and difficulty scheduling an operating room. For blind guidewire placement the principal advantages are that the catheter may be placed by a nephrologist and the equipment is simple and relatively inexpensive. However, blind guidewire placement may lead the catheter into a position between bowel loops rather than against the parietal peritoneum, and there is approximately a 1% risk of perforation of bowel or blood vessels by the introducing the needle since the needle is quite sharp. These disadvantages of blind guidewire placement are obviated by use of the minitrocar/peritoneoscopy (YTEC) setup, where there is direct visualization of the site where the Tenckhoff catheter tip will reside and that makes use of a small-diameter minitrocar and dilatable guide, which creates a tight fit of the abdominal wall around the Tenckhoff catheter and cuff, reducing the chance of leakage.

3.   Anticipatory implantation of a chronic catheter: The Moncrief–Popovich method. This technique is a method of "burying" the external portion of the catheter under the skin at the time of placement, to minimize risk of infection and catheter care while the catheter incisions are healing and fibrous tissue is growing into the cuffs. When the catheter is first implanted it is tunneled to an exit site as usual. After 1,000 units of heparin is instilled into the catheter, the external segment, the external tip, is sealed and then buried subcutaneously and the exit site is closed. The catheter remains "buried" for a period of 2–8 weeks or longer to allow tissue ingrowth into the external cuff in a sterile environment. Subsequently, a small incision is made in the skin through which the external segment of the catheter is brought out. The external portion of any peritoneal dialysis catheter may be similarly buried, but Moncrief and Popovich did design a catheter similar to the standard swan-neck Tenckhoff, except that the external cuff was much longer for the purpose of greater stability of this cuff (Fig. 20-4).

4.   Prophylactic antimicrobial drugs. A cephalosporin should be administered orally 1–2 hours before or parenterally 30 minutes before chronic catheter placement using any of the above methods. Follow-up doses do not appear to be necessary. Alternatives for patients with cephalosporin allergy include vancomycin, carbapenem, and quinolone antibiotics. If prophylactic antimicrobials are accidentally omitted, the risk of early infection for catheters placed with suitable caution is low.

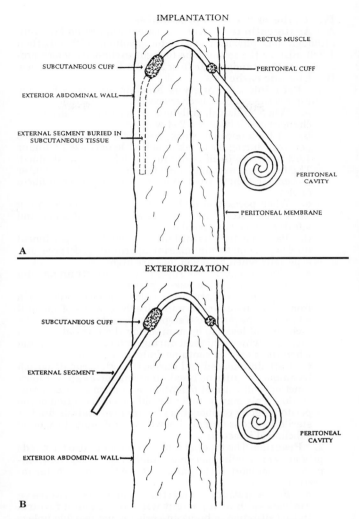

IMPLANTATION

RECTUS MUSCLE

SUBCUTANEOUS CUFF

PERITONEAL CUFF

EXTERIOR ABDOMINAL WALL

EXTERNAL SEGMENT BURIED IN
SUBCUTANEOUS TISSUE

PERITONEAL
CAVITY

PERITONEAL MEMBRANE

A

EXTERIORIZATION

SUBCUTANEOUS CUFF

EXTERNAL SEGMENT

PERITONEAL
CAVITY

EXTERIOR ABDOMINAL WALL

B

Figure 20-4.   Technique of peritoneal catheter implantation advocated by Moncrief et al. (1993). A: Initially, there is no exit site. B: Two to eight weeks later, the external end of the catheter is exteriorized.

IV.   Catheter break-in procedures

A.   Acute catheters. Acute catheters require no break-in, although some physicians use reduced volumes (500 mL, then 1,000 mL) for the initial four to eight exchanges before proceeding to the standard 2,000- or 2,500-mL exchange volumes.

B.   Chronic catheters

1.   Principles. A variety of break-in strategies for new chronic catheters have been proposed. These include:

a.   When practical, full-volume peritoneal dialysis exchanges are delayed for 2–4 weeks.

b.   At least once per week and preferably up to 3 times per week during the break-in period, heparinized saline or 1.5% dialysate is infused into the abdomen and drained. The first such exchange may be performed the day after placement, to help avoid occlusion of the catheter by fibrin or clot.

c.   When peritoneal dialysis has to be started within a week of catheter placement, the abdomen is drained and left dry for part of each day.

d.   Patient activity is initially restricted when peritoneal fluid is present, to minimize intraperitoneal (IP) pressure, especially when fluid volumes are high.

e.   The patient is instructed to avoid straining and coughing during the break-in period.

The purpose of step b is to clear IP blood and fibrin from the catheter and to minimize the chances of omental adhesion. The purpose of steps a, c, d, and e is to reduce the incidence of leakage by minimizing the intra-abdominal pressure, which is highest during ambulation or straining when the abdomen contains dialysis solution.

f.   Catheters placed and buried (the Moncrief–Popovich technique) require no break-in technique at all, yet most function well without omental obstruction after exteriorization. This may be due to avoidance of irritation of the peritoneum by components of peritoneal dialysis fluid or sterile solutions that are known to be inflammatory, or by subclinical infection.

2.   Practice. The type of break-in procedure used depends primarily on whether peritoneal dialysis is needed for treatment and support of the patient at the time of catheter insertion.

a.   For a patient requiring immediate, intensive dialysis such as a patient with acute renal failure. In this situation, a break-in period is not feasible unless temporary hemodialysis is used. However, because such a patient is usually at bed rest, the intra-abdominal pressure rise during peritoneal dialysis is limited, and leakage is not usually a problem. Some nephrologists set the exchange volume at 500 mL for the first four exchanges and 1,000 mL for the next four, and then proceed to the desired exchange volume, if tolerated. Others proceed directly to 2,000-mL exchanges in patients who are supine and inactive. Heparin (500 units/L) is added to each solution bag for the first few exchanges if the peritoneal fluid is pink or bloody. Once the need for acute dialysis has subsided, break-in can be instituted according to the most appropriate option described below.

b. For a patient requiring maintenance dialysis, already trained for continuous ambulatory peritoneal dialysis (CAPD) or cycler therapy

(1) **First 24 hours.** Immediately after catheter insertion, 2 L of 1.5% dextrose dialysis solution containing 500 units per L heparin may be infused and immediately drained, or the catheter may merely be injected with 100 mL of normal saline (especially if the catheter is placed by peritoneoscopy or guidewire techniques). Rapid drainage of a small amount of fluid out of the catheter tip by gravity and observation of respiratory variation of an air–fluid column within the catheter confirms adequate location and function of the catheter.

(2) **Days 2–14 (or less).** Manual or automated nocturnal intermittent peritoneal dialysis (NIPD) is begun using a schedule such as the following. The typical manual schedule is three exchanges per 24 hours using 2-L volumes, with inflow at about 5 P.M., exchange at 8 P.M., another exchange at 11 P.M., and outflow in the morning. The abdomen is left dry during the day. Activity is forbidden while the abdomen contains dialysis solution. NIPD using a cycler can be performed with exchange volume of 2 L, three to five exchanges during 8 hours overnight. The abdomen is drained in the morning and left dry during the day. Heparin is optional.

3. For a patient requiring maintenance dialysis, not yet trained for CAPD

a. First 24 hours. Same as described in Section b (1) above.

b. Days 2–14 (or less). There are three options:

(1) **NIPD using a cycler.** This option is possible if the patient is hospitalized.

(2) **Intermittent peritoneal dialysis.** This consists of rapid exchanges in a dialysis unit using a cycler for 8–12 hours, 3 days per week.

(3) **Hemodialysis.** This is performed as needed using a temporary vascular access. At least weekly, an in–out exchange is performed using 1 L of normal saline containing 500 units/L heparin.

c. For a patient not yet requiring maintenance dialysis

(1) **First 24 hours.** Same as Section b (1) above.

(2) **Day 2 until the start of maintenance dialysis.** At least once per week, an in–out exchange (zero dwell time) using 1 L of sterile saline solution containing 500 units/L heparin is performed.

V. Complications of peritoneal catheters. The three major catheter-related complications are pericatheter leak, outflow failure due to migration and omental attachment, and infection of the exit site or catheter. With Tenckhoff double-cuff catheters, these complications occur with incidence rates of 7%, 17%, and 14% of insertions, respectively, during the first year.

A. Pericatheter leak. This complication usually presents in the first weeks after insertion but may not become apparent until after the patient begins CAPD. In addition to overt leakage at the skin exit site, leaks may manifest more subtly as asymmetrical subcutaneous swelling and edema, weight gain, and diminished outflow volume. The risk of leakage is increased if there is little or no break-in period. Management of leaks is discussed in Chapter 25. Diagnosis may be aided by ultrasound examination of the deep cuff and surrounding subcutaneous tissues. As leaks are often a complication of late or early cuff infection, peritoneal cell counts and culture and careful physical examination for redness or tenderness are important. Ultrasound of the cuffs and tunnel may also be helpful in detecting fluid surrounding the catheter in these locations, often a sign of infection.

B. Outflow failure. Outflow failure is usually detected when the drainage volume is substantially less than the inflow volume and there is no evidence of pericatheter leakage. It usually occurs soon after catheter placement, but it may also commence during or after an episode of peritonitis, or at any time during the life of the catheter. Outflow failure is often preceded by irregular drainage, increased fibrin in the dialysate, or constipation.

There are several approaches to treatment, which vary according to whether peritonitis is present. The management strategy includes the following:

1. Check for kinking. Kinking of the catheter outside the skin exit site is made apparent by removal of the exit site bandage. Kinking of the catheter in the subcutaneous tunnel sometimes occurs with double-cuff catheters when the cuffs have been implanted too close to each other or the catheter was twisted during the tunneling procedure. Obstruction due to kinking usually becomes apparent soon after catheter placement. Functional obstruction is present during both inflow and outflow. The degree of obstruction may be variable, depending on patient position. Pressing the subcutaneous tunnel may increase flow.

Management consists of catheter replacement, redirection of the catheter in the subcutaneous space, or removal of the superficial cuff, which allows the external portion to extend outward through the exit site, correcting the kink. The latter can be accomplished as described in Section IV D 1, below.

2. Treatment of constipation. Constipation due to decreased bowel motility is a common cause of outflow obstruction. Thus, a logical early step in treatment of outflow obstruction is to administer a laxative (either a single 10-mg bisacodyl suppository or two 5-mg bisacodyl tablets). If necessary, these may be repeated or a saline enema can be given. Laxatives containing magnesium and enemas containing phosphate, such as the Fleet enema, should be avoided in renal failure patients. After a bowel movement is achieved, outflow is again attempted. Correction of constipation resolves approximately 50% of catheter outflow obstructions.

3. Heparin. Heparin should be added to peritoneal fluid (250–500 units/L) whenever fibrin plugs, strands of fibrin, or blood is visible in the outflow fluid. Heparin is more useful prophylactically than therapeutically; once outflow obstruction is established, irrigation of the catheter with heparin is usually unsuccessful in relieving the obstruction.

4. Thrombolytic agents. If heparin is ineffective, the next step is to try a thrombolytic agent. Tissue plasminogen activator and streptokinase are both available. Urokinase is temporarily not available in the United States, but the imminent availability of recombinant urokinase is anticipated. Streptokinase is the least expensive but entails a slight risk of inducing an anaphylactic reaction. Protocols for using these agents are in Table 20-2.

5. Catheter reposition. If obstruction is not relieved by any of the above techniques, it is likely to be due to attachment of omentum or other tissues to the catheter tip. Catheters that have migrated and show poor outflow after some time of successful use are usually tightly attached to omentum, and it is the omental attachment rather than the actual migration that is the principal cause of the outflow obstruction.

The position of the Tenckhoff catheter tip can be determined by an abdominal radiograph and should vary <4 cm in 1 month. All recently manufactured catheters incorporate a radiopaque stripe. If the catheter does not have such a stripe, a very low x-ray dose will usually allow visualization of a plain silicone catheter as will catheter injection with radiopaque dye (keep osmolality <300 mOsm per kg).

Whether or not the catheter has migrated, the next step in the attempt to relieve obstruction is to move the catheter to a different location in the abdomen, in the process attempting to free it of its omental attachments. There are three methods of relocating the catheter tip: (a) blind techniques (radiographic monitoring is desirable but not essential), (b) peritoneoscopic techniques, and (c) surgical "stripping."

a. Blind or fluoroscopic techniques. These are feasible with all types of Tenckhoff catheters but are easier in catheters without a sharp subcutaneous bend (nonarcuate catheters). The abdomen, if not already distended, is filled with dialysis solution. The patient is premedicated because IP manipulation of a catheter is often painful. A sterile, malleable metal rod, bent into a curve to facilitate passage through the catheter, is advanced to within 4 cm of the catheter tip. Using the skin site as a fulcrum, the catheter is rotated gently until the distal tip lies in another IP location. The function of the catheter in the new position can be tested by infusing and draining heparinized saline or dialysis solution.

Even though the catheter can be moved by this technique, breaking omental adhesions to the catheter is difficult, and catheter outflow is restored only about 30% of the time.

b. Reposition using peritoneoscopy. Microfiltered air (about 600 mL) is insufflated into the abdomen through the obstructed Tenckhoff catheter, which is then sealed. Using the Y-TEC minitrocar and plastic catheter guide, the abdomen is punctured about 5–10 cm from the malfunctioning catheter. Ideally, the puncture site position is such that it would be appropriate for a new catheter so that, if repositioning of the existing catheter is unsuccessful, a new one can be placed through this puncture site. The minitrocar is removed and the IP position of the cannula is confirmed by insertion of the

---

Table 20-2. Protocols for streptokinase, urokinase, or tissue plasminogen activator infusion for treatment of peritoneal catheter outflow obstruction

A. **Streptokinase**
1. *Testing for streptokinase allergy.* Because of the slight risk of an anaphylactic reaction, a scratch test, followed by an intradermal test, should be performed prior to intraperitoneal (IP) infusion. A 100 IU/mL solution is prepared. After the skin has been scratched with a 25-gauge needle, a drop of solution is placed over the scratch. If no wheal and flare appear within 15 minutes, then 0.1 mL of the same solution is injected intradermally. If no wheal and flare appear, then immunoglobulin E (IgE)-mediated allergy to streptokinase is unlikely. (From Dykewicz et al., 1986).
2. *Infusion protocol.* Streptokinase is available as a lyophilized powder in both 250,000- and 750,000-IU vials. We reconstitute 750,000 IU (with sterile saline), dilute it to 30–100 mL in 0.9% saline, inject the total volume into the peritoneal catheter, clamp the catheter, wait 2 hours, and assess drainage. If drainage is still poor, repeat the protocol once.

B. **Urokinase**
Urokinase is available as a lyophilized powder in vials containing 250,000 IU (reconstitute using sterile water) and also in liquid form as vials of 5,000 IU/mL. Both 75,000 IU diluted to 40 mL in 0.9% saline and 5,000 IU diluted to 40 mL in 0.9% saline, injected into the peritoneal catheter as described above for streptokinase, have been used successfully. As in the case of streptokinase, the treatment can be repeated if initially unsuccessful, using a larger dose of urokinase if desired.

C. **Tissue plasminogen activator**
Introduction into the catheter lumen of a concentration of 1 mg/mL for a period of 1 or more hours has been effective (according to Sahani MM, et al. Tissue plasminogen activator can effectively declot peritoneal dialysis catheters [Letter]. *Am J Kidney Dis* 2000;36:675). Administration of 10 mL saline with tissue plasminogen activator at a concentration of 0.1 mg/mL is also effective.

peritoneoscope. The catheter and attached omentum are inspected. A sterile, malleable, curved metal rod (such as a Foley catheter guide) is inserted into the catheter, which is then moved to a location free of adhesions, under observation through the peritoneoscope. If the catheter cannot be freed from the attached omentum, it can be further manipulated by advancing the peritoneoscope underneath the catheter, between the adhesion and the peritoneal penetration point, and rotating the peritoneoscope into the contralateral quadrant while avoiding contact of its tip with visceral or parietal peritoneum. This movement displaces the catheter and attached omentum. The catheter is then reinspected to determine its position and to ascertain if the omentum has been removed. In our experience, reposition using peritoneoscopy is successful in relieving outflow obstruction about 50% of the time, with the best results being for straight Tenckhoff catheters. If repositioning is unsuccessful, a new catheter can be placed through the catheter guide that was inserted along with the minitrocar, as already described, and the old dysfunctional catheter can then be removed.

c. Surgical stripping of the catheter. It is possible surgically to remove omentum from a catheter while leaving the catheter in place. Under general anesthesia, a 3- to 5-cm incision is made in the midline or next to the site of the deep cuff. The catheter is identified and the attached omentum is removed, using a specially designed stripping tool if desired. Performing a local omentectomy at the same time diminishes the chances of reocclusion. The procedure can also be performed effectively during laparoscopic techniques. All of these strategies to correct outflow failure result in a success rate at 1 month of only about 50% of cases.

6. Catheter replacement. If attempts to restore outflow of a peritoneal catheter fail, the only remaining option is to surgically remove the obstructed catheter and replace it with a new one.

7. Treating peritonitis. Outflow obstruction is sometimes a consequence of acute peritonitis, leading to omental irritation and attachment to the catheter. Peritonitis changes the management of outflow obstruction for several reasons. In the presence of peritonitis, obstruction is unlikely to be due to kinking or constipation. Manipulation of the catheter can be especially painful and should not be tried until the infection has mostly resolved. Finally, rapid correction of catheter obstruction is desirable because IP administration of antimicrobials is preferable when treating peritoneal dialysis–associated peritonitis, especially during the initial few days. The following management plan is proposed:

a. Infuse a loading dose of antimicrobials IP (see Chapter 24) mixed with dialysis solution. The volume of solution given should depend on the degree of abdominal distention. Also, add 1,000 units of heparin to the initial exchange and after any exchange in which fibrin is seen.

b. Infuse streptokinase, urokinase, or tissue plasminogen activator as described in Table 20-1.

c. If adequate outflow is not established within 24 hours (after two infusions of thrombolytic agent), place an acute peritoneal catheter, or a second chronic catheter, by peritoneoscopy (with or without an attempt at reposition). Treat peritonitis promptly with IP antimicrobials. Add heparin 500 units/L to all subsequent exchanges. The obstructed chronic catheter can be left in place if tunnel infection does not appear to be present.

d. After 2–3 days, when symptoms have subsided and fluid is clearing, if an acute catheter was inserted it should be removed. Repositioning of the chronic catheter can then be attempted using either fluoroscopy or peritoneoscopy to guide the manipulation, but a low success rate should be anticipated. If function of the original catheter can be restored, continue to treat peritonitis as usual. If repositioning fails and fluid is clear or nearly clear, catheter removal and placement of a new catheter can be performed in the same operative setting without persistence of the peritonitis in many cases.

e. If peritonitis fails to clear in 2 or 3 days, or if fungal or pseudomonal organisms or *Staphylococcus aureus* is cultured, remove the peritoneal dialysis catheter and wait 2 weeks or more before placement of a new catheter (see Chapter 24).

C. Catheter infection

1. Exit site infection. This presents as redness, swelling, and tenderness at the exit site, sometimes with a large amount of crusting or purulent exudate. Treatment is discussed in Chapter 24.

2. Tunnel infection. Tunnel infection can present as an extension of skin exit site infection, with pain, swelling, nodularity, and redness over the subcutaneous portion of the catheter. Systemic signs, such as fever, may also be present. Alternatively, tunnel infection can result in "relapsing" peritonitis caused by the same organism. Cuff or tunnel infection may be confirmed by ultrasonography; a lucent space completely surrounding either the cuff or the tunnel of the catheter usually indicates infection. Management of tunnel infection is discussed in Chapter 24.

D. Other complications related to peritoneal catheters. Other catheter-related complications include cuff erosion, pain on dialysis solution inflow, and abdominal wall hernias.

1. Cuff erosion. The superficial cuff can erode through the skin because of exit site infection or because it initially was located too close to the skin exit site. Late erosion of the superficial cuff can also occur if the deep cuff separates from the abdominal musculature. The entire catheter can then be extruded outward, pushing the superficial cuff through the skin. Treatment consists of removal of the superficial cuff, which should be done as soon as inflammation appears around the cuff. A double-cuff catheter is thus converted to a single-cuff catheter. External cuff removal is done by anesthetizing the exit site, widening it with a scalpel, and separating the cuff from the subcutaneous tissues. The cuff is then trimmed with a cold-sterilized single-sided safety razor and forceps are used to remove the fragments. If a subcutaneous tunnel infection subsequently becomes apparent, the catheter must be removed.

2. Pain during dialysis solution inflow and outflow. Infusion pain is less common than drain pain, affecting about 5% of patients. It is often related to the low dialysis solution pH or to abnormally high dialysis solution temperature, and less often to omental attachment to the catheter or to pressure created in a neighboring structure (rectum, vagina, spermatic cord) during inflow. It is typically worse with more hypertonic glucose solutions. If the symptom is related to low pH, it can be solved by using new normal pH solutions based on multicompartmental bags, with or without bicarbonate buffer (see Chapter 19). However, these are not available in some countries, including the United States. Addition of sterile pyrogen-free sodium bicarbonate to the dialysis solution is an alternative option. The titratable acid in the dialysis solution reacts with some of the bicarbonate added to generate PCO_2, which acts to increase the acidity of the dialysis solution, so limiting the rise in pH. Thus, addition of the usual amount of bicarbonate (4–5 mEq/L) does not neutralize the pH of the dialysis solution completely, but overalkalinization is avoided. If the infusion pain is related to placement of the catheter, reposition may be required to cure the condition.

Pain during outflow is more common, especially toward the end of the drain, and is especially frequent in the early days after initiation of peritoneal dialysis. It is thought to be related to negative pressure or irritation created in neighboring structures during outflow. It sometimes resolves with time or with treatment of associated constipation. If persistent, it can sometimes be managed by avoiding complete drainage of the peritoneal effluent. In cycler patients, this can be achieved by doing some degree of tidal peritoneal dialysis. In resistant cases of drain pain, repositioning of the catheter may be required and even this does not always resolve the problem.

3. Abdominal and pericatheter hernias. These are discussed in Chapter 25.

VI. Care of peritoneal catheters. The exit site and related incisions should be cared for in the same manner as other fresh surgical wounds. For the first few days after placement, the exit site should be covered by gauze bandages and the bandages changed whenever they are noted to be discolored by exudate or blood. Occlusive, air-impermeable coverings should never be used, nor should ointments. The dressing should immobilize the catheter against the skin.

The patient should be instructed to avoid catheter movement at the exit site as much as possible because movement delays healing and can lead to infection. When necessary, the catheter can be anchored to the skin at a second site to minimize motion at the exit site. As the patient begins to care for the catheter, bandage changes may be made less frequently. After a few weeks, the catheter exit site may be left unprotected and open to the air, but it is generally preferable to cover it with gauze dressing to minimize irritation. The optimal method of exit site care is controversial. By 1–2 months after insertion, the general consensus is that the least exit site treatment is the best. However, one randomized study showed that thrice-weekly applications of a povidone–iodine solution followed by a dry gauze dressing reduced exit site infection compared with a daily wash with nonbacterial soap (Luzar et al., 1991). Training patients to observe their catheters regularly for signs of exit site and tunnel infection is important. The role of *S. aureus* nasal carriage and exit site infection is discussed in Chapter 24.

CAPD patients may shower a few weeks after catheter placement if the catheter site is well sealed. The exit site should be dried thoroughly after a shower. Baths are also allowed if the catheter exit site is only briefly wetted. Patients typically are not permitted to swim. The risk of infection increases with the bacterial count of the water.

VII.   Catheter removal and replacement

A.   Acute catheters. As noted above, acute uncuffed catheters should be removed within 3, or at most 4, days of insertion. After the abdomen has been drained and the sutures removed, the catheter is gently pulled out. It is best to let the peritoneum rest for a day or so before inserting a new catheter, if possible. The replacement catheter should be inserted at least 2–3 cm from the original site, preferably alternating medial and lateral locations.

B.   Chronic catheters. Chronic catheters that have been in place for more than 3 months should be removed by surgical dissection in either an outpatient surgical suite or an operating room. With some types of catheters (Table 20-1) dissection down to the deep cuff to free it from the abdominal musculature is required. In all cases, any defect left in the abdominal wall after removal of the catheter should be repaired carefully to avoid subsequent hernia or leakage.

SELECTED READINGS

Ash SR. Chronic peritoneal dialysis catheters: overview of design, placement, and removal procedures. *Semin Dial* 2003;16(4): 323–334.

Ash SR. Chronic peritoneal dialysis catheters: procedures for placement, maintenance, and removal. *Semin Nephrol* 2002;22(3): 221–236.

Asif A, et al. Modification of the peritoneoscopic technique of peritoneal dialysis catheter insertion: experience of an interventional nephrology program. *Semin Dial* 2004;17:171–173.

Chadha V, et al. Tenckhoff catheters prove superior to Cook catheters in pediatric acute peritoneal dialysis. *Am J Kidney Dis* 2000;35:1111–1116.

Dykewicz MS, et al. Identification of patients at risk for anaphylaxis due to streptokinase. *Arch Intern Med* 1986;146:305–307.

Flanigan M, Gokal R. Peritoneal catheters and exit-site practices toward optimum peritoneal access: a review of current developments. *Perit Dial Int* 2005;25(2):132–139.

Gadallah MF, et al. Peritoneoscopic versus surgical placement of peritoneal dialysis catheters: a prospective randomized study on outcome. *Am J Kidney Dis* 1999;33:118–122.

Gokal R, et al. Peritoneal catheters and exit-site practices: toward optimum peritoneal access: 1998 update. *Perit Dial Int* 1998;18:11–33.

Luzar MA. Exit-site infection in continuous ambulatory peritoneal dialysis: a review. *Perit Dial Int* 1991;11:330–340.

Moncrief JW, et al. The Moncrief–Popovich catheter: a new peritoneal access technique for patients on peritoneal dialysis. *ASAIO J* 1993;39:62–65.

Nicholson ML, et al. The role of omentectomy in continuous ambulatory peritoneal dialysis. *Perit Dial Int* 1991;11:330–332.

Ozener C, Bihorac A, Akoglu E. Technical survival of CAPD catheters: comparison between percutaneous and conventional surgical placement techniques. *Nephrol Dial Transplant* 2001;16:1893–1899.

Park MS, et al. Effect of prolonged subcutaneous implantation of peritoneal catheter on peritonitis rate during CAPD: a prospective, randomized study. *Blood Purif* 1998;16:171–178.

Prischl FC, et al. Initial subcutaneous embedding of the peritoneal dialysis catheter: a critical appraisal of this new implantation technique. *Nephrol Dial Transplant* 1997;12:1661–1667.

Sahani MM, et al. Tissue plasminogen activator can effectively declot peritoneal dialysis catheters [Letter]. *Am J Kidney Dis* 2000;36:675.

Song JH, et al. Clinical outcomes of immediate full-volume exchange one year after peritoneal catheter implantation for CAPD. *Perit Dial Int* 2000;20:194–199.

Twardowski ZJ. Peritoneal access: the past, present, and the future. *Contrib Nephrol.* 2006;150:195–201.

Twardowski ZJ, et al. Six-year experience with swan neck presternal peritoneal dialysis catheter. *Perit Dial Int* 1998;18:598–602.

WEB REFERENCES

Peritoneal catheter insertion methods: http://www.hdcn.com/pd/cath

Peritoneoscopic placement of peritoneal dialysis catheters: www.medigroupinc.com and asdin.org

Acute Peritoneal Dialysis Prescription

Stephen M. Korbet

I. Introduction. Acute peritoneal dialysis provides the nephrologist with a nonvascular alternative for dialysis. Peritoneal dialysis, like other continuous renal replacement therapies used in the intensive care setting, is acutely less efficient than conventional hemodialysis. However, because of its continuous nature, its efficiency may ultimately be comparable or superior to that of hemodialysis (depending on the regimens being used) in the management of acute renal failure, as well as toxic/metabolic, electrolyte, or volume problems in critically ill patients. Recently, the effectiveness of acute peritoneal dialysis as a treatment for sepsis-associated acute renal failure (mostly due to malaria) in adults has been questioned, because of a randomized trial from Vietnam showing superior survival with continuous hemofiltration (Phu, 2002). However, the generalizability of these findings is not clear, and acute peritoneal dialysis continues to be widely used in children and in developing countries where its simplicity and lower cost makes it attractive. It is now much less commonly used in adults in wealthier, developed countries where hemodialysis and hemofiltration technologies are widely available.

A. Advantages. The performance of peritoneal dialysis is technically simpler than that of hemodialysis or other forms of continuous renal replacement therapy, as peritoneal dialysis does not require highly trained personnel or expensive, complex equipment. As a result, peritoneal dialysis can be instituted quickly. Acute peritoneal dialysis is usually performed manually but can be done with the assistance of a cycler (see below). It avoids the potential problems related to vascular access (hemorrhage, air embolism, thrombosis, infection) and does not require anticoagulation. The gradual but continuous nature of the procedure results in effective removal of fluid and solute with less hemodynamic instability. Lack of a blood–hemodialyzer interaction and the lower likelihood of hypotensive episodes may lessen ongoing insults to the already acutely damaged kidneys.

B. Disadvantages. Peritoneal dialysis is less efficient than hemodialysis in the treatment of acute problems (i.e., flash pulmonary edema, poisonings or drug overdose, acidosis, and hyperkalemia) and may not be the dialytic therapy of choice for extremely catabolic patients when daily hemodialysis or continuous renal replacement therapy is feasible. Protein losses can be substantial in peritoneal dialysis and could complicate the care of already malnourished, critically ill patients. Serious morbidity (30%) and mortality (5%) attributed to the use of acute peritoneal dialysis and hemodialysis are similar.

Concerns have also been expressed about the substantial amount of glucose absorption and about the effect of dialysate-induced increases in intraperitoneal pressure on ventilation.

C. Indications. Acute peritoneal dialysis is most often used in the setting of acute renal failure, but it is also beneficial in the control of volume overload states in patients with cardiovascular compromise, such as those with congestive heart failure, and in the treatment of hypothermia or hemorrhagic pancreatitis (where peritoneal lavage may be beneficial). It is most beneficial in the treatment of hemodynamically unstable patients or patients in whom vascular access is problematic.

D. Contraindications. There are few absolute contraindications to the use of peritoneal dialysis, but the most obvious are recent surgery requiring abdominal drains; known fecal or fungal peritonitis (the catheter acts as a foreign body, delaying therapeutic response); and a known pleuroperitoneal fistula. Relative contraindications for peritoneal dialysis include severe hypercatabolic states where clearance may not be sufficient, abdominal wall cellulitis (may lead to peritonitis), adynamic ileus (results in technical problems that decrease the efficiency of peritoneal dialysis), and a new aortic prosthesis (may result in infection of the prosthesis). The presence of abdominal adhesions or fibrosis is often considered a relative contraindication as it decreases the efficiency of peritoneal dialysis. Peritoneal dialysis can complicate the care of patients with underlying respiratory failure as it may mechanically interfere with respiration and may increase the production of carbon dioxide resulting from the metabolism of absorbed glucose.

II. Peritoneal catheter. For many patients, such as those with multiorgan system failure, a prolonged period of renal failure can be anticipated, and initial insertion of a Tenckhoff catheter (rather than use of an uncuffed temporary catheter, which will have to be replaced after 3 days) is recommended. If a shorter course is expected or if peritoneal dialysis must be started before such a catheter can be placed, a temporary stylet catheter is a reasonable choice (see Chapter 20).

III. Use of automated cyclers. Acute peritoneal dialysis has traditionally been done using manual exchanges. Increasingly, automated cyclers are being used instead, with considerable savings in nursing time, especially when a short (30–60 minutes) exchange time is required. However, temporary peritoneal catheters sometimes function erratically with cyclers, triggering the cycler alarm system and causing frequent interruptions of dialysis. Some degree of tidal peritoneal dialysis is particularly helpful in this situation. Also, the problem is less likely to occur with Tenckhoff catheters.

IV. Prescribing acute peritoneal dialysis

A. Session length. In the setting of acute renal failure, continuous removal of fluids and solutes is required in a patient who often is catabolic, oliguric, and in need of ongoing nutritional and therapeutic support. This commonly results in the need for hourly exchanges on a continuous basis for days or weeks. As the dialysis requirements of a patient may change from day to day, it is prudent to write peritoneal dialysis orders for only 24 hours at a time, reassessing and altering the prescription as indicated. A standardized form with "Acute Peritoneal Dialysis Orders" is helpful in ensuring that the specifications of the procedure are complete and clear for the nursing staff responsible for its delivery (Table 21-1).

B.   Exchange volume. Choice of exchange volume is dictated primarily by the size of the peritoneal cavity. An average-sized adult can usually tolerate 2-L exchanges, but in smaller patients, those with pulmonary disease (in whom a large exchange volume might contribute to respiratory difficulty), and those with abdominal wall or inguinal hernias, the exchange volume should be reduced.

Some nephrologists prefer to start with smaller volumes (1–1.5 L) for the first few exchanges for all patients in the hope of minimizing the risk of leaks. Otherwise, one should not reduce the exchange volume without good reason as the larger the volume is, the greater the clearance and ultrafiltration rates that can be achieved. In large or very catabolic patients, an exchange volume of 2.5–3 L can be used if tolerated to augment the efficiency of dialysis.

C.   Exchange time. This is the combined time required for inflow, dwell, and drain. To maximize dialysis efficiency in acute peritoneal dialysis, the exchange time most commonly used is 1 hour, although 2-hour exchange times also are commonly used in patients who are not overly catabolic.

1.   Inflow time. Inflow is by gravity and usually requires about 10 minutes (200 mL per minute). Inflow time is dictated by the volume to be infused and the height of the dialysis solution above the patient's abdomen (when using the manual method). It may be prolonged due to kinking of the tubing or increased inflow resistance by intra-abdominal tissues in close proximity to the catheter tip. On initiation of acute peritoneal dialysis, some patients may experience pain or cramping with inflow of dialysis solution. This may result from the hypertonic and acidic nature of the peritoneal dialysis fluid or distention of tissues around the catheter by rapidly inflowing fluid. These problems often improve with time but when severe may be relieved by slowing the dialysate inflow rate for several exchanges. Otherwise, inflow time should be kept to a minimum to maximize dialysis efficiency. Cold dialysate solution also results in discomfort, and for this reason, the solution should be warmed to 37°C before infusion.

2.   Dwell time. The dwell period is the time during which the total exchange volume is present in the peritoneal cavity (i.e., the time from the end of inflow to the beginning of outflow).

a.   Standard dwell period. When initiating peritoneal dialysis in acutely ill and catabolic patients, the usual dwell time is 30 minutes to achieve an exchange time of 60 minutes. With a 2-L exchange volume, 48 L of fluid will thus be exchanged daily. Given a peritoneal membrane with average transport characteristics, the urea concentration in the drained dialysate will be approximately

Table 21-1. Acute Peritoneal Dialysis Orders

A. Nursing orders:
 1. Dialysis to run____hours
 2. Exchange volume:____L
 3. Warm dialysis fluid to 37°C.
 4. Exchange time: Inflow 10 minutes
    Dwell____minutes
    Outflow 20 minutes or as long as fluid drains freely
    DO NOT LEAVE FLUID IN ABDOMEN
 5. Strict intake and output to be kept on fluid
    intake–output record.
 6. Dialysate balance to be recorded on peritoneal dialysis
    record.
 7. Dialysis fluid running balance to be maintained at:____L.
 8. Dialysate solution:____%
 9. Additives to dialysate:
    Medication Dose Frequency
    ____ ____/2 L q exchange **or** × ____exchanges
    ____ ____/2 L q exchange **or** × ____exchanges
 10. Heparin: 1,000 units per 2 L q exchange: yes/no
 11. Turn and position patient PRN for optimum outflow.
 12. Vital signs q____hours
 13. Catheter care and dressing change every day.
 14. Withdraw 15 mL dialysis fluid from catheter port every
     morning during dialysis and send for cell count with
     differential, and culture and sensitivity: yes/no
B. Blood draw orders:
 1. BUN, creatinine, HCO_3, Na, K, Cl, and glucose 8 A.M. and
    6 P.M. EACH DAY DURING DIALYSIS
C. Notify physician immediately for:
 1. Poor dialysate flow
 2. Severe abdominal pain or distention
 3. Bright red blood or cloudy dialysate drain
 4. Dialysate leak or purulent drainage around catheter exit
    site
 5. Blood pressure of <____ mm Hg systolic
 6. Respiration rate of >____ per minute, or severe shortness
    of breath
 7. Temperature of >____°C
 8. Two consecutive positive exchanges
 9. Single positive exchange balance (dialysate-IN –
    dialysate-OUT) of ≥1,000 mL
 10. If negative balance exceeds ____ L over ____ hours

BUN, blood urea nitrogen.

50%–60% of that in the plasma. Thus, with an aggressive dialysis exchange rate of 2 L per hour, the plasma urea clearance could approximate 24–29 L per day (0.5–0.6 × 48 L per day), or 168–202 L per week. This is at the lower end of the clearances normally obtained with blood-based continuous renal replacement therapies.

b. Dwell period for more stable patients. If the patient is not extremely catabolic, a longer dwell time (e.g., 1.5–5 hours) can often be used. With a 4-hour exchange time (dwell time 3.5 hours), the dialysate urea concentration is, on average, 90% of that in the plasma. This leads to a plasma urea clearance of at least 11 L per day (0.9 × 12 L per day), or 77 L per week. In terms of weekly ($K \times t$)/V, the weekly clearance of 77 L is the ($K \times t$) term. For a 72-kg patient with a V of 38 L, weekly ($K \times t$)/V would be 77/38, or 2.0.

3. Outflow time. Outflow of spent dialysate is by gravity and usually requires 20–30 minutes. Outflow time depends on the total volume to be drained, the resistance to outflow, and the difference in height between the patient's abdomen and the drainage bag. In many patients, particularly those with large abdomens, the first exchange may not drain completely (often only 1–1.5 L is retrieved) due to initial filling of poorly draining areas of the abdomen. As long as marked abdominal distention is not present, a second exchange of 2 L can be cautiously instilled. Subsequent drainage usually proceeds normally. If outflow continues to be poor, then outflow obstruction should be managed according to the guidelines described in Chapter 20. Pain during outflow is unusual, but localized pain may occasionally be noted at the end of a drain due to a siphoning effect of the catheter on the peritoneum.

D. Continuous equilibration peritoneal dialysis (CEPD). An alternative approach to providing peritoneal dialysis in acute renal failure is to prescribe a modified version of continuous ambulatory peritoneal dialysis. This involves a standard manual exchange every 3 to 6 hours, depending on the patient's clearance and fluid removal requirements. This is sometimes described as CEPD to emphasize the point that almost complete equilibration for small solutes will occur, in contrast to the situation with conventional acute peritoneal dialysis. The advantages of CEPD are its simplicity, its lower cost, and its less labor-intense nature. The disadvantage is that clearances are less with this approach and may not be adequate in more catabolic patients. It is popular in the developing world because of the low costs and in pediatrics because the smaller size of patients allows adequate normalized clearances.

E. Choosing the dialysis solution dextrose concentration

1. Standard 1.5% dextrose (glucose monohydrate). This concentration of dextrose (approximately 1,360 mg glucose per dL [75 mM]) will exert an osmotic force sufficient to remove 50–150 mL of fluid per hour when using a 2-L exchange volume and a 60-minute exchange time

Table 21-2. Estimated ultrafiltrate volume during acute peritoneal dialysis

Dextrose[a]	Glucose			Solution Osmolarity[b]	Ultrafiltrate Volume[c]	
g/dL	g/dL	mg/dL	mmol/L	(mOsm/L)	mL per exchange	L per day
1.5	1.36	1,360	76	346	50–150	1.2–3.6
2.5	2.27	2,270	126	396	100–300	2.4–7.2
4.25	3.86	3,860	215	485	300–400	7.2–9.6

[a]Glucose monohydrate, weighing 10% more than anhydrous glucose.
[b]Solution osmolarity = electrolyte osmolarity (270 mOsm per L) + glucose osmolarity.
[c]2–L exchange volume, 60-minute exchange time.

(Table 21-2). That is, the volume drained exceeds the volume instilled by 50–150 mL. (The mechanism of osmotic ultrafiltration during peritoneal dialysis is discussed in Chapters 18 and 23.) This ultrafiltration rate translates into fluid removal of 1.2–3.6 L per day.

2. Higher concentrations of dextrose. Greater fluid removal can be achieved with higher dextrose concentrations (Table 21-2). A 4.25% dextrose solution can result in an ultrafiltration rate of 300–400 mL per hour. Acutely, this degree of fluid removal can be required for the treatment of congestive heart failure. However, continued use of the 4.25% solution could theoretically result in the removal of 7.2–9.6 L per day and cause marked hypernatremia. In practice, this degree of fluid removal is not often required. Available dextrose solutions used alone or in combination (i.e., either 1.5% or 2.5% exchanges used continuously or some combination of 1.5% and 4.25% exchanges) can be adjusted to provide the level of ultrafiltration desired. Once the patient is euvolemic, one can resume using 1.5% solution for all exchanges.

3. When very rapid fluid removal is required. The osmotic effect of a high-dextrose dialysis solution diminishes rapidly as the glucose is absorbed and as the glucose concentration is further diluted by fluid movement into the peritoneal space. Thus, high-dextrose dialysis solution is most effective during the initial 15–30 minutes. Occasionally, a patient in severe pulmonary edema will require very rapid fluid removal. Such patients can be treated initially with two or three in–out (zero dwell time) 2-L exchanges of 4.25% solution. Each exchange will still remove approximately 300 mL of fluid, so that almost 1 L may be removed over a 1-hour period.

4. Effect of peritonitis. During peritonitis, inflammation of the peritoneum leads to enhanced absorption of glucose from the dialysate, rapidly reducing the osmotic gradient. In such patients, maintaining the efficiency of ultrafiltration may require that the exchange time be reduced and/or that more hypertonic exchanges (2.5% or 4.25%) be used.

F.   Dialysis solution additives. When injecting any additive into dialysis solution containers, meticulous sterile technique must be followed to prevent bacterial contamination of the dialysis solution and peritonitis.

  1.   Potassium. Standard peritoneal dialysis solutions contain no potassium, but when the patient is hypokalemic, potassium chloride (3–5 mEq/L) can be added. Even in normokalemic patients, failure to add potassium chloride may result in hypokalemia (especially with 60-minute exchanges) if the patient's total-body potassium content is normal or low and the oral intake is poor. It must also be remembered that glucose absorption and correction of acidosis with peritoneal dialysis promotes a shift of extracellular potassium into cells, lowering the serum concentration. If moderate to severe metabolic acidosis is being corrected, addition of even 5 mEq/L of potassium to dialysis solutions may not prevent hypokalemia, and parenteral supplementation may be required. Higher concentrations of potassium in the dialysis solution have been used on a short-term basis, but caution is advised.

  2.   Heparin. Sluggish dialysate flow from catheter obstruction by fibrin clots may occasionally be seen in acute peritoneal dialysis. This is usually a result of the slight bleeding that may accompany catheter insertion or irritation of the peritoneum by the catheter. Heparin (1,000 units/2 L) added to the dialysis solution can be helpful in preventing or treating this problem. Because heparin is not absorbed through the peritoneum, there is no increased risk of bleeding.

  3.   Insulin. Because glucose is absorbed from the dialysis solution, supplemental insulin administration may be required for the diabetic patient undergoing acute peritoneal dialysis. Regular insulin may be added to the dialysis solution (Table 21-3) before infusion. The blood glucose level must be monitored closely and the dose of insulin tailored to the needs of the patient. To minimize the risk of hypoglycemia after dialysis has been stopped, insulin should not be added to the last exchange of a treatment session.

  4.   Antibiotics. Intraperitoneal administration of antibiotics is efficient and provides an alternative route for patients with poor vascular access and for those with peritonitis (see Chapter 24). Intraperitoneal administration or

Table 21-3.   Insulin addition to peritoneal dialysis solutions

Dialysate Dextrose Conc. (%)	Amount of Regular Insulin to Add (units/2 L)
1.5	8–10
2.5	10–14
4.25	14–20

more frequent IV or PO dosing may be required for antibiotics (e.g., aminoglycosides) whose clearances are enhanced by peritoneal dialysis (see Chapter 33).

V. Monitoring fluid balance. Monitoring fluid balance during acute peritoneal dialysis can be difficult. However, it is important to maintain an accurate flow sheet of all fluid intake and output (Table 21-4) to determine not only the adequacy of dialysate drainage during each exchange, but also the patient's overall fluid balance. Weighing the patient daily is helpful but should be done in the same phase of the fill–drain cycle (preferably at the end of drainage). Because neither the fluid balance nor the weight is completely reliable, the nephrologist must use both along with clinical assessment to monitor the patient for signs of fluid overload and dehydration.

VI. Monitoring clearance. It is important to ensure that acute peritoneal dialysis is delivering adequate clearance to the patient with acute renal failure. There are, however, no validated definitions of what adequate clearance is in this context. In general, the blood urea nitrogen level should be maintained below 80 mg/dL (29 mmol/L). Formal clearance measurements are not practical, but clearance can be estimated by measuring the urea nitrogen concentration in representative samples of dialysate and plasma in order to calculate a D:P ratio for urea. This is multiplied by the total daily dialysate drain volume to give daily urea clearance. This should be at least 10 mL per minute (14 L per day) and may need to be 20–30 mL per minute (28–42 L per day) in larger, highly catabolic patients. Clearance can be raised by increasing dwell volumes to 2.5–3 L or by decreasing dialysis exchange time as described above.

VII. Complications. A number of problems may arise during the course of acute peritoneal dialysis. To minimize the potential for complications, clearly defined indications for immediate physician notification should be provided in the nursing orders (Table 21-1).

A. Abdominal distention. Incomplete drainage may lead to progressive intraperitoneal accumulation of dialysate, with attendant discomfort, distention, and even respiratory compromise. Thus, one should observe the drainage cycle and make sure that the patient is emptying completely during the allowed drainage period. An experienced nurse will know this, but for extra security, the dialysis orders should require the nephrologist to be called immediately for any technical problems related to the dialysis procedure.

B. Peritonitis. Peritonitis may complicate acute peritoneal dialysis in up to 12% of cases. This occurs most often within the first 48 hours. Although infections from Gram-positive organisms dominate (more than 50%), there is a higher incidence of fungal-related peritonitis in acute peritoneal dialysis. This may be a reflection of the severity of illness in patients requiring acute peritoneal dialysis as well as predisposing factors, such as the prolonged use of multiple antibiotics.

C. Hypotension. Rapid removal of large amounts of fluid can lead to hypovolemia with consequent hypotension, arrhythmia, and even death. In some patients (e.g., those with

Table 21-4. Peritoneal dialysis record

	Intake (mL)											Output (mL)								Totals	
	Dialysis Solution											Dialysis Solution									
				Time IN								Time OUT									
Date	Ex #	Sol, %	Medications	Start	End	PD vol.	Oral	IV	Other	Total IN		Start	End	PD vol.	Urine	Other	Total OUT	Exchange balance		Running balance	Weight (kg)

hypoproteinemia), large amounts of fluid can be removed even when using exclusively 1.5% dextrose solutions. Immediate administration of intravenous fluid (0.9% normal saline) to correct hypotension, along with decreasing the dextrose concentration of the dialysate and/or increasing the dwell time to limit ongoing excess fluid removal, is indicated in this setting. To avoid such catastrophes when using high-dextrose solutions, it is best to write orders for a period of only a few hours at a time, reassessing and adjusting the dialysis solution concentration depending on the patient's condition.

D.   Hyperglycemia. In the diabetic or prediabetic patient, the high-dextrose solutions used for peritoneal dialysis can result in hyperglycemia. Blood glucose levels should therefore be monitored closely in such patients and treated with insulin accordingly. Intraperitoneal instillation of regular insulin may enhance the ease of glucose management (Table 21-3; see Chapter 30).

E.   Hypernatremia. Due to the low sieving coefficient for sodium (ultrafiltrate concentration/plasma concentration = 0.5), the ultrafiltrate generated in peritoneal dialysis has a sodium concentration of approximately 70 mEq/L (0.5×140 mEq/L). Increased losses of water associated with frequent hypertonic exchanges can therefore lead to hypernatremia. Implementing intravenous replacement of losses with 0.45% normal saline or replacing half of the losses with 5% dextrose water prevents the development of hypernatremia.

F.   Hypoalbuminemia. With the frequent exchanges utilized in acute peritoneal dialysis, protein loss via the dialysate can be as high as 10–20 g per day and up to twice this amount if peritonitis supervenes. Thus, oral or parenteral hyperalimentation should be instituted early. Metabolism of carbohydrate absorbed from the dialysis solution combined with metabolism of carbohydrate supplied by hyperalimentation can lead to excessive generation of carbon dioxide, which can be problematic for patients with respiratory compromise or failure. Intensive peritoneal dialysis coupled with hyperalimentation can result in hypophosphatemia, hyperglycemia, hypokalemia, or hypomagnesemia.

SELECTED READINGS

Ash S. Peritoneal dialysis in acute renal failure of adults: the underutilized modality. *Contrib Nephrol* 2004;144:239–254.

Chitalia VC, et al. Is peritoneal dialysis adequate for hypercatabolic acute renal failure in developing countries? *Kidney Int* 2002;61:747–757.

Leblanc M, Tapolyai M, Paganini EP. What dialysis dose should be provided in acute renal failure? *Adv Ren Replace Ther* 1995;2:255–264.

Phu NH, et al. Hemofiltration and peritoneal dialysis in infection-associated acute renal failure in Vietnam. *N Engl J Med* 2002;347:895–902. Commentary 2002;347:933–935. Correspondence 2003;348:858–860.

Reznick VM, et al. Peritoneal dialysis for acute renal failure in children. *Pediatr Nephrol* 1991;5:715–717.

Valeri A, et al. The epidemiology of peritonitis in acute peritoneal dialysis: a comparison between open- and closed-drainage systems. *Am J Kidney Dis* 1993;21:300–309.

Adequacy of Peritoneal Dialysis and Chronic Peritoneal Dialysis Prescription

Peter G. Blake

The prescription of chronic peritoneal dialysis (PD) involves a number of elements. Initially, there is the choice of peritoneal dialysis modality between continuous ambulatory peritoneal dialysis (CAPD) and cycler or automated peritoneal dialysis (APD) and their variants. Then there is the selection of a specific prescription based on clearance, ultrafiltration, and nutritional requirements. The term "adequacy" is often used in this context and usually refers specifically to the quantity of clearance delivered but can also be used in a broader sense to reflect the quality of the dialysis prescription as a whole. Additional issues are the choice of the giving set (for CAPD), the cycler (for APD), and the composition of the dialysis solution with particular reference to calcium concentration, the osmotic agent, and the buffer used; however, these have already been dealt with in Chapter 19 and will not be further addressed here.

I. Choice of a PD treatment modality (Table 22-1; Fig. 22-1)

A. Modalities of peritoneal dialysis therapy

1. CAPD. The simplicity of CAPD, its relatively low cost, and the associated freedom from dialysis machinery have combined to make it historically the most popular chronic peritoneal dialysis modality. It provides continuous therapy and a steady physiologic state. Control of body fluid volume can usually be achieved, and normalization of blood pressure is possible in most patients. Reasonable glycemic control in diabetic patients can be obtained in a relatively physiologic manner with the use of intraperitoneal insulin, though many units and patients prefer to stay with the more familiar subcutaneous injections.

The principal disadvantage of CAPD for many patients is the requirement for multiple procedural sessions (usually four per day), each taking up 30–40 minutes of patient time. While these can be done away from home, the requirement for sterility and access to supplies usually means that the patient has to return to his or her home, and so this may constrain daily activities somewhat. Frequency of procedures may also be an issue where relatives or other caregivers are carrying out the exchanges for the patient. Other factors are limitations on dwell volumes due to increased intraperitoneal pressure and a limited range of solute clearance. Episodes of peritonitis occurring as often as once every

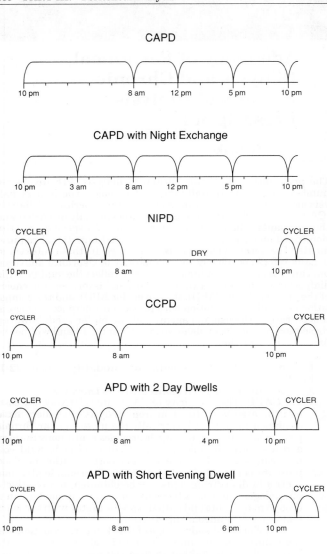

CAPD

CAPD with Night Exchange

NIPD

CCPD

APD with 2 Day Dwells

APD with Short Evening Dwell

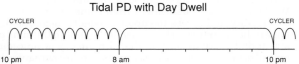

Tidal PD with Day Dwell

Figure 22-1. Diagrammatic representation of various continuous ambulatory peritoneal dialysis and automated peritoneal dialysis prescriptions.

Table 22-1. Comparison of typical CAPD and APD prescriptions

	CAPD	CCPD	NIPD
PD solution used (L per week)	56–72	70–120	84–120
Dialysis time (hours per week)	168	168	70
Time on machine (hours per week)	0	63–70	63–70
Number of procedures per week	28	14	14
Kt/V urea per week	1.5–2.4	1.5–2.6	1.2–2.0
CrCl (L per week)	40–70	40–70	25–50

CAPD, continuous ambulatory peritoneal dialysis; APD, automated peritoneal dialysis; CCPD, continuous cycling peritoneal dialysis; NIPD, nocturnal intermittent peritoneal dialysis; CrCl, creatinine clearance.

12 months were a significant disadvantage in the past; however, with improved transfer sets and connecting devices, such occurrences have been markedly reduced and successful programs report rates of one every 3 years or better.

2. APD. This has become very popular in recent years and in many wealthier countries is being used in the majority of peritoneal dialysis patients. It has classically been divided into continuous cycling peritoneal dialysis (CCPD) and nocturnal intermittent peritoneal dialysis (NIPD) (Fig 22-1). These modalities have already been described in Chapter 19.

The main advantage of CCPD is the ability to provide continuous therapy without the need for on–off procedures during the day. All connections and preparation of equipment usually take place at bedtime in the privacy of the home, so that psychological adjustment is facilitated and patient fatigue and "burnout" may be reduced. CCPD is an attractive treatment option for active individuals who are being inconvenienced by the interruptions in daily routine that are required with CAPD. It is also the therapy of choice for most patients who require assistance in carrying out their dialysis (e.g., children, the dependent elderly, nursing home residents).

The main disadvantages of CCPD are the need for a cycler, the slightly greater complexity and cost, and the complications associated with a prolonged day dwell, which may result in excessive resorption of dialysate. Variants of CCPD in which the day dwell is only kept in place for part of the day are useful in such cases, as is the polyglucose solution icodextrin, which still provides net ultrafiltration, even after 16-hour dwells. Shorter day dwells may also be helpful in patients with mechanical symptoms such as back pain or abdominal fullness or in those with a history of leaks or hernias.

NIPD is similar to CCPD, except that there is no dialysis fluid in the abdomen during the daytime. Ideally, the number of cycled exchanges done at night is increased to compensate for the lack of a day dwell, and cycler dwell times are correspondingly shorter; however, in practice, the cycler prescriptions used are often no different from those in CCPD. NIPD is particularly suitable for patients with good residual renal function who do not need the greater amount of clearance provided by CCPD. It also may be useful in those with high peritoneal transport status who have problems with ultrafiltration due to rapid absorption of glucose (see Chapter 23). It is also helpful, either temporarily or permanently, in those with mechanical complications (e.g., hernias, leaks, back pain) that prevent them from having fluid in their abdomen while they are ambulatory. Generally, patients tend to prefer NIPD to CCPD because the absence of the day dwell often leads to a decrease in the sensation of abdominal fullness that many report on CCPD. Other theoretical benefits of NIPD include a lower overall glucose absorption rate, due to the absence of a day dwell, and better peritoneal immunologic defenses, due to the lack of peritoneal lavage during the day.

The main disadvantages of NIPD, just as for CCPD, are complexity and cost. More important is its inability in most patients to provide adequate small solute clearance because of the absence of a day dwell.

An alternative form of APD is tidal peritoneal dialysis (TPD), which is described in Chapter 19 (Fig. 22-1). This modality uses an initial fill volume followed by partial drainage at periodic intervals. As explained in Chapter 19, the principal purpose of TPD is to enhance clearance of small solutes by avoiding the normal loss of dialytic time that is associated with inflow and drainage of solution on standard APD. However, in terms of clearance, the advantage of TPD over standard APD is not seen unless very large quantities of dialysis solution are used, which then increases cost as well as complexity. The main use of TPD nowadays is to minimize drain pain during nighttime cycling.

3. Hybrid forms of peritoneal dialysis. Hybrid forms between CAPD and APD have become popular in recent years, principally to achieve higher clearances and better ultrafiltration (Fig 22-1). These hybrid forms can be divided as follows:

a. CAPD with automated nocturnal exchanges. This is done with a night exchange device that can be set up at bedtime to do an exchange while the patient sleeps. It has the advantage of breaking up the long nocturnal dwell, thus increasing ultrafiltration as well as clearance. The disadvantage is that it increases both the cost and the complexity of CAPD and requires the patient to be attached to a device while sleeping.

b. APD with additional exchanges during the day. This is a strategy to break up the long diurnal dwell of APD with a view to improving both clearance and ultrafiltration. Typically, the first day dwell is delivered by the cycler as a last exchange ("last-bag option"). The second diurnal exchange can either be a manual CAPD-type exchange or can be done with the cycler tubing and large-volume solution bags, using the cycler as a "docking station." The advantage of this strategy is that it maximizes the clearances and ultrafiltration that can be achieved on peritoneal dialysis. The disadvantages are that it requires more procedures than standard CCPD and is more costly. The use of the docking-station approach rather than manual exchanges can, however, decrease this extra cost.

4.   Intermittent peritoneal dialysis (IPD). This PD modality is now almost extinct. It typically involved 12–24 hours of frequent peritoneal dialysis exchanges, usually delivered by a cycler in a hospital or in-center setting, two to three times weekly. It provides inadequate clearances because of its very intermittent nature, it is inefficient in terms of the time it consumes, and it is expensive because it is hospital based. Its only role nowadays is to provide temporary dialytic support for patients not capable of doing their own treatments at home.

B.   CAPD or APD: Which modality to choose? This should take into consideration both patient preferences and the need to provide a medically optimal peritoneal dialysis prescription. Patient preferences may be based on lifestyle, employment, place of residence, ability to perform the various modalities of PD, comfort with the cycler technology, and family and social support.

Medical requirements of the prescription typically include the provision of adequate clearances and fluid removal. In the past, medical factors and, in particular, peritoneal transport status and its influence on clearance and fluid removal were thought to be critical in choosing between CAPD and the different types of APD, but there is now an increasing sense that these aspects were overstated and that lifestyle factors should be given more emphasis.

APD was previously thought to be better than CAPD for managing volume status. However, the phenomenon of sodium sieving (see Chapter 18) is more apparent with the short cycled dwell times of APD and this, along with the risk of net fluid resorption with long day dwells, has led to concerns about adequacy of sodium removal with APD. One recent study suggests less salt removal and a higher prevalence of systolic hypertension with APD versus CAPD, but this was not a randomized trial and there is no consensus that these findings are generalizable. As is discussed further in Chapter 23, salt and water removal require close attention on both CAPD and APD, but there is insufficient evidence to justify it being a factor in initial modality selection.

Risk of peritonitis is another medical factor that may arise when deciding between CAPD and the variants of APD. One randomized trial done over a decade ago showed less peritonitis on APD, but both modalities have changed since then and there is now no consensus that one or the other is more likely to predispose to peritonitis.

A third consideration, in addition to patient preference and medical factors, is the relative cost of CAPD and of the variants of APD, as programs have to deal with financial constraints and, in some settings, patients may have to bear some or all of the costs.

Overall, if economic factors are not predominant, the choice between CAPD and APD should be made on lifestyle criteria by the patient and his or her family, but the exact prescription, especially in APD, should also be driven by medical factors such as clearance and volume status and so should be determined by the physician.

II.   Choice of a prescription

A.   Clearance targets. A critical issue in selection of a peritoneal dialysis prescription is the clearance requirements of the patient. In general, optimal clearance can be defined as that clearance above which further increments do not lead to clinically significant improvements in patient outcome. Such clearances should allow the patient to be maintained in reasonably good health without significant uremic symptoms and with patient outcomes at least as good as those associated with well-prescribed chronic hemodialysis.

These target clearances have been a source of great controversy. The key point is that greater residual renal clearance has repeatedly been shown to be associated with superior patient survival but that it has been difficult to show a similar effect for peritoneal clearance, at least within the range of prescriptions in typical clinical use. One should also keep in mind that increasing clearance in PD may come at the cost of increasing the total amount of glucose given to the patient; one needs to balance the potential benefits of increased clearance versus the disadvantages of a higher metabolic glucose load. Randomized, controlled trials published in recent years have shown that previous higher clearance targets advocated by the National Kidney Foundation's (NKF) Kidney Disease Outcome Quality Initiative (KDOQI) and other guideline bodies are not justified, and a more conservative approach is now being taken, with guidelines being adjusted accordingly. In particular, the excellent ADEMEX study involving almost 1,000 Mexican CAPD patients, randomized to either standard 4×2 L CAPD or to a high peritoneal clearance regimen and followed for at least 2 years, showed absolutely no difference in technique, patient survival, or quality-of-life between the two groups. The mean peritoneal Kt/V received by the two groups in this study was 1.62 and 2.12 per week, respectively. A smaller study from Hong Kong randomizing patients to three different levels of Kt/V was also essentially negative.

A consensus target Kt/V for all modalities of PD is now 1.7 per week instead of the previous 2.0 because levels above this have not been shown to improve outcomes whereas the evidence is less clear for lower levels. Recent European guidelines suggest that this target should be met by peritoneal clearance alone and that residual renal clearance should be treated as a precious bonus. New KDOQI guidelines suggest that peritoneal and renal Kt/V can be added to achieve the target, even though it is clear that the latter has a much greater impact on outcomes than the former. Allowing the addition of residual renal clearance permits incremental strategies whereby patients with significant residual renal function can use less onerous, lower clearance prescriptions, such as NIPD or CAPD with three dwells daily.

The previous idea that target clearances for APD should be higher than those for CAPD because APD is somewhat more intermittent is now thought to be unjustified and to introduce unnecessary complexity. Similarly, creatinine clearance targets have not been shown to be of any additional value over Kt/V targets and are probably not worth measuring. There is also no evidence to support differential targets for those with different peritoneal transport status.

Finally, a Kt/V on peritoneal dialysis of 1.7 per week may seem low compared to the target Kt/V of 1.2 three times weekly on hemodialysis. However, it is well recognized that clearance delivered continuously as in CAPD and CCPD is more efficient than the same amount of clearance delivered intermittently as in hemodialysis, and so the Kt/V figures are not comparable.

B.   Measurement of clearance (Table 22-2). Clearance in peritoneal dialysis is typically measured either by Kt/V or CrCl. Both comprise a peritoneal and a residual renal component. The latter is frequently very important in peritoneal dialysis as residual renal function usually accounts for a greater proportion of total clearance.

Table 22-2.   Formulas for calculating clearance indices in peritoneal dialysis

---

Kt/V:
Kt = Total Kt = peritoneal Kt + renal Kt
Peritoneal Kt = 24-hour dialysate urea nitrogen content/serum urea nitrogen
Renal Kt = 24-hour urine urea nitrogen content/serum urea nitrogen

V (by Watson formula):
V = 2.447 − 0.09516 A + 0.1704 H + 0.3362 W (in males)
V = −2.097 + 0.1069 H + 0.2466 W (in females)

where A = age (years); H = height (cm), and W = weight (kg)[a]

CrCl (creatinine clearance)
CrCl = total **CrCl** corrected for 1.73 m^2 body surface area
Total **CrCl** = peritoneal **CrCl** + renal **CrCl**
Peritoneal **CrCl** = 24-hour dialysate creatinine content/serum creatinine
Renal **CrCl**[b] = 0.5 [24-hour urine creatinine content/serum creatinine + 24-hour urine urea nitrogen content/serum urea nitrogen]

Body surface area (duBois formula):
BSA (m^2) = 0.007184 × W$^{0.425}$ × H$^{0.725}$

where BSA = body surface area (m^2), W = weight (kg)* and H = height (cm)

---

[a]Desirable instead of actual body weight may be used for calculation of V or BSA.
[b]For PD adequacy purposes, renal "CrCl" is the average of the creatinine and urea clearances.

1.   Measurement of *Kt/V*. *Kt/V* was originally conceived for hemodialysis and is a dimensionless index that measures fractional urea clearance. Peritoneal *Kt/V* is calculated by performance of a 24-hour collection of dialysate effluent and measurement of its urea content. This is then divided by the average plasma urea level for the same 24-hour period to give a clearance term, *Kt*. The timing of the plasma urea sample is not critical in CAPD because it is relatively constant over time. In CCPD and, especially, NIPD, blood urea is not constant throughout the day; an average value is best estimated from a sample drawn between 1:00 and 5:00 PM on a noncycling day.

Residual renal *Kt* is calculated in the same way using a 24-hour collection of urine. The two *Kt* terms are then combined to give total *Kt* and are normalized to *V*, which represents total-body water. It is recommended that *V* be estimated using one of the standard formulas for total-body water, such as those of Watson or of Hume-Weyers. These are based on the age, sex, height, and weight of the patient (Table 22-3). This normalization will give a daily *Kt/V*, which is then multiplied by 7 to give a weekly value because this is how clearance is conventionally expressed in peritoneal dialysis. Normalization to the patient's desirable (see Tables A-8 and A-9 in Appendix A) rather than actual body weight is increasingly recommended. This makes it easier to achieve targets in obese patients and is appropriate in that most do not believe that clearance requirements should rise in proportion to body fat. Conversely, wasted malnourished patients will require more dialysis to achieve targets if clearance is corrected to their desirable weight. Desirable weight is calculated from anthropometric tables, based on age, sex, height, and body frame (see Chapter 28).

2.   CrCl. The measurement of CrCl is similar to that of *Kt/V* (Table 22-2). Again, the peritoneal component is calculated by measuring creatinine content of a 24-hour collection of dialysate effluent, and this is then divided by the serum creatinine. The residual renal CrCl is known to markedly overestimate true glomerular filtration rate in most patients; therefore, it is conventional to add the mean of the urinary urea and creatinine clearances to the peritoneal clearance to give the total creatinine clearance. This is then corrected for 1.73 m^2 body surface area, with the latter estimated using the formula of DuBois (Table 22-2).

The high glucose levels found in dialysate artifactually elevate the measurement of creatinine in some biochemical assays, and each laboratory should make a correction for this based on its own experience. This may be done by measuring the apparent creatinine content after adding various test concentrations of creatinine powder to unused bags of dialysis solution with different dextrose concentrations, so that a correction factor can be calculated for whatever local assay method is being used. In the future, it is likely that CrCl measurements will be less widely performed as there is no evidence that they add anything

Table 22-3.   Examples of clearance calculations in CAPD and APD

EXAMPLE 1: A 50-year-old man weighing 66 kg has no residual renal function. He is on CAPD with four 2.5-L exchanges daily, and his net UF is 1.5 L. His V by the Watson formula is 36 L, and his BSA by the DuBois formula is 1.66 m^2. Serum urea nitrogen is 70 mg/dL (25 mmol/L), and serum creatinine is 10 mg/dL (885 mcmol/L). The urea nitrogen and creatinine (after correction for glucose) levels in the 24-hour dialysate collection are 63 mg/dL (22.5 mmol/L) and 6.5 mg/dL (575 mcmol/L), respectively. Calculate his Kt/V and CrCl.

Calculations using mg:
Kt urea per day = 24-hour drain volume × D/P urea = 11.5 L × 63/70 = 10.35 L per day. Daily Kt/V = 10.35 L/36 L = 0.288 L. Weekly Kt/V = 0.288 × 7 = 2.02 L.
Creatinine clearance per day = 24-hour drain volume × D/P creatinine = 11.5 L × 6.5/10 = 7.48 L per day. Corrected for 1.73 m^2 BSA = 7.48 × 1.73/1.66 = 7.80 L per day. Weekly CrCl = 7.8 × 7 = 55 L per week.

Calculations using SI units:
Kt urea per day = 24-hour drain volume × D/P urea = 11.5 L × 22.5/25 = 10.35 L per day. Daily Kt/V = 10.35 L/36 L = 0.288 L. Weekly Kt/V = 0.288 × 7 = 2.02 L.
Creatinine clearance per day = 24-hour drain volume × D/P creatinine = 11.5 L × 575/885 = 7.48 L per day. Corrected for 1.73 m^2 BSA = 7.48 × 1.73/1.66 = 7.80 L per day. Weekly CrCl = 7.8 × 7 = 55 L per week.

EXAMPLE 2: A 48-year-old woman on APD weighs 63 kg and does five 2.4-L cycles nightly plus a 6-hour 2-L day dwell. Her V by Watson is 32 L, and her BSA by DuBois is 1.60 m^2. Her 24-hour dialysate drain volume is 15 L, indicating 1 L net UF. Her pooled dialysate collection has a urea nitrogen level of 48 mg/dL (17.1 mmol/L) and a creatinine level (after correction for glucose) of 4.5 mg/dL (398 mcmol/L). Her midafternoon serum urea nitrogen is 65 mg/dL (23.2 mmol/L), and serum creatinine is 9 mg/dL (796 mcmol/L). Her urinary urea and creatinine clearance are 2 and 4 mL/minute, respectively. Calculate her total weekly Kt/V and creatinine clearance.

Calculations using mg:
Peritoneal Kt = daily drain volume × D/P urea = 15 L × 48/65 = 11.1 L
Peritoneal Kt/V = 11.1 L/32 L = 0.35 per day = 2.45 per week
Renal urea clearance = renal Kt urea = 2 mL per minute = 20 L per week.
Renal Kt/V = 20/32 = 0.63 perweek
Total Kt/V = peritoneal plus renal Kt/V = 2.45 + 0.63 = 3.08 per week
Peritoneal creatinine clearance = daily drain volume × D/P creatinine = 15 L × 4.5/9 = 7.5 L. Corrected for 1.73 m^2 BSA = 7.5 × 1.73/1.60 = 8.1 L per day = 57 L per week.

continued

Table 22-3. *Continued.*

Calculations using SI units:
Peritoneal Kt = daily drain volume × D/P urea = 15 L × 17.1/23.2 = 11.1 L
Peritoneal Kt/V = 11.1 L/32 L = 0.35 per day = 2.45 per week.
Renal urea clearance = renal Kt urea = 2 mL per minute = 20 L per week
Renal Kt/V = 20/32 = 0.63 per week.
Total Kt/V = peritoneal plus renal Kt/V = 2.45 + 0.63 = 3.08 per week
Peritoneal creatinine clearance = daily drain volume × D/P creatinine = 15 L × 398/796 = 7.5 L. Corrected for 1.73 m² BSA = 7.5 × 1.73/1.60 = 8.1 L per day = 57 L per week

For both mg and SI units:
Renal creatinine clearance (for this purpose) = mean of renal urea and renal creatinine clearance = mean of 2 and 4 mL/minute = 3 mL per minute = 30 L per week. Corrected for 1.73 m² BSA = 30 × 1.73/1.60 = 32.4 L per week
Total creatinine clearance = 57 + 32.4 = 89.4 L per week

CAPD, continuous ambulatory peritoneal dialysis; APD, automated peritoneal dialysis; UF, ultrafiltration; BSA, body surface area; D/P, dialysate/plasma.

useful to Kt/V measurements. Peritoneal CrCl is less than peritoneal urea clearance because creatinine has a higher molecular weight and diffuses more slowly.

3. Frequency of measurements. It is recommended by the KDOQI that in peritoneal dialysis patients' Kt/V should be measured within 1 month of initiating peritoneal dialysis and every 4 months subsequently, as well as after every significant change in the peritoneal dialysis prescription or in the patient's clinical status. Urinary clearance should be measured every 2 months if an incremental approach to peritoneal dialysis is being used (see Section II E). Some will find these requirements unduly onerous, and a compromise in more stable patients who have been achieving their targets would be to measure clearances every 3 months.

4. Examples of clearance calculations. See Table 22-3.

5. Discordance between Kt/V and CrCl. A frequent finding when measuring clearances in patients on peritoneal dialysis is that the Kt/V target is being achieved but not the CrCl one, or vice versa. The first scenario is most common and typically occurs in patients who have lost residual renal function, which contributes disproportionately to creatinine clearance as compared with urea clearance. This is because in the failing kidney a significant proportion of urinary creatinine comes from tubular secretion in addition to glomerular filtration, whereas in the case of urea urinary clearance is less than glomerular filtration because there is ongoing tubular resorption.

The same discordance between Kt/V and CrCl is frequently seen in patients on APD because the short dwells contribute disproportionately to urea clearance as compared

Table 22-4. Factors determining clearance in peritoneal dialysis patients

1. **Nonprescription factors**
   Residual renal function
   Body size
   Peritoneal transport characteristics
2. **Prescription factors**
   (a) CAPD:
   Frequency of exchanges
   Dwell volume
   Tonicity of dialysis solution
   (b) APD:
   Number of day dwells
   Volume of day dwells
   Tonicity of day dwells
   Time on cycler
   Cycle frequency
   Cycler dwell volumes
   Tonicity of cycler solution

CAPD, continuous ambulatory peritoneal dialysis; APD, automated peritoneal dialysis.

with creatinine clearance. As explained in Chapter 18, this is because creatinine has a higher molecular weight than urea and so diffuses more slowly. It may also be seen in low transporters where creatinine equilibration is disproportionately low in comparison with urea equilibration. The opposite situation, where CrCl, but not Kt/V, targets are achieved is most commonly seen in patients who have substantial residual renal function. The issue that arises in all of these cases is whether it is important to achieve both targets, or whether one suffices. In general, more emphasis is now being given to Kt/V.

C. **Determinants of clearance** (Table 22-4). The total weekly Kt/V achieved on standard peritoneal dialysis prescriptions typically varies from as little as 1.2 to as much as 3.0 a week. Similarly, CrCl can vary from as little as 30 L per week to as much as 150 L per week. The major source of this variation is residual renal function. This and the other determinants of clearance are now reviewed.

1. **Residual renal function.** This typically accounts for as much as 50% of total clearance at the initiation of peritoneal dialysis, especially with the move in recent years to earlier initiation of dialysis. Studies that have shown a correlation between total clearances achieved and subsequent patient outcome have been somewhat confounded, because residual renal function is a much more potent predictor of outcome than peritoneal clearance per se. There is now evidence that residual renal function can be preserved in patients on CAPD by treatment with angiotensin-converting enzyme inhibitors or angiotensin receptor blockers. One also should minimize exposure to potentially nephrotoxic

agents, including aminoglycosides, radiocontrast dyes, and nonsteroidal anti-inflammatory drugs. It has been suggested that preservation of residual function is better on CAPD than on APD, but this is not a consistent finding.

2.   Peritoneal transport status. This is an important determinant of clearances, especially in APD where the short duration cycles limit solute equilibration between plasma and dialysate. Peritoneal transport is measured by the peritoneal equilibration test (PET), as discussed in Chapter 18. In general, low transporters achieve greater clearances with high-volume, long-duration dwells, whereas high transporters do well with short-duration dwells. However, these differences are less pronounced for urea as compared to creatinine because the lower molecular weight leads to relatively rapid diffusion, even in low transporters. What determines baseline transport status is not well understood and is discussed in Chapter 18. Transport status is now recognized as a determinant of patient and technique survival on CAPD, with low transporters doing best despite clearances that tend to be lower than those their high-transport counterparts achieve. It is likely that the patient survival effect is related to the critical importance of ultrafiltration and its interaction with cardiovascular morbidity; also, high transporters receive a higher glucose load and absorb more glucose, although a direct link between glucose load and survival in PD patients has not been documented.

3.   Body size. Given that clearance indices are normalized to body surface area or total-body water, this is an important determinant. Its effect is less if normalization is done using desirable rather than actual measures of body size (see II B 1 above). While large body size makes it harder to achieve higher clearance targets, there is controversy about whether larger patients have worse outcomes.

D.   Prescription. If clearance targets are not being achieved, a prescription change needs to be considered. A number of different strategies are available with both CAPD and APD. The choice of strategy should take into account the increment in clearance required, the patient's transport status, volume and nutritional considerations, and, perhaps most importantly, the likely effect on lifestyle for the patient and his or her caregivers, as a disruptive prescription may lead to noncompliance or burnout and consequent technique failure.

In the past, much emphasis was given to transport status in deciding whether a patient should do CAPD or APD with high transporters being directed to the former and low transporters to the latter. With lower clearance targets, more emphasis on Kt/V over CrCl, and a greater focus on lifestyle factors in determining modality and prescription, this approach is now less common.

1.   CAPD. The typical initial CAPD prescription continues to be 4×2 L daily. Some centers will start with 4×2.5 L in larger patients, especially if residual renal function is small. Some use 3×2 L if patients are small or residual renal function is substantial. In Hong Kong, where mean body weight is less than in western countries, good results have been reported using 3×2 L initially in almost all patients. A few centers use icodextrin routinely for the nocturnal dwell, but it is expensive, and others never use it at all or use it only in high transporters or in patients in whom fluid resorption at night becomes a clinical problem.

In attempting to increase peritoneal Kt/V in CAPD patients, there are three options (Table 22-4). One is to increase the frequency of daily exchanges, the second is to increase the individual dwell volumes, and the third is to increase the tonicity of the solutions, thereby augmenting ultrafiltration.

a. Increasing exchange volumes. This increases clearance because the total volume of solution delivered daily rises and the larger dwell volume leads to only a small decrease in urea and creatinine equilibration. So, the percentage increase in Kt/V and CrCl will be close to the percentage increase in the exchange volume, especially in larger patients; for example, a switch from 4×2 L to 4×2.5 L CAPD involves a 25% increase in instilled volume and will typically raise peritoneal Kt/V by 18%–20%. However, in smaller patients, and especially when 3-L dwell volumes are used, there may be greater fall-off in equilibration. To achieve clearance targets it is typically necessary to use at least 2.5-L dwell volumes in anuric patients who weigh more than 75 kg. Some programs prefer to initiate such patients on the larger dwell volumes. The lower Kt/V targets mean that fewer patients will require 3-L volumes.

The main disadvantage of increasing exchange volumes is that a minority of patients may complain of back pain, abdominal distention, and even shortness of breath. This can be minimized if the increased volumes are introduced at the time of initiation of peritoneal dialysis, before the patient becomes accustomed to smaller volumes. Studies show only a small increase in the risk of hernias and leaks with the associated rise in intraperitoneal pressure. This rise in pressure may also impair ultrafiltration, but this effect is partly offset by the longer persistence of the glucose osmotic gradient when higher volumes are used.

b. Increasing the frequency of daily exchanges. Most CAPD patients do four exchanges daily. Some smaller patients with significant residual renal function are commenced on three exchanges daily; this has become less common in North America but is frequent practice in other countries. Increasing the number of exchanges from four to five per day generally does not have a major effect on urea equilibration, which remains at approximately 90% in patients with average transport characteristics. However, this will not be the case if patients do not ensure that the five daily exchanges are well spaced, with at least a 4-hour dwell time for each. For creatinine, however, there will be a noticeable drop in creatinine equilibration in the drained effluent because the equilibration curve for creatinine is typically still rising 4 hours after the dwell commences. Thus, increasing the frequency of exchanges is less effective than increasing dwell volumes, especially where CrCl is concerned.

An additional disadvantage of increasing the frequency of exchanges to five daily is that it may interfere with a patient's lifestyle and lead to noncompliance or burnout. However, night exchange devices make a fifth exchange more practical. These devices can be set up before the patient goes to bed and will deliver the additional exchange halfway through the night. This strategy has the added advantage of increasing net ultrafiltration, as well as clearance.

Finally, it should be noted that five exchanges a day is 25% more costly than four daily, whereas 2.5-L bags are not usually much more expensive than 2-L ones.

c. Increasing the tonicity of the dialysis solutions. This strategy increases both ultrafiltration and clearance. It is used in some centers, but there are increasing concerns that it may lead to a higher incidence of hyperglycemia, hyperlipidemia, obesity, and long-term peritoneal membrane damage. The introduction of icodextrin-based dialysis solution (see Chapter 19) for long dwells is a simpler way to increase both ultrafiltration and clearance, although the effect on the latter is usually modest.

2. APD. The initial APD prescription is quite variable across centers. A typical starting volume is 10 or 12 L daily but some use 15 L, especially in larger patients. Some start with NIPD, if the patient has good residual renal function and/or is small. Others use a day dwell from the start but may shorten it to avoid fluid resorption, especially in higher transporters, and then either leave the patient "dry" for part of the day or add a second dwell. If icodextrin is available, some centers will use it routinely for the day dwell or will prescribe it only in high transporters or only in patients who have fluid resorption problems and/or in those in whom there are metabolic concerns about excess glucose absorption (e.g., diabetic or obese patients).

Typical cycler time is 8–10 hours and dwell volumes on the cycler and in the daytime are usually 2 L or, in larger patients, 2.5 L.

Peritoneal clearance in APD can be increased using a number of different strategies (Table 22-4). In order of importance, these are:

a. Introduction of a day dwell. In NIPD patients, the best way to increase clearance is to add a day dwell. This raises both Kt/V and CrCl, but the effect on CrCl is greater because creatinine equilibration is more dependent on longer dwell times. Typically, adding a day dwell in an NIPD patient will increase daily peritoneal Kt/V and CrCl by 25%–50% and so is very cost effective. The main disadvantage is that the long day dwell frequently results in net fluid resorption, particularly in high and high-average transporters. This can be dealt with by introducing icodextrin or by shortening the day dwell from 16 hours to 2–8 hours, depending on membrane characteristics, perhaps using the docking-station approach mentioned above. Thus, the day dwell can be done in the first part of the day (i.e., directly after coming off the cycler) or, alternatively, in the evening, before using the cycler. This allows both clearance and ultrafiltration to be maintained.

Further increases in clearance can be achieved by adding a second or even a third day dwell, although this is less likely to be required with the new lower clearance targets. Again, these can be done using the docking-station approach or, if it suits the patient better, using manual CAPD tubing in the conventional way. These strategies are relatively cost effective in increasing clearance but do have the disadvantage of requiring patients to do more procedures and to have fluid in their peritoneal cavity for at least part of the day. Day dwell volumes can be titrated to maximize clearance while minimizing mechanical symptoms.

b.   Increase dwell volumes on cycler. This increases clearance in APD, just as it does in CAPD. Because patients are supine during cycling, they can usually tolerate larger dwell volumes more easily. Greater clearances will be achieved if the same total amount of dialysis solution is delivered in a smaller number of larger aliquots (i.e., 4×2.5 L per session is better than 5×2 L per session). In some patients, however, the rise in intraperitoneal pressure with increased dwell volume may impair ultrafiltration, but this is not usually clinically significant because its effect is offset by the longer-lasting glucose osmotic gradient.

c.   Time on cycler. In general, the longer the time the patient spends on APD, the better the clearance because individual dwell times are longer, allowing more complete equilibration. However, this is limited by patient willingness to stay hooked up to the cycler.

d.   Increasing frequency of cycles. In general, doing more frequent cycles increases clearances on APD because it maximizes the concentration gradient between blood and dialysate. However, when the number of cycles in a given time period is increased, a greater proportion of that period is spent draining and filling, and as a result some dialysis time is lost. Thus, there is a point beyond which increasing the number of cycles further is counterproductive in terms of cost and clearance achieved, and this is in the range of six to nine cycles per 9-hour cycling session. It tends to be higher in high transporters and lower in low transporters and is higher for urea than for creatinine. It may also be influenced by catheter function. To get around this problem, a small degree of TPD (e.g., 80%) can be used to minimize downtime.

e.   Increasing dialysis solution tonicity. As in CAPD, clearance can be augmented in APD by increasing daytime or nighttime ultrafiltration. Again, however, the same concerns about glucose-related complications arise and the use of icodextrin for the APD day dwell may be a better approach.

E.   Incremental versus maximal prescription. There are two distinct approaches to prescription of peritoneal dialysis when clearance targets are being considered. The incremental approach, which is particularly suitable when dialysis is being initiated early, suggests that peritoneal dialysis should be used to make up the difference between residual renal clearances and targeted clearances. Thus, patients may initially require only two or three CAPD exchanges daily or a low-volume, day-dry APD prescription. The alternative is the so-called maximal approach in which patients are at the outset given a sufficient prescription to meet their targets with peritoneal dialysis alone. This approach considers residual renal function as a temporary bonus that inevitably deteriorates with time.

The advantages of the incremental approach are that it is initially less costly and less onerous for the patient, and it may decrease total glucose exposure and risk of peritonitis, in so far as less procedures are required. A disadvantage is that it requires regular monitoring of residual function to ensure that the total clearance achieved does not fall below target levels. The topic of incremental dialysis is particularly important because of recommendations in recent years to initiate dialysis earlier and because of the relative ease of taking this approach with peritoneal dialysis.

F.   Empirical versus modeled approach. Another decision when prescribing peritoneal dialysis is whether to use commercially available software programs for modeling appropriate prescriptions or whether to proceed in an empirical manner. The modeled approach involves collecting patient anthropometric data, measuring peritoneal transport with a PET, and quantifying residual renal function. It also typically involves collection of 24-hour dialysate effluent to make particular calculations about peritoneal fluid removal and absorption. The computer program uses the data to predict, with reasonable accuracy, the clearances that will be achieved with various potential prescriptions. The program can also suggest appropriate prescriptions to achieve the desired clearances. With this approach, the actual clearances still have to be measured as there is sometimes a discrepancy between the modeled and actual clearances achieved.

The alternative approach is empirical, in which the physician uses knowledge of the patient's size, residual renal function, and peritoneal transport status to choose a reasonable prescription. This is then tested, clearances are assessed, and the prescription is adjusted if necessary. The modeled approach has the advantage that it may involve less trial and error and so result in earlier identification of an appropriate prescription for the patient, with consequent decreases in cost as well as inconvenience to the patient. However, even with the modeled approach, the initial prescription has to be selected empirically because peritoneal transport status will not yet have been determined. The empirical method has a theoretical advantage that it focuses the physician's attention on the patient rather than on purely numerical data. In practice, a combination of both approaches is frequently used, with the modeled approach being of particular use in complex cases and in patients on APD.

G. Glucose-sparing strategies. As will be discussed in more detail in Chapter 23, there is increasing concern about the deleterious effects of hypertonic glucose solutions on the peritoneal membrane and on the cardiovascular risk profile of patients. This needs to be taken into account in choosing PD prescriptions. Avoiding long glucose dwells and considering nonglucose solutions are two such approaches.

H. Prescription pitfalls in peritoneal dialysis. There are a number of common pitfalls that physicians face in attempting to achieve adequate clearances and fluid removal on peritoneal dialysis.

1. Loss of residual renal function. A common problem is that residual renal function is not monitored closely enough and drops to a very low level without the physician being aware. Thus, the patient is left on an inadequate prescription for a significant period of time. This is best avoided by measuring residual clearance every 2–3 months or by adopting a maximal prescription approach that gives sufficient peritoneal clearance independent of residual function.

2. Noncompliance. A chronic peritoneal dialysis patient may sometimes appear uremic or have unexpectedly high blood levels of urea and potassium despite measured clearances that exceed recommended targets. A strong possibility here is noncompliance. On the day that collections are performed, the patient is fully compliant with the prescription and appears to have excellent clearances. On other days, however, the patient is omitting exchanges or shortening time on the cycler. There is no single test that identifies this particular problem, and a high index of suspicion is required. Serial measurements of 24-hour dialysate plus urinary creatinine excretion may help identify the problem. Patients in whom the total creatinine excretion has increased in comparison with a baseline value should be suspected of noncompliance. The rationale here is that on the day of the collection, creatinine that has accumulated on previous noncompliant days is being dialyzed out, giving an artificially high value. The alternative explanation for an increase in total creatinine excretion is a gain in lean body mass, but this does not often occur in chronic dialysis patients. There are a number of patterns of noncompliance in peritoneal dialysis patients that should be borne in mind. These include:

    a. Skipping CAPD exchanges

    b. Having inadequate spacing of CAPD exchanges

    c. Reducing the dwell volume of CAPD exchanges by flushing fresh dialysis solution directly into the drain bag

    d. Shortening of cycler time in APD

    e. Skipping or shortening day dwells in APD

3. High serum creatinine despite good clearances. This is a common scenario. The patient has a Kt/V well in excess of 1.7 per week but the serum creatinine is over 12–15 mg/dL (1,060–1,330 mcmol/L). There are a number of possibilities here. One is noncompliance with the prescription (see II G 2 above). If this is the case, then blood urea and potassium may also be high. A second possibility is that this is an example of discordance between Kt/V, which is high, and CrCl, which is low. As discussed above (see II B 5), this is most often seen once residual renal function fades away in low transporter patients or in those on APD with one or no day dwell. This can be confirmed by measuring the CrCl. The third possibility, also common, is that the serum creatinine is markedly elevated, not because of particularly low clearance, but rather because of high creatinine generation, indicating a higher percent of lean body mass. This can be demonstrated by measuring CrCl and showing it to be at or above 50 L per week per 1.73 m^2 and by showing that the percent of lean body mass is high relative to what might be predicted (see III A 5 below). Such patients are not necessarily overtly muscular and indeed may be somewhat thin. Identification of this situation is helpful because patients with high creatinine generation or percent of lean body mass have a good prognosis on PD and it would be a mistake for the elevated serum creatinine to trigger a diagnosis of inadequate clearance and a switch to hemodialysis.

4. Prescriptions with "dry" time. Patients with good residual renal function are often prescribed NIPD or APD with very short day dwells. Such prescriptions can give good clearance and are often preferred by patients. Once residual function falls off, a full day dwell is typically added. However, there are some patients who, even when residual function is lost, can achieve a Kt/V above 1.7 per week with prescriptions that leave them "dry" for all or most of the day. Such patients are typically smaller in body size and/or high or high-average transporters. This creates a concern because while Kt/V is above target, middle molecule clearance in the absence of residual function is dependent on dialysis time and so will be low. There is no recommended target for middle molecule clearance in either peritoneal or hemodialysis and no high-level clinical evidence that it is important. However, there has always been a viewpoint that it is important and that it may be better in CAPD or CCPD because they are continuous modalities compared to NIPD and conventional hemodialysis. There is no answer to this dilemma, but it should at least be kept in mind when prescribing "day dry" APD.

5. Inappropriate switch from CAPD to APD. It is sometimes presumed that APD is a panacea for inadequate dialysis on CAPD, but the problem can actually become worse on APD if prescriptions are inappropriate. This is particularly likely in low transporters who are unlikely to achieve higher clearances on APD than CAPD, unless two separate daytime dwells are prescribed. It should be remembered that CrCl targets in particular may be difficult to achieve in APD. The point here is that creatinine equilibration is much more time dependent than urea equilibration; therefore, the shorter-duration dwells of APD typically lead to a fall in creatinine relative to urea clearance. Thus, a patient who has the same Kt/V urea after a switch from CAPD to APD will have a lower CrCl. This effect is most marked in low transporters and in NIPD. It may, however, be less important with the tendency to emphasize CrCl less.

6. Inadequate attention to fluid removal. Fluid removal is frequently neglected in prescriptions for peritoneal dialysis. Prescriptions that yield good clearances may not give sufficient ultrafiltration to keep the patient euvolemic and free from hypertension. This is particularly so in high and high-average transporters, especially if long dwells that result in net fluid resorption are used. The use of icodextrin for the long dwell in both CAPD and APD and the prescription of short day dwells in APD are two strategies that may be useful. This is discussed in detail in Chapter 23.

III. Nutritional issues in peritoneal dialysis. Nutritional measures in peritoneal dialysis patients have been repeatedly shown to predict patient survival and other outcomes. It is recommended that a number of these be routinely monitored to identify high-risk patients with a view to appropriate interventions.

Indices followed include normalized protein equivalent of nitrogen appearance (nPNA), serum albumin, subjective global assessment, and lean body mass as estimated from creatinine excretion.

A. Nutritional indices

1. nPNA. This is easily measured using the same 24-hour collections of dialysate and urine as are used to calculate Kt/V. The rationale is that, in steady state, nitrogen excretion is proportional to protein intake. A variety of formulas have been derived to estimate nPNA from nitrogen and protein excretion, but there is evidence that the best of these may be those of Bergström (see Table 22-5 for formula and sample calculation). Previously, PNA estimates were normalized to actual body weight, but this can lead to misleadingly high nPNA values in wasted malnourished patients and to inappropriately low values in obese patients. Normalization to desirable or ideal weight based on anthropometric tables (see Tables A-8 and A-9 in Appendix A) is now preferred. Recommended target nPNA for peritoneal dialysis patients is 1.2 g/kg per day, but this may be unnecessarily and unrealistically high for many patients who achieve nitrogen balance at lower intakes. However, a falling nPNA or a level less than 0.8–0.9 g/kg per day should be a cause for concern, especially if accompanied by other evidence of poor nutrition.

2. Caloric intake. This is sometimes neglected in dialysis patients because it cannot be as easily measured as protein intake and there are no data correlating it to outcome. In peritoneal dialysis, caloric intake is a combination of dietary intake plus calories from the glucose absorbed from the dialysis solution.

The suggested target is 35 kcal/kg per day; typically, 10%–30% of this comes from the glucose, with the exact amount depending on the tonicity, dwell times, and volume of

Table 22-5. Calculation of nPNA with example

Bergström formulas
(1) PNA (g per day) = 20.1 + 7.5 UNA (g per day)
or
(2) PNA (g per day) = 15.1 + 6.95 UNA (g per day) + dialysate protein losses (g per day)
UNA (g per day) = urinary urea nitrogen losses (g per day) + dialysate urea nitrogen losses (g per day)
Use formula (1) if dialysate protein losses are unknown and formula (2) if they are known.
Normalization of PNA to body weight gives nPNA. Actual body weight, if used, can give a misleadingly high value in malnourished patients and a misleadingly low one in obese patients.
Normalization to standard body weight based on anthropometric tables (see Tables A-8 and A-9 in Appendix A) is preferable.

Example using mg:
A 60-kg man on CAPD 4 × 2.5 L daily has 24-hour dialysate effluent volume of 12 L, which contains 58.3 mg/dL urea nitrogen so that total content = 12 × 58.3 × 10 = 7,000 mg = 7 g of urea nitrogen.
The 24-hour urine has a 500-mL volume and contains 560 mg per dL = 2,800 mg = 2.8 g of urea nitrogen.
Total UNA = 7 + 2.8 = 9.8 g per day
Dialysate protein losses are measured at 8 g per day.
Thus,
PNA = 15.1 + 6.95 (9.8) + 8 = 91.2 g per day
nPNA based on actual weight = 91.2/60 = 1.52 g/kg per day
Patient has lost weight, however, and anthropometric tables suggest that his standard weight is 72 kg.
nPNA based on this weight is 91.2/72 = 1.27 g/kg per day

Bergström formulas (SI units):
(1) PNA (g per day) = 20.1 + 210 UA (mol per day)
or
(2) PNA (g per day) = 15.1 + 194.6 UA (mol per day) + dialysate protein losses (g per day)

Example in SI units:
A 60-kg man on CAPD 4 × 2.5 L daily has 24-hour dialysate effluent volume of 12 L, which contains 20.8 mmol/L urea so that total content = 12 × 20.8 = 250 mmol = 0.25 mol of urea per day.
The 24-hour urine has a 500-mL volume and contains 0.20 mol/L = 0.10 mol of urea per day.
Total UA = 0.25 + 0.10 = 0.35 mol per day
Dialysate protein losses are measured at 8 g per day.
Thus,
PNA = 15.1 + 194.6 (0.35) + 8 = 91.2 g per day
nPNA based on actual weight = 91.2/60 = 1.52 g/kg per day
Patient has lost weight, however, and anthropometric tables suggest that his standard weight is 72 kg.
nPNA based on this weight is 91.2/72 = 1.27 g/kg per day

PNA, protein nitrogen appearance; UNA, urea nitrogen appearance; nPNA, normal protein nitrogen appearance; CAPD, continuous ambulatory peritoneal dialysis; UA, urea appearance rate.

solutions used and on the patient's PET characteristics, which also influence the percentage of infused glucose absorbed (see Table 28-3). Measurement requires dietary assessment plus quantification of the glucose absorbed, reached by subtraction of the amount of glucose in the effluent from the amount delivered.

3. Serum albumin. This is one of the strongest predictors of patient survival on peritoneal dialysis. It has become apparent that it is mainly influenced by peritoneal transport status, which influences dialysate albumin losses, and by the presence of systemic illness or inflammation, as judged by the serum levels of acute-phase reactants, such as C-reactive protein. Compared with these factors, dietary protein intake has only a minor effect on serum albumin. Thus, serum albumin is a marker of more than nutritional status only.

4. Subjective global assessment. This simple clinical tool has become popular because it is easily done at the bedside, promotes history taking and physical examination, and has been shown to predict patient outcome. It is described in both the KDOQI and Canadian Society of Nephrology references (see Selected Readings).

5. Creatinine excretion. The total creatinine content measured in the same 24-hour urine and dialysate collections done to calculate clearance can be used to estimate lean body mass using the method of Keshaviah et al, 1995 (see Selected Readings). These estimates are predictive of patient outcome, and a low or falling value identifies a patient at risk.

B. Treatment of malnutrition. This is reviewed in detail in Chapter 28. However, there are some points specific to peritoneal dialysis.

1. Dietitian support. Regular review of patients by an experienced renal dietitian to ensure adequate protein intake as well as avoidance of excessive salt and caloric intake is important

2. Nutritional supplements. It is common practice to prescribe oral protein supplements, some of which are specifically designed for renal failure patients, for those with persistent low protein intake. There is no high-level clinical evidence that these supplements are effective, but, surprisingly, no good randomized studies have been done. In the absence of better alternatives they will continue to be prescribed.

3. Promotility agents. There is evidence that gastric emptying is impaired in peritoneal dialysis patients, especially diabetics, and there are some data suggesting a beneficial role for agents such as domperidone in improving nutrition.

4. Anabolic steroids. One randomized, controlled trial, including both peritoneal and hemodialysis patients, shows that nandrolone 100 mg given intramuscularly weekly for 6 months improves lean body mass, walking, and stair-climbing ability. Concerns about side effects have limited the use of this approach.

5. Amino acids. Intraperitoneal amino acids have long been studied and are available in many countries, though not in the United States. They are typically administered as one 2-L dwell given during the daytime on either CAPD or APD using the "last-bag option." About 85% of the amino acid content of the bag will be absorbed if it is left in place for 6 hours. Food should be taken at the time to maximize utilization of the absorbed amino acids. This strategy does improve nitrogen balance but there is little evidence of a dramatic effect on important clinical outcomes. The best randomized study to date suggests that intraperitoneal amino acids are associated with better long-term maintenance of nutritional indices, particularly in women, but no study has been large enough to detect any beneficial effect on quality-of-life or survival.

SELECTED READINGS

Bergström J, et al. Calculation of the protein equivalent of total nitrogen appearance from urea appearance. Which formulas should be used? *Perit Dial Int* 1998;18:467–473.

Bernardini J, et al. Pattern of noncompliance with dialysis exchanges in peritoneal dialysis patients. *Am J Kidney Dis* 2000;35:1104–1110.

Blake PG, et al. Canadian Society of Nephrology clinical practice guidelines for adequacy and nutrition in peritoneal dialysis. *J Am Soc Nephrol* 1999;10(Suppl 13):S311–S321.

Blake PG, et al. Recommended clinical practices for maximizing peritoneal clearances. *Perit Dial Int* 1996;16:448–456.

Churchill DN, et al. Adequacy of dialysis and nutrition in continuous peritoneal dialysis. *J Am Soc Nephrol* 1995;7:198–207.

Diaz-Buxo JA. Enhancement of peritoneal dialysis: the "PD Plus" concept. *Am J Kidney Dis* 1996;27:92–98.

Durand PY. APD schedules and clinical results. *Contrib Nephrol* 2003;140:272–277.

Harty JC, et al. The normalized protein catabolic rate is a flawed marker of nutrition in CAPD patients. *Kidney Int* 1994;45:103–109.

Johansen KL, et al. Anabolic effects of nandrolone decanoate in patients receiving dialysis: a randomized controlled trial. *JAMA* 1999;281:1275–1281.

Keshaviah PR, et al. Lean body mass estimation by creatinine kinetics. *J Am Soc Nephrol* 1995;4:1475–1485.

Keshaviah PR, et al. The peak concentration hypothesis: a urea kinetic approach to comparing the adequacy of continuous ambulatory peritoneal dialysis and hemodialysis. *Perit Dial Int* 1989;9:257–260.

Li FK, et al. A 3 year prospective randomized controlled study on amino acid dialysate in patients on CAPD. *Am J Kidney Dis* 2003;42:173–183.

Li PK, et al. Effects of an ACEI on residual renal function in patients receiving CAPD: a randomized controlled trial. *Ann Intern Med* 2003;139:105–112.

Lo WK, et al. Effect of Kt/V on survival and clinical outcome in CAPD patients in a randomized prospective study. *Kidney Int* 2003;64:649–656.

National Kidney Foundation. K/DOQI clinical practice guidelines for peritoneal dialysis adequacy: update 2000. *Am J Kidney Dis* 2001;37(Suppl 1):S65–S136.

National Kidney Foundation. K/DOQI clinical practice guidelines and clinical practice recommendations for peritoneal dialysis adequacy: 2006 updates. *Am J Kidney Dis* 2006;48(Suppl 1):S1–S322.

Paniagua R, et al. Effect of increased peritoneal clearance on mortality rates in peritoneal dialysis: ADEMEX, a prospective randomized controlled trial. *J Am Soc Nephrol* 2002;13:1307–1320.

Perez RA, et al. What is the optimal frequency of cycling in APD? *Perit Dial Int* 2000;20:548–556.

Rodriguez-Carmona A, et al. Compared time profiles of ultrafiltration, sodium removal and renal function in incident CAPD and APD patients. *Am J Kidney Dis* 2004;44:132–145.

Sarkar S, et al. Tolerance of large exchange volumes by peritoneal dialysis patients. *Am J Kidney Dis* 1999;33:1136–1141.

Woodrow G, et al. Comparison of icodextrin and glucose solutions for daytime dwell in APD. *Nephrol Dial Transplant* 1999;14:1530–1535.

Yeun JY, et al. Acute phase proteins and peritoneal dialysate albumin loss are the main determinants of serum albumin in peritoneal dialysis patients. *Am J Kidney Dis* 1997;30:923–927.

WEB REFERENCES

Peritoneal dialysis adequacy KDOQI guidelines: http://www.kidney.org

Peritoneal dialysis adequacy links: http://www.hdcn.com/pd/adequacy

Standardized weight tables: http://www.hdcn.com/ch/nutri/stdwt.htm

Volume Status and Fluid Overload in Peritoneal Dialysis

Neil Boudville and Peter G. Blake

Fluid overload can manifest in obvious fashion as hypertension or edema in peritoneal dialysis (PD) patients, but may also present in more subtle fashion, making it difficult to diagnose clinically. Chronic hypervolemia can lead to left ventricular hypertrophy, and may be a major contributor to cardiovascular disease in PD patients with attendant morbidity and mortality. In addition, fluid overload with peritoneal membrane dysfunction is a common cause for technique failure.

I. Assessment of fluid status. This is based primarily on clinical examination, which gives at best a crude estimation. More precise predictions using laboratory investigations have so far not proven clinically useful. The target body weight for PD is that which gives a well-tolerated normotensive, edema-free state, and, just as in hemodialysis, it is determined by trial and error. Since PD patients tend to be seen less frequently than those on hemodialysis, there is a risk that fluid status assessment will be more protracted and less well done.

II. Mechanisms of fluid overload. Fluid overload often reflects a combination of inappropriate prescription, noncompliance, loss of residual renal function, mechanical problems, and peritoneal membrane dysfunction (Table 23-1). It is important to avoid thoughtlessly attributing fluid overload to membrane-related ultrafiltration failure only.

III. Diagnosis of ultrafiltration failure (UFF). UFF is defined as fluid overload in association with an ultrafiltration volume <400 mL in a modified peritoneal equilibration test (PET) (Ho-dac-Pannakeet et al., 1997). The modified PET uses a 4.25% dialysate dwell instead of the usual 2.5% bag used in the standard PET (described in Chapter 18). UFF should not be diagnosed if the ultrafiltration volume exceeds 400 mL or if there is no clinical evidence of significant volume overload. *Finally, UFF should not be diagnosed unless catheter malfunction and leaks have been excluded.* If fluid overload is present and the ultrafiltration volume is >400 mL by modified PET, normal peritoneal membrane function is implied, and closer attention needs to be paid to potential nonmembrane causes listed in Table 23-1.

If UFF has been diagnosed, the next step is to review the patient's solute transport characteristics, which can be done using the results of the modified (4.25%) PET or the standard PET; the findings are very similar.

A. High transporter with UFF (type I). In this situation the dialysate dextrose concentration falls rapidly after infusion, resulting in loss of the concentration gradient that drives

Table 23-1. Causes of fluid overload in PD patients

Inappropriate bag selection
Inappropriate prescription for membrane transport status
  Long, dextrose-containing daytime or nocturnal dwells
  Failure to optimize APD regimen for transport status
  Failure to use icodextrin-containing solutions
Noncompliance with PD prescription
Noncompliance with salt and water restriction
Loss of residual renal function
Abdominal leak
Catheter malfunction
Poor blood glucose control
Peritoneal membrane dysfunction

PD, peritoneal dialysis; APD, automated peritoneal dialysis.

fluid removal. This is the most common cause and is often called type I UFF. It typically develops after 3 or more years on PD. It is believed to reflect an increase in the effective peritoneal surface area consequent to increased membrane vascularity that occurs with time on PD, to a greater extent in some patients than in others. Causes of increased effective surface area may include cumulative exposure of the membrane to high glucose loads and, possibly, to other bioincompatible elements of PD solutions including low pH, lactate, and toxic glucose degradation products. Other cases may be related to cumulative episodes of peritonitis or to systemic inflammation seen in uremia generally. Type I UFF may also occur transiently in some patients during and after peritonitis due to acute inflammation of the membrane.
  B. Low transporter with UFF (type II). This group of patients has reduced small solute clearance by PET, a normal or reduced glucose absorption profile, and reduced fluid removal. This is also called type II UFF and is much less common. It reflects decreased membrane surface area and is most often due to adhesions and scarring after a severe peritonitis or other intra-abdominal complication. Peritoneal sclerosis is also a cause. It is difficult to maintain these patients on PD unless they have significant residual renal function.
  C. UFF with transport in the "normal" range (usually high average or low average). Here the cause may or may not be membrane related, and especially diligent effort should be made to exclude leaks and catheter malfunction as causes for the abnormal test as well as for poor fluid removal.
    1. Increased lymphatic absorption of peritoneal fluid is the apparent cause in some patients with this pattern, and it has been given a name: **type III UFF.** The amount of lymphatic absorption can be quantified by measuring the disappearance rate of dextran-70 from the peritoneal cavity, but this is rarely done in clinical practice and the diagnosis is one of exclusion.
    2. Aquaporin deficiency. UFF with normal transport characteristics on PET can also be seen with aquaporin deficiency. This can be diagnosed by measuring the decrease in

dialysate sodium concentration as measured 30–60 minutes into a 2-L dialysis dwell using 4.25% dextrose. As a control, the sodium concentration is also measured 30–60 minutes into a 2-L dwell using 1.5% dextrose, and the two sodium values are subtracted from one another. Why does the dialysate sodium level fall during the early part of an exchange? When dialysate glucose levels are high, osmotically driven ultrafiltration occurs primarily via aquaporin channels, which pass water but no sodium; this results in a transient initial lowering of the dialysate sodium concentration. As the dwell continues, diffusion of sodium from blood to the relatively hyponatric dialysate acts to raise the dialysate sodium level back toward the serum level. If the difference between the sodium level of the 4.25% and 1.5% dextrose dwell samples taken at 30–60 minutes is <5 mmol/L, this suggests that very little aquaporin-mediated convective transport is occurring, and that aquaporin-mediated water transport is impaired (Ni et al., 2006).

IV.   Management of fluid overload. Often multiple causes of fluid overload coexist in an individual patient. As an example, elements of UFF often are present together with high salt intake or poor glucose control. A global approach to solving the problem is best.

A.   General measures

   1.   Sodium restriction. It is vital that patients receive education on sodium and fluid restriction, with the emphasis on sodium. An intake of <100 mmol (2.3 g) a day, consistent with the Joint National Committee on Prevention, Evaluation, and Treatment of High Blood Pressure (JNC) guidelines, is recommended, and for those with difficult hypertension or volume control problems, nutritional intake usually can be maintained on an even lower level of daily sodium intake.

   2.   Patient education regarding when to select higher dextrose solutions. Normally patients have some leeway regarding what concentrations of dextrose to use for a given day. Regular selection of high-concentration dextrose solutions, however, should not be the preferred method of fluid volume control over sodium restriction. Overuse of the high-concentration dextrose solutions may affect peritoneal membrane function, increase glucose absorption, worsen blood sugar and lipid control, and promote obesity.

   3.   Good blood glucose control. A lower serum glucose level will help maintain the glucose concentration gradient across the peritoneal membrane required for fluid removal.

   4.   Preserve residual renal function. This is important for both clearance and fluid removal. There is clinical trial evidence that angiotensin-converting enzyme inhibitors and angiotensin receptor blockers preserve residual renal function, which has a beneficial impact on both clearance and on volume control, as a higher urine volume is then maintained. Use of high-dose loop diuretics in patients with residual renal function, with or without metolazone, will also increase urine volume and so fluid removal. Avoidance of nephrotoxins and intravascular volume depletion both serve to protect residual renal function.

5. Abdominal leaks. See Chapter 25.

6. Catheter malfunction. See Chapter 20.

7. Preservation of peritoneal membrane function. Reduction in episodes of peritonitis will assist in preserving membrane function. Avoidance of high dextrose concentration PD fluid may also help to preserve long-term peritoneal membrane function. Biocompatible PD solutions based on multipouched bag technology allow sterilization of glucose to occur at very low pH and so minimize generation of glucose degradation products (GDPs). The final infused solution has normal pH and this, along with the low GDPs, may lessen damage to the membrane; definitive clinical studies proving a benefit of the newer solutions in terms of lowering the risk of type I UFF have not yet been done, however.

B. Measures according to the type of UFF identified

    1. High transport status (type 1). Short dwell times are required to maintain the dialysate dextrose concentration gradient and so automated peritoneal dialysis (APD), programmed for short 1- to 1.5-hour dwells, may be best. For both continuous ambulatory peritoneal dialysis (CAPD) and APD, long-duration dwells containing dextrose must be avoided. In APD, short dextrose day dwells can be used. In CAPD, the nocturnal dwell should be shortened either by draining in the middle of the night or by using a night exchange device. In this type of UFF, an especially attractive approach is the use of icodextrin for the long dwell in both CAPD and APD.

        a. Icodextrin. This is a large carbohydrate polymer that is used in the place of dextrose to produce a concentration gradient for ultrafiltration. Icodextrin is not absorbed across the membrane, although it is slowly taken up by lymphatics. Accordingly, a concentration gradient is better maintained throughout exchange with long dwell times, allowing ongoing ultrafiltration. An icodextrin-containing exchange is ideal for the 14- to 16-hour day dwell in APD and for the long nocturnal dwell in CAPD. Use of icodextrin has been shown to prolong technique survival substantially in patients with UFF characterized by high transport status. It has also been shown to reduce the extracellular fluid–to–intracellular fluid ratio as documented by bioimpedance analysis (Woodrow et al., 2004).

        b. Resting the peritoneum. There have been documented cases of improved peritoneal membrane function in type I UFF following a temporary cessation of PD. The mechanism of this is unclear; presumably resting improves peritoneal membrane inflammation and hypervascularity, resulting in a return to more normal transport characteristics.

    2. UFF with low transport status. These patients are not likely to do much better on APD or with icodextrin. Transfer to hemodialysis is generally required.

3. **UFF with average transport status.** There is no tested, reliable method to either reduce lymphatic absorption or to correct a transport deficiency due to impaired function of aquaporin channels. Generally this type of UFF is managed by salt and water restriction, diuretics, and general measures to increase total ultrafiltration volume to compensate for the increased volume reabsorbed. This approach may include shortening dwell times and using icodextrin for long dwells.

V. **Glucose-sparing strategies.** In laboratory animal studies, hypertonic glucose exposure leads to neovascularization of the peritoneal membrane and to a functional pattern analogous to UFF with high transport status. Clinical studies have now shown that patients using a greater amount of hypertonic glucose are more likely to develop high transport characteristics than those who receive less glucose (Davies et al., 2003). Systemically, glucose loading is also undesirable, as detailed in Chapter 26. The widespread availability of icodextrin allows reduction of daily glucose exposure, and there are studies showing that patients using this solution have more stable long-term membrane function. Intraperitoneal amino acids can also be substituted for one daily dextrose dwell.

VI. **Hypertension and hypotension in PD**

A. **Hypertension.** PD was initially advocated as providing better blood pressure control than hemodialysis because of its continuous nature. This was certainly demonstrated in early reports on PD populations. More recently, concern has been raised about blood pressure control with CAPD. It has been demonstrated that antihypertensive medication requirements increase with duration on CAPD, to the point that more are required than on hemodialysis (Enia et al., 2001). This, however, has been refuted by other studies. It seems likely therefore that differences in blood pressure control with CAPD reflect differences in case mix and dialysis practices (Wong et al., 2004).

1. **Sodium sieving and removal and hypertension using APD.** Sodium removal tends to be reduced during APD, given that the dialysate is drained early into an exchange, at a time when its sodium concentration has been reduced due to the effects of aquaporin-mediated sieving (see above). Studies to date, however, have not shown a consistent pattern of impaired blood pressure control in APD, and differences in blood pressure control between CAPD with APD identified in some studies most likely reflect variations in case mix and dialysis practice.

2. **Management.** One should focus initially on volume control, and antihypertensives (other than cardioprotective drugs) should be introduced only if this approach has been unsuccessful. Preference should be given to agents that have a beneficial effect on residual renal function, such as loop diuretics, angiotensin-converting enzyme inhibitors, and angiotensin receptor blockers. The choice of agent in many patients may be driven by coexisting medical conditions such as ischemic heart disease.

B. Hypotension. Hypotension is not uncommon in PD populations, with one cohort study (Malliara et al., 2002) detecting it in 13% of patients. The cause of hypotension is sometimes unclear but approximately 20% of cases are secondary to heart failure. An additional 40% may be due to hypovolemia, and it is important to recognize this as it typically responds to volume repletion that may also improve residual renal function. Patients with hypotension due to cardiac causes and cases in which no cause could be identified have a poor prognosis, with a high early mortality rate. Agents such as midodrine and fludrocortisone have been used but with no proven benefit. Hypotension can also be the initial presenting symptom of covert sepsis in PD patients, and this diagnosis should be considered as part of the differential diagnosis.

VII. Simple peritoneal sclerosis and sclerosing peritonitis

A. Description. Simple peritoneal sclerosis is a mild fibrosing condition of the peritoneal membrane that appears in most patients after several years of peritoneal dialysis. Histologically, mesothelial cells lose microvilli, and submesothelial tissue becomes thickened. This slight thickening appears to occur in the majority of patients being treated with PD (Garosi, 2000). In a small minority, these sclerotic changes are magnified so that the visceral organs are encased in a thick, fibrotic, abdominal cocoon. The more severe condition has been termed **sclerosing peritonitis,** although no infectious agent has been implicated. Estimated prevalence of sclerosing peritonitis is between 0.5 and 0.9% of PD patients. In this more aggressive condition the tissue contains inflammatory cells as well as calcifications, and ossification of the peritoneum has been observed. While bioincompatible PD solutions have been speculated to cause simple peritoneal sclerosis, the etiology of sclerosing peritonitis is unknown. Use of acetate, chlorhexidine, and repeated episodes of peritonitis all have been implicated. Diagnosis can be made by ultrasound or by CT scanning. Whether use of more biocompatible solutions will prevent sclerosing peritonitis is unknown. Cessation of PD when peritoneal biopsy shows a >40 micrometer thick PD membrane has been recommended (Garosi, 2000). A number of pharmacologic drug treatment options have been tried, including steroids, cytotoxic drugs, and octreotide.

B. Peritoneal transport. Patients with sclerosing peritonitis almost invariably develop low rates of diffusive and convective peritoneal transport, and this should be suspected in any patient in whom a rapid deterioration of clearance develops. Peritoneal dialysis should be stopped and transfer to hemodialysis is the only practical option. Specific therapy at this point in time remains undefined.

SELECTED READINGS

Ateş K, et al. Effect of fluid and sodium removal on mortality in peritoneal dialysis patients. *Kidney Int* 2001;60(2):767–776.

Clerbaux G, et al. Evaluation of peritoneal transport properties at onset of peritoneal dialysis and longitudinal follow-up. *Nephrol Dial Transplant* 2006;21(4):1032–1039.

Davies SJ, et al. Icodextrin improves the fluid status of peritoneal dialysis patients: results of a double-blind randomized controlled trial. *J Am Soc Nephrol* 2003;14(9):2338–2344.

Ellis KJ, et al. Bioelectrical impedance methods in clinical research: a follow-up to the NIH technology assessment conference. *Nutrition* 1999;15:874–880.

Enia G, et al. Long-term CAPD patients are volume expanded and display more severe left ventricular hypertrophy than haemodialysis patients. *Nephrol Dial Transplant* 2001;16:1459–1464.

Garosi G, et al. Peritoneal sclerosis: one or two nosological entities. *Semin Dial* 2000;13:297–308.

Ho-dac-Pannakeet MM, et al. Analysis of ultrafiltration failure in peritoneal dialysis patients by means of standard peritoneal permeability analysis. *Perit Dial Int* 1997;17:144–150.

La Milia V, et al. Peritoneal transport assessment by peritoneal equilibration test with 3.86% glucose: a long-term prospective evaluation. *Kidney Int* 2006;69(5):927–933.

Li PK, et al. Effects of an angiotensin-converting enzyme inhibitor on residual renal function in patients receiving peritoneal dialysis: a randomized, controlled study. *Ann Intern Med* 2003;139:105–112.

Malliara M, et al. Hypotension in patients on chronic peritoneal dialysis: etiology, management, and outcome. *Adv Perit Dial* 2002;18:49–54.

McCafferty K, Fan SL. Are we underestimating the problem of ultrafiltration in peritoneal dialysis patients? *Perit Dial Int* 2006;26(3):349–352.

Mujais S, et al. Evaluation and management of ultrafiltration problems in peritoneal dialysis. International Society for Peritoneal Dialysis Ad Hoc Committee on ultrafiltration management in peritoneal dialysis. *Perit Dial Int* 2000;20(Suppl 4):S5–21.

Ni J, et al. Aquaporin-1 plays an essential role in water permeability and ultrafiltration during peritoneal dialysis. *Kidney Int* 2006;69(9):1518–1525.

Rodriguez-Carmona A, et al. Compared time profiles of ultrafiltration, sodium removal and renal function in CAPD and APD patients. *Am J Kidney Dis* 2004;44:132–145.

Sharma AP, Blake PG. Should fluid removal be used as an index of adequacy in PD? *Perit Dial Int* 2003;23:107–108.

Smit W, et al. Quantification of free water transport in peritoneal dialysis. *Kidney Int* 2004;66:849–854.

Tonbul Z, et al. The association of peritoneal transport properties with 24-hour blood pressure levels in CAPD patients. *Perit Dial Int* 2003;23:46–52.

Twardowski ZJ. Pathophysiology of peritoneal transport. *Contrib Nephrol* 2006;150:13–19.

Wang AY, Lai KN. The importance of residual renal function in dialysis patients. *Kidney Int* 2006;69(10):1726–1732.

Wong PN, et al. Factors associated with poorly-controlled hypertension in continuous ambulatory peritoneal dialysis patients. *Singapore Med J* 2004;45(11):520–524.

Woodrow G, et al. Abnormalities of body composition in peritoneal dialysis patients. *Perit Dial Int* 2004;24(2):169–175.

Peritonitis and Exit Site Infection

David J. Leehey, Cheuk-Chun Szeto, and Philip K-T Li

I. Peritonitis

A. Incidence. Peritonitis remains the Achilles heel of peritoneal dialysis (PD). The overall incidence of peritonitis in continuous ambulatory peritoneal dialysis (CAPD) patients during the 1980s and early 1990s had averaged 1.1–1.3 episodes per patient per year in the United States, but the introduction of Y-set and double-bag disconnect systems (see Chapter 19) has reduced this to approximately one episode per patient every 24 months (Gahrmani et al., 1995; Monteon et al., 1998, Li et al., 2002). The incidence rate in CAPD patients in the United States is now comparable to that seen in automated peritoneal dialysis (APD) patients. The same flush-before-fill methodology used in CAPD Y sets may also be used effectively in APD. Patients on APD going "dry" during the day (i.e., no daytime dwell) may have a decreased risk of infection compared to continuous cycling peritoneal dialysis (CCPD) patients. Double-cuffed catheters are clearly superior to single-cuffed catheters in decreasing the risk of peritonitis. It is now recommended by the International Society for Peritoneal Dialysis (ISPD) Ad Hoc Advisory Committee on Peritoneal Dialysis–Related Infections (Piraino et al., 2005) that all centers calculate and track their peritonitis rates.

B. Pathogenesis

    1. Potential routes of infection

        a. Intraluminal. Peritonitis is thought to occur most often because of improper technique in making or breaking a transfer set–to–bag or catheter–to–transfer set connection. This allows bacteria to gain access to the peritoneal cavity via the catheter lumen.

        b. Periluminal. Bacteria present on the skin surface can enter the peritoneal cavity via the peritoneal catheter tract.

        c. Transmural. Bacteria of intestinal origin can enter the peritoneal cavity by migrating through the bowel wall. This is the usual mechanism of peritonitis associated with diarrheal states and/or instrumentation of the colon and may be seen also with strangulated hernia.

        d. Hematogenous. Less commonly, peritonitis is due to bacteria that have seeded the peritoneum from a distant site by way of the bloodstream.

        e. Transvaginal. Little is known about the possibility of ascending infection reaching the peritoneum from the vagina by way of the uterine tubes, but it may explain some instances of *Candida* peritonitis.

2. **Bacteria-laden plaque.** Within several months, the intraperitoneal (IP) portion of almost all permanent peritoneal catheters becomes covered with a bacteria-laden slime or plaque. It is unknown whether such plaque has an important role in the pathogenesis of peritonitis.

3. **Role of host defenses.** The peritoneal leukocytes are critical in combating bacteria that have entered the peritoneal space by any of the routes mentioned above. A number of factors are now known to alter their efficacy in phagocytosing and killing invading bacteria.

   a. **Dialysis solution pH and osmolality.** Some peritoneal dialysis solutions have a pH close to 5.0 and the osmolality of most ranges from 1.3–1.8 times that of normal plasma, depending on the glucose concentration used. These unphysiologic conditions greatly inhibit the ability of peritoneal leukocytes to phagocytose and kill bacteria. High osmolality, low pH, and the presence of the lactate anion combine to cause inhibition of superoxide generation by neutrophils (Yu et al., 1992). Whether newer, pH-corrected and/or bicarbonate-buffered solutions will lower the peritonitis risk remains to be determined.

   b. **Peritoneal dialysis solution calcium levels.** The antimicrobial actions of peritoneal macrophages are enhanced by both calcium and cholecalciferol. Use of a 1.25 mM (2.5 mEq/L) calcium concentration in peritoneal dialysis solution has gained popularity (see Chapter 19). However, an increased risk of *Staphylococcus epidermidis* peritonitis has been associated with use of such low-calcium dialysis solutions, presumably because peritoneal macrophage function is impaired in the reduced calcium environment (Piraino et al., 1992).

   c. **Peritoneal fluid immunoglobulin G (IgG) levels.** The level of IgG in the peritoneal fluid correlates with the ability of peritoneal leukocytes to phagocytose bacteria. Patients with abnormally low levels may be prone to having more frequent episodes of peritonitis.

   d. **Human immunodeficiency virus (HIV) infection.** The overall incidence of peritonitis does not appear to be higher in HIV-infected patients (Kimmel et al., 1993); however, infection with fungal species is probably more common.

C. **Etiology.** Using appropriate culture techniques, an organism can be isolated from the peritoneal fluid in over 90% of cases in which symptoms and signs of peritonitis and an elevated peritoneal fluid neutrophil count are present. The responsible pathogen is almost always a bacterium, usually of the Gram-positive variety (Table 24-1). The occurrence of fungal peritonitis (e.g., *Candida*) is uncommon but by no means rare. Infections with *Mycobacterium tuberculosis* or other type of mycobacteria have been reported but are unusual.

D. **Diagnosis**

1. **Diagnostic criteria for peritonitis.** At least two of the following three conditions should be present: (a) symptoms and signs of peritoneal inflammation, (b) cloudy peritoneal fluid with an elevated peritoneal fluid cell count

Table 24-1. Frequency of organisms isolated in patients with peritonitis

Organism	Frequency (%)
Bacteria	80–90
Staphylococcus epidermidis	30–45
Staphylococcus aureus	10–20
Streptococcus sp.	5–10
Coliforms	5–10
Klebsiella and *Enterobacter*	5
Pseudomonas	3–8
Others	<5
Mycobacterium tuberculosis	<1
Candida and other fungi	<1–10
Culture negative	5–20

(more than 100/mcL) due predominantly (more than 50%) to neutrophils, and (c) demonstration of bacteria in the peritoneal effluent by Gram stain or culture.

a. Symptoms and signs. The most common symptom of peritonitis is abdominal pain. However, peritonitis should be suspected whenever a chronic peritoneal dialysis patient suffers from generalized malaise, particularly if nausea, vomiting, or diarrhea is also present. The usual manifestations of peritonitis are listed in Table 24-2. Not all abdominal pain in a patient receiving PD is peritonitis, and a broad differential diagnosis should always be kept in mind. Strangulated hernia is a common mimic for peritonitis. We encountered a patient who presented with typical symptoms 2 months after starting PD; his transplant had recently failed and his steroids had been tapered. Abdominal pain in that instance was a manifestation of Addison disease due to steroid withdrawal.

Table 24-2. Symptoms and signs of peritonitis

	Percentage
Symptoms	
Abdominal pain	95
Nausea and vomiting	30
Feverish sensation	30
Chills	20
Constipation or diarrhea	15
Signs	
Cloudy peritoneal fluid	99
Abdominal tenderness	80
Rebound tenderness	10–50[a]
Increased temperature	33
Blood leukocytosis	25

[a] Highly variable, depending on the severity of infection and the amount of time elapsed between onset and medical evaluation.

b.   Peritoneal fluid

(1)   Cloudiness of the fluid. The peritoneal fluid generally becomes cloudy when the cell count exceeds 50–100/mcL ($50–100 \times 10^6$/L). In most patients, sudden onset of cloudy fluid with appropriate abdominal symptoms is sufficient evidence of peritonitis to warrant initiation of antimicrobial therapy. However, peritoneal fluid cloudiness may be due to other factors (e.g., fibrin, blood, or, rarely, malignancy or chyle) rather than to an increase in the white blood cell (WBC) count, and therefore a cell count should be obtained whenever feasible. Occasionally, fluid drained after a prolonged dwell period (such as after the daytime dwell in APD patients) appears cloudy in the absence of peritonitis. On the other hand, a relatively translucent peritoneal fluid does not completely exclude the possibility that peritonitis is present; occasionally, early in the course of peritonitis, the cell count may be only modestly elevated (not enough to cause marked cloudiness of the fluid), but the percentage of peritoneal fluid neutrophils will be increased.

(2)   Importance of performing a differential count of peritoneal fluid cells. Peritonitis is usually associated with an increase in the absolute number and percentage of peritoneal fluid neutrophils. On some occasions, a high peritoneal fluid cell count (causing cloudy fluid) will be present due to an increase in the number of peritoneal fluid monocytes or eosinophils (see below). Most such cases are not associated with peritonitis and do not require antimicrobial treatment. For this reason, one should perform a differential cell count on the peritoneal fluid sample. Prior to counting, the fluid is spun in a special centrifuge (e.g., Cytospin, Shandon, Inc., Pittsburgh, PA) and the sediment colored with Wright stain. The number of cells in the effluent will vary depending on the length of the preceding dwell and patients with a "dry" abdomen will have higher absolute cell counts than those with instilled dialysate. Thus, the percentage of polymorphonuclear neutrophils (PMNs) and not the absolute number of WBCs should be used to diagnose peritonitis.

(3)   Obtaining the specimen

(a)   CAPD patients. After disconnecting the drain bag full of peritoneal effluent, the bag is inverted several times to mix its contents. A sample (7 mL) is aspirated from the port of the drain bag and transferred to a tube containing ethylenediamine tetraacetic acid (EDTA).

(b)   APD patients. In CCPD patients, a representative cell count can be obtained easily from the daytime dwell by first draining the abdomen and taking the sample from the drainage bag. In nocturnal intermittent peritoneal dialysis (NIPD) patients who go "dry" during the day, there will often be some residual fluid present in the abdomen at the time the patient is seen. In these patients, the peritoneal fluid sample can be obtained directly via the peritoneal catheter. After careful cleaning of the catheter with povidone–iodine, a syringe is attached using meticulous sterile technique and the 2- to 3-mL of fluid in the catheter lumen is withdrawn and discarded. The peritoneal fluid sample (7 mL) is then withdrawn from the catheter using a second syringe. The sample is injected into a tube containing EDTA. If insufficient fluid is obtained in this manner, one can infuse 1 L of dialysis solution and drain the abdomen, obtaining a sample from the effluent. Although the absolute peritoneal fluid cell count will be lower in this diluted specimen, the differential will be similar to that in a sample obtained directly via the catheter.

(c) Storage time. Morphologic identification of the various cell types can become quite difficult in peritoneal effluent samples that have been stored for more than 3–5 hours prior to injection into the EDTA-containing sample tube.

(4) Normal peritoneal fluid cell count values and criteria for peritonitis. The absolute peritoneal fluid cell count in CAPD patients is usually <50 cells/mcL and is often <10 cells/mcL. In NIPD patients going "dry" during the day, the absolute cell count may be much higher, especially in specimens obtained directly via the catheter when the residual peritoneal fluid volume is small. Normally, the peritoneal fluid contains predominantly mononuclear cells (macrophages, monocytes, and, to a lesser extent, lymphocytes). Eosinophils and basophils are usually absent. The percentage of neutrophils does not normally exceed 15% of the total nonerythrocyte cell count and a value >50% strongly suggests peritonitis, whereas one >35% should raise suspicion. The percentage of neutrophils will be increased with both bacterial and fungal peritonitis, and even in many cases of tuberculous peritonitis.

The percentage of neutrophils in the peritoneal fluid is rarely elevated in the absence of peritonitis, but there are exceptions: In patients with infectious diarrhea or active colitis, in those with pelvic inflammatory disease, and in women who are menstruating or ovulating or who have recently had a pelvic examination. Pseudoperitonitis (elevated cell count, negative peritoneal fluid cultures, and benign course) has even been reported in CAPD patients who travel long distances over bumpy mountain roads (Katirtzoglou et al., 1985).

(5) Peritoneal fluid monocytosis. Tuberculous peritonitis is rare in peritoneal dialysis patients. Nevertheless, in the presence of persistent peritoneal fluid monocytosis, a diagnostic evaluation to exclude this diagnosis is warranted. Peritoneal fluid monocytosis may also occur in conjunction with peritoneal fluid eosinophilia.

(6) Peritoneal fluid eosinophilia. The peritoneal fluid eosinophil count may become elevated in peritoneal dialysis patients, causing cloudy fluid and leading to a suspicion of peritonitis (Humayun et al., 1981). Usually, the peritoneal fluid monocyte number is elevated also. Peritoneal fluid eosinophilia/monocytosis occurs most often soon after peritoneal catheter insertion. The irritant effect of peritoneal air (e.g., introduced at time of laparotomy) and possibly of plasticizers leached into the peritoneum from peritoneal dialysis solution containers and tubings is a suspected cause. In such cases, the eosinophilia most often resolves spontaneously within 2–6 weeks. Peritoneal fluid eosinophilia can also occur (uncommonly) during the treatment phase of peritonitis; in other patients it occurs episodically for unknown reasons. There have been several case reports of its occurring in association with fungal and parasitic infections of the peritoneum, including *Aspergillus niger, Paecilomyces variotii,* and *Strongyloides stercoralis.*

c. **Culture of peritoneal fluid**

(1) Technique. The incidence of positive peritoneal fluid cultures in patients suspected of having peritonitis depends on culture technique.

(a) Storage. Peritoneal fluid should be cultured promptly; however, infected fluid kept at room temperature or refrigerated for a period often grows pathogenic organisms on subsequent culture.

(b) Sample volume. The volume of peritoneal effluent sent for culture should be at least 50 mL because larger volumes increase the yield of positive culture results.

(c) Sample preparation. The aliquot is centrifuged (e.g., at 3,000 g for 15 minutes) to concentrate the organisms. The supernatant is decanted off and the pellet resuspended in 3–5 mL of sterile saline and inoculated into standard blood culture media (aerobic and anaerobic). Rapid culture techniques (e.g., Septi-chek, BACTEC) may be utilized.

(2) Yield of positive cultures. Seventy percent to ninety percent of dialysate samples obtained from patients with clinical peritonitis yield positive cultures for a specific micro-organism within 24–48 hours. A more prolonged incubation period may be needed for more fastidious organisms.

(3) Improving culture yield. The yield of positive cultures may be improved by hypotonic lysis. The centrifuged sediment is resuspended in 100 mL of sterile water to cause osmotic lysis of its cellular elements. This may induce release of intracellularly located bacteria from peritoneal leukocytes, thus increasing the recovery rate and allowing earlier microbiologic diagnosis. Washing the sediment with sterile saline and/or using an antibiotic-removing resin may result in positive cultures in patients receiving antibiotics.

(4) Incidence of false-positive results. When such sensitive culture methods are used, approximately 7% of cultures may be positive (sometimes prolonged incubation is required), even in asymptomatic peritoneal dialysis patients. Whether such "false-positive" cultures represent contamination or subclinical peritonitis is not known.

(5) Gram stain. Gram stain of the peritoneal fluid sediment is useful but positive in less than half of cases of culture-proven peritonitis. Gram stain is also useful for making the diagnosis of fungal peritonitis. Staining with fluorescent acridine orange dye has been reported to increase the visibility of bacterial organisms.

(a) Necessity of performing blood cultures. Routine blood cultures are unnecessary; however, they should be performed if a patient appears septic, especially if an acute abdominal source (such as appendicitis, cholecystitis, perforated viscus, etc.) is suspected.

E. Treatment

1. Initial management of peritonitis

a. Choice of antimicrobial therapy. Vancomycin or a first-generation cephalosporin such as cefazolin or cephalothin is used in combination with an antibiotic to cover Gram-negative organisms such as ceftazidime. For the cephalosporin-allergic patient, aztreonam is an alternative to ceftazidime for Gram-negative coverage. It is now recommended that aminoglycosides be avoided if possible in patients with residual renal function because of their nephrotoxicity (Shemin et al., 1999), although short courses of aminoglycosides probably do not harm residual renal function. Aminoglycosides may be used in patients without residual renal function, although one still must be wary of otovestibular toxicity (see below).

(1) Gram positive. First-generation cephalosporins (e.g., cefazolin) rather than vancomycin are often preferred because of the emergence of vancomycin-resistant organisms. Intraperitoneal cefazolin can be conveniently administered in a single daily dose of 15 mg/kg, although a 25% increase in dose is recommended in patients with substantial residual renal function (Manley et al., 1999). Alternatives to cephalosporins include nafcillin and clindamycin. Vancomycin can be used as first-line treatment or reserved for patients harboring β-lactam–resistant organisms, especially methicillin-resistant *Staphylococcal aureus* (MRSA), or with penicillin/cephalosporin allergy. Ciprofloxacin alone is not recommended to treat Gram-positive infections (Waite et al., 1993).

(2) Gram negative, indeterminate, or not done. In many instances, it may be impractical or impossible to perform a prompt Gram stain of the peritoneal fluid effluent. Moreover, Gram stain is positive in only 9%–40% of peritonitis episodes and treatment usually is begun without the assistance of Gram stain results.

Table 24-3. Sample prescriptions for initial treatment of peritonitis with unknown organism type

CAPD (continuous dosing method)
1. Drain abdomen and obtain cell count and culture from drainage bag. Change the transfer set.
2. Loading dose: Infuse 2 L of 1.5% dextrose dialysis solution containing:
   1 g ceftazidime
   1 g cefazolin
   1,000 units/L heparin
   Allow to dwell for 3–4 hours. In patients who appear septic, administer loading doses IV rather than IP.
3. Continue regular CAPD schedule, using normal exchange volume if tolerated. Add 125 mg per L ceftazidime, 125 mg/L cefazolin, and 1,000 units/L heparin to each dialysis solution bag.

CAPD (intermittent dosing method)
1. Drain abdomen and obtain cell count and culture from drainage bag. Change the transfer set.
2. Loading dose: Infuse 2 L of 1.5% dextrose dialysis solution containing:
   1.0 g ceftazidime
   1.0 g cefazolin
   1,000 units/L heparin
   Allow to dwell for 3–4 hours. In patients who appear septic, administer loading doses IV.
3. Continue regular CAPD schedule, using normal exchange volume if tolerated. Administer 1.0 g ceftazidime and 1.0 g cefazolin into each nocturnal exchange. If there is fibrin or blood in dialysate, add heparin to every exchange.

APD (continuous dosing method)
Severe cases: Administer the loading doses of antimicrobials IV. Place on cycler for 24–48 hours continuously, using a 1- to 4-hour dwell time. Add maintenance doses of antimicrobials and heparin to each bag of dialysis solution as for CAPD.
Mild to moderate cases: Loading doses optional. Continue on usual CCPD or NIPD schedule; add maintenance doses of antimicrobials and heparin to each dialysis solution bag.

APD (intermittent dosing method)
Severe cases: Not recommended
Mild to moderate cases: Treat with CCPD schedule; add 1.0 g ceftazidime and 1.0 g cefazolin to daytime dwell.
CAPD, continuous ambulatory peritoneal dialysis; APD, automated peritoneal dialysis; CCPD, continuous cycling peritoneal dialysis; NIPD, nocturnal intermittent peritoneal dialysis.

See text for alternative drugs.

Therefore, it is usual practice to use an additional antibiotic to cover Gram-negative organisms (usually ceftazidime) until culture results are known. Table 24-3 lists sample prescriptions based on use of cefazolin in combination with ceftazidime.

(3) Fungal organisms seen on Gram stain. Strategies for treatment of fungal peritonitis are discussed later in this chapter.

b. Delivery methods and schedules for antimicrobial drugs

(1) IP versus oral (PO) or intravenous (IV) antimicrobial therapy. IP dosing of antibiotics is preferable to PO or IV dosing when possible in order to ensure adequate drug levels in the dialysate. This remains the accepted approach, although some antimicrobials are more appropriately administered either IV (if the patient appears septic) or PO initially.

(2) The loading dose. A loading dose of antimicrobials is usually given IP when CAPD is the treatment modality (Table 24-4). If a patient appears toxic, we recommend giving a single loading dose IV (note that for aminoglycosides, we generally give 1.5 mg/kg [gentamicin, tobramycin] or 5 mg/kg [amikacin] IV). Because many patients with peritonitis are in substantial pain, they may be unable to tolerate their usual exchange volume; in such instances the IP loading dose can be administered in a bag containing only 1 L of dialysis solution. If the patient is to be treated for peritonitis while on APD, IP administration of the loading dose is less convenient. In APD patients we generally administer the loading dose IV (Table 24-5).

(3) Maintenance antimicrobial dose. After the loading dose has been given, a CAPD or CCPD schedule is continued, with maintenance doses of antimicrobials added to each exchange (Table 24-4). One-liter exchange volumes may be used for several days to reduce patient discomfort. We prefer to use a CAPD regimen because of ease of antibiotic administration; however, this may result in fluid retention in rapid transporters. Alternatively, maintenance antibiotics in CAPD patients could be administered as an intermittent IP dose once daily. For patients on a CCPD schedule, antibiotics can be conveniently added to the daytime dwell only. In APD patients, antibiotic half-lives are shorter during the cycler exchanges due to greater peritoneal clearance; to ensure maximal bioavailability, the antibiotic-containing dialysate must dwell at least 4 hours to ensure an adequate antibiotic depot in the body (Manley and Bailie, 2002). An even longer dwell time (e.g., 6–8 hours) is probably preferable.

(4) Antimicrobial dosing guidelines. Suggested loading and maintenance doses for a number of antimicrobial drugs are listed in Table 24-4. For maintenance doses added to the dialysis solution, there are two strategies. The first is to add the same dose to each dialysis solution bag. An alternative strategy is to add a larger dose to one bag only, every 12 or 24 hours (or, in the case of vancomycin, every 4–5 days). A recent randomized trial in children found that intermittent vancomycin dosing was as effective as continuous dosing (Schaefer et al., 1999). Single-daily-dose

Table 24-4.   Loading and maintenance doses of antimicrobials for peritonitis (CAPD)

	Intermittent: per Exchange, Once Daily	Continuous: per L, All Exchanges
Aminoglycosides		
Amikacin	2 mg/kg	LD 25, MD 12
Gentamicin	0.6 mg/kg	LD 8, MD 4
Netilmicin	0.6 mg/kg	LD 8, MD 4
Tobramycin	0.6 mg/kg	LD 8, MD 4
Cephalosporins		
Cefazolin	15 mg/kg	LD 500, MD 125
Cefepime	1 g	LD 500, MD 125
Cephalothin	15 mg/kg	LD 500, MD 125
Cephradine	15 mg/kg	LD 500, MD 125
Ceftazidime	1,000–1,500 mg	LD 500, MD 125
Ceftizoxime	1,000 mg	LD 250, MD 125
Penicillins		
Azlocillin	ND	LD 500, MD 250
Ampicillin	ND	MD 125
Oxacillin	ND	MD 125
Nafcillin	ND	MD 125
Amoxicillin	ND	LD 250–500, MD 50
Penicillin G	ND	LD 50,000 units, MD 25,000 units
Quinolones		
Ciprofloxacin	ND	LD 50, MD 25
Others		
Vancomycin	15–30 mg/kg q5–7d	LD 1,000, MD 25
Aztreonam	ND	LD 1,000, MD 250
Antifungals		
Amphotericin	NA	1.5
Combinations		
Ampicillin/ sulbactam	2 g q12h	LD 1,000, MD 100
Imipenem/ cilastatin	1 g b.i.d.	LD 500, MD 200
Quinupristin/ dalfopristin	25 mg/L in alternate bags[a]	

CAPD, continuous ambulatory peritoneal dialysis; LD, loading dose in mg; MD, maintenance dose in mg; NA, not applicable; ND, no data; b.i.d., two times per day.

[a] Given in conjunction with 500 mg IV twice daily.

Dosing of drugs with renal clearance in patients with residual renal function (defined as more than 100 mL per day urine output) should be increased by 25%.

Source: Piraino B, et al. Peritoneal dialysis-related infections recommendations: 2005 update. *Perit Dial Int* 2005;25:107–131.

Table 24-5.   Loading and maintenance doses of antimicrobials for peritonitis (APD)

Drug	Intraperitoneal Dose
Vancomycin	Loading dose 30 mg/kg IP in long dwell; repeat dosing 15 mg/kg IP in long dwell every 3–5 days, following levels (limited data)
Cefazolin	20 mg/kg IP every day in long day dwell
Tobramycin	Loading dose 1.5 mg/kg IP in long dwell, then 0.5 mg/kg IP each day in long day dwell
Fluconazole	200 mg IP in one exchange per day every 24–48 hours
Cefepime	1 g IP in one exchange per day (unpublished data)

APD, automated peritoneal dialysis; IP, intraperitoneally.
Source: Piraino B, et al. Peritoneal dialysis-related infections recommendations: 2005 update. *Perit Dial Int* 2005;25:107–131.

aminoglycoside therapy has several advantages, including ease of administration (especially for outpatient therapy), increased efficacy (especially for organisms with relatively high mean inhibitory concentrations [i.e., >2 mcg/mL]), and potentially less toxicity. Increased bacterial killing rates associated with prolonged postantibiotic effect are obtained using once-daily dosing. However, trough concentrations of antibiotic (i.e., 24 hours after a dose) will be low. The fact that the exact duration of the postantibiotic effect is unknown has led to some concern about the advisability of this type of regimen, especially in patients with residual renal function (Low et al., 1996).

There has been interest in once-daily cefazolin dosing. Doses of 1.0–2.0 g IP daily have been utilized (Vas et al., 1997; Lai et al., 1997; Troidle et al., 1997). However, intraperitoneal cephalosporin levels may fall below the minimal inhibitory concentration (MIC) of most organisms. As there is no postantibiotic effect with cephalosporins as there is with aminoglycosides, there is some concern that once-daily dosing may lead to more treatment failures than intermittent dosing (Fielding et al., 2002). Therefore, adding cephalosporins to every exchange is preferred.

(5)   Stability of antibiotics in dialysis solution. Vancomycin, aminoglycosides, and cephalosporins can be mixed in the same dialysis solution bag; however, aminoglycosides are incompatible with penicillins. Vancomycin (25 mg/L) is stable for 28 days in dialysate stored at room temperature, although high ambient temperatures will reduce the duration of stability. Gentamicin (8 mg/L) is stable for 14 days, but the duration of stability is decreased if heparin is added. Cefazolin (500 mg/L) is stable for at lest 8 days at room temperature or for 14 days if refrigerated; addition of heparin does not impair stability. Ceftazidime is less stable; concentrations of 125 mg/L are stable for 4 days at room temperature or 7 days if refrigerated and 200 mg/L is stable for 10 days if refrigerated.

c.   Heparin. Peritonitis is often associated with formation of fibrinous clots in the peritoneal fluid, and the risk of catheter obstruction is high. For this reason, most care providers add heparin (500–1,000 units/L) to the dialysis solution until signs and symptoms of peritonitis have resolved and until fibrinous clots are no longer visible in the peritoneal effluent.

d.   Alterations in schedule for CAPD and APD. CAPD patients can generally continue their normal schedule of exchanges, unless, as discussed below, ultrafiltration becomes inadequate. Some physicians prefer to treat moderate to severe peritonitis in both CAPD and APD patients for the initial 24–48 hours with a series of 1- to 4-hour exchanges containing antimicrobials administered via a cycler. In CCPD patients with mild to moderate peritonitis, the usual CCPD schedule can be continued unchanged with antibiotics administered either continuously (added to all exchanges) or intermittently (added only to the daytime dwell). Alternatively, the patient can temporarily be converted to CAPD. Doses of selected antimicrobials in patients who remain on APD during treatment of peritonitis are given in Table 24-5. The decision to hospitalize a patient depends on many factors, including patient reliability, severity of peritonitis, and the type of treatment schedule chosen. In most centers, the majority of cases are now managed on an outpatient basis.

e.   Consideration of secondary peritonitis. In a small but significant proportion of patients with peritonitis, a serious, underlying intra-abdominal disease process (e.g., perforated gastric or duodenal ulcer, pancreatitis, appendicitis, or diverticulitis) may be present. The presence of peritoneal fluid in the abdomen may mask the local tenderness commonly associated with some of these conditions. There is no easy method to detect these conditions at initial presentation. The presence of free IP air on upright chest radiograph is an unusual finding in CAPD patients, provided recent laparotomy or transfer set change has not been performed, and may suggest the presence of a perforated viscus. However, free IP air may occur more commonly in patients being treated with cyclers. A very high peritoneal fluid amylase level suggests pancreatitis or other serious intra-abdominal pathology. The interpretation of plasma amylase and lipase levels in dialysis patients with suspected pancreatitis is discussed in Chapter 29.

f.   Consequence of changes in peritoneal permeability. During peritonitis the permeability of the peritoneum to water, glucose, and proteins is increased. Rapid glucose absorption from the dialysis solution reduces the amount of ultrafiltration and can result in fluid overload. Higher dialysis solution glucose levels and shorter dwell times may be needed to maintain adequate ultrafiltration. Because glucose absorption is more rapid during peritonitis, hyperglycemia can result and may be severe in diabetics unless plasma glucose values are monitored with appropriate adjustments to the insulin dosage.

Protein losses during peritonitis are increased and should be dealt with by increasing dietary protein intake.

g. Constipation. Constipation is a common associated complaint during peritonitis episodes. If present, calcium-containing phosphate binders (which sometimes can cause constipation) should be temporarily discontinued.

2. Initial management of peritoneal contamination without peritonitis. After bacterial contamination of the peritoneal cavity, the incubation period for most organisms is about 12–48 hours. If a break in sterile technique has occurred, then it is advisable to institute antimicrobial therapy promptly in order to prevent peritonitis. The transfer set should be changed and the peritoneal cavity flushed with Ringer's lactate solution containing an antistaphylococcal antibiotic. A short (1- to 2-day) course of oral antimicrobial therapy may also be given; however, there is no documentation that these procedures are effective in preventing peritonitis.

3. Change in management of peritonitis based on patient course and initial culture results. With effective treatment, the patient should begin to improve clinically within 12–48 hours, and the total cell count and percentage of neutrophils in the peritoneal fluid should begin to decrease. Often visual inspection of the effluent will suffice, but if there is no improvement within 48 hours, repeat cell count and culture is necessary. Isolation of causative bacteria and determination of their antimicrobial sensitivity can generally be performed within 2–3 days. Longer growth periods may be needed for certain fastidious organisms (e.g., gentamicin- and methicillin-resistant *S. aureus*). A single organism is isolated in 70%–90% of cases (Table 24-1).

a. Gram-positive organism cultured. If *S. aureus, S. epidermidis,* or a *Streptococcus* species is identified, then continued therapy with a single antimicrobial agent is recommended. If an aminoglycoside was given initially, it can now be stopped. Many *S. epidermidis*–like organisms reported to be resistant to first-generation cephalosporins are sensitive to the levels achieved in the peritoneal cavity. Thus, if the patient is clinically responding to treatment, there is usually no need to change the antibiotic regimen. If an *Enterococcus* species is cultured, ampicillin or vancomycin plus an aminoglycoside are generally employed, unless sensitivity testing indicates vancomycin resistance, in which case linezolid or quinupristin/dalfopristin is needed.

(1) Duration of therapy. If patient improvement is prompt, antimicrobial therapy should be continued for a total of 14 days. If a cephalosporin is being used, then some physicians will switch to PO therapy after the first 5 days. Severe *S. aureus* infections require antimicrobials for 3 weeks, and treatment with one IP antistaphylococcal drug plus PO rifampin is recommended (except in areas in which *M. tuberculosis* is endemic).

(2)   Nasal carriage and *S. aureus* infection. Patients in whom *S. aureus* peritonitis develops not uncommonly are found to carry this organism in the nose. Eradication of nasal carriage may help prevent further peritoneal infections by this bacterium. This can be accomplished with intranasal mupirocin (b.i.d. for 5 days every 4 weeks) or oral rifampin (300 mg b.i.d. for 5 days every 3 months). Nevertheless, resistance to mupirocin and rifampicin are increasingly common. Eradication of the carrier state should be documented by repeating appropriate cultures after antibacterial treatment.

b.   Gram-negative organism cultured. Recovery of a Gram-negative organism, even in a patient who is improving clinically, has several important implications: (a) Gram-negative infections (especially *Pseudomonas* species) are hard to eradicate and may require treatment with several antimicrobial drugs for a prolonged duration, (b) Gram-negative peritonitis may be a sign of unsuspected intra-abdominal pathology, and (c) prolonged treatment with aminoglycosides engenders the risk of otovestibular toxicity.

If a single, non-*Pseudomonas* species is recovered, the peritonitis can usually be treated by continuation of the initial IP third-generation cephalosporin or aminoglycoside alone, or by another single appropriate antibiotic. If a *Pseudomonas* species is recovered, then two antimicrobials are mandatory. The IP aminoglycoside should be continued with the addition of a third-generation cephalosporin administered IP or semisynthetic penicillin with anti-*Pseudomonas* activity (e.g., piperacillin) administered IV. Semisynthetic penicillins can inactivate aminoglycosides in vitro and thus should not be coadministered IP. Other alternatives are ciprofloxacin (or another quinolone), aztreonam, imipenem, and trimethoprim–sulfamethoxazole. *Pseudomonas* peritonitis requires catheter removal in up to two thirds of cases (Bunke et al., 1995). Fluoroquinolones (such as ciprofloxacin and ofloxacin) have the advantage that effective dialysate levels can usually be achieved after PO dosing; however, concurrent administration with phosphate-binding antacids should be avoided to ensure adequate absorption from the gastrointestinal tract. Often catheter removal is required.

(1)   Duration of therapy. In uncomplicated cases, duration of therapy for Gram-negative peritonitis should be 21 days. If the peritoneal catheter is removed, appropriate antipseudomonal antibiotics should be continued (either PO or IV) for another 2 weeks.

(2)   IP aminoglycoside toxicity. To treat Gram-negative peritonitis, a prolonged course (2 weeks) of aminoglycosides may be required. In the usual dosing strategy (after the loading dose), 4–6 mg/L of gentamicin, tobramycin, or netilmicin is added to the peritoneal dialysis solution. This results in constant serum drug levels, which may cause otovestibular toxicity. Adding a higher dose to a single bag only every 24 hours (e.g., 20 mg/L of gentamicin or tobramycin) avoids constant serum levels above 2 mg/L and might reduce the toxicity of IP aminoglycosides.

(3)   Alternative agents. Many Gram-negative organisms are sensitive to aztreonam, newer cephalosporins, quinolones, imipenem, or the semisynthetic penicillins. Use of these alternative agents should be considered both initially and when prolonged therapy of Gram-negative peritonitis is required.

(4)   Infection with *Pseudomonas cepacia*. A report of peritonitis with this agent traced the cause to contaminated povidone–iodine solutions (Panlilio et al., 1992). If this organism is cultured and if povidone–iodine was being used, contamination of the solution should be suspected.

(5)   Infection with *Stenotrophomonas* (formerly called *Xanthomonas*) species. The major risk factor for infection with *Stenotrophomonas maltophilia* is the previous use of broad-spectrum antibiotics. These are usually very resistant organisms. Medical therapy requires two antibiotics, usually including cotrimoxazole, and must be extended to a minimum of 3–4 weeks, and catheter removal is usually required (Szeto et al., 1997).

(6)   Infection with *Campylobacter* species. *Campylobacter* is an unusual cause of peritonitis. There is a strong association with acute enterocolitis, which may precede the onset of cloudy dialysate by many days. The method of spread of these organisms from the gastrointestinal tract to the peritoneal cavity is unknown. Treatment can include an IP aminoglycoside in combination with PO erythromycin (Wood et al., 1992).

(7)   Infection with *Pasteurella multocida*. This is a Gram-negative bacterium that resides in the upper respiratory tracts of animal hosts, especially dogs and cats. Peritonitis has been described after cat bites of the dialysis tubing.

c.   Polymicrobial peritonitis. Occasionally, more than one organism is recovered on culture. In general, peritonitis due to multiple Gram-positive organisms will respond to antibiotic therapy. About 60% of these infections can be resolved without catheter removal (Holley et al., 1992). Surgical evaluation is not routinely required.

(1)   Secondary peritonitis. When one of the organisms recovered is Gram negative or an anaerobe such as *Clostridium* or *Bacteroides,* this is a poor prognostic sign, suggestive of the presence of an intra-abdominal abscess or a perforated abdominal viscus. Perforated diverticulum, tubo-ovarian abscess, cholecystitis, appendicitis, perforated ulcer, and pancreatitis must all be included in the differential diagnosis. The occurrence of an abdominal catastrophe in PD patients is associated with a high mortality (Kern et al., 2002).

Management of secondary peritonitis must be individualized. Initial management can be accomplished by triple-antibiotic therapy aimed at Gram-positive, Gram-negative, and anaerobic organisms. Use of an IP aminoglycoside, IP vancomycin, and PO metronidazole is one possible strategy. If multiple enteric organisms are grown, particularly in association with anaerobic bacteria, the risk of death is increased and a surgical evaluation should be obtained.

d.   Culture-negative peritonitis. If the culture results are negative at 24 hours, then the most likely explanation is that a bacterial infection was present but that the responsible organisms failed to grow in the culture sample. Sometimes growth appears only after 5–7 days, and cultures should be incubated for this length of time. Management depends on whether the patient is improving clinically. Although some continue both the initial aminoglycoside and cephalosporin for a full 14 days, many recommend discontinuing the aminoglycoside after 3 days if the patient is improving in order to limit the side effects.

Infection with *M. tuberculosis* or with nontuberculous mycobacteria sometimes presents as culture-negative peritonitis. The differential cell count cannot be used to differentiate mycobacterial peritonitis from other forms. When mycobacterial peritonitis is suspected, special attention must be paid to culture techniques. Diagnostic sensitivity can be improved by culturing the sediment after centrifugation of a large volume of effluent (50–100 mL) using a solid medium (such as Lowenstein Jensen agar) and a fluid medium (Septi-chek, BACTEC, etc). Catheter removal is usually required but is not mandatory provided prompt therapy is carried out. This consists of a multiple-drug regimen (usually isoniazid, rifampin, ofloxacin, and pyrazinamide). Streptomycin and ethambutol are generally not recommended in dialysis patients.

Patients with culture-negative peritonitis who do not improve should be recultured using special culture techniques to look for unusual organisms such as yeast, mycobacteria, Legionella, Campylobacter, Ureaplasma, Mycoplasma, enteroviruses, and fungi. As an example, *Histoplasma capsulatum* peritonitis requires special staining and fungal culture media (Marcic et al., 2006).

e.   Fungal peritonitis. Factors predisposing to fungal peritonitis include prior antibiotic use, immunosuppression (e.g., immunosuppressive therapy, HIV infection), and malnutrition, especially a low serum albumin level. A variety of fungi are sometimes cultured; *Candida* is the most prevalent species, but many types of fungi can be responsible. Cases due to *Paecilomyces* species may occur (Wright et al., 2003). Previous antibiotic therapy and diabetes mellitus are predisposing factors. In the past, some recommended that selected patients could be treated with antifungal agents without catheter removal. However, the ISPD now recommends prompt removal of the catheter as soon as fungi are identified by Gram stain or culture in addition to treatment for at least 10 days with antifungal agents after catheter removal. The patient is then maintained on hemodialysis. In some patients, a new catheter can be inserted 4–6 weeks later, and at least 1 week after all clinical evidence of peritonitis has subsided.

In an attempt to limit adhesion formation, in addition to catheter removal, prolonged PO administration of antifungal drugs, such as flucytosine, miconazole, fluconazole, ketoconazole, itraconazole, or voriconazole, has been employed. The recommended dosages of these agents are the same as for patients with normal renal function, with the exception of flucytosine, for which the dosage must be reduced (see Chapter 33). However, penetration of many antifungal drugs (e.g., amphotericin B, ketoconazole) into the peritoneum after other than IP administration is poor. Penetration of flucytosine is relatively good, and a reduced incidence of peritoneal adhesion formation has been claimed after its use in fungal peritonitis. Recently voriconazole has been utilized as an alternative to amphotericin B for *Candida* peritonitis.

4. Refractory peritonitis and indications for catheter removal. Refractory peritonitis is defined as peritonitis treated with appropriate antibiotics for 5 days without resolution. Catheter removal is indicated in such cases in order to reduce morbidity and preserve the peritoneum. Ultrasonography, computed tomography, or gallium scan is indicated if an intra-abdominal abscess is suspected, since in such cases surgical exploration and drainage may be needed at the time of catheter removal.

In general, it is preferable to remove the PD catheter in patients who do not promptly respond to antimicrobials rather than subject the patient to a long period of exposure to antibiotics (with increased risk of superinfection and morbidity) and of damage to the peritoneal membrane, precluding future peritoneal dialysis. Increased age and duration of peritonitis are associated with both requirement for PD catheter removal and prolonged postoperative hospitalization (Choi et al., 2004). PD catheter removal is also more likely when the causative organism is Gram-negative, possibly because of difficulty in obtaining adequate drug concentrations in the biofilm (Sepandj et al., 2004). After catheter removal, the safe time interval before a new catheter can be reinserted is a matter of controversy; it probably depends on the severity of the underlying peritonitis and whether fungal peritonitis or tunnel infection was present. A conservative approach is to wait 4–6 weeks. Resumption of PD is possible in approximately one half of patients, but may necessitate a change in dialysis prescription to achieve adequate dialysis and ultrafiltration (Szeto et al., 2002).

5. Relapsing peritonitis. Relapsing peritonitis is defined as peritonitis with the same organism within 4 weeks of stopping antimicrobial therapy. *S. epidermidis* or a Gram-negative organism is usually involved, but "relapsing" culture-negative peritonitis is also common. In the case of relapsing Gram-negative peritonitis, catheter removal with or without surgical exploration should be strongly considered, especially in patients with *Pseudomonas* infection. If it is elected to treat the patient medically, because of the dangers of prolonged aminoglycoside therapy, either the IP maintenance aminoglycoside dose should be administered intermittently or an alternative agent should be employed. With less serious infections, it may be possible to insert a new catheter simultaneously with removal of the old catheter, obviating the need for hemodialysis. The new catheter should be inserted as far as possible from the old skin exit site. This approach has been especially useful in the management of relapsing peritonitis due to coagulase-negative staphylococci.

    a. Treatment with fibrinolytic enzymes. Streptokinase and urokinase have been used by some investigators in the treatment of relapsing peritonitis. These agents are utilized in an attempt to release bacteria entrapped in fibrin within the peritoneum or along the catheter, thus making it possible to eradicate the infection. Controlled studies on the use of such agents in the treatment of relapsing peritonitis are warranted.

6. Peritonitis with catheter obstruction. Catheter obstruction frequently accompanies peritonitis. Management is discussed in Chapter 20.

7. Prophylactic antibiotic use. Prophylactic antibiotic use does not prevent peritonitis; this is probably true even for patients with exit site infections. However, short-term prophylactic antibiotics may be beneficial in the following settings: (a) before catheter placement (vancomycin or cefazolin); (b) after a technique break (vancomycin); (c) to prevent bacteremia during invasive procedures, such as dental procedures (amoxicillin 2.0 g) or colonoscopic polypectomy (ampicillin plus an aminoglycoside); and (d) to prevent exit site infection in the presence of *S. aureus* nasal carriage. Based on a recent controlled trial, vancomycin 1.0 g IV at the time of PD catheter placement is preferable to cefazolin (Gadallah et al., 2000).

II. Exit site infection. Approximately one fifth of peritonitis episodes are temporally associated with exit site and tunnel infections (Piraino et al., 2005).

A. Incidence. The incidence of exit site infections is approximately one episode every 24–48 patient-months. Patients with previous infections tend to have a higher frequency of occurrence.

B. Etiology and pathogenesis. Exit site infections are predominantly due to *S. aureus* or Gram-negative organisms, particularly *Pseudomonas*. In contrast to peritonitis, *S. epidermidis* is the causative organism in <20% of patients. *S. aureus* infections appear to have a distinct pathogenesis as they are associated with nasal and/or skin carriage of the organism (Luzar et al., 1990a,b). Therefore, eradication of the carrier state is very helpful to effective management.

C.   Therapy. Treatment is dependent on whether there is erythema alone or erythema in conjunction with purulent drainage. In the former case, topical treatment with hypertonic saline compresses, hydrogen peroxide, or mupirocin 2% ointment is usually sufficient. Mupirocin ointment should not be used with polyurethane catheters (e.g., many catheters made by Vas-Cath or the Cruz catheter from Corpak) because the polyethylene glycol in mupirocin ointment will degrade the polyurethane and destroy the catheter. Ciprofloxacin otologic solution can be used with polyurethane catheters, but efficacy in treating exit site infection is unknown.

Treatment is more problematic and more prone to failure when there is purulent drainage. Moreover, some exit site infections extend into the subcutaneous tunnel, which may be evident only on ultrasonographic examination of the tunnel tract (Vychytil et al., 1999). Therapy for purulent exit site infection should be based on results of Gram stain and culture. If Gram-positive organisms are found, a cephalosporin or an antistaphylococcal penicillin PO is first-line treatment; IP vancomycin should be avoided unless necessary. If no improvement occurs after 1 week despite appropriate treatment based on culture and sensitivity, rifampin 600 mg/day PO may be added. If the infection has not resolved in 2 weeks, a surgical approach (deroofing, outer-cuff shaving, or catheter removal) is necessary. In the presence of tunnel infection, early cuff excision in combination with antibiotic administration results in a substantial rate of catheter salvage (Suh et al., 1997), although catheter removal is sometimes required, especially when there is coexisting peritonitis.

If Gram-negative organisms are present, treatment should be based on sensitivity results. Oral quinolones are useful, though care must be taken to avoid ingestion of multivalent cations (calcium, iron, zinc, antacids) within 2 hours of drug ingestion. With more serious pseudomonal infections, IP ceftazidime or aminoglycoside may be necessary. Therapy should be continued until the exit site appears normal. If the exit site infection has not improved substantially within 4 weeks, catheter removal is generally required. *Pseudomonas* exit site infections often require catheter removal. With any organism, if prolonged therapy with appropriate antibiotics fails to resolve the infection, removal of the catheter with replacement at a different site as a single procedure is recommended. Table 24-6 lists appropriate oral antimicrobial doses for treatment of exit site infections.

D.   Prevention. The major risk factor for exit site infection is staphylococcal nasal carriage. Persistently positive nasal cultures are associated with a threefold to fourfold increased risk of staphylococcal exit site infection. Therefore, it is logical to attempt to eradicate nasal carriage to prevent these infections. Protocols used include rifampin (600 mg PO for 5 days), mupirocin (2% ointment twice daily for 5 days every 4 weeks), and trimethoprim–sulfamethoxazole (one

Table 24-6. Oral Antimicrobial doses for exit site and tunnel infections

Amoxicillin	250–500 mg b.i.d.
Cephalexin	500 mg b.i.d.
Ciprofloxacin	250–500 mg b.i.d.
Clarithromycin	250–500 mg b.i.d.
Dicloxacillin	250–500 mg b.i.d.
Fluconazole	200 mg q.day
Flucloxacillin	500 mg b.i.d.
Flucytosine	2-g load, then 1 g PO, q.day
Isoniazid	300 mg q.day
Linezolid	600 mg b.i.d.
Metronidazole	400 mg b.i.d. for <50 kg
	400–500 t.i.d. for >50 kg
Ofloxacin	400 mg first day, then 200 mg q.day
Pyrazinamide	35 mg/kg q.day (given as b.i.d. or once daily)
Rifampin	450 mg q.day for <50 kg
	600 mg q.day for >50 kg
Trimethoprim/ sulfamethoxazole	80/400 mg q.day

b.i.d., two times per day; q.day, every day; PO, orally; t.i.d., three times per day. Source: Piraino B, et al. Peritoneal dialysis-related infections recommendations: 2005 update. *Perit Dial Int* 2005;25:107–131.

single-strength tablet three times weekly). In a randomized, controlled trial, rifampin 600 mg PO for 5 days given every 3 months was effective in decreasing catheter infections (Zimmerman et al., 1991). In a multicenter randomized trial (Mupirocin Study Group, 1996), use of nasal mupirocin using the regimen stated above in *S. aureus* nasal carriers resulted in a significant decline in exit site infections from this organism; however, the overall incidence of exit site infections was not decreased due to an increase in Gram-negative infections, and rates of tunnel infection and peritonitis were not affected. In other trials, mupirocin ointment applied daily to the exit site decreased the rate of both exit site infections and peritonitis in comparison with a historical control group (Bernardini et al., 1996; Thodis et al., 1998).

Gentamicin cream has been shown to be as effective as mupirocin in preventing *S. aureus* infections and also reduced catheter infections due to *P. aeruginosa* and other Gram-negative organisms (Bernardini et al., 2005); peritonitis, particularly that caused by Gram-negative organisms, was reduced by 35%. Because of its efficacy against both Gram-positive and Gram-negative infections, daily gentamicin cream at the exit site may be the prophylaxis of choice.

There does not appear to be a difference in the incidence of exit site infections between double-cuff and single-cuff catheters, although the method of catheter placement may be important. The Moncrief technique (see Chapter 20) of leaving the catheter subcutaneously for several weeks after placement and then exteriorizing it prior to use may reduce the rate of exit site infection. Use of chlorhexidine versus povidone–iodine solution is associated with a significant decrease in exit site infections in children (Jones et al., 1995). Use of protective dressings incorporating povidone iodine may also be of benefit (Luzar et al., 1990a).

SELECTED READINGS

Bernardini J, et al. A randomized trial of *Staphylococcus aureus* prophylaxis in peritoneal dialysis patients; mupirocin calcium ointment 2% applied to the exit site versus cyclic oral rifampin. *Am J Kidney Dis* 1996;27:695–700.

Bernardini J, et al. Randomized, double-blind trial of antibiotic exit site cream for prevention of exit site infection in peritoneal dialysis patients. *J Am Soc Nephrol* 2005;16:539–545.

Bunke M, et al. *Pseudomonas* peritonitis in peritoneal dialysis patients: the Network 9 Peritonitis Study. *Am J Kidney Dis* 1995;25:769–774.

Choi P, et al. Peritoneal dialysis catheter removal for acute peritonitis: a retrospective analysis of factors associated with catheter removal and prolonged postoperative hospitalization. *Am J Kidney Dis* 2004;43:103–111.

Daugirdas JT, et al. Induction of peritoneal fluid eosinophilia and/or monocytosis by intraperitoneal air injection. *Am J Nephrol* 1987;7:116–120.

Fielding RE, et al. Treatment and outcome of peritonitis in automated peritoneal dialysis, using a once-daily cefazolin-based regimen. *Perit Dial Int* 2002;22:345–349.

Gadallah M, et al. Role of preoperative antibiotic prophylaxis in preventing postoperative peritonitis in newly placed peritoneal dialysis catheters. *Am J Kidney Dis* 2000;36:1014–1019.

Gahrmani N, et al. Infection rates in end-stage renal disease patients treated with CCPD and CAPD using the UltraBag system. *Adv Perit Dial* 1995;11:164–167.

Goldie SJ, et al. Fungal peritonitis in a large chronic peritoneal dialysis population: a report of 55 episodes. *Am J Kidney Dis* 1996;28:86–91.

Holley JL, et al. Polymicrobial peritonitis in patients on continuous peritoneal dialysis. *Am J Kidney Dis* 1992;19:162–166.

Humayun HM, et al. Peritoneal fluid eosinophilia in patients undergoing maintenance peritoneal dialysis. *Arch Intern Med* 1981;141:1172–1173.

Jones LL, et al. The impact of exit-site care and catheter design on the incidence of catheter-related infections. *Adv Perit Dial* 1995;11:302–305.

Katirtzoglou A, et al. "Pseudoperitonitis" in CAPD patients during travel. *Perit Dial Bull* 1985;5:140.

Kern EO, et al. Abdominal catastrophe revisited: the risk and outcome of enteric peritoneal contamination. *Perit Dial Int* 2002;22:323–324.

Kimmel PL, et al. Continuous ambulatory peritoneal dialysis and survival of HIV infected patients with end-stage renal disease. *Kidney Int* 1993;44:373–378.

Lai MN, et al. Intraperitoneal once-daily dosing of cefazolin and gentamicin for treating CAPD peritonitis. *Perit Dial Int* 1997;17: 87–89.

Li PKT, et al. Comparison of clinical outcome and ease of handling in two double-bag systems in continuous ambulatory peritoneal dialysis—a prospective randomized controlled multi-center study. *Am J Kidney Dis* 2002;40:373–380.

Low CL, et al. Pharmacokinetics on once-daily IP gentamicin in CAPD patients. *Perit Dial Int* 1996;16:379–384.

Luzar MA, et al. Exit-site care and exit-site infection in continuous ambulatory peritoneal dialysis (CAPD): results of a randomized multicenter trial. *Perit Dial Int* 1990a;10:25–29.

Luzar MA, et al. *Staphylococcus aureus* nasal carriage and infection in patients on continuous ambulatory peritoneal dialysis. *N Engl J Med* 1990b;322:505–509.

Manley HJ, et al. Pharmacokinetics of intermittent intraperitoneal cefazolin in continuous ambulatory peritoneal dialysis patients. *Perit Dial Int* 1999;19:67–70.

Manley HJ, Bailie GR. Treatment of peritonitis in APD: pharmacokinetic principles. *Semin Dial* 2002;15:418–421.

Marcic SM, et al. 'Culture-negative' peritonitis due to histoplasma capsulatum. *Nephrol Dial Transplant* 2006, Jun 17 (Epub).

Monteon F, et al. Prevention of peritonitis with disconnect systems in CAPD: a randomized controlled trial. The Mexican Nephrology Collaborative Study Group. *Kidney Int* 1998;54:2123–2138.

Mupirocin Study Group. Nasal mupirocin prevents *Staphylococcus aureus* exit-site infection during peritoneal dialysis. *J Am Soc Nephrol* 1996;7:2403–2408.

Panlilio AL, et al. Infections and pseudoinfections due to povidone–iodine solution contaminated with *Pseudomonas cepacia. Clin Infect Dis* 1992;14:1078–1083.

Piraino B. A review of *Staphylococcus aureus* exit-site and tunnel infections in peritoneal dialysis patients. *Am J Kidney Dis* 1990;16:89–95.

Piraino B, et al. Increased risk of *Staphylococcus epidermidis* peritonitis in patients on dialysate containing 1.25 mmol/L calcium. *Am J Kidney Dis* 1992;19:371–374.

Piraino B, et al. Peritoneal dialysis-related infections recommendations: 2005 update. *Perit Dial Int* 2005;25:107–131.

Posthuma N, et al. Simultaneous peritoneal dialysis catheter insertion and removal in catheter-related infections without interruption of peritoneal dialysis. *Nephrol Dial Transplant* 1998;13:700–703.

Schaefer F, et al. Intermittent versus continuous intraperitoneal glycopeptide/ceftazidime treatment in children with peritoneal dialysis-associated peritonitis. *J Am Soc Nephrol* 1999;10:136–145.

Sepandj F, et al. Minimum inhibitory concentration versus minimum biofilm eliminating concentration in evaluation of antibiotic sensitivity of Gram negative bacilli causing peritonitis. *Perit Dial Int* 2004;24:65–67.

Shemin D, et al. Effect of aminoglycoside use on residual renal function in peritoneal dialysis patients. *Am J Kidney Dis* 1999;34: 14–20.

Suh H, et al. Persistent exit-site/tunnel infection and subcutaneous cuff removal in PD patients. *Adv Perit Dial* 1997;13:233–236.

Szeto CC, et al. Feasibility of resuming peritoneal dialysis after severe peritonitis and Tenckhoff catheter removal. *J Am Soc Nephrol* 2002;13:1040–1045.

Szeto CC, et al. Xanthomonas maltophilia peritonitis in uremic patients receiving continuous ambulatory peritoneal dialysis. *Am J Kidney Dis* 1997;29:91–96.

Teitelbaum I. Cloudy peritoneal dialysate: it's not always infection. *Contrib Nephrol* 2006;150:187–194.

Troidle L, Finkelstein F. Treatment and outcome of CPD-associated peritonitis. *Ann Clin Microbiol Antimicrob* 2006;5:6.

Vas S, et al. Treatment in PD patients of peritonitis caused by gram-positive organisms with single daily dose of antibiotics. *Perit Dial Int* 1997;17:91–94.

Vychytil A, et al. Ultrasonography of the catheter tunnel in peritoneal dialysis patients: what are the indications? *Am J Kidney Dis* 1999;33:722–727.

Waite NM, et al. Poor response to oral ciprofloxacin in the treatment of peritonitis in patients on intermittent peritoneal dialysis. *Perit Dial Int* 1993;13:50–54.

Wood CJ, et al. *Campylobacter* peritonitis in continuous ambulatory peritoneal dialysis: report of eight cases and a review of the literature. *Am J Kidney Dis* 1992;19:257–263.

Wright K, et al. Paecilomyces peritonitis: case report and review of the literature. *Clin Nephrol* 2003;59:305–310.

Yu AW, et al. Neutrophilic intracellular acidosis induced by conventional lactate-containing peritoneal dialysis solutions. *Int J Artif Organs* 1992;15:661–665.

Zimmerman SW, et al. Randomized controlled trial of prophylactic rifampin for peritoneal dialysis–related infections. *Am J Kidney Dis* 1991;18:225–231.

Mechanical Complications of Peritoneal Dialysis

Joanne M. Bargman

The instillation of dialysis fluid into the peritoneal cavity is accompanied by an increase in intra-abdominal pressure (IAP). The two principal determinants of the magnitude of the increased IAP are dialysate volume and the position of the patient during the dwell. The supine position is associated with the lowest IAP for a given dialysate volume; sitting entails the highest. Furthermore, actions such as coughing, bending, or straining at stool transiently cause very high levels of IAP. The increased IAP in peritoneal dialysis can lead to a variety of mechanical complications.

I. Hernia formation
A. Incidence and etiologic factors. The incidence and prevalence of hernias are difficult to assess. Hernias can be asymptomatic and difficult to diagnose on cursory examination. It has been suggested that as many as 10%–20% of patients may develop a hernia at some time on peritoneal dialysis.

Potential risk factors are listed in Table 25-1 and include large dialysate volumes and activities that involve isometric straining or the Valsalva maneuver. Furthermore, deconditioning of the musculature of the abdominal wall increases wall tension and predisposes to hernia formation.

B. Types of hernia. Many different types of hernias have been described in the peritoneal dialysis patient. These are listed in Table 25-2.

Indirect inguinal hernias are the result of bowel and/or dialysate tracking through the processus vaginalis, which has remained patent rather than obliterating normally. It is much more common in males. In boys, it is very likely that if one processus vaginalis is patent (causing inguinal hernia), then the other side is patent also, and repair (see below) should be done bilaterally.

C. Diagnosis. As mentioned above, hernias can be clinically occult. It is often better to have the patient stand and "bear down" as this increases IAP and makes a hernia even more obvious.

Pericatheter hernias need to be differentiated from masses caused by a hematoma, seroma, or abscess. Ultrasonography can distinguish the solid-appearing hernia from the fluid collections characterizing these other conditions. The scrotal fullness of an indirect inguinal hernia has in its differential diagnoses hydrocele (fluid/dialysate alone seeping through a patent processus vaginalis) and intrinsic scrotal or testicular pathology.

Table 25-1. Potential risk factors for hernia formation

Large dialysis solution volumes
Sitting position
Isometric exercise
Valsalva maneuver (e.g., coughing, chopping wood)
Recent abdominal surgery
Pericatheter leak or hematoma
Obesity
Deconditioning
Multiparity
Congenital anatomical defects

Delineation of a hernia can be aided by computed tomography (CT) scanning. One hundred milliliters of Omnipaque 300 (an iohexol preparation manufactured by Amersham Health, Amersham, UK) is added to a 2-L bag of dialysis solution and then infused into the patient. **It is important that the patient then be as active and ambulatory as possible for the next 2 hours to facilitate the entry of dye into hernia sacs.** CT scanning is then performed. In the case of inguinal hernias, it is important that the genitalia be scanned. The CT scan can indicate whether scrotal edema is the result of fluid tracking along a patent processus vaginalis or along the anterior abdominal wall (see below). This procedure can also help delineate anterior abdominal wall hernia from isolated leaks. In other types of hernia, such as umbilical hernia, CT scanning is not necessary because the diagnosis is usually obvious.

Early experience with magnetic resonance imaging suggests that it may be useful in the diagnosis of abdominal wall and genital leaks. The dialysate itself is used as the "dye," and therefore it may be helpful in patients with allergy to conventional radiologic dye.

D. Treatment. Small hernias pose the greatest risk of incarceration or strangulation of bowel. These should be repaired surgically. The patient should be warned that if a hernia stops being reducible, and especially if it becomes tender, medical consultation should be sought immediately. **Any patient**

Table 25-2. Types of hernias reported in peritoneal dialysis patients

Ventral
Epigastric
Pericatheter
Umbilical
Inguinal (direct and indirect)
Femoral
Spigelian
Richter
Foramen of Morgagni
Cystocele
Enterocele

presenting with peritonitis should be examined for the presence of small strangulated hernias, as these can lead to transmural leakage of bacteria and peritonitis. Large hernias can also be repaired surgically, as can cystocele and enterocele. Uterine prolapse (not really a hernia) can sometimes be managed with a pessary, but ultimately hysterectomy may be necessary.

After surgical repair of a hernia, IAP must be kept as low as possible to facilitate healing. If the patient has significant residual renal function (e.g., 10 mL per minute or more), it may be possible to stop dialysis altogether for a week and then recommence with small volumes (e.g., 1 L) for another week. With less residual renal function, it may still be possible to hold dialysis for one or two days and then recommence PD with smaller volumes. The patient must be watched for the development of uremic symptoms or hyperkalemia. If continuous cycling peritoneal dialysis (CCPD) is available, then the patient can dialyze supine and hence with lower IAP. If there is little or no renal function, low-volume peritoneal dialysis should be started postoperatively. An alternative is to hemodialyze the patient until wound healing is more complete (2–3 weeks).

Options for the patient with recurrent hernias include a reduction in physical activities (e.g., stop chopping wood), more frequent dialysis exchanges with lower volumes (e.g., 5 × 1.5 L), CCPD with a small (e.g., 1-L) or short-duration day dwell, or transfer to hemodialysis.

If the patient is too ill or refuses surgery, mechanical support of the hernia can be effected with a corset or truss. The patient should be warned about symptoms of incarceration and strangulation.

II. Abdominal wall and pericatheter leak. The incidence of these complications is also unknown, but they are less common than hernias. Risk factors are similar to those outlined in Table 25-2, and surgical technique may play a role in the development of pericatheter leak.

A. Diagnosis. Abdominal wall leak may be difficult to diagnose clinically. It may be mistaken for ultrafiltration failure when dialysate returns are less than the instilled volume (Chapter 23). Weight gain is common as the dialysate accumulates in the tissues of the abdominal wall. The diagnosis should be considered with decreased effluent volumes, weight gain, protuberant abdomen, and absence of generalized edema. The patient should stand during the examination as this may reveal asymmetry of the abdomen. The abdominal wall itself may have a "boggy" look, with deep impressions made by waist bands, dialysate tubing, etc.

Pericatheter leak is usually diagnosed by wetness (dialysate) on the exit site dressing. Diagnosis can be proven using contrast CT scanning as described under "Hernia formation" (Section I C). Again, it is important to make sure that the patient is ambulatory for at least 2 hours after instillation of the dye to facilitate its movement into the abdominal wall.

B. Treatment. Pericatheter leak usually occurs as a postoperative complication of catheter implantation. It is not helpful to place pursestring sutures in response to the leak because the dialysate will then be diverted into the intervening tissue rather than exit around the catheter site. The patient should be drained and peritoneal dialysis stopped for at least 24–48 hours. The longer the patient can be left dialysate-free, the greater the chance that the leak will seal. If necessary, the patient should receive hemodialysis, and peritoneal dialysis can be recommenced several days later. In most cases, the leak seals spontaneously. If it persists, the catheter should be removed and reinserted at another site.

In contrast to pericatheter leaks, abdominal wall leaks can occur early or late. CCPD in the supine position usually allows the dialysate accumulation to resolve. If the leak is the result of disruption of abdominal wall integrity, the patient should be converted to a nocturnal intermittent peritoneal dialysis (NIPD) regimen or to hemodialysis. Sometimes the abdominal wall defect heals after a transient course of NIPD, and continuous ambulatory peritoneal dialysis (CAPD) can then be resumed. Sometimes surgical repair is feasible. Antibiotic prophylaxis is not usually necessary for pericatheter leak unless there are obvious signs of infection.

Vaginal leaks can also occur. Some may result from tracking of dialysate through the fallopian tubes and may resolve with tubal ligation. Other incidents are due to dissection of dialysate through fascial defects and require patients to convert to NIPD or hemodialysis.

III. Genital edema

A. Pathogenesis. Dialysate can reach the genitalia by two routes: One is by traveling through a patent processus vaginalis to the tunica vaginalis, resulting in hydrocele. In this first route, the dialysate can also dissect through the tunica vaginalis, causing edema of the scrotal wall itself. The second route is through a defect in the abdominal wall, often associated with the catheter. In this instance, the dialysate tracks inferiorly along the abdominal wall and leads to edema of the foreskin and scrotum.

B. Diagnosis. This complication is often painful and distressing to the patient who is quick to bring it to medical attention. CT peritoneography should be performed to distinguish which route has led to the genital swelling (i.e., anterior abdominal wall or processus vaginalis). Alternatively, 3–5 mCi of technetium-labeled albumin colloid can be injected into the dialysate and infused into the patient, and the route of leakage traced by scintigraphy.

C. Treatment. Peritoneal dialysis should be temporarily stopped. Bed rest and scrotal elevation are helpful. Depending on the need, temporary CCPD with low volumes and with the patient supine can often be used without causing reaccumulation of genital edema. Hemodialysis can be used temporarily.

A leak via a patent processus vaginalis can be repaired surgically. If the leak is through the anterior abdominal wall, replacement of the catheter can be helpful. One needs to allow time for healing of the previous defect with hemodialysis support. CCPD in the supine position allows lower IAP and decreases the chances of recurrent leakage.

IV.   Respiratory complications

A.   Hydrothorax. Under the influence of raised IAP, dialysate can travel from the peritoneal to the pleural cavity, leading to a pleural effusion composed of dialysis effluent. This complication is termed hydrothorax.

1.   Incidence and etiologic factors. The incidence of hydrothorax is unknown because the pleural effusion may be small and asymptomatic. It is less common than hernia.

There are defects in the hemidiaphragm that allow passage of dialysate. These defects may be congenital, in which case hydrothorax can occur with the first dialysis exchange, or acquired, whereby hydrothorax can be a late complication. They occur almost exclusively on the right side, probably because the left hemidiaphragm is mostly covered by heart and pericardium.

2.   Diagnosis. Symptoms of hydrothorax range from asymptomatic pleural effusion to severe shortness of breath. Such symptoms may worsen with administration of hypertonic dialysate, which raises IAP.

Thoracentesis can be done for diagnosis or to relieve symptoms. The most diagnostic feature of the pleural fluid is the very high glucose level, although this is not always a consistent finding. It is otherwise typically transudative, with variable numbers of leukocytes.

Radionuclide scanning with technetium is also helpful. Technetium-labeled albumin colloid (5 mCi) is added to a dialysis solution bag, which is then infused into the patient. Posterior views are taken at 0, 10, 20, and 30 minutes and an anterior view at 30 minutes. It is important that the patient be ambulatory while the instilled tracer is dwelling to increase IAP and flux into the pleural cavity. Late (2–3 hours) views may be necessary if the movement of tracer into pleural cavity is not detected by gamma camera in earlier shots.

3.   Treatment. If there are respiratory symptoms, peritoneal dialysis should be stopped immediately. Thoracentesis may be necessary; in which case the diagnosis can be made by measuring glucose in the pleural fluid.

Definitive treatment entails repair of defects in the hemidiaphragm or obliteration of the pleural space (pleurodesis). Rarely, the dialysate itself acts as an irritant in the pleural cavity and causes pleurodesis, so that peritoneal dialysis can be resumed 1–2 weeks later. Peritoneal dialysis with low IAP (small volumes, supine position) can

Table 25-3.   Surgical options for treatment of hydrothorax

Pleurodesis
    Talc
    Oxytetracycline
    Autologous blood
    Aprotinin–fibrin glue
Repair of hemidiaphragm
    Oversewing defects
    Reinforcement with patches

sometimes be carried out without recurrence. Surgical options for treatment of hydrothorax are listed in Table 25-3.

B. Altered mechanics of breathing. Pulmonary function is unchanged with peritoneal dialysis, except for a mildly decreased functional residual capacity. Arterial oxygenation has been observed to decrease slightly and transiently with the start of CAPD.

Peritoneal dialysis does not worsen respiratory symptoms in patients with obstructive airway disease. The tonic stretch placed on the diaphragm by the raised IAP may actually facilitate the mechanics of breathing in these patients.

V. Back pain

A. Pathogenesis. The presence of dialysate in the peritoneal cavity both raises IAP and swings the center of gravity forward, producing lordotic stress on the lumbar vertebrae and paraspinal muscles. In predisposed individuals, the altered spinal mechanics can lead to exacerbation of sciatica or posterior facet symptoms. Lax anterior abdominal musculature will exacerbate this effect.

B. Treatment. Bed rest and analgesia are important when symptoms are acute. Some patients benefit from the performance of more frequent exchanges with smaller dialysate volumes. If possible, CCPD with a small day dwell is advisable for these patients in order to dialyze supine and so remove the lordotic stress on the lumbar spine. Ideally, the patient should undertake abdomen and back strengthening exercises, but this is not always feasible.

SELECTED READINGS

Chow KM, et al. Management options for hydrothorax complicating peritoneal dialysis. *Semin Dial* 2003;16:389–394.

Cochran ST, et al. Complications of peritoneal dialysis: evaluation with CT peritoneography. *Radiographics* 1997;17:869–878.

Derici U, et al. Dialysate leakage in CAPD patients. *EDTNA ERCA J* 2005;31(1):13–14.

Garcia-Urena MA, et al. Prevalence and management of hernias in peritoneal dialysis patients. *Perit Dial Int* 2006;26(2):198–202.

Juergensen PH, et al. Value of scintigraphy in chronic peritoneal dialysis patients. *Kidney Int* 1999;55:1111–1119.

Litherland J, et al. Computed tomographic peritoneography: CT manifestations in the investigation of leaks and abnormal collections in patients on CAPD. *Nephrol Dial Transplant* 1994;9:1449–1452.

Mak SK, et al. Long-term follow-up of thoracoscopic pleurodesis for hydrothorax complicating peritoneal dialysis. *Ann Thorac Surg* 2002;74:218–221.

Morris-Stiff GJ, et al. Management of inguinal herniae in patients on continuous ambulatory peritoneal dialysis: an audit of current UK practice. *Postgrad Med J* 1998;74:669–670.

Prischl F, et al. Magnetic resonance imaging of the peritoneal cavity among peritoneal dialysis patients, using the dialysate as "contrast medium." *J Am Soc Nephrol* 2002;13:197–203.

Wanke T, et al. Diaphragmatic function in patients on continuous ambulatory peritoneal dialysis. *Lung* 1994;172:231–240.

Metabolic Complications of Peritoneal Dialysis

Sarah S. Prichard

Peritoneal dialysis (PD) is generally well tolerated and serves as an effective form of renal replacement therapy for most patients. However, PD can be associated with a number of metabolic abnormalities that warrant attention and appropriate intervention.

   I.   Glucose absorption. Glucose remains the standard agent added to PD fluid as an osmotic agent, although amino acids and polyglucose solutions have become available as alternatives. Glucose has the advantage of being cheap, stable, and relatively nontoxic to the peritoneum. However, it is easily absorbed across the peritoneal membrane. This is measured in the standard peritoneal equilibration test (PET), which demonstrates that there is variability from patient to patient depending on peritoneal transport characteristics, but as much as 60%–80% of the dialysis solution glucose can be absorbed with each continuous ambulatory peritoneal dialysis (CAPD) exchange. Since automated peritoneal dialysis (APD) cycles tend to be shorter than in CAPD, the percent of glucose absorbed with each exchange will be less, but is still significant. Depending on the glucose concentration of solutions used and the length of the exchanges, up to 100–150 g per day of glucose may be absorbed, which represents 500–800 kcal per day. This constitutes a significant portion of the recommended total energy intake of about 2,500 kcal per day (35 kcal/kg per day) in a 70-kg patient. In some patients, this provides a welcome source of calories since achieving the nutritional recommendation for PD is often difficult. The caloric loading is also in part responsible for the 5%–10% weight gain frequently seen during a patient's first year on PD. In patients who start PD obese, the glucose loading from PD may contribute to further weight gain.
   There are, however, disadvantages to dialysis solution glucose absorption. It results in increased insulin secretion, which together with insulin resistance (a common feature of chronic renal failure) results in plasma insulin levels that are persistently high. Hyperinsulinemia may be an independent risk factor for the development of atherosclerosis. In certain patients, the glucose loading can result in hyperglycemia severe enough to require the initiation of oral hypoglycemics or insulin therapy. Patients who were previously well controlled on oral hypoglycemics often require increased doses of these medications, and they may even require a change to insulin therapy after the initiation of PD. Patients should be advised of this possibility prior to starting PD (see Chapter 30 regarding

management of diabetes in PD patients). The hypertriglyceridemia found in PD patients is at least in part related to glucose absorption.

To minimize glucose absorption, patients should be advised on appropriate salt and water management, which will diminish the need for hypertonic solutions to maintain fluid balance. When available, non–glucose-based solutions such as polyglucose or amino acids solutions can be prescribed as a glucose-sparing strategy. In fact, recent evidence suggests that use of icodextrin solutions improves the plasma lipid profile and function of adipocytes (Furuya et al., 2006).

II. Lipid abnormalities. Patients on PD have a variety of lipid abnormalities. Typically, they have high total and low-density lipoprotein (LDL) cholesterol, high triglycerides, low high-density lipoprotein (HDL) cholesterol, high apolipoprotein B (apoB), low apoA-I, and high lipoprotein(a) (Lp[a]) levels. Compared with hemodialysis patients, the most striking differences are the high apoB protein and LDL cholesterol levels, which are usually normal in hemodialysis patients. Levels of oxidized LDL and antibodies to oxidized LDL are elevated in end-stage renal disease (ESRD). These abnormalities are summarized in Table 26-1.

This lipid/lipoprotein profile of PD is markedly atherogenic. The LDL particles are small and dense, indicated by the high apoB protein levels with modest elevations of LDL cholesterol. Small, dense LDL particles are particularly atherogenic in that they cross the endothelium with greater ease and are oxidized more readily than larger LDL particles. The pathogenesis of the overproduction of LDL particles in PD remains obscure. Hypoalbuminemia secondary to peritoneal protein loss may at least partly contribute to the abnormality.

The hypertriglyceridemia seen in PD results largely from the overproduction of the very low-density lipoproteins and a deficiency in lipoprotein lipase. There may also be a partial deficiency of hepatic lipase. The pathogenesis of these abnormalities is not understood, but the use of glucose-based PD solutions and a variety of drugs, such as beta-blockers,

Table 26-1. Lipid abnormalities in end-stage renal disease

Factor	PD	HD
Total cholesterol	↑	Normal
LDL cholesterol	↑	Normal
HDL cholesterol	↓	↓
Triglycerides	↑↑	↑
ApoA1 protein	↓	↓
ApoB protein	↑↑	Normal
Lp(a)	↑↑	↑↑
LDL oxidation	↑	↑

PD, peritoneal dialysis; HD, hemodialysis; LDL, low-density lipoprotein; HDL, high-density lipoprotein; Lp(a), lipoprotein(a); Apo, apolipoprotein.

aggravate the problem. The usual level of triglycerides seen in PD patients is 220–400 mg/dL (2.5–4.5 mmol/L), but levels >530 mg/dL (6 mmol/L) are not unusual.

A. Treatment for the dyslipidemia of PD

1. Elevated LDL cholesterol/apoB protein. In the nonuremic population, there is compelling evidence that treatment that reduces elevated LDL cholesterol levels is associated with a significant reduction in the progression of coronary artery disease and a decrease in cardiac clinical events and deaths. Even patients with "normal" cholesterol and preexisting coronary artery disease benefit from treatment that reduces LDL cholesterol. Specifically, the hydroxymethylglutaryl coenzyme A reductase group of drugs, also known as statins, has been shown to be very efficacious.

No equivalent studies have been done in PD. However, statins have been demonstrated to be effective in reducing LDL cholesterol and apoB protein in this population. Current recommendations from the National Kidney Foundation's (NKF) Kidney Disease Outcome Quality Initiative (KDOQI) and the International Society for Peritoneal Dialysis are to treat PD patients with elevated LDL cholesterol whether or not coronary artery disease (CAD) or other risk factors for CAD are present. These recommendations consider PD patients with dyslipidemia as being equivalent to nonuremic patients with known CAD. This is considered reasonable in light of the extraordinarily high incidence of fatal and nonfatal CAD events in this population.

The statins, which are recommended as first-line therapy, are generally safe in patients with renal disease. However, they can cause rhabdomyolysis and muscle enzymes should be followed. Ezetimibe, a new drug that reduces the small bowel absorption of cholesterol, is also reported to be safe in renal failure. It reduces LDL levels by about 20% in most patients. It may be a good drug to add to a statin to reach treatment goals or may be an alternative to statins if the patient is intolerant of that class of drug. However, experience with ezetimibe remains somewhat limited. The phosphate binder sevelamer also significantly reduces LDL.

2. Elevated triglycerides. Triglyceride (Tg) elevation alone is a very weak independent risk factor for the development of CAD. However, in PD patients, hypertriglyceridemia is almost always found in association with other lipid and lipoprotein abnormalities. Extreme elevations in Tg in PD patients may predispose to pancreatitis. Carbohydrate loading from the dialysis solution, a factor that contributes to the hypertriglyceridemia, cannot be avoided altogether in the PD patients, although the use of polyglucose and amino acid–based solutions may help. Sodium and water management to minimize the use of hypertonic solutions is advisable in the face of severe hypertriglyceridemia. As in the nonuremic population, ingestion of alcohol should be avoided because it can markedly increase triglycerides. Drugs known to exacerbate hypertriglyceridemia should also be avoided. There is no evidence in dialysis patients that treatment of hypertriglyceridemia is associated with improved clinical outcomes, although many physicians feel that treatment of levels >350 mg/dL (4 mmol/L) is advisable. As noted, hypertriglyceridemia is usually associated with other abnormalities such as high LDL and apoB levels for which therapy is recommended. Statins will often reduce triglyceride levels, although high doses are often required. The fibrate drugs (benzofibrate, fenofibrate, gemfibrozil) also effectively reduce triglyceride levels. These drugs have a renal route of excretion, and the dosage therefore must be reduced by at least 25%. The major side effect is muscle toxicity, and muscle enzymes should be followed. There are also reports of loss of renal function with the use of fibrates. They should therefore be used with caution, and the use of fibrates together with statins is generally not recommended.

3. Low HDL cholesterol. The fibrate class of drugs raises HDL cholesterol levels. However, the value of raising HDL in reducing cardiac morbidity and mortality in ESRD has not been established, and as noted above, these drugs have risks for patients on PD.

4. Antioxidants. In nonuremic patients, vitamin E, which is an effective antioxidant, has not proven to be an effective therapy to reduce cardiovascular events. There is one trial in hemodialysis patients that showed benefit of vitamin E for patients with known CAD. No trials have been done in PD and currently there is no recommendation to use antioxidant therapy in PD.

5. Lp(a). There is no known treatment for the elevated Lp(a) seen in PD patients. In some patients it may be elevated as part of an inflammatory response.

III. Protein loss. PD is associated with significant loss of protein across the peritoneum. This loss is about 0.5 g/L of dialysate drainage, but may be higher and account for as much as 10–20 g per day. The major component of the protein losses is albumin, but immunoglobulin G (IgG) accounts for up to 15%. These losses are likely the main reason why PD patients tend to have lower serum albumin levels than their hemodialysis counterparts, with typical values being 3.3–3.6 g/dL (33–36 g/L). Protein losses are greatest in high and high-average transporters. Amino acid losses of approximately 2–3 g per day also occur. Acute peritoneal inflammation is associated with substantially greater protein losses, and a rapid reduction in serum albumin is common during episodes of peritonitis. Unresolving peritonitis is associated with protracted and exaggerated protein losses causing protein malnutrition. The protein loss itself may become an indication to terminate peritoneal dialysis temporarily or, on occasion, permanently. In addition, inasmuch as PD may preserve residual renal function, in patients with nephrotic syndrome, this preserved renal function may be at the cost of ongoing protein losses. Therefore, measurements of both peritoneal and urinary protein losses need to be evaluated in PD patients, and appropriate dietary adjustments should be made.

IV. Hyponatremia/hypernatremia. Peritoneal dialysis solutions typically contain 132 mM of sodium. Most patients maintain a normal serum sodium on PD.

A. Hyponatremia. Patients who are excessive water drinkers can get a dilutional hyponatremia. In patients with marked hyperglycemia, translocational hyponatremia may be seen as a result of water shifting into the extracellular fluid. Typically, the serum sodium falls about 1.3 mmol/L for each 100 mg/dL (5.6 mmol/L) rise in blood glucose. Similarly, the use of icodextrin is associated with a small translocation reduction in serum sodium levels. Finally, severe hypertriglyceridemia can also give hyponatremia (when serum sodium is measured by flame photometry), which is classified as factitious since it is caused by a reduction in the amount of water per liter of plasma rather than a true reduction of sodium per unit of plasma water.

B. Hypernatremia. With rapid ultrafiltration using hypertonic solutions, hypernatremia may occur due to the sieving effect of the peritoneal membrane on sodium. More water than salt convects across the membrane, and so the serum sodium rises due to loss of sodium-free water from the blood. As the dwell time proceeds and ultrafiltration decreases, diffusion of sodium from serum to dialysate corrects the hypernatremia. However, with the short dwells of APD, there is maximal ultrafiltration and less time for diffusion, and so hypernatremia is more likely. It is also more pronounced in low transporters where ultrafiltration is greater and diffusion is less.

V. Hypokalemia/hyperkalemia. Standard PD solution contains no potassium. Potassium is removed during PD by diffusion and convection; after a 4- to 6-hour exchange, the dialysate potassium level is usually close to that of plasma. In renal failure, gastrointestinal secretion of potassium is enhanced. Usually only patients who are noncompliant in performing their dialysis exchanges or who have excessive potassium intake have ongoing problems with hyperkalemia. However, hypokalemia has been reported in 10%–30% of CAPD patients. These cases are usually associated with poor nutritional intake, and most can be managed by liberalizing the diet, but persistent levels lower than 3 mmol/L should be managed with potassium supplementation orally, or by adding potassium chloride to the dialysis solution. When adding potassium chloride to dialysis solution, 2–4 mM is commonly used.

VI. Hypocalcemia/hypercalcemia

A. Dialysis solution calcium level. As discussed in Chapter 19, PD solutions are available with 1.25 mM (2.5 mEq/L) or 1.75 mM (3.5 mEq/L) calcium concentrations. The 1.75 mM (3.5 mEq/L) dialysis solution keeps the patient in positive calcium balance unless there is very high ultrafiltration. This explains why low turnover bone disease has been frequently observed in PD patients on these solutions. The standard solution is now considered to be the 1.25 mM (2.5 mEq/L) calcium solution. This solution may put the patient in slightly negative balance for calcium with respect to the dialysis itself, but the patient will remain in neutral or positive balance for calcium overall because of the high oral intake of calcium from diet and calcium-based phosphate binders. Current concerns about widespread vascular calcification in dialysis patients and the new KDOQI guidelines on calcium/phosphate/vitamin D and bone disease make the use of the lower, physiologic calcium PD dialysis solution the appropriate first-line solution for the vast majority of patients.

B.   Hypocalcemia is not common in patients on PD because of the widespread use of calcium-based phosphate binders and vitamin D. Even on non-calcium based phosphate binders, such as sevelamer, serum calcium levels stay normal but PTH levels can rise. However, when it does occur, it can be easily managed with calcium and vitamin D supplements together with the 1.75 mM calcium dialysis solution. This high-calcium dialysis solution brings about a net positive transfer of calcium to the patient except in patients with a continuous high ultrafiltration.

C.   Hypercalcemia is common in PD patients who are taking large doses of calcium-containing phosphate binders. Switching to non–calcium-based phosphate binders may be required, and vitamin D supplementation may also have to be stopped (see Chapter 35). PD has been used occasionally in the treatment of severe hypercalcemia using either the standard 1.25 mM (2.5 mEq/L) solution or a locally prepared calcium-free dialysis solution.

VII.   Magnesium and vascular calcification

A.   Magnesium depletion has been linked to increased risk of atherosclerosis and risk of cardioevents in nonuremic populations. Because magnesium is excreted renally, a common assumption has been that dialysis patients have magnesium excess, rather than deficiency.

Magnesium tends to oppose calcium-induced vascular calcification, and a recent review has found an inverse relationship between serum magnesium levels and vascular calcification in PD patients (Wei et al., 2006). Higher dialysis solution magnesium can suppress parathyroid hormone and be associated with adynamic bone disease. The optimum peritoneal dialysis solution magnesium levels and the potential adjunct use of magnesium as a phosphorus binder remain unknown.

VIII.   Hypophosphatemia/hyperphosphatemia.   See Chapter 35.

IX.   Acidosis/alkalosis. Adequately dialyzed PD patients will usually maintain a serum bicarbonate that is normal. As the quantities of calcium carbonate used for phosphate binding decrease and the use of sevelamer increases, there may be a fall in serum bicarbonate levels since the latter agent has chloride as its anion. Amino acid–based dialysis solution has been reported to lower the serum bicarbonate level in some patients, which is predictable, given that metabolism of many amino acids generates protons. This usually can be managed by increasing the dialysis dose or by prescribing an oral base (e.g., bicarbonate) supplement.

SELECTED READINGS

Fernstrom A, et al. Increase of intra-abdominal fat in patients treated with continuous ambulatory peritoneal dialysis. *Perit Dial Int* 1998;18(2):166–171.

Fried L, et al. Recommendations for the treatment of lipid disorders in patients on peritoneal dialysis. ISPD guidelines/recommendations. International Society for Peritoneal Dialysis. *Perit Dial Int* 1999;19(1):7–16.

Furuya R, et al. Beneficial effects of icodextrin on plasma level of adipocytokines in peritoneal dialysis patients. *Nephrol Dial Transplant* 2006;21(2):494–498.

Holmes CJ, Shockley TR. Strategies to reduce glucose exposure in peritoneal dialysis patients. *Perit Dial Int* 2000;20(S2):S37–41.

Little J, et al. Longitudinal lipid profiles on CAPD: their relationship to weight gain, comorbidity, and dialysis factors. *J Am Soc Nephrol* 1998;9(10):1931–1939.

McDonald SP, Collins JF, Johnson DW. Obesity is associated with worse peritoneal dialysis outcomes in the Australia and New Zealand patient populations. *J Am Soc Nephrol* 2003;14(11):2894–2901.

Moberly JB, et al. Alterations in lipoprotein composition in peritoneal dialysis patients. *Perit Dial Int* 2002;22(2):220–228.

National Kidney Foundation. K/DOQI Clinical Practice Guidelines for managing dyslipidemias in chronic kidney disease. *Am J Kidney Dis* 2003;41:S1–S91.

Nutescu EA, Shapiro NL. Ezetimibe: a selective cholesterol absorption inhibitor. *Pharmacotherapy* 2003;23(11):1463–1474.

Prichard SS. Impact of dyslipidemia in end-stage renal disease. *J Am Soc Nephrol* 2003;14:S315–320.

Shahab I, Nolph KD. MIA syndrome in peritoneal dialysis: prevention and treatment. *Contrib Nephrol* 2006;150:135–143.

Stenvinkel P, et al. Malnutrition, inflammation, and atherosclerosis in peritoneal dialysis patients. *Perit Dial Int* 2001;21(S3):S157–162.

Wei M, et al. Relationship between serum magnesium, parathyroid hormone, and vascular calcification in patients on dialysis: a literature review. *Perit Dial Int* 2006;26(3):366–373.

Clinical Problem Areas

Psychosocial Issues in End-stage Renal Disease Patients

Scott D. Cohen and Vicenzio Holder-Perkins and Paul L. Kimmel

Patients with chronic kidney disease (CKD) are affected by numerous psychosocial stressors. These include effects of illness and treatment, including functional limitations and sexual dysfunction, dietary restrictions, time constraints, and fear of death. In addition, there may be marital conflict, strained interpersonal relationships with family and administrative or medical personnel, and socioeconomic concerns regarding costs of treatment and unemployment.

Approximately 10% of end-stage renal disease (ESRD) patients who are hospitalized have an underlying psychiatric disorder. Hospitalization rates for psychiatric disorders are high relative to other chronically ill patients. Common problems include depression, dementia and delirium, psychosis, personality and anxiety disorders, and substance abuse.

I. Psychologic problems in the ESRD population

A. Depression. Depression is the most common problem, as well as the most important, because of the risk of resulting noncompliance with the dialysis and/or medication regimen and the risk of suicide. Depression may be widely underdiagnosed and untreated. A major depressive disorder should be diagnosed if, during a period of at least 2 weeks, a patient experiences depressed mood or loss of interest in usual activities and at least five of the following symptoms: (a) depressed mood most of the day, (b) diminished interest or pleasure in most activities for most of the day, (c) significant weight loss or weight gain or appetite disturbance, (d) change in sleep pattern including insomnia or hypersomnia, (e) psychomotor retardation, (e) fatigue, (f) feelings of worthlessness or excessive guilt, (g) decreased concentration, or (h) recurring thoughts of death or suicide. The last criterion (h) is probably the most specific, as some of the others are associated with uremia per se.

Some investigators have estimated that depression occurs in as many as 10%–50% of dialysis patients. Screening tools include the Beck Depression Inventory (BDI) and the Hamilton Rating Scale for Depression. In patients with no underlying medical problems, a BDI score <9 suggests no or minimal depression, 10–18 indicates mild to moderate depression, 19–29 moderate to severe depression, and ≥30 severe depression.

Screening for underlying depression in the dialysis population is an important element of the treatment plan. Depressive affect can influence medical outcomes in several ways. In addition to the risk of suicide, depression may lead to poor compliance with the dialysis prescription, to abnormal immunologic function, or to anorexia and poor nutritional status. Depressive affect has also been linked to a higher incidence of peritonitis. Whether depression increases mortality risk is controversial. Some studies have suggested that baseline depressive symptomatology is associated with increased mortality, even after the multiple medical risk factors have been accounted for in analyses.

1. Suicide. ESRD patients can display suicidal behavior differently from patients with other chronic illnesses. Their rate of suicide is higher than in the general U.S. population. Important risk factors include a previous history of mental illness, recent hospitalization, age >75, male gender, white or Asian race, and alcohol or drug dependence. ESRD patients presumably can commit or attempt suicide more easily through either noncompliance with their medical regimen or by manipulating their dialysis access sites.

2. Treatment options. Treatment options for depression include pharmacotherapy, psychotherapy, and electroconvulsive therapy (ECT).

   a. Pharmacotherapy

      (1) Selective serotonin reuptake inhibitors (SSRIs) and tricyclic antidepressants (TCAs). Treatment with SSRIs should be continued for at least 4–6 weeks before deciding whether there has been a therapeutic benefit. If efficacy is not achieved, then a switch to another antidepressant of the same class or a different class is a reasonable step. SSRIs are advantageous because they typically cause fewer anticholinergic symptoms than TCAs, and are not associated with cardiac conduction abnormalities. Furthermore, TCAs can cause death if taken in large doses and hence pose a potential suicide risk.

      SSRIs are typically cleared by the liver. Despite this, it has been recommended that the dose of SSRI should be reduced to two thirds of the usual dose for patients with ESRD. SSRIs may have an additional benefit of reducing postural and intradialytic hypotension through effects on vascular tone. Fluoxetine, the first available SSRI, is the best studied drug in this family. A dose of 20 mg of fluoxetine daily is usually well tolerated, although data are limited to the short term. Other medications in this same family include paroxetine, sertraline, and citalopram.

      (2) Selective norepinephrine reuptake inhibitors (SNRIs). Venlafaxine and bupropion hydrochloride are examples of a different class of antidepressants called SNRIs. The SNRIs should be used with caution in ESRD patients, since these drugs are primarily renally excreted. Bupropion has active metabolites that are almost completely removed by the kidney. These metabolites may accumulate in dialysis patients, predisposing them to developing seizures.

(3) Monoamine oxidase inhibitors (MAOIs).
MAOIs have numerous side effects and should be avoided if possible in ESRD patients, because of their potential to cause hypotension.

b. Non-pharmacologic options. There are several forms of psychotherapy (cognitive-behavioral, interpersonal, supportive, and group therapy) that might be effective in managing psychological distress. There are few data on such treatments in patients with chronic kidney disease (CKD). Individual psychotherapy (cognitive-behavioral, interpersonal, and supportive) is useful when the patient has identified that there is a problem and has accepted encouragement by the clinician to seek treatment. Denial is common and is a way of coping with uncomfortable thoughts or feelings related to being a "dialysis patient." When a patient is noncompliant with treatment, denial might play a part in such behavior. Such patients may benefit from psychiatric interventions. However, these patients may resist treatment, as the implication is that "there is something wrong" with them. Motivating a patient to accept these forms of therapy may be difficult. Introducing therapy as a stress management approach to living with ESRD might be one approach to ease the patient into appropriate treatment. Supportive psychotherapy in conjunction with pharmacologic treatment is important for decreasing the rate of relapse. Group therapy may also have a positive impact. One uncontrolled study showed participation in group therapy sessions at the dialysis unit was associated with improved patient survival. Finally, electroconvulsive therapy (ECT) may be used for patients with severe refractory depression, provided that there are no contraindications.

B. Dementia/delirium. Neurocognitive disorders are common in ESRD patients. Cognitive deficits may be related to underlying uremia or other coexistent underlying medical conditions, as described in more detail in Chapter 42. Physicians should initiate discussions with the family about cessation of dialysis in patients with progressive dementia. Withdrawal from dialysis is relatively common, especially in elderly patients or patients who fail to thrive. Advanced directives should be offered to patients at the initiation of renal replacement therapy, ideally before the onset of any disease that would impair the capacity for decision making. The guidelines regarding shared decision making endorsed by the U.S. Renal Physicians Association are a helpful resource.

C. Anxiety and behavior disorders. Disruptive behavior directed toward the dialysis staff occurs in a minority of patients, but nevertheless can be a disturbance to all those in the dialysis unit. It is important to try to understand why the patient is angry and to explore potential solutions. Anxiety states should be treated through psychotherapy and behavioral techniques. Setting limits or establishing boundaries is paramount when hostility or aggression poses a threat of harm to the patient or to others. Hostility and aggressive behaviors might be manifestations of an underlying psychiatric symptom, such as paranoia, referential thinking, or even conditions associated with delirium. If doubt about a particular patient exists, consultation with a psychiatrist should be sought. If these measures are not effective, short-acting benzodiazepines such as lorazepam or alprazolam may be prescribed for limited periods. These benzodiazepines are metabolized by the liver. Nevertheless, as with the SSRIs, it is prudent to start with lower doses. The use of diazepam and chlordiazepoxide should be avoided in dialysis patients, due to their metabolism to pharmacologically active metabolites. Barbiturates should not be used in place of benzodiazepines, since the long-acting ones are removed by hemodialysis. For the acutely agitated patient, antipsychotic medications, such as haloperidol, are sometimes required. Haloperidol is not renally cleared; therefore, no dose adjustment is usually necessary. Little is known about the effects of other atypical antipsychotics, such as risperidone or olanzapine, in this patient population. Gabapentin is currently used to treat anxiety, but it does not have U.S. Food and Drug Administration approval for this indication. Gabapentin is eliminated by renal excretion as an unchanged drug. In patients with ESRD, the plasma clearance of gabapentin is reduced. ESRD and CKD patients with bipolar disorders requiring lithium should have serum lithium levels checked frequently. Lithium is cleared by dialysis; therefore, the dose should be given after each dialysis treatment. Valproic acid is another mood stabilizer sometimes used to treat bipolar disorder. Free serum levels of this drug have been observed to be elevated in patients with impaired renal function. Caution should be exercised in the administration of glucocorticoids to potential renal transplant patients with a history of psychosis, because of the risk of steroid-induced psychosis. Other steroid-sparing agents should be used if clinically feasible.

II. Other psychosocial issues in the ESRD population

A. Marital issues. There have been only a few studies that assess marital relationships in ESRD patients. One study found that more than 50% of couples that included a patient with ESRD experienced marital discord. Perception of marital conflict may be an important stressor for ESRD patients. Marital conflict may be associated with a patient's perception of burden of illness and the degree to which a patient does not adhere to the dialysis prescription. Marital satisfaction and conflict may be particularly salient for female patients. One study showed that female ESRD patients treated with hemodialysis with higher levels of marital satisfaction had improved survival. Marital satisfaction was not associated with differential outcomes in men.

B. Sexual dysfunction. ESRD patients have a high prevalence of sexual dysfunction, due to the effects of uremia, neuropathy, autonomic dysfunction, vascular disease, depression, and medications. Disturbances in the hypothalamic–pituitary–gonadal axis are also frequently encountered in ESRD patients. Sexual disturbances in this patient population include decreased libido, erectile dysfunction, menstrual disorders, and infertility. Impotence is believed to occur in roughly

70% of men treated with dialysis. Therefore, all males about to initiate dialysis should be counseled regarding the possibility of erectile dysfunction. This may lead to better communication with the physician and therefore reduce the possibility of depression. Women treated with dialysis commonly have disturbances in fertility and menstruation. Irregular menstrual cycles are common after the initiation of hemodialysis treatment. The most common menstrual disorder in women with ESRD is anovulation. For information about treatment see Chapter 40.

C. Socioeconomic issues. More than half of ESRD patients do not continue working after beginning renal replacement therapy. Those holding professional occupations may have greater flexibility in their work schedules and may be more likely to continue employment. Unemployment can have a significant psychologic impact on the individual, possibly contributing to a greater likelihood of depression.

D. Rehabilitation. Exercise may play an important role in improving a patient's overall sense of well-being. Specially designed exercise programs are available for those with physical impairments, and these should be promoted at the dialysis center or during routine physician visits. Other therapeutic modalities to consider are stress reduction/relaxation exercises and biofeedback, which have been successfully used, especially in managing disruptive and unstable patients.

E. Quality-of-life (QOL). It is essential for the medical staff and family to address the patient's perception of QOL. This is especially important when making decisions regarding the initiation or withdrawal of dialysis. Patients who rate their QOL higher and have an increased sense of well-being may be more likely to comply with their dialysis prescription. There are several different scales that have been used to assess QOL in ESRD patients, including the SF-36, Illness Effects Questionnaire, Karnofsky Scale, Satisfaction with Life Scale, and the KD-QOL, or Kidney Disease Quality-of-Life Scale. These scales primarily use subjective measures. Therapy with erythropoietin has improved QOL for dialysis patients. ESRD patients with successful renal transplants tend to rate their QOL higher than those with failed transplants or those treated with dialysis. Physicians should strongly consider the impact their medical decisions have on a patient's QOL, and discuss these issues in depth with patients and their families. In addition, patient satisfaction with care is an important aspect of QOL that should be evaluated.

SELECTED READINGS

Blumenfield M, et al. Fluoxetine in depressed patients on dialysis. *Int J Psychiatry Med* 1997;27:71–78.

Castaneda C, et al. Resistance training to reduce the malnutrition-inflammation complex syndrome of chronic kidney disease. *Am J Kidney Dis* 2004;43:607–616.

Daneker B, et al. Depression and marital dissatisfaction in patients with end-stage renal disease and in their spouses. *Am J Kidney Dis* 2001;38:839–846.

Dheenan S, et al. Effect of sertraline hydrochloride on dialysis hypotension. *Am J Kidney Dis* 1998;31:624–630.

Dogan E, et al. Relation between depression, some laboratory parameters, and quality-of-life in hemodialysis patients. *Ren Fail* 2005;27:695–699.

Finkelstein FO, et al. Depression in chronic dialysis patients: assessment and treatment. *Nephrol Dial Transplant* 2000;15:1911–1913.

Friend R, et al. Group participation and survival among patients with end-stage renal disease. *Am J Public Health* 1986;76:670–672.

Gee CB, et al. Couples coping in response to kidney disease: a developmental perspective. *Semin Dial* 2005;18:103–108.

Holley JL. Palliative care in end-stage renal disease: focus on advance care planning, hospice referral, and bereavement [Review]. *Semin Dial* 2005;18:154–156.

Kimmel PL, et al. Depression in end-stage renal disease patients treated with hemodialysis: tools, correlates, outcomes, and needs. *Semin Dial* 2005;18:73–79.

Kimmel PL. Just whose quality-of-life is it anyway? Controversies and consistencies in measurements of quality-of-life. *Kidney Int* 2000;57(Suppl 74):113–120.

Kimmel PL, et al. Marital conflict, gender and survival in urban hemodialysis patients. *J Am Soc Nephrol* 2000;11:1518–1525.

Kimmel PL, et al. Multiple measurements of depression predict mortality in a longitudinal study of chronic hemodialysis patients. *Kidney Int* 2000;57:2093–2098.

King K, et al. The frequency and significance of the "difficult" patient: the nephrology community's perceptions. *Adv Chronic Kidney Dis* 2004;11:234–239.

Kolewaski CD, et al. Quality-of-life and exercise rehabilitation in end stage renal disease. *CANNT J* 2005;15:22–29.

Kouidi E, et al. Exercise renal rehabilitation program: psychosocial effects. *Nephron* 1997;77:152–158.

Kurella M, et al. Chronic kidney disease and cognitive impairment in the elderly: the Health, Aging and Body Composition Study. *J Am Soc Nephrol* 2005;16:2127–2133.

Kurella M, et al. Suicide in the end-stage renal disease program. *J Am Soc Nephrol* 2005;16:774–781.

Lopes AA, et al. Depression as a predictor of mortality and hospitalization among hemodialysis patients in the United States and Europe. *Kidney Int* 2002;62:199–207.

Moss AH, et al. Palliative care [Review]. *Am J Kidney Dis* 2004; 43:172–173.

Painter P. Physical functioning in end-stage renal disease patients: update 2005 [Review]. *Hemodial Int* 2005;9:218–235.

Patel SS, et al. Psychosocial variables, quality of life and religious beliefs in end-stage renal disease patients treated with hemodialysis. *Am J Kidney Dis* 2002;40:1013–1022.

Patel S, et al. The impact of social support on end-stage renal disease. *Semin Dial* 2005;18:89–93.

Renal Physicians Association. *Shared decision making (guideline regarding withdrawal from dialysis and palliative care)*. Available at http://www.renalmd.org/. Accessed September 12, 2006.

Shidler NR, et al. Quality-of-life and psychosocial relationships in patients with chronic renal insufficiency. *Am J Kidney Dis* 1998;32:557–566.

Snow V, et al. Pharmacologic treatment of acute major depression and dysthymia. American College of Physicians-American Society of Internal Medicine. *Ann Intern Med* 2000;132:738–742.

Tawney K. Developing a dialysis rehabilitation program. *Nephrol Nurs J* 2000;27:524–539.

Turk S, et al. Treatment with antidepressive drugs improved quality-of-life in chronic hemodialysis patients. *Clin Nephrol* 2006;65:113–118.

Unruh ML, et al. Health-related quality-of-life in nephrology research and clinical practice. *Semin Dial* 2005;18:82–90.

Watnick S, et al. The prevalence and treatment of depression among patients starting dialysis. *Am J Kidney Dis* 2003;41:105–110.

Wilson B, et al. Screening for depression in chronic hemodialysis patients: comparison of the Beck Depression Inventory, primary nurse, and nephrology team. *Hemodial Int* 2006;10:35–41.

Wu AW, et al. Changes in quality-of-life during hemodialysis and peritoneal dialysis treatment: generic and disease specific measures. *J Am Soc Nephrol* 2004;15:743–753.

Wuerth D, et al. Chronic peritoneal dialysis patients diagnosed with clinical depression: results of pharmacologic therapy. *Semin Dial* 2003;16:424–427.

Wuerth D, et al. The identification and treatment of depression in patients maintained on dialysis. *Semin Dial* 2005;18:142–146.

Nutrition

Michael V. Rocco and T. Alp Ikizler

I. Causes of kidney disease wasting (KDW) in chronic dialysis patients. Kidney disease wasting affects approximately one third of hemodialysis or peritoneal dialysis patients (Pupim, 2006). Malnutrition can be secondary to poor nutritional intake, to increased losses (via dialysate), and/or to an increase in protein catabolism (Table 28-1). The sequelae of kidney disease wasting are numerous and include malaise, fatigue, poor rehabilitation, impaired wound healing, increased susceptibility to infection, and increased rates of hospitalization and mortality. Serum levels of inflammatory markers are increased, and numerous causes of chronic inflammation may be present (Kaysen, 2001). Proinflammatory cytokines can cause anorexia with suppression of nutrient intake (Kaizu, 2003). Chronic inflammation also is associated with cytokine-mediated hypermetabolism. Disruption of the growth hormone (GH) and insulin-like growth factor-1 (IGF-1) axis leads to decreased protein synthesis. Increased leptin concentrations may worsen anorexia due to central effects (Don, 2001).

A. Obesity. Concern has always focused on wasting in chronic kidney disease (CKD) patients, because the death rate increases steeply with evidence of skeletal muscle loss, weight that is below peer weight, or body mass index. There is, however, an increasing incidence of obesity among patients initiating hemodialysis therapy (Kramer, 2006). Patients beginning hemodialysis who tend to be overweight or frankly obese, regardless of its cause (i.e., increased adiposity and/or lean body mass), appear to have some survival advantage over underweight patients, although their physical functioning is still impaired (Johansen et al., 2006). While the exact mechanism underlying this association have not been elucidated, it may well be that obesity is a marker of resistance to catabolic consequences of advanced kidney disease, or else of a better antecedent nutritional state. In peritoneal dialysis patients obesity is associated with both decreased patient survival and with increased risk of technique failure (Collins, 2005 oral presentation). Also the rate of new-onset diabetes is high. So once end-stage renal disease (ESRD) has been reached in hemodialysis patients, unless the patient is markedly obese, the benefits of weight reduction are not clear. In peritoneal dialysis patients, dietary restriction and, especially, carbohydrate restriction to control both weight and hypertriglyceridemia (see below), may be indicated.

II. Nutritional assessment

A. Patient interview. Symptoms of nausea, vomiting, and anorexia, as well as recent changes in body weight, should be carefully evaluated to ascertain cause. Nonuremic causes

Table 28-1. Causes of kidney disease wasting

Decreased nutritional intake
Overzealous dietary restrictions
Delayed gastric emptying and diarrhea
Other medical comorbidities
Intercurrent illnesses and hospitalizations
Decrease in food intake on hemodialysis days
Medications causing dyspepsia (phosphate binders, iron
  preparations)
Suppression of oral intake by peritoneal dialysate glucose load
Inadequate dialysis
Monetary restrictions
Depression
Altered sense of taste

Increased losses
Gastrointestinal blood loss (100 mL blood = 14–17 g protein)
Intradialytic nitrogen losses (hemodialysis 6–8 g amino acid
  per procedure; peritoneal dialysis 8–10 g protein per day)

Increase in protein catabolism
Intercurrent illnesses and hospitalizations
Other medical comorbidities
Metabolic acidosis (promotes protein catabolism)
Catabolism associated with hemodialysis (controversial)
Dysfunction of the growth hormone–insulin growth factor
  endocrine axis
Catabolic effects of other hormones (parathyroid hormone,
  cortisol, glucagon)

must be kept in mind, including severe congestive heart failure, diabetes, various gastrointestinal diseases, and depression. Phosphate binders or oral iron preparations can cause dyspepsia, and prednisone can increase the protein catabolic rate.

B. Assessment of food intake. Patient recall of food intake should be determined on both dialysis and nondialysis days; intake on dialysis days typically is about 20% lower (Burrowes et al., 2003). Food frequency questionnaires may also provide useful information (Kalantar-Zadeh et al., 2002).

C. Physical examination, including anthropometry. One should compare ideal or average "peer" weight (see Tables A-8 and A-9 in Appendix A) to actual body weight. Comparison to prior values is important as both body weight and V decrease over time in hemodialysis patients (DiFilippo, 2006; Rocco, 2006). Skinfold thickness measured at the biceps or triceps provides an estimate of body fat, whereas midarm circumference can be used to estimate muscle mass. These measures can be compared to reference ranges established in well-nourished dialysis patients (Chumlea et al., 2003, Nelson et al., 1990). Patients with values below the 25th percentile for either middle upper arm circumference or triceps skinfold thickness are likely to be malnourished.

D.   Subjective global assessment. Subjective global assessment (SGA) is a clinical method for evaluating nutritional status that includes history, symptoms, and physical parameters (Baker 1982; Detsky, 1987). The history component focuses on five areas: (a) percentage of body weight lost in the previous 6 months; (b) dietary nutrient intake; (c) the presence of anorexia, nausea, vomiting, diarrhea, or abdominal pain; (d) functional capacity; and (e) metabolic demands in view of underlying disease state. Physical parameters focus on assessment of subcutaneous fat; muscle wasting in the temporal area, deltoids, and quadriceps; the presence of ankle or sacral edema; and the presence of ascites. The SGA has a good reproducibility and correlates strongly with outcomes in ESRD patients (Duerksen et al., 2000). Other scoring systems utilizing components of the conventional SGA have been suggested (Kalantar-Zadeh et al., 2001); they are associated with morbidity and mortality but have not been tested in terms of their relationship to other nutritional markers or response to feeding.

E.   Bioimpedance. Bioimpedance analysis is based on the measurement of resistance and reactance when a constant alternating electrical current is applied to a patient. Empirical equations are used to predict total-body water from resistance and total-body mass from the ratio of resistance to reactance or from its geometrical derivative, the phase angle. **Phase angle** correlates strongly with anthropometric measures of nutritional status and with serum albumin levels. For reproducibility, bioimpedance measurements should be performed within 120 minutes of the end of a dialysis treatment (Di Iorio et al., 2004). Low phase angle measurements are associated with an increased risk of mortality (Chertow et al., 1997; Mushnick et al., 2003).

F.   Dual energy x-ray absorptiometry (DEXA). This test was developed to measure bone density, but later was adapted to quantify soft tissue composition, including body fat. A DEXA scan takes only 6–15 minutes, involves minimal radiation exposure, and hence can be used serially to follow changes over time (Wang, 2001). It is costly, however, and there are no data relating DEXA results to outcome in patients with advanced kidney disease. DEXA findings must be evaluated with hydration status in mind (Dumler, 1997).

G.   Laboratory tests
  1.   Serum albumin. Low levels are a strong predictor of mortality and hospitalization; risk rises dramatically and logarithmically as levels decline below 4.0 g/dL (40 g/L). The assay method used can change results by as much as 20%. Serum albumin levels correlate poorly with other nutritional measures, especially in continuous ambulatory peritoneal dialysis (CAPD) patients. Serum level of acute-phase proteins, such as C-reactive protein (CRP) and serum amyloid A, have a greater impact on serum albumin levels than the protein catabolic rate. Low serum albumin levels also have been shown to predict coronary calcification (Joki et al., 2006). Despite this, albumin, or alternatively, prealbumin, levels provide a consistent assessment of visceral protein stores (Pupim et al., 2004). Furthermore, serum

albumin levels do decline in patients who manifest other signs of kidney disease wasting and increase with feeding.

2. **Predialysis serum urea nitrogen (SUN).** The predialysis SUN level reflects the balance between urea generation and removal. Thus, a low SUN level could occur in a very well-dialyzed patient with good protein intake, or in an inadequately dialyzed patient with poor protein intake. Therefore, it is difficult to infer the level of protein intake from the SUN directly.

3. **Urea nitrogen appearance (g).** This measurement can be used to estimate protein intake. This is because, when patients are in nitrogen balance, the **g** is closely similar to the urea nitrogen intake (from which protein intake can be estimated). In catabolic or anabolic patients, protein intake will be over- or underestimated, respectively. As discussed in Chapter 3, in hemodialysis patients, the **g** can be computed using either a pre- and postdialysis SUN, or a set of three values: a pre-, post-, and next predialysis SUN. Another method used in computing the **g** for both hemodialysis and peritoneal dialysis patients is to collect aliquots of the spent dialysate, measure the amount of urea nitrogen, and use this information to estimate weekly dialytic removal.

4. **Protein equivalent of total nitrogen appearance (PNA).** Several formulas are available for the calculation of PNA from **g**, given that, on average, the percent of nitrogen from protein that winds up as urea is known. Dialysis modeling programs usually normalize the PNA to the "kinetic" body weight; the latter is estimated as urea distribution volume divided by 0.58. The kinetic weight (which usually is an internal number and is not reported) is usually, but not always, close to actual body weight. Dividing PNA by the kinetic weight gives a "normalized" PNA, or nPNA.

5. **Clinical utility of the nPNA.** The utility of the PNA in terms of predicting outcomes has been questioned. In the HEMO trial, as well as in observational data sets, once serum albumin and creatinine were controlled for, the PNA had little if any additional predictive power in terms of outcome. The issue of coupling between Kt/V and PNA has not yet been definitively settled, and some reports continue to suggest that this is a problem (Cano et al., 2006a). In the HEMO trial, PNA was a very poor predictor of dietary protein intake. It was assumed that the dietary recall method used was not sufficiently sensitive to show a relationship, but alternative explanations are possible as well. Perhaps it is best not to divide PNA by body weight at all. In one study, the PNA correlated reasonably well with the serum albumin concentration, but when it was "normalized" to body weight, the association with serum albumin was no longer present (Beddhu et al., 2005).

6. **Other laboratory findings. Serum transferrin** is low in almost all dialysis patients and is influenced by changes in iron stores, presence of inflammation, and changes in volume status; it is not a good indicator of nutritional status. **Serum prealbumin** levels may be elevated due to interaction of prealbumin with retinol-binding

protein and decreased renal clearance. **C-reactive protein** (CRP) is an acute phase reactant that correlates negatively with visceral protein concentrations. When serum levels of albumin or prealbumin are low, it is appropriate to check CRP levels to help uncover potential covert inflammation, although CRP levels are highly variable in ESRD patients, reducing their practical utility. Some evidence does suggest serial CRP measurements are valuable.

III. Dietary requirements. The recommended average levels of nutritional intake are listed in Table 28-2 and include recommendations that are generally consistent with the National Kidney Foundation's (NKF) Kidney Disease Outcome Quality Initiative (KDOQI) 2001 guidelines on nutrition and the European best practice guidelines for nutrition (Dombros, 2005).

A. Need for individualization. A "renal" diet has numerous restrictions, and so adherence to such a diet can be difficult and stressful. Prescribed diets should be individualized to help accommodate each patient's unique circumstances in terms of palatability, cost, comorbid medical conditions, and cultural eating habits. Specific nutritional issues in the diabetic dialysis patient are discussed in Chapter 30. Too many restrictions should be avoided as they may lead to poor intake. The nutritional recommendations need to be reinforced by all members of the health care team. Compliance should be assessed on a regular basis, even monthly at the initiation of dialysis or for those with a previous history of noncompliance.

B. Peer rather than actual body weight. One problem with dietary intake recommendations for dialysis patients, who often are malnourished, is the choice of weight to use in the denominator. For example, if a patient has lost body mass such that his or her weight is now 50 kg versus a premorbid weight of 90 kg, ingestion of an "adequate" amount of protein or calories based on actual weight may maintain the patient at that lower body weight, but may not be optimal for regaining lost weight, assuming that this is desired. Protein and caloric recommendations should be based on the peer body weight (see Tables A-8 and A-9 in Appendix A) for healthy subjects of the same sex, height, age, and body frame size as the patient.

Example: A severely malnourished 35-year-old male hemodialysis patient weighs 60 kg. Using an Internet calculator for ideal body weight, we find that the peer weight for this medium-frame patient (were he healthy) given his height of 183 cm (72 in.) would be about 84 kg. Our urea kinetic modeling program had reported that his nPNA of was 1.2 g/kg per day. As discussed above, this nPNA is based on the patient's "kinetic" weight. Is this patient ingesting an adequate amount of protein?

We can recover the value for modeled V from the program and divide this by 0.58 to find the "kinetic" weight that was used by the program. Assume that this turns out to be 60 kg. Then 1.2 g/kg per day = $1.2 \times 60 = 72$ g per day for his PNA, which means that estimated protein intake is also 72 g per day. To compute PNA normalized to this patient's

Table 28-2. Daily dietary recommendations for dialysis patients[a]

Nutrient or Substance	Hemodialysis	Peritoneal Dialysis
Protein (g/kg)	1.2	1.2–1.3
Calories (sedentary, kcal/kg)	30–35[b]	30–35[b,c]
Protein (%)	15–25	
Carbohydrate (%)	50–60[d]	50–60[c,d]
Fat (%)	25–35	
Cholesterol	<200 mg (0.52 mmol)	
Saturated fat (%)	<7	
Crude fiber (g)	20–30	
Sodium	<2.0 g (<87 mmol)[e]	
Potassium	2.0 g (50 mmol) + 1 g (25 mmol)/LUO	4.0 g (100 mmol) + 1 g (25 mmol)/ LUO
Calcium	2.0 g (50 mmol)[f]	
Phosphorus	0.8–1.0 g (26–32 mmol)[g]	
Magnesium	0.2–0.3 g (8–12 mmol)	
Iron	See Chapter 32	
Vitamin A	None	
β-carotene	None	
Retinol	None	
Thiamine (mg)	1.5	
Riboflavin (mg)	1.7	
Vitamin B$_6$ (mg)	10	
Vitamin B$_{12}$ (mg)	0.006	
Niacin (mg)	20	
Folic acid (mg)	>1.0	
Pantothenic acid (mg)	10	
Biotin (mg)	0.3	
Vitamin C (mg)	60–100	
Vitamin E	None	
Vitamin D	See Chapter 35	
Vitamin K	See text	

LUO, liters of urine output per day.

[a] All intakes calculated on the basis of normalized body weight (i.e., the average body weight of normal persons of the same age, height, and sex as the patient).

[b] 35 kcal/kg body weight per day if <60 years of age; 30–35 kcal/body weight per day if >60 years of age.

[c] Includes glucose absorbed from dialysis solutions.

[d] Carbohydrate intake should be decreased in patients with hypertriglyceridemia.

[e] Lower sodium intakes, in the range of 1.0–1.5 g (43–65 mmol), may result in better control of blood pressure in peritoneal dialysis patients and a lower dialysis solution glucose load, and are recommended if this can be done while maintaining energy intake.

[f] The total dose of elemental calcium provided by the calcium-based phosphate binders should not exceed 1,500 mg (37 mmol) per day, and the total intake of elemental calcium (including dietary calcium) should not exceed 2,000 mg (50 mmol) per day.

[g] For patients with serum phosphorus level >5.5 mg/dL (1.8 mmol/L).

peer weight, we divide 72 by 84 kg. Now his PNA/peer weight is only $72/84 = 0.86$ g/kg per day, which may be suboptimal.

C.　Adequacy of dialysis. The delivery of a dialysis dose that is less than adequate can adversely affect appetite, nutrient intake, and measures of nutrition. Provision of adequate dialysis corrects subtle uremia and thus mitigates uremia-associated anorexia, and may improve hypercatabolism as well. Having said this, in the HEMO study, there was no improvement in either protein or energy intake in patients randomized to high-dose ($spKt/V \sim 1.65$) compared to patients randomized to standard-dose ($spKt/V \sim 1.25$) dialysis. Weight declined similarly in both groups of patients, although the decreases in some anthropometric parameters were somewhat less for patients assigned to the higher dialysis dose (Rocco et al., 2004). Assignment to the high-flux group had little measurable nutritional advantage. Despite this disappointing data, evidence continues to accumulate from smaller, observational studies that moving to a more frequent dialysis schedule, and, especially, markedly increasing weekly dialysis time using a five to six times/week nocturnal schedule, is followed by gain in flesh weight and improvement in serum albumin and other nutritional measures (see Chapter 14). Claims have also been made of nutritional improvement in patients receiving intermittent hemofiltration or hemodiafiltration (see Chapter 15), although the evidence there is not as strong.

D.　Protein. KDOQI guidelines recommend that both hemodialysis and peritoneal dialysis patients should ingest 1.2 g of protein/kg (using peer body weight) per day. At least 50% of the protein ingested should be of high biologic value. This level of protein intake is often difficult to achieve in practice, however, and 30%–50% of hemodialysis patients report intakes of <1.0 g of protein/kg per day (Rocco et al., 2004). For peritoneal dialysis patients who are protein depleted, some physicians recommend protein intakes as high as 1.5 g of protein/kg per day, the higher level designed to compensate for substantial (10–20 g per day) losses into the dialysate.

E.　Energy. KDOQI guidelines recommend that all dialysis patients younger than 61 years ingest 35 kcal/kg per day. For patients older than 60 years, the recommended intake is 30–35 kcal/kg per day. Higher levels of caloric intake may be required for patients who perform strenuous labor, for patients who are well below their desired weight, and for patients who are hospitalized, have peritonitis, or have other causes of catabolic stress. This recommended level of caloric intake is difficult to achieve in practice; as an example, in the HEMO study, intake based on dietary recall averaged 23–27 kcal/kg. The data correlates with an observed mean resting energy expenditure of 24.6 kcal/kg/day in Japanese hemodialysis patients (Kogirima, 2006). While this may be related to the usual underreporting observed in dietary recalls, the KDOQI recommended levels of dietary protein and energy intake have been achieved in patients receiving more frequent hemodialysis (McPhatter, et al., 1999; Galland, 2004).

In both hemodialysis and peritoneal dialysis patients, a substantial amount of glucose absorbed from the dialysate

Table 28-3. Estimated kilocalories of glucose absorbed as instilled volume varies in CAPD and CCPD patients

Instilled Volume	%D Daytime	%D Overnight	kcal Absorbed
CAPD			
4 × 2.0 L	1.5% D	2.5% D	332
4 × 2.5 L	1.5% D	7.5% Icodextrin	187
4 × 2.5 L	1.5% D	2.5% D	386
4 × 3.0 L	1.5% D	2.5% D	432
CCPD[a]			
3 × 2.0 & 2.0	2.5% D	1.5% D	299
3 × 2.5 & 2.5	2.5% D	1.5% D	350
3 × 3.0 & 3.0	2.5% D	1.5% D	396
3 × 2.5 & 2.5 + 2.5	Both 1.5% D	1.5% D	342
3 × 2.5 & Ico	7.5% Icodextrin	1.5% D	144

D, % dextrose of instilled solution; CCPD, continuous ambulatory peritoneal dialysis.
[a] CCPD using 9 hours overnight and three exchanges per night and a last-bag-fill for CCPD regimens 1, 2, 3, and 5. CCPD regimen 4 includes a last-bag-fill and midday exchange.
Adapted from Burkart J. Metabolic consequences of peritoneal dialysis. *Semin Dial* 2004;17:498–504. These estimates do not take into account glucose losses during icodextrin dwells or kcal gained from the metabolism of polyglucose.

contributes to total energy intake. In hemodialysis this amounts to about 400 kcal/treatment when dialysis solution glucose concentration is 200 mg/dL (11 mM), but this is a factor only three times/week. In peritoneal dialysis the amount of glucose absorption is substantially greater (Table 28-3) as it occurs daily; the amount depends on the percent dextrose used for each dwell, the length of each exchange, the volume of each dwell, the number of exchanges, and peritoneal membrane transport properties.

    1. Percent carbohydrates. Table 23-2 reflects the conventional wisdom that 50%–60% of dietary intake (including glucose absorbed from dialysate) should be carbohydrates. This would represent 1,000 kcal, or 250 g of carbohydrates for a 2,000-kcal diet. Given that 300–400 kcal of glucose is normally absorbed with most peritoneal dialysis regimens, in peritoneal dialysis patients the percent carbohydrates ingested as food needs to be reduced by a similar amount. Hypertriglyceridemia and impaired glucose tolerance are common in peritoneal dialysis patients (see Chapter 26) and are not rare in those being treated with hemodialysis. For such patients, the percent carbohydrates may need to be further reduced, with the caloric deficit being made up primarily by increased intake of both protein and monounsaturated fats (Arora, 2005).

    F. Lipids. The therapeutic goal should be to achieve a low-density lipoprotein (LDL) cholesterol of <100 mg/dL (2.6 mmol/L) and a fasting triglyceride level of <500 mg/dL (5.7 mmol/L). Therapeutic lifestyle changes include diet, weight reduction, increased physical activity, abstinence from alcohol, and treatment of hyperglycemia, if present. The diet should contain <7% saturated fat, with polyunsaturated fat <10% of total calories and monounsaturated fat <20% of total calories, and with total fat at 25%–35% of total calories. Carbohydrates should not exceed 50%–60% of total calories in hemodialysis patients but should likely be less in peritoneal dialysis patients. In all dialysis patients, 20–30 g of fiber per day should be consumed to help reduce dyslipidemia. Drug therapy for hypercholesterolemia and hypertriglyceridemia is discussed in Chapter 26 for peritoneal dialysis patients, and in Chapter 37 for CKD patients in general.

G.   Sodium and water. Most excess fluid intake is driven by ingestion of excess sodium and dietary counseling needs to address other, non–salt-driven causes of fluid ingestion as well; however, emphasis always should be on educating patients and their families about the importance of limiting sodium. Regulatory bodies now suggest that healthy (nonuremic) persons limit dietary sodium intake to 2 g (87 mmol) per day, and for older persons, African Americans, or patients with kidney disease, a restriction to 1.5 g (65 mmol) per day, or even to 1.2 g (52 mmol) per day, is now being suggested (Institute of Medicine, 2004). Dialysis patients are mostly elderly, many are African American, and they by definition have kidney disease; most of them also suffer from heart disease, so one would assume that sodium recommendations for this group would be in the 1.2–1.5 g (52–65 mmol) per day range. In fact, KDOQI guidelines suggest a slightly higher amount: 2 g (87 mmol) per day, with the recognition that each additional dietary restriction may serve to limit intake of key nutrients and to worsen kidney disease wasting. Having said this, in programs where long dialysis sessions are combined with careful attention to sodium restriction (e.g., Tassin, France), the incidence of hypertension is low and patient survival is excellent. Therefore, especially in patients with limited residual renal function, limiting sodium intake to 1.2–1.5 g (52–65 mmol) per day may be helpful, provided that this does not adversely affect food intake. In peritoneal dialysis, although one can remove sodium-stimulated fluid ingestion using higher glucose dwells, this comes at the cost of glucose loading, with potentially adverse effects on the peritoneal membrane as well as on lipids and triglyceride levels, so a lower sodium intake is also desirable for peritoneal dialysis patients. A low sodium intake should assist patients with limiting their fluid intake. In patients who are anuric, fluid intake should be limited to about 1.0–1.5 L per day. Additional fluid can be consumed in patients with residual renal function, with the amount based on the typical daily urinary output.

H.   Potassium. Mild potassium restriction (4 g or 100 mmol per day) is usually all that is needed in patients with a moderate degree of residual renal function. Hyperkalemia sometimes becomes an issue in the presence of acidemia or hypoaldosteronism, or with the administration of nonsteroidal anti-inflammatory drugs (NSAIDs), potassium-sparing diuretics, angiotensin-converting enzyme inhibitors, angiotensin blockers, aldosterone receptor antagonists, or β-receptor blockers.

Hyperkalemia in anuric peritoneal dialysis patients is unusual because the dialysate contains no potassium and almost all of these patients require either a modest potassium restriction (4 g or 100 mmol per day) or no restriction at all. In hemodialysis patients with limited residual renal function, a lower intake of potassium (2 g or 50 mmol per day) often is required to prevent hyperkalemia.

I. Calcium and phosphorus. The dietary intake of calcium and phosphorus and management of hyperphosphatemia are discussed in Chapter 35.

J. Vitamins

   1. Water-soluble vitamins. Dialysis patients may develop deficiencies of water-soluble vitamins unless supplements are given. Vitamin deficiencies are caused by poor intake, interference with absorption by drugs or uremia, altered metabolism, and losses to the dialysate. All dialysis patients should receive supplementary folic acid and B vitamins in the doses listed in Table 28-2 (Rocco et al., 1997). B-vitamin replacement may need to be more intensive in patients undergoing high-flux dialysis due to increased losses (Kasama et al., 1996). High levels of folate supplementation, however, do not result in a significant decrease in homocysteine levels (Ghandour et al., 2002). Ascorbic acid supplementation should be limited to 60–100 mg per day as higher doses can result in the accumulation of its metabolite, oxalate.

   2. Fat-soluble vitamins. Fat-soluble vitamins cannot be removed effectively by either hemodialysis or peritoneal dialysis. Multivitamin supplementation in these patients should not include fat-soluble vitamins. The dosing of vitamin D is discussed in Chapter 35. Vitamin E has been promoted as an antioxidant in chronic dialysis patients and additional studies are currently being performed to determine the risk/benefit ratio of this therapy. Vitamin K deficiency can occur in patients receiving antibiotics that suppress the production of vitamin K by intestinal bacteria. Under these circumstances, supplementation with 7.5 mg of vitamin K per week may be beneficial. High levels of vitamin A can result in multiple, serious adverse effects in nonuremic individuals. Hypervitaminosis A in dialysis patients can also cause anemia and abnormalities of lipid and calcium metabolism.

IV. Nutrient requirements with acute kidney failure

A. Energy requirements in hospitalized dialysis patients. In general, most patients with acute renal failure requiring dialysis have energy needs between 30 and 40 kcal/kg. Higher levels of nutrient intake have not been shown to be beneficial from a nutritional standpoint and can cause hypercapnia, especially if patients have impaired pulmonary function. A simple method is to assume a baseline requirement of 30 or 35 kcal/kg per day, and then multiply by one or more adjustment factors, which range from 1.1 to 1.7, and are used when hypermetabolism is likely to be present (Table 28-4).

Table 28-4.   Adjustment factors for determination of energy requirements

Clinical Condition	Adjustment Factor
Mechanical ventilation	
Without sepsis	1.10–1.20
With sepsis	1.25–1.35
Peritonitis	1.15
Infections	
Mild	1.00–1.10
Moderate	1.10–1.20
Sepsis	1.20–1.30
Soft tissue trauma	1.10
Bone fractures	1.15
Burns (% of body surface area)	
0%–20%	1.15
20%–40%	1.50
40%–100%	1.70

Recommendations adapted from Blackburn GL, et al. Nutritional and metabolic assessment of the hospitalized patient. *J Parenter Enteral Nutr* 1977;1:11–22; Bouffard Y, et al. Energy expenditure in the acute renal failure patient mechanically ventilated. *Intens Care Med* 1987;13:401–404; Schneeweiss B, et al. Energy metabolism in acute and chronic renal failure. *Am J Clin Nutr* 1990;52:596-601; Soop M, et al. Energy expenditure in postoperative multiple organ failure with acute renal failure. *Clin Nephrol* 1989; 31:139–145.

Apart from these adjustment factors, energy expenditure in acutely ill patients with acute renal failure has been shown to be somewhat lower than in similar patients with normal renal function (Soop et al., 1989).

B.   Protein requirements. Amino acids are infused to help prevent protein breakdown, not to provide an additional source of calories; hence, they are not counted as part of the daily energy intake. The amino acid intake for patients with acute or chronic renal failure undergoing either chronic dialysis or one of the continuous renal replacement therapies should be in the range of 1.1–2.0 g/kg per day. There appears to be no benefit in using higher levels of protein supplementation, even in the face of very high nitrogen losses. When higher levels are given, there does not appear to be any additional improvement in nitrogen balance (Feinstein et al., 1983), and there is enhanced formation of urea and other nitrogenous waste products.

C.   Lipid requirements. Energy requirements cannot usually be achieved by the administration of glucose infusions alone. The daily amount of glucose administered should not exceed 5 g/kg body weight as supplementation above this level results in incomplete oxidation of glucose and conversion of glucose to fat. The balance of energy requirements is provided by lipids. Lipids have a high specific energy content as well as a low osmolality. The provision of 1.0 g/kg body weight or less usually prevents the development of an essential fatty acid deficiency while decreasing the risk of hypertriglyceridemia.

V. Treatment

A. General comments. Reversible causes of poor nutritional status should be diligently pursued and corrected. The provision of adequate dialysis is a crucial first step in improving nutritional status. Other medical conditions should also be identified and treated if possible. Social considerations include access and preparation of food, consideration of ethnic and personal food preferences, and assessment for the need for or repair of dentures and/or bridges. Endurance exercise has been associated with an improvement in the rate of glucose disappearance and a reduction in fasting plasma insulin levels; in addition, plasma triglyceride values decrease and high-density lipoprotein (HDL) cholesterol concentrations increase. Other benefits of exercise include an increase in muscle size and strength and improvement in endurance. Once reversible causes of poor nutritional status have been identified and corrected, intervention in the form of oral or parenteral supplements should be considered.

B. When to initiate nutritional supplements. The available studies suggest that the benefits of nutritional supplementation are most significant in patients with the highest degree of kidney disease wasting, but no specific cutoff has been established. In the authors' opinion, it is reasonable to consider subjects with serum albumin <3.9 g/dL (39 g/L) and serum prealbumin <32 mg/dL (320 mg/L) as potentially suffering from malnutrition. A continuous decline in these parameters despite aggressive efforts to improve dietary nutrient intake should prompt consideration of nutritional supplementation. In patients with minimal to no residual function, serum creatinine concentrations can provide a reasonable estimate of somatic protein stores and time-dependent changes in this marker can be utilized to assess the patients' nutritional status. If the goal is to precisely and longitudinally follow changes in body composition, one may want to use anthropometry, DEXA, or bioelectrical impedance analysis. For all methods, repeated measures and technical standardization are the key to reduce variability of results.

Once supplementation has been initiated, the same markers that were used to justify initiation of therapy should be monitored for improvement. If catabolic stimuli can be identified, it is reasonable to continue the therapy until this stimulus subsides.

The gastrointestinal tract is preferred over the parenteral route; intradialytic parenteral nutrition (IDPN) should be reserved for patients who cannot tolerate or do not respond to oral intake or use of a feeding tube. (Cano, 2006b)

C. Oral supplements. Oral amino acid supplementation, given either during hemodialysis or three times a day, has been shown to improve whole-body protein metabolism in the short term and SGA, serum albumin, and serum prealbumin in the long term (Caglar et al., 2002). This and similar studies remain preliminary, and larger, randomized clinical trials are needed to establish a definite benefit.

A number of different enteral formulas specifically formulated for chronic dialysis patients are available; some of the more common products available in the United States are summarized in Table 28-5. Other considerations in the choice of oral nutritional supplements include cost, palatability, and lactose tolerance. Preliminary data from the HEMO study and our own experience suggest that supplements given to take home are generally consumed as a substitute for regular meals, leading to a limited effectiveness. Offering them around the hemodialysis procedure may provide significant logistical and therapeutic advantage.

D.   Intradialytic total parenteral nutrition (IDPN) in hemodialysis patients

   1.   Indications and benefits. IDPN is indicated in the adequately dialyzed hemodialysis patient who has malnutrition and is unable to ingest or absorb sufficient food via the gastrointestinal tract. IDPN promotes protein anabolism in the acute setting; in one larger study, IDPN treatments were associated with decreased mortality in patients with an initial serum albumin level of <3.4 g/dL (34 g/L) (Chertow et al., 1994).

   2.   Composition, infusion and complications. The IDPN solution is usually composed of an 8.5% amino acid solution mixed with 250 mL of 50% dextrose and is infused in the venous drip chamber for the entire duration of the hemodialysis procedure. Additional energy can be provided by also infusing a lipid emulsion; patients receiving lipids should be monitored closely for hypertriglyceridemia, changes in liver function tests, or compromise of the reticuloendothelial system. A typical composition of IDPN is outlined in Table 28-6.

   Painful arm cramps can occur when a high-osmolality IDPN solution is infused too rapidly (the dialysis session may need to be lengthened). Hypoglycemia can occur when a rapid infusion of glucose-containing IDPN solution is suddenly discontinued. Patients should consume some carbohydrate within the last 30 minutes of the IDPN infusion to prevent hypoglycemia. Likewise, if patients dialyze against a glucose-free dialysate, the IDPN should not be discontinued until the conclusion of the hemodialysis procedure.

   3.   Potential risks of IDPN. Hypo- and hyperglycemia, especially in patients with diabetes mellitus, should be anticipated and appropriately treated. Prolonged use of IDPN may lead to increased risk of infections, abnormalities in lipid profile, and accumulation of fat tissue rather than muscle. When amino acids are given as part of IDPN, there typically will be about a 0.2 decline in the treatment Kt/V (McCann et al., 1999). This decline in Kt/V is due to the sudden increase in urea generation associated with amino acid infusion, which elevates the postdialysis SUN level.

E.   Continuous total parenteral nutrition (TPN). TPN is used in patients with severe nutritional deficits who cannot receive adequate nutritional intake from oral supplements, intraperitoneal amino acids, or IDPN. General guidelines for the formulation of a typical TPN solution are outlined in Table 28-7.

Table 28-5. Composition of enteral products commonly prescribed as an oral supplement for poorly nourished dialysis patients

Source	Calorie Density	Protein	CHO	Fat	Osmolality	Sodium	Potassium	Phosphorus	Calcium
Novartis Med. Nutrition	0.68	34	131	0	900–930	210	970	1,480	630
Novartis Med. Nutrition	1.5	59	200	58	720	720	1,610	1,310	1,390
Novartis Med. Nutrition	1	61	139	23	540–610	720	1,610	1,310	1,390
Novartis Med. Nutrition	1	43	178	18	480	720	1,610	1,310	1,390
Novartis Med. Nutrition	1.6	47	223	61		845	1,690	1,352	1,690
Novartis Med. Nutrition	1.5	60	180	61	460	1,200	1850	1,200	1,200
Novartis Med. Nutrition	2.0	75	200	101	640	800	1,690	1,010	1,010
Ross Laboratories	1.5	55	212	48	680	800	1,860	845	845
Ross Laboratories	1.5	62	200	50	650	1,014	1,817	1,057	1,057
Novartis Med. Nutrition	1.5	68	170	65	650	1,290	2,250	1,070	1,070
Novartis Med. Nutrition	2.0	75	200	101	570	800	1,270	800	1,010
Ross Laboratories	2.0	70	223	96	665	845	1,055	695	1,370
Novartis Med. Nutrition	2.0	74	200	100	700	900	810	650	1,300
Nestle Nutrition	1	40	209	1.8	990	307	307	1,018	509
Nestle Nutrition	1.5	35	132	37	620	876	1,248	500	500
Nestle Nutrition	2.0	70	205	104	650	740	1,256	700	1,400
Ross Laboratories	1.1	37	151	35	300	640	1,020	535	535
Nestle Nutrition	2.0	34	290	82	600	N/A	N/A	N/A	N/A
Nutra/Balance	1.7	68	262	93	N/A	N/A	N/A	507	
Nutra/Balance	1.9	76	194	93	N/A	N/A	126.8	304	
Novartis Med. Nutrition	1.1	38	230	0	750	<340	<85	680	42
Ross Laboratories	2.0	30	255	96	600	790	1120	730	1,390
Mead Johnson	1.5	40	125	37	630–670	559	974	559	
	Amount of powder								
Novartis Med. Nutrition	5.4 g	2.5	7.4	0.1	64	19	56	25	29
Global Health Products	6.6 g	5	<1	0.5	N/A	10	35	27	N/A
Ross Laboratories	6.6 g	5.0	0.67	0.6	30	25	45	33	65
Novartis Med. Nutrition	7.0 g	6.0	0.0	0.0	N/A	15	35	17	40

Nutrient content based on 1 L for liquids/pudding or on the listed amount of powder for protein powders. Data obtained from manufacturer Web sites during December 2004. Caloric density expressed in kcal/mL. Protein, carbohydrate (CHO), and fat content expressed in grams. Osmolality expressed in mosm/kg H_2O. Electrolyte content expressed in mg.

Table 28-6.   Composition of a "typical" solution for intradialytic parenteral nutrition

Component	Amount
50% dextrose (D-glucose)	125 g (250 mL)
8.5% crystalline amino acids (essential and nonessential)	42.5 g (500 mL)
20% lipids	50 g (250 mL)
Electrolytes:	Sodium, phosphate, potassium sulfate, chloride, and magnesium with amount per IDPN bag adjusted for serum electrolyte levels
Vitamins	See text and Table 28-2
Insulin, regular	Adjusted/blood glucose levels
Caloric content	
50% dextrose	425 kcal/treatment
20% lipid emulsion	500 kcal/treatment
Total	925 kcal/treatment

IDPN, intradialytic parenteral nutrition.

1.   Carbohydrates. Approximately 50%–70% of nonprotein calories in TPN are provided from glucose. Glucose is usually provided as 70% D-glucose to minimize the amount of fluid administered. The precise amount of D-glucose given is dependent on the calculated energy intake indicated for an individual patient. Each milliliter of 70% dextrose provides 2.38 kcal.

2.   Amino acids. There is much controversy regarding the optimal mix of essential and nonessential amino acids used in TPN solutions. Some authors report that essential amino acids can be used more efficiently than larger quantities of essential and nonessential amino acids, whereas others report the development of nausea, vomiting, and metabolic acidosis when only essential amino acids are administered. Most commercial crystalline amino acid solutions provide a mix of essential and nonessential amino acids.

3.   Lipids. Lipids can provide up to 50% of the nonprotein calories in TPN solutions. Lipid emulsions are usually available in 10% and 20% solutions; the latter provides 2.0 kcal/mL. Lipids should be given over a 12- to 24-hour period to decrease the risk of decreased functioning of the reticuloendothelial system. Some authors recommend decreasing the amount of lipids given by 50% if the patient is septic or is at a high risk for sepsis. There is some controversy regarding the ratio of polyunsaturated to saturated fatty acids that is preferable in acutely ill dialysis patients, with most authors recommending a ratio between 1.0 and 2.0. If patients develop marked hypertriglyceridemia, lipid infusions can be provided once or twice weekly instead of daily.

Table 28-7. Composition of "typical" total parenteral nutrition solutions for hospitalized renal failure patients

Component	Amount
70% dextrose (D-glucose)	350 g (500 mL)
8.5% crystalline amino acids (essential and nonessential)	42.5 g (500 mL)
20% lipids or 10% lipids	100 g or 50 g (in 500 mL)

Electrolytes (general guidelines)[a]

Sodium	40–80 mM
Chloride	25–35 mM
Potassium	<35 mmol per day
Acetate	35–40 mmol per day
Calcium	5 mmol per day
Phosphorus	5–10 mmol per day
Magnesium	2–4 mmol per day
Iron	2 mg per day
Vitamins	See text and Table 28–2

Caloric content

Solution Administration Rate:	40 mL per hour or 960 mL per day	60 mL per hour or 1,440 mL per day
70% dextrose	762 kcal per day	1,142 kcal per day
20% lipid emulsion	640 kcal per day	960 kcal per day
Total	1,402 kcal per day	2,102 kcal per day
70% dextrose	762 kcal per day	1,142 kcal per day
10% lipid emulsion	352 kcal per day	528 kcal per day
Total	1,114 kcal per day	1,670 kcal per day

[a]The specific amount of electrolytes given should be modified based on the patient's clinical condition and serum concentration of electrolytes. The guidelines listed include electrolytes contributed by the infusion of amino acids. Use of a total parenteral nutrition sodium level of about 140 mmol/L will prevent hyponatremia but requires either daily dialysis or continuous renal replacement therapy for adequate volume control.

4. **Electrolytes.** The amount of sodium and chloride, the two principal ions, depends on whether continuous renal replacement therapy (CRRT) or intermittent hemodialysis (IHD) is being done. With CRRT, the TPN solutions, as well as most other infusates, should have a sodium level close to 140 mM. With IHD, a lower serum sodium level is used (40–80 mM) in order to minimize the risk of causing volume overload and pulmonary edema. Acetate, which is metabolized to bicarbonate, is traditionally added to TPN solutions when alkalinization of the serum is desired. The high glucose load plus the anabolism induced by TPN solutions can result in hypokalemia, hypophosphatemia, and

hypomagnesemia due to intracellular shifts of these ions. Therefore, blood levels of these electrolytes should be monitored frequently and they should be added to the TPN solution or infused separately, as needed.

5.   Vitamins. Little research has been performed on vitamin requirements in patients with acute renal failure. In general, vitamin supplementation during TPN should be similar to that provided to chronic dialysis patients (Table 28-2).

6.   Minerals and trace elements. Iron should be supplemented to help provide for effective erythropoiesis. Zinc is sometimes given based on some evidence that it accelerates wound healing. Other trace elements probably need not be supplemented unless the patient receives TPN for more than 3 weeks.

F.   Intraperitoneal infusion of amino acids in peritoneal dialysis patients

1.   Indications and benefits. The utilization of amino acid dialysate in place of glucose-based dialysate has been proposed as a means to replace proteins lost in the dialysate and to help minimize complications associated with use of glucose-based dialysate solutions, including weight gain, hyperlipidemia, and glucose intolerance. In CAPD patients, the replacement of one or two of the four daily glucose dialysate exchanges with glucose-free, amino acid dialysate results in an improvement in nitrogen balance, greater net protein anabolism, and a significant increase in serum transferrin and total protein levels (Kopple, 1995).

2.   Composition, infusion, and complications. Usually, the amino acid dialysate solution consists of both essential and nonessential amino acids. It is given as the overnight exchange in CAPD patients or as the long daytime dwell in continuous cycling peritoneal dialysis patients in order to maximize protein absorption. The osmotic effect of a 1.0% amino acid dialysate solution is similar to that of a 2.0% dextrose solution. Complications of utilizing amino acid dialysate solutions include anorexia, nausea, vomiting, and an increase in SUN levels, and are more common when patients receive two amino acid dialysate dwells per day versus one per day.

SELECTED READINGS

Arora SK, McFarlane SI. The case for low carbohydrate diets in diabetes management. *Nutr Metab (Lond)* 2005;2:16.

Baker JP, et al. Nutritional assessment: a comparison of clinical judgment and objective measurements. *N Engl J Med* 1982;306:969–972.

Beddhu S, Ramkumar N, Pappas LM. Normalization of protein intake by body weight and the associations of protein intake with nutritional status and survival. *J Ren Nutr* 2005;15(4):387–397.

Burrowes JD, et al. Effects of dietary intake, appetite, and eating habits on dialysis and non-dialysis treatment days in hemodialysis patients: cross-sectional results from the HEMO study. *J Ren Nutr* 2003;13:191–198.

Caglar K, et al. Therapeutic effects of oral nutritional supplementation during hemodialysis. *Kidney Int* 2002;62:1054–1059.

Cano F, et al. Kt/V and nPNA in pediatric peritoneal dialysis: a clinical or a mathematical association? *Pediatr Nephrol* 2006a;21(1): 114–118.

Cano N, et al. ESPEN guidelines on enteral nutrition: adult renal failure. *Clin Nutr* 2006b;25:295:310.

Chertow GM, et al. Phase angle predicts survival in hemodialysis patients. *J Ren Nutr* 1997;7:204–207.

Chertow GM, et al. The association of intradialytic parenteral nutrition with survival in hemodialysis patients. *Am J Kidney Dis* 1994;24:912–920.

Chumlea WC, et al. Nutritional status assessed from anthropometric measures in the HEMO study. *J Ren Nutr* 2003;13:31–38.

Detsky AS, et al. What is subjective global assessment of nutritional status? *J Parenter Enteral Nutr* 1987;11:8–13.

Di Filippo S, et al. Reduction in urea distribution volume over time in clinically stable dialysis patients. *Kidney Int* 2006;69(4):754–59.

Di Iorio BR, et al. A systematic evaluation of bioelectrical impedance measurement after hemodialysis session. *Kidney Int* 2004;65:2435–2440.

Dombros N, et al. for the EBPG Expert Group on Peritoneal Dialysis. European best practice guidelines for peritoneal dialysis. 8 Nutrition in peritoneal dialysis. *Nephrol Dial Transplant* 2005;20(Suppl 9):ix28–ix33.

Don BR, et al. Leptin is a negative acute phase protein in chronic hemodialysis patients. *Kidney Int* 2001;59:1114–1120.

Duerksen DR, et al. The validity and reproducibility of clinical assessment of nutritional status in the elderly. *Nutrition* 2000;16:740–744.

Dumler F. Use of bioelectric impedance analysis and dual-energy x-ray absorptiometry for monitoring the nutritional status of dialysis patients. *ASAIO J* 1997;43:256–260.

Feinstein EI, et al. Total parenteral nutrition with high and low nitrogen intakes in patients with acute renal failure. *Kidney Int* 1983;24(Suppl 16):S319–S323.

Galland R, Traeger J. Short daily hemodialysis and nutritional status in patients with chronic renal failure. *Semin Dial* 2004;17:104–108.

Ghandour H, et al. Distribution of plasma folate forms in hemodialysis patients receiving high daily doses of L-folinic or folic acid. *Kidney Int* 2002;62:2246–2249.

Institute of Medicine. Dietary reference intakes: water, potassium, sodium, chloride, and sulfate. National Academy Press, Washington, DC, 2004.

Johansen KL, et al. Association of body size with health status in patients beginning dialysis. *Am J Clin Nutr* 2006;83(3):543–549.

Joki N, et al. Relationship between serum albumin level before initiating haemodialysis and angiographic severity of coronary atherosclerosis in end-stage renal disease patients. *Nephrol Dial Transplant* 2006;21(6):1633–1639.

Jones M, et al. Treatment of malnutrition with 1.1% amino acid peritoneal dialysis solution: results of a multicenter outpatient study. *Am J Kidney Dis* 1998;32:761–769.

Kaizu Y, et al. Association between inflammatory mediators and muscle mass in long-term hemodialysis patients. *Am J Kidney Dis* 2003;42:295–302.

Kalantar-Zadeh K, et al. A modified, quantitative, subjective, global assessment of nutrition for dialysis patients. *Nephrol Dial Transplant* 1999;14:1732–1738.

Kalantar-Zadeh K, et al. A malnutrition-inflammation score is correlated with morbidity and mortality in maintenance hemodialysis patients. *Am J Kidney Dis* 2001;38:1251–1263.

Kalantar-Zadeh K, et al. Food intake characteristics of hemodialysis patients as obtained by food frequency questionnaire. *J Ren Nutr* 2002;12:17–31.

Kasama R, et al. Vitamin B_6 and hemodialysis: the impact of high flux/high-efficiency dialysis and review of the literature. *Am J Kidney Dis* 1996;8:680–686.

Kaysen GA. The microinflammatory state in uremia: causes and potential consequences. *J Am Soc Nephrol* 2001;12:1549–1557.

Kogirima M, et al. Low resting energy expenditure in middle-aged and elderly hemodialysis patients with poor nutritional status. *J Med Invest* 2006;53(1-2):34–41.

Kopple JD, et al. Treatment of malnourished CAPD patients with an amino acid based dialysate. *Kidney Int* 1999;55:1961–1969.

Kramer HJ, et al. Increasing body mass index and obesity in the incident ESRD population. *J Am Soc Nephrol* 2006;17(5):1453–1459.

McCann L, et al. Effect of intradialytic parenteral nutrition on delivered Kt/V. *Am J Kidney Dis* 1999;33:1131–1135.

McPhatter LL, et al. Nightly home hemodialysis: improvement in nutrition and quality-of-life. *Adv Ren Replace Ther* 1999;6:358–365.

Mushnick R, et al. Relationship of bioelectrical impedance parameters to nutrition and survival in peritoneal dialysis patients. *Kidney Int* 2003;87(Suppl):S53–S56.

National Kidney Foundation. *K/DOQI clinical practice guidelines for nutrition in chronic renal failure.* New York: National Kidney Foundation, 2001.

Nelson E, et al. Anthropometric norms for the dialysis population. *Am J Kidney Dis* 1990;16:32–37.

Pupim RB, et al. Intradialytic parenteral nutrition improves protein and energy homeostasis in chronic hemodialysis patients. *J Clin Invest* 2002;110:483–492.

Pupim LB, Cuppari L, Ikizler TA. Nutrition and metabolism in kidney disease. *Semin Nephrol* 2006;26(2):134–157.

Pupim LB, et al. Uremic malnutrition is a predictor of death independent of inflammatory status. *Kidney Int* 2004;66(5):2054–2060.

Rocco MV, et al. Intake of vitamins and minerals in stable hemodialysis patients as determined by 9-day food records. *J Ren Nutr* 1997;7:17–24.

Rocco MV, et al. Nutritional status in the HEMO study cohort at baseline. *Am J Kidney Dis* 2002;39:245–256.

Rocco MV, et al. for the HEMO Study Group. The effect of dialysis dose and membrane flux on nutritional parameters in hemodialysis patients: results of the HEMO study. *Kidney Int* 2004;65:2321–2334.

Soop M, et al. Energy expenditure in postoperative multiple organ failure with acute renal failure. *Clin Nephrol* 1989;31:139–145.

Wang J, et al. Anthropometry in body composition. An overview. *Ann N Y Acad Sci* 2001;904:317–326.

WEB REFERENCES

National Kidney Foundation KDOQI Clinical Guidelines: http://www.kidney.org/professionals/kdoqi/guidelines.cfm

Nutritional guidelines, tables, and links: http://www.hdcn.com/ch/nutri

Serum Enzyme Levels

N. D. Vaziri and D. Kayichian

The concentrations of a number of serum enzymes commonly measured for diagnostic purposes can be abnormal in asymptomatic patients with end-stage renal disease (Table 29-1).

I. Acute myocardial infarction (MI). In dialysis patients undergoing acute MI, the time course of elevations in serum levels of creatine kinase (CK), aspartate aminotransferase (AST), and lactate dehydrogenase (LDH) is presumably similar to that in nonuremic patients, although no data to this effect have been published. It is of note that measurements of total CK and LDH are no longer recommended for the diagnosis of MI (Alpert et al., 2000).

A. Creatine kinase

1. Elevated baseline serum total CK level. Baseline serum total CK values are elevated persistently in 10%–50% of dialysis patients (Lal et al., 1987). When elevation is present, it is usually mild (e.g., to values less than three times the upper limit of normal). Occasionally, CK levels of 5–10 times the upper limit of normal are encountered.

The reason for the persistent elevation of total serum CK levels in some dialysis patients is unknown. CK levels are more often elevated in hemodialysis patients than in those treated with continuous ambulatory peritoneal dialysis (CAPD). CK levels are higher in males than in females and higher in blacks than in whites; they correlate with arm circumference. Postulated causes for high levels include intramuscular injection of androgens or other drugs. Other potential causes include subclinical myopathies, vitamin D deficiency, carnitine deficiency, and reduced degradation of enzyme. One should also consider drug toxicity in those receiving statins, fibrates, antiviral agents, etc. After renal transplantation, elevated serum CK levels return to the normal range.

2. Elevated percentage of CK-MB. In nonuremic patients, up to 5% of total serum CK is the MB isoenzyme. In the appropriate clinical circumstances, when serum total CK levels are elevated, a concomitant rise in the percentage of the MB isoenzyme is a highly specific indicator of myocardial damage. However, some of the methods used for quantitation of the MB isoenzyme may yield falsely elevated CK-MB values. From 3% to 30% of dialysis patients without evidence of myocardial ischemia have been reported to have an elevated percentage of CK-MB in their sera. Some of the higher numbers reported may have been due to methodologic problems; the more recent studies report an increase in the CK-MB percentage in 5% or less of dialysis patients. When the CK-MB percentage is increased in dialysis

Table 29-1. Alterations of baseline serum enzyme levels in dialysis patients

Enzyme	Serum Level
CK	Increased in 10%–50%
CK-MM	Increased in up to 40%
CK-MB	Increased in 3%–30%
Cardiac troponin	
Troponin T	Increased in up to 71%
Troponin I	Increased in up to 9%
LDH	Increased in about 35%
LDH isoenzymes (1–5)	Isomorphic pattern
Aspartate aminotransferase	Decreased in 10%–90%
Alkaline phosphatase	
Total	Increased in about 50%
Intestinal isoenzyme	Increased in about 50%
Bone isoenzyme	Increased in about 50%
Glutamyl transpeptidase	Increased in 10%–15%
Amylase	Increased in about 50%
Lipase	Increased in about 50%
Trypsin(ogen)	Increased in up to 100%
Elastase	Increased in up to 43%
Phospholipase A_2	Increased in up to 100%

CK, creatine kinase; LDH, lactic dehydrogenase.

patients without MI, the elevation is slight (e.g., usually to <8% of the total CK value).

3. Elevated percentage of CK-BB and CK-MM in acute renal failure. Serum levels of these isoenzymes are reportedly increased in patients with acute renal failure, possibly due to their release from damaged renal tubular tissue. In some assays, the CK-BB and CK-MB isoenzymes are not well separated. In stable hemodialysis patients, the serum CK-BB concentration is usually in the normal range.

B. Aspartate aminotransferase. See Section II A.

C. Lactic dehydrogenase

1. Increased baseline serum LDH level. Serum levels of LDH may be elevated (to three times the upper limit of normal) in as many as 35% of patients with renal insufficiency, due either to a reduced elimination rate or to increased release from damaged renal tissue in patients with acute renal failure. The elevation is characterized by an "isomorphic" pattern; the LDH-1:LDH-5 ratio is <1, and there is a nearly proportional increase in the activities of the various LDH isoenzymes (Vaziri et al., 1990). Serum LDH levels also may increase acutely in the course of hemodialysis, consistent with a hemoconcentration effect, as well as release from leukocytes. For this reason, predialysis samples should always be used for evaluation of serum LDH (and other enzyme) levels.

2. Human cardiac myosin light chain 1. Enzyme immunoassay of cardiac myosin light chains has been proposed as a sensitive test for MI. Unfortunately, in dialysis patients, serum levels of this compound are elevated 40-fold over control values (Nakai et al., 1992); accordingly, this test is not useful in the end-stage renal disease population.

D. Cardiac troponins

1. Cardiac troponin T is a regulatory contractile protein that is normally absent in blood, and its detection serves as a specific and sensitive indicator of myocardial damage (Hamm et al., 1992). However, blood troponin T is elevated in over 80% of dialysis patients with no clinical evidence of acute myocardial injury (Apple et al., 2002). Elevation of troponin T level in this population is probably due to its impaired renal clearance (Diris et al., 2004), as well as endothelial dysfunction and left ventricular hypertrophy. Blood troponin T levels are not altered by hemodialysis. Interestingly, chronic elevation of troponin T (>0.1 ng/mL) has been shown to be of prognostic value in predicting mortality and cardiac events in otherwise asymptomatic dialysis patients (Iliou et al., 2003; Porter et al., 2000) and those exhibiting intradialytic hypotension (Hung et al., 2004).

2. Cardiac troponin I is another cardiac specific regulatory contractile protein, elevated blood levels of which are a specific indicator of cardiac injury. However, elevated troponin I levels occur in up to 8%–9% of patients with advanced renal failure in the absence of clinical evidence of myocardial injury (Apple et al., 2002). Nonetheless, troponin I has been shown to be a reasonably accurate predictor of myocardial injury in renal failure patients (Martin et al., 1998) and to be a more specific marker of acute MI than troponin T and CK-MB in this population (McCullough et al., 2002). Hemodialysis does not significantly change the serum levels of troponin I.

II. Enzymes associated with hepatic disease

A. Alanine and aspartate aminotransferases (ALT and AST)

1. Low baseline serum ALT and AST levels. Serum aminotransferase values are sometimes depressed (e.g., by 20%–50%) in 10%–90% of dialysis patients (Cohen et al., 1976). The reason is unknown. Many explanations have been advanced, including inhibition of transaminase activity in the serum by uremic toxins. When ALT and AST levels are measured by an ultraviolet method using the SMA 12/60 autoanalyzer, some degree of factitious underestimation may result due to the presence of materials in uremic serum that absorb ultraviolet light. Serum AST values have been shown to increase after dialysis; the increase is presumably due to (a) removal of a dialyzable inhibitor, (b) increased release of the enzyme from erythrocytes in the extracorporeal circuit, and/or (c) ultrafiltration-induced hemoconcentration.

Because of the low baseline serum aminotransferase levels in dialysis patients, the finding of a value slightly above the upper limits of normal or of a substantial rise within the normal range should alert the clinician to a possible underlying disease process. In fact, comparison of HbsAg-positive and -negative dialysis patients has shown higher values in the former than in the latter group without exceeding the upper limit of normal range (Fabrizi et al., 2003). Similar findings were reported when patients with persistent hepatic C viremia were compared with those exhibiting intermittent viremia (Fabrizi et al., 2000). These observations have led to a call for reduction of the upper limits of normal to 18 IU/L for AST and 16 IU/L for ALT in the dialysis population (Herrine et al., 2002).

2. Causes of mildly elevated serum aminotransferase levels. A common clinical problem is to evaluate the importance of mildly elevated aminotransferase levels (ALT, AST, or both) in a dialysis patient. The frequency with which acute viral hepatitis B or C becomes chronic is increased in dialysis patients, and an elevated serum ALT level must be considered to reflect possible hepatitis (especially hepatitis C infection) until proven otherwise (Mondelli et al., 1991). Herpes simplex hepatitis and cytomegalovirus hepatitis also present with elevated aminotransferases (AST > ALT). Other causes of elevated serum aminotransferase levels in dialysis patients include the effects of hepatotoxic drugs and iron overload (hemosiderosis).

B. Alkaline phosphatase

1. Sites of alkaline phosphatase production. Alkaline phosphatase is normally produced by cells lining the biliary tree. In obstructive jaundice, the serum level of alkaline phosphatase is increased. However, alkaline phosphatases are produced by many other tissues as well, including bone, intestine, lung, kidney, some hepatic and extrahepatic tumors, white blood cells, and placenta.

2. Elevated serum levels of bone- or intestine-derived alkaline phosphatase. Both bone and liver disease are common in dialysis patients; hence, an elevated unfractionated serum alkaline phosphatase level is often difficult to interpret. The cause of alkaline phosphatase elevation in a given patient can usually be at least partially resolved by determination of the heat stability of the enzyme in the serum specimen (the bone-derived enzyme loses its activity after exposure to heat). In addition, concomitant elevation of other hepatobiliary enzymes (see below) increases the likelihood that an elevated serum alkaline phosphatase value is of hepatic origin.

C. Other hepatobiliary enzymes. Serum levels of 5'-nucleotidase, leucine aminopeptidase (LAP), and γ-glutamyl transpeptidase (GGT) are also increased in the presence of active hepatobiliary disease. Elevated serum values of these enzymes reflect hepatobiliary dysfunction somewhat specifically. One exception is pregnancy, in which serum concentrations of 5'-nucleotidase and LAP may be increased. Elevation of the serum GGT level can be caused by ingestion of certain drugs that induce hepatic microsomal enzymes (e.g., phenytoin and phenobarbital).

1. Levels of other hepatobiliary enzymes in dialysis patients. Reliable data concerning baseline serum levels of 5'-nucleotidase and LAP in dialysis patients are lacking. For reasons that are not entirely clear, serum GGT levels

may be significantly elevated (two to three times the upper limit of normal) in about 10%–15% of end-stage renal
disease patients who do not abuse alcohol, who exhibit no
clinical evidence of liver disease, and who are not known
to be using drugs that affect hepatic microsomal enzymes
(Fine and McIntosh, 1975).

III.   Enzymes associated with pancreatitis

A.   Amylase

1.   Elevated baseline levels of serum amylase. In most
dialysis patients, due to the loss of urinary excretion, serum
total amylase activity is elevated up to three times the upper limit of normal, even in the absence of clinical evidence
of pancreatitis. The magnitude of elevation is greater in
patients with acute renal failure than in chronic dialysis
patients. Serum amylase activity may be spuriously low
(by 90%) in peritoneal dialysis patients using icodextrin-
containing dialysis solutions (Schoenicke et al., 2002). This
phenomenon has been attributed to the interference of
icodextrin with serum amylase activity assay (Anderstam
et al., 2003). Serum concentrations of the pancreas-specific
P_3 isoenzyme have been variably reported to be increased or
normal in asymptomatic dialysis patients. In fact, P_3 values
exceeding three times the upper limit of normal are seen in
up to 18% of asymptomatic dialysis patients. In contrast, in
the nonuremic population, the P_3 amylase fraction is consistently absent in the serum and appears only with acute
pancreatitis.

**2.   Question of occult pancreatitis in dialysis pa-
tients.** Autopsy studies of largely asymptomatic dialysis
patients have revealed a high incidence of pancreatic abnormalities, including chronic pancreatitis. In addition, examination of pancreatic exocrine function has revealed
significant reduction of fecal chymotrypsin in hemodialysis
patients with no evidence of significant ultrasonographic
abnormalities (Ventrucci et al., 1995). The extent to which
persistent elevations of the serum amylase levels are due to
decreased catabolism of the enzyme versus low-grade pancreatitis is not known.

**3.   Serum and peritoneal fluid amylase levels during
pancreatitis in dialysis patients.** In a dialysis patient
suspected of having pancreatitis, the finding of a serum total amylase value in excess of three times the upper limit
of normal suggests that pancreatitis is present. Unfortunately, very severe pancreatitis can be present in dialysis
patients with only slight, and therefore nondiagnostic, elevations in the serum total amylase level. We have found
elevation of the plasma P_3 isoenzyme level to be a reliable
indicator of pancreatitis in dialysis patients (Vaziri et al.,
1988).

The peritoneal fluid amylase concentration, easily obtainable in patients receiving peritoneal dialysis, is not a sensitive indicator of pancreatitis because the peritoneal fluid
amylase levels can be only slightly elevated in the presence
of severe pancreatitis. Nevertheless, an effluent amylase

level >100 units/dL is suggestive of pancreatitis or some other intra-abdominal catastrophe (Caruana et al., 1987; Gupta et al., 1992).

B. Lipase

1. Elevated baseline serum lipase levels in dialysis patients. Serum lipase activity is elevated (as high as twice the upper limit of normal) in about 50% of dialysis patients. Serum lipase activity rises following hemodialysis due to (a) heparin-induced release of endothelium-bound lipoprotein lipase and (b) presumably, ultrafiltration-induced hemoconcentration. Therefore, predialysis samples should be used for this test. In peritoneal dialysis patients using icodextrin-based peritoneal dialysis solutions, measurement of lipase is superior to amylase for diagnosis of acute pancreatitis.

C. Serum pancreatic secretory trypsin inhibitor (PSTI). The plasma concentration of this inhibitory peptide (MW 6,000) is increased in acute pancreatitis. Unfortunately, PSTI is also markedly elevated in dialysis patients in the absence of discernible pancreatic pathology. Reduced renal degradation, possibly with increased pancreatic or extrapancreatic production, is involved.

D. Serum trypsin(ogen) rises in pancreatitis in concert with other pancreatic enzymes. However, trypsinogen level may be elevated in up to 100% of dialysis patients (Seno et al., 1995; Kimmel et al., 1995). The magnitude of elevation is greater in hemodialysis than in peritoneal dialysis patients.

E. Elastase I and phospholipase A$_2$ are two other pancreatic enzymes whose serum concentrations rise in acute pancreatitis. However, a large percentage of dialysis patients show marked elevations of these enzymes as well in the absence of clinical evidence of pancreatitis (Seno et al., 1995).

SELECTED READINGS

Alpert JS, et al. Myocardial infarction redefined, a consensus document of the Joint European Society of Cardiology/American College of Cardiology Committee for the redefinition of myocardial infarction. *J Am Coll Cardiol* 2000;36:959–969.

Anderstam B, et al. Determination of alpha-amylase activity in serum and dialysate from patients using icodextrin-based peritoneal dialysis fluid. *Perit Dial Int* 2003;23:146–150.

Apple FS, et al. Predictive value of cardiac troponin I and T for subsequent death in end-stage renal disease. *Circulation* 2002;106:2941–2945.

Caruana RJ, et al. Serum and peritoneal fluid amylase levels in CAPD: normal values and clinical usefulness. *Am J Nephrol* 1987;7:169–172.

Cohen GA, et al. Observations on decreased serum glutamic oxalacetic transaminase (SGOT) activity in azotemic patients. *Ann Intern Med* 1976;84:275–280.

Diris JH, et al. Impaired renal clearance explains elevated troponin T fragment in hemodialysis patients. *Circulation* 2004;109:23–25.

Fabrizi F, et al. Biological dynamics of viral load in hemodialysis patients with hepatitis C virus. *Am J Kidney Dis* 2000;35:122–129.

Fabrizi F, et al. Influence of hepatitis B virus viremia upon serum aminotransferase activity in dialysis population. *Int J Artif Organs* 2003;26:1048–1055.

Fine A, McIntosh, WB. Elevation of serum gamma-glutamyl transpeptidase in end-stage chronic renal failure. *Scott Med J* 1975; 20:113–115.

Gupta A, et al. CAPD and pancreatitis: no connection. *Perit Dial Int* 1992;12:309–316.

Hamm CW, et al. The prognostic value of serum troponin T in unstable angina. *N Engl J Med* 1992;327:146–150.

Herrine SK, et al. Development of an HCV infection risk stratification algorithm for patients on chronic hemodialysis. *Am J Gastroenterol* 2002;97:2619–2622.

Hung SY, et al. Cardiac troponin I and creatine kinase isoenzyme MB in patients with intradialytic hypotension. *Blood Purif* 2004;22:338–343.

Iliou MC, et al. Prognostic value of cardiac markers in ESRD: Chronic Hemodialysis and New Cardiac Markers Evaluation (CHANCE) study. *Am J Kidney Dis* 2003;42:513–523.

Kimmel PL, et al. Trypsinogen and other pancreatic enzymes in patients with renal disease: a comparison of high efficiency hemodialysis and continuous ambulatory peritoneal dialysis. *Pancreas* 1995;10:325–330.

Lal SM, et al. Total creatine kinase and isoenzyme fractions in chronic dialysis patients. *Int J Artif Organs* 1987;10:72–76.

Martin GC, et al. Cardiac troponin-I accurately predicts myocardial injury in renal failure. *Nephrol Dial Transplant* 1998;13:1709–1712.

McCullough PA, et al. Performance of multiple cardiac biomarkers measured in the emergency department in patients with chronic kidney disease and chest pain. *Acad Emerg Med* 2002;9:1389–1396.

Mondelli MU, et al. Abnormal alanine aminotransferase activity reflects exposure to hepatitis C virus in haemodialysis patients. *Nephrol Dial Transplant* 1991;6:480–483.

Nakai K, et al. Increased serum levels of cardiac myosin light chain-1 in patients with renal failure. *Rinsho Byori* 1992;40:529–534.

Porter GA, et al. Long term follow up of the utility of troponin T to assess cardiac risk in stable chronic hemodialysis patients. *Clin Lab* 2000;46:469–476.

Roppolo LP, et al. A comparison of troponin T and troponin I as predictors of cardiac events in patients undergoing chronic dialysis at a veteran's hospital: a pilot study. *J Am Coll Cardiol* 1999;34:448–454.

Schoenicke G, et al. Dialysis with icodextrin interferes with measurement of serum alpha-amylase activity. *Nephrol Dial Transplant* 2002;17:1988–1992.

Seno T, et al. Serum levels of six pancreatic enzymes as related to the degree of renal dysfunction. *Am J Gastroenterol* 1995;90:2002–2005.

Tibi L, et al. Multiple forms of alkaline phosphatase in plasma of hemodialysis patients. *Clin Chem* 1991;37:815–820.

Vaziri ND, et al. Pancreatic enzymes in patients with end-stage renal diseases maintained on hemodialysis. *Am J Gastroenterol* 1988;83:410–412.

Vaziri ND, et al. Serum LDH and LDH isoenzymes in chronic renal failure: effect of hemodialysis. *Int J Artif Organs* 1990;13:223–227.

Ventrucci M, et al. Alterations of exocrine pancreas in end-stage renal disease. Do they reflect a clinically relevant uremic pancreopathy? *Dig Dis Sci* 1995;40:2576–2581.

Diabetes

Antonios H. Tzamaloukas, David J. Leehey, and Eli A. Friedman

More than 40% of all new patients starting dialysis are diabetic. Provision of maintenance dialysis for this group can be a challenging task. Morbidity and mortality are substantially higher in diabetic patients maintained on dialysis than in their non-diabetic counterparts, with cardiovascular disease and infection being the leading causes of death.

I. **When to initiate dialysis.** Early referral to nephrologists of diabetic patients with renal failure reportedly improves outcomes. Current guidelines emphasize initiation of dialysis prior to the appearance of frank uremic manifestations (at an estimated glomerular filtration rate [eGFR] of ≤ 15 mL per minute per 1.73 m^2 for a 70-kg patient) to prevent insidious malnutrition. There are several reasons for starting dialysis in diabetic patients at an eGFR at or above 15 mL per minute per 1.73 m^2. Renal function deteriorates rapidly in this group. Hypertension, which is associated with rapid acceleration of diabetic retinopathy, is often difficult to control when the eGFR falls below this level. Anecdotally, uremic symptoms may manifest at a less advanced degree of renal insufficiency in diabetic patients than in nondiabetic patients.

II. **Hemodialysis versus peritoneal dialysis.** The problems with each form of dialysis are listed in Table 30-1. Long-term peritoneal dialysis in diabetic patients may complicate control of blood sugar because deranged glucose homeostasis is stressed further by the large amount of glucose administered via the dialysis solution. In addition, glucose absorption from the abdominal cavity decreases appetite. Many peritoneal dialysis patients have great difficulty ingesting the recommended amount of protein (1.2 g/kg daily). On the other hand, the incidence and severity of hypoglycemic episodes is reduced in continuous ambulatory peritoneal dialysis (CAPD) compared to that in hemodialysis patients due to the constant presence of glucose in the abdomen. Rates of infection (peritonitis, exit site and tunnel infections) and rates of catheter replacement are similar between diabetics and nondiabetics on peritoneal dialysis. Administration of insulin intraperitoneally appears to increase slightly the risk of peritonitis only in continuous ambulatory peritoneal dialysis. With hemodialysis, coexisting blood vessel disease often hinders creation of an adequate, long-lasting vascular access. The survival rates of both arteriovenous (AV) fistulas and grafts are substantially reduced in diabetics. A small fraction of diabetic patients develop severe hand ischemia after creation of an ipsilateral AV fistula and may lose their arms to gangrene. Because of autonomic nervous system dysfunction or cardiac diastolic

Table 30-1. Dialysis modalities for diabetics

Modality	Advantages	Disadvantages
Hemodialysis	Very efficient Frequent medical follow-up (in-center) No protein loss to dialysate Less need for leg amputation (?)	Risky for patients with advanced cardiac disease Multiple arteriovenous access surgeries often required; risk of severe hand ischemia High incidence of hypotension during dialysis session Predialysis hyperkalemia Prone to hypoglycemia
CAPD	Good cardiovascular tolerance No need for arteriovenous access Good control of serum potassium Good glucose control, particularly with use of intraperitoneal insulin; less severe hypoglycemia	Peritonitis, exit site infection, and tunnel infection risks similar to those in nondiabetic dialysis patients Protein loss to dialysate Increased intra-abdominal pressure effects (hernias, fluid leaks, etc.) Schedule not convenient for helper if one is required (e.g., some blind patients)
CCPD	Good cardiovascular tolerance No need for arteriovenous access Good control of serum potassium Good glucose control with use of intraperitoneal insulin Good for blind diabetics	Protein loss to dialysate Peritonitis risk slightly less than for CAPD

CAPD, continuous ambulatory peritoneal dialysis; CCPD, continuous cycling peritoneal dialysis.

dysfunction, diabetics are at increased risk for hypotension during hemodialysis. The poor vascular access and risk of hypotension may cause diabetics to receive a lesser amount of dialysis (in terms of fractional urea clearance [Kt/V]) than their nondiabetic counterparts.

Lower extremity amputations are frequent in diabetic patients on either hemodialysis or peritoneal dialysis. The rate of progression of retinopathy is also apparently similar between patients treated with hemodialysis and those treated with peritoneal dialysis. Although visual impairment impedes training for CAPD and makes it difficult for the patient to perform the exchange procedure properly, blind diabetics can be trained to perform CAPD without a helper. When properly instructed, their risk of developing peritonitis is only slightly greater than the risk in sighted diabetics. A number of devices are available to help visually impaired patients connect the dialysis solution container to the peritoneal transfer set (see Chapter 19). Continuous cycling peritoneal dialysis (CCPD) is a good therapeutic choice for blind diabetic patients because it requires the performance of only one "on" and one "off" procedure daily.

Reports from the U.S. Renal Data System (USRDS) suggested that mortality is higher in diabetic subjects, and especially diabetic women, on peritoneal dialysis than in those on hemodialysis. Results from the Canadian Organ Replacement Registry did not support this finding. Patient selection biases may have affected these observations. Comorbidity and malnutrition have much larger effects on mortality than the dialysis modality. Meticulous management and prevention of cardiovascular and infectious morbidity may lead to substantial improvement in patient survival. There is evidence suggesting that aggressive cardiac revascularization procedures are effective in diabetics on chronic dialysis (Aoki et al., 2002).

III.   Diet. Whatever the mode of dialysis therapy, diabetic patients generally show evidence of wasting and malnutrition. Many factors contribute, including chronic inflammation, inadequate food intake, diabetic gastroparesis and enteropathy, and the catabolic stress associated with frequent intercurrent illness. In the event of serious illness, diabetic dialysis patients often require early and intensive nutritional support.

A.   Routine dietary prescription. The diets advocated for nondiabetic hemodialysis and CAPD patients in Chapter 28 also apply to diabetics. In an anuric diabetic patient being treated with hemodialysis, the stringent sodium, potassium, and fluid restrictions listed in Table 28-2 should be applied. Special effort should be made to limit intake of simple sugars and saturated fats. Hypolipidemic drugs should be used if lipid control is not adequate based on diet and insulin schedule alone. In malnourished patients, nutrition can improve with the use of intradialytic parenteral nutrition in hemodialysis or one exchange per day with amino acid–containing dialysate in peritoneal dialysis.

1.   Carbohydrates percentage. The general recommendation for a diabetic diet is for 50%–60% of intake to be carbohydrates, with an emphasis on lower glycemic index foods. There is some interest in using a lower carbohydrate diet in diabetics (Arora et al., 2005), although such approaches remain experimental. In patients undergoing peritoneal dialysis, the glucose calories supplied from the peritoneal dialysis regimen (usually around 400 kcal) should be subtracted from the dietary carbohydrate prescription, and perhaps in selected patients with hypertriglyceridemia, a focus on avoiding all high-glycemic-index carbohydrates might be of benefit.

Table 30-2. Toronto western hospital protocol for intraperitoneal insulin administration in CAPD patients

Goals of therapy: Fasting blood glucose <140 mg/dL (7.8 mmol/L)
1-hour postprandial: <200 mg/dL (11 mmol/L)
  1. Hospitalize patient.
  2. The protocol is based on use of four 2-L exchanges per day (adapt if necessary).
  3. First three exchanges are performed 20 minutes before each of the major meals, and the fourth exchange at approximately 11 p.m. A snack, consisting of a sandwich and small glucose-containing soft drink, is given at that time.
  4. Target total caloric intake (diet + dialysate) is 35 kcal/kg per day. Target oral caloric intake is 25–30 kcal/kg per day, depending on the expected amount of glucose absorption from dialysis solution.
  5. Measure blood glucose four times a day: Fasting in the morning, 1 hour after breakfast, 1 hour after lunch, and 1 hour after supper.

Day 1: To each 2-L dialysis solution container, add the following amounts of regular insulin:
  a. One fourth of the total number of insulin units (all types of insulin) ordinarily given subcutaneously daily prior to starting peritoneal dialysis. (However, all units added to the bag are regular insulin.) This amount of insulin is designed to help metabolize the dietary carbohydrate intake.
  b. To each bag, in addition to the insulin dose in a, add an insulin supplement to help metabolize the glucose present in the dialysis solution. This supplemental regular insulin dose is as follows:
      To each 2-L 1.5% dextrose bag: 2 units
      To each 2-L 2.5% dextrose bag: 4 units
      To each 2-L 4.25% dextrose bag: 6 units

EXAMPLE
Patient previously receiving 20 units of NPH insulin plus 10 units of regular insulin in the morning and 10 units of NPH insulin in the evening:
    Total daily SC insulin dose is 40 units
If CAPD schedule is to use three 2-L 1.5% exchanges during the day and one 2-L 4.25% exchange at night, then:
    To each 2-L 1.5% container add 10 + 2 = 12 units regular insulin
    To the 2-L 4.25% container add 10 + 6 = 16 units regular insulin

Day 2: Adjust amount of insulin added to the dialysis solution containers according to serum glucose levels obtained the previous day. The fasting blood sugar will reflect the insulin dose added to the solution infused at 11 P.M. The postprandial serum glucose concentrations will reflect the insulin added to the solutions administered 20 minutes prior to the respective meals. The adjustment is made according to the table below, using columns 1 versus 3 to adjust the nocturnal exchange and columns 2 versus 3 to adjust each of the daytime exchanges.

continued

Table 30-2. *Continued.*

EXAMPLE
On day 1, the serum glucose values were:

1 hour after breakfast	220 mg/dL	12 mmol/L
1 hour after lunch	350 mg/dL	19.4 mmol/L
1 hour after supper	300 mg/dL	16.7 mmol/L
Fasting (day 2)	160 mg/dL	8.9 mmol/L

One could now add an extra 2 units to the first daytime exchange and an extra 4 units to each of the second and third daytime exchanges, and leave the insulin dose for the nocturnal exchange the same.

Fasting Serum Glucose Level (mg/dL)	1-hour Post-Prandial Serum Glucose Level (mg/dL)	Fasting Serum Glucose Level (mmol/L)	1-hour Post-Prandial Serum Glucose Level (mmol/L)	Amount of Insulin Change (units/2-L bag)
<40	<40	<2.2	<2.2	−6
<40	40–80	<2.2	2.2–4.4	−4
40–80	80–120	2.2–4.4	4.4–6.7	−2
80–180	120–180	4.4–10	6.7–10	No change
180–240	180–240	10–13.3	10–13.3	+2[a]
240–400	240–300	13.3–22	13.3–16.7	+4[a]
>400	>300	>22	>16.7	Variable

CAPD, continuous ambulatory peritoneal dialysis; SC, subcutaneous.
[a]In type 1 diabetics, substantially less additional insulin may be required.
Modified from Amair P, et al. Continuous ambulatory peritoneal dialysis in diabetics with end-stage renal disease. *N Engl J Med* 1982;306:625.

2. **Dietary "glycotoxins" from advanced glycosylation end products (AGEs)**. Levels of AGEs are increased in food that has been cooked at high temperature, especially if food contains a high proportion of fat (Goldberg et al., 2004). Dietary AGE ingestion has been linked to adverse lipid profiles and inflammatory markers in diabetics (Cai et al., 2004; Uribarri et al., 2005) and to increased serum levels of AGEs in end-stage renal disease (ESRD) patients, with perhaps increased risk of access thrombosis (Uribarri et al., 2003; Cai et al., 2006). Any reason to additionally restrict food in ESRD patients should be done with caution, given the high prevalence of malnutrition; however, some attention to food preparation with focusing on formation of AGEs (deep frying, extensive heating) might be a consideration.

B. **Diabetic gastroparesis and enteropathy.** The diagnosis of diabetic gastroparesis is often made based on symptoms of nausea, vomiting, early satiety, and postprandial fullness.

However, since other treatable conditions can have similar symptoms, an esophagogastroduodenoscopy (EGD) should be performed before symptoms are ascribed to gastroparesis alone. The traditional "gold standard" to establish the diagnosis of gastroparesis is scintigraphic measurement of gastric emptying. However, a drawback is that scintigraphy exposes patients to radiation and is therefore not ideally suited for repeated investigations (to monitor the response to therapy). This problem can be overcome by 13C-labeled acetate and octanoic acid breath tests. Diabetic gastroparesis can be associated with poor food intake and unpredictable nutrient absorption; the result can be hypoglycemia alternating with hyperglycemia. In such patients, small, frequent (up to six times per day) feedings may improve symptoms. The pharmacologic treatment of gastroparesis in diabetics on dialysis is unsatisfactory. Metoclopramide in a small starting dose (5 mg before meals), with small increments until results are seen, is usually the first drug prescribed. However, this drug is associated with a high incidence of extrapyramidal complications in dialysis patients, particularly at higher doses, and its effects are often temporary. Other "prokinetic" gastrointestinal motility drugs, such as domperidone, motilin agonists, or ondansetron, may be tried. Intraperitoneal ondansetron in a dose of 16 mg twice a day stopped the intractable nausea and vomiting in a peritoneal dialysis patient who had failed all other treatments (Amin et al., 2002).

Diabetic enteropathy results from functional impairment of the enteric nervous system and can result in disordered motility of the small bowel and the colon, resulting in either delayed or accelerated bowel transit times. Diabetic enteropathy with resulting diarrhea can complicate alimentation, causing debilitation, poor food intake, and hypoglycemia. Severe cases of diabetic enteropathy can be treated with a trial of a broad-spectrum antimicrobial (e.g., doxycycline in a dose of 50 or 100 mg daily) to combat bacterial overgrowth in the intestine. Loperamide hydrochloride (up to 10 mg daily) to decrease bowel motility is also useful.

IV. Control of blood sugar
A. Alteration in insulin metabolism.
In uremic patients (both diabetic and nondiabetic), insulin secretion by the β cells of the pancreas is reduced and the responsiveness of peripheral tissues (e.g., muscle) to insulin is depressed. On the other hand, the rate of insulin catabolism (renal and extrarenal) is decreased, and therefore, the half-life of any insulin present in the circulation is prolonged. All of these abnormalities are only partially corrected after institution of maintenance dialysis therapy. The newer, faster, insulin forms (e.g., lispro insulin) have a faster onset of action in uremic patients as well as subjects with normal renal function (Czock et al., 2003).

1. Abnormal glucose tolerance tests in all dialysis patients.
The glucose tolerance test cannot be used to diagnose diabetes in dialysis patients because the rise in serum glucose concentration will be greater and more prolonged than normal in all dialysis patients as a result of uremia-induced insulin resistance. However, fasting serum glucose

concentrations are normal in nondiabetic hemodialysis patients; a high level suggests the presence of diabetes. In CAPD patients, a true fasting state is never achieved due to constant absorption of glucose from the dialysis solution. In this group, unless peritonitis is present, the "fasting" serum glucose value rarely exceeds 160 mg/dL (8.9 mmol/L), even when using 4.25% dextrose dialysis solution; higher levels suggest that the patient has diabetes. In CAPD patients using icodextrin, serum glucose values may be spuriously overestimated by auto-analyzers that use the glucose dehydrogenase method of sample analysis (Wens et al., 1997).

2. Increased sensitivity to insulin. In diabetic dialysis patients being treated with exogenous insulin, the importance of reduced insulin catabolism overrides the impact of insulin resistance; when exogenous insulin is administered, its effect may be intensified and prolonged. Thus, smaller-than-usual doses should be given. Bolus administration of moderately large intravenous doses (e.g., 15 units of regular insulin), even when ketosis is present, can result in severe hypoglycemia. Hypoglycemia can also occur after administration of the longer-acting insulins, such as isophane insulin (NPH) and insulin glargine.

3. Hyperglycemia. The clinical presentation of hyperglycemia is modified when renal function is absent. The absence of the "safety valve" effect of glycosuria may result in the development of severe hyperglycemia (serum glucose level >1,000 mg/dL [56 mmol/L]). Severe hyperosmolality with accompanying alteration of mental status is unusual because of the absence of water loss induced by osmotic diuresis. Indeed, even extreme hyperglycemia is often asymptomatic in dialysis patients (Al-Kudsi et al., 1982). However, manifestations can include thirst, weight gain, and, on occasion, pulmonary edema or coma (Tzamaloukas et al., 2004). Also, diabetic ketoacidosis, frequently accompanied by severe hyperkalemia and coma, can develop in insulin-dependent dialysis patients. Management of hyperglycemia with or without ketoacidosis differs from that in patients without renal failure in that administration of large amounts of fluid is unnecessary and generally contraindicated. All of the clinical and laboratory abnormalities of hyperglycemia are corrected by insulin administration, which is often the only treatment needed. To manage severe hyperglycemia, one can administer a continuous infusion of low-dose insulin (starting at 2 units per hour) with close clinical monitoring and measurement of serum glucose and potassium concentrations at 2- to 3-hour intervals. If severe hyperkalemia is present, electrocardiography should also be done. Emergency dialysis may be needed in patients with hyperglycemia and either severe pulmonary edema or life-threatening hyperkalemia.

4. Hypoglycemia. Hypoglycemia can develop in diabetic patients treated with either hemodialysis or peritoneal dialysis; it is usually due to reduced insulin catabolism and to reduced intake and absorption of food. The risk of hypoglycemia is increased in malnourished diabetic patients with diminished glycogen stores and in diabetics receiving beta-blocking drugs (which impair glycogenolysis). In diabetic patients, hemodialysis solution should always contain about 200 mg/dL (11 mM) glucose; if glucose is not added, then severe hypoglycemia during or soon after the hemodialysis session can result.

B. Insulin therapy. Tight control of the serum glucose concentration is difficult to achieve in dialysis patients, primarily because of variations in dietary intake and food absorption and the confounding effect of dialysis therapy. Nevertheless, good glucose control is worthwhile. Prolonged hyperglycemia leads to the development and progression of all diabetic complications, which become irreversible only in their later stages. Irreversibly and slowly formed compounds that are the result of nonenzymatic glycosylation of proteins, the so-called AGEs, alter the structure and function of vascular basement membranes, stimulate the production of growth factors, and alter the function of intracellular proteins (Brownlee, 1997). In peritoneal dialysis patients, AGE deposition in the peritoneal membrane is associated with an increase in peritoneal permeability and excessive protein losses in the dialysate (Nakamoto et al., 2002). Many of the changes associated with AGEs (e.g., vascular changes) may have reached an irreversible stage by the time patients start dialysis. However, it is conceivable that good glycemic control will prevent some of these changes because the morbidity and mortality of diabetics with good glycemic control are lower than those of subjects with poor control. A fasting serum glucose level of <140 mg/dL (7.8 mmol/L), a postprandial value of <200 mg/dL (11 mmol/L), and a glycosylated hemoglobin level in the range of 100%–120% of the normal range are reasonable therapeutic goals.

Hypoglycemia must be avoided. Regular verification of glycemic control is important. Usually, patients are taught to prick their fingers and impregnate a piece of test paper with their blood. An automated device can then estimate the serum glucose concentration. The serum glucose level is checked in this manner at least once daily, usually two or three times a day. For peritoneal dialysis patients, measuring capillary blood glucose concentration at various levels of glucose absorption from the abdominal cavity during a peritoneal equilibration test may help determination of the proper insulin dose (Thorp et al., 2004).

Glycosylated hemoglobin values can be used to follow the degree of glycemia; however, a method of determination of glycosylated hemoglobin not receiving interference from uremic compounds should be used in dialysis patients (Little et al., 2002). Newer methods of assessing glycemic control by continuous monitoring of glucose concentration in the interstitial fluid (Marshall et al., 2003) may improve monitoring and control of glycemia in the future.

1. Regimens for hemodialysis patients. Because of its prolonged half-life in dialysis patients, initial insulin doses should be decreased to 25%–50% of the usual starting dose. Insulin is not significantly removed by hemodialysis. The amount of insulin per day required for patients receiving maintenance hemodialysis is usually small; optimum control of glycemia is achieved by administration of long-acting insulin at two separate times during the day (split dosing) and by supplementing with short-acting insulin for meals as needed. The proportions of long-acting and short-acting insulin, as well as the total insulin doses, vary widely among different patients. There is little published experience with long-acting insulins such as insulin glargine in dialysis patients (see Table 30-3).

2. Regimens for peritoneal dialysis patients. Insulins may be administered by the usual subcutaneous route in peritoneal dialysis patients. Insulin is not significantly removed by peritoneal dialysis. Another option is to administer insulin in the peritoneal dialysis solution. This has the advantages that the dose can be easily titrated and that the insulin will be administered simultaneously with the glucose present in the solution. Despite the fact that variable amounts of insulin are adsorbed to the dialysis solution container and infusion lines, control of the serum glucose level can be readily obtained by addition of regular insulin to peritoneal dialysis solutions. Relatively long (3.8-cm, or 1.5-in.) needles should be used to ensure that the full dose of insulin is injected into the dialysis solution container rather than being trapped in the infusion port. After injection, the dialysis solution container should be inverted several times to ensure proper mixing. The absorption of insulin from the abdominal cavity varies greatly between individuals, and therefore, the dose of insulin needs to be determined in each individual.

a. CAPD patients

(1) Intraperitoneal regimen. The total dose of intraperitoneal insulin added daily to all dialysis solution containers will often be two to three times the previous daily subcutaneous dose. A number of regimens have been proposed, one of which, the Toronto Western Hospital Protocol, is reproduced in Table 30-2. Other approaches have been described by Beardsworth et al. (1988), Flynn (1981), and Legrain and Rottembourg (1981).

(2) Subcutaneous regimen. Although some reports suggest that use of intraperitoneal insulin is associated with an increased incidence of peritonitis, intraperitoneal insulin should be tried first under ordinary circumstances because of the good control of glycemia that it can provide. If intraperitoneal insulin fails, subcutaneous injection can provide a satisfactory alternative in a schedule similar to that described for hemodialysis.

b. CCPD or nocturnal intermittent peritoneal dialysis (NIPD) regimen

(1) Intraperitoneal regimen. The intraperitoneal insulin dose is added as regular insulin to any one of the nocturnal dialysis solution containers attached to the cycler. Initially, the amount added will usually be equal to the total amount of insulin (regular plus long acting) previously given subcutaneously. In cyclers that

Table 30-3.   Agents for diabetes mellitus in chronic kidney disease

Drug	Usual Nonuremic Dose	Dialysis Patient Dose (% of Nonuremic Dose)
Insulins		
Short-acting		
Regular	0.2–1 units/kg per day SC b.i.d.–q.i.d.	Decrease dose (25%–50%)
Lispro	0.2–1 units/kg per day SC b.i.d.–q.i.d.	Decrease dose (25%–50%)
Aspart	0.2–1 units/kg per day SC b.i.d.–q.i.d.	Decrease dose (not defined)
Intermediate–acting		
NPH	0.2–1 units/kg per day SC q24h–b.i.d.	Decrease dose (not defined)
Long-acting		
Glargine	0.1–1 units/kg per day SC q24h	Decrease dose (not defined)
Detemir	0.1–1 units/kg per day SC q24h	Decrease dose (not defined)
Sulfonylureas		
Glipizide	2.5–20 mg PO q24h–b.i.d.	2.5–10 mg PO q24h–b.i.d. (50%)
Glimeperide	1–8 mg PO q24h	1–4 mg PO q24h (50%)
Tolbutamide	250–3,000 mg PO q24h	Same (100%)
Glyburide	1.25–10 mg PO q24h	Avoid in renal failure
Thiazolidinediones[a]		
Rosiglitazone	4–8 mg PO q24h–b.i.d.	Same (100%)
Pioglitazone	15–30 mg PO q24h	Same (100%)
α-Glucosidase inhibitors		
Acarbose	50–100 mg PO t.i.d.	Not recommended in renal failure
Miglitol	50–100 mg PO t.i.d.	Not recommended in renal failure
Meglitinides		
Repaglinide	0.5–8 mg PO t.i.d.	0.5–4 mg PO tid (50%)

continued

Table 30-3. *Continued.*

Drug	Usual Nonuremic Dose	Dialysis Patient Dose (% of Nonuremic Dose)
Nateglinide	60–120 mg PO t.i.d.	Same?
Biguanides		
Metformin	850–2,550 mg PO q24h–b.i.d.	Avoid in renal failure
Amylin analogues		
Pramlintide	30–120 mcg SC q.a.c.	Same?
Incretin mimetics: glucagons-like peptide-1 (GLP-1)		
Exenatide	5–10 mcg SC b.i.d.	Not recommended in renal failure

SC, subcutaneously; b.i.d., two times per day; q.i.d., four times per day; q24h, daily; PO, by mouth; t.i.d., three times per day; q.a.c., before meals.
[a]May cause fluid retention in chronic kidney disease patients not on dialysis.

infuse the "final" long-dwell daytime exchange from a separate container, regular insulin should be added to the latter as well. The amount of insulin added to the nocturnal dialysis solution container subsequently can be adjusted as guided by the fasting morning serum glucose level. A supplemental subcutaneous insulin dose may be required during the day to help metabolize carbohydrate absorbed with meals.

(2) Subcutaneous regimen. An alternative strategy is to give subcutaneous insulin in the evening to help metabolize the nocturnal glucose load.

C. Oral hypoglycemic agents. A common problem for all oral hypoglycemic agents is that there are no appropriate studies of their use in dialysis patients. Nevertheless, these agents are useful adjuncts in the treatment of diabetics and are used by many nephrologists. Suggested agents and appropriate doses are listed in Table 30-3.

1. Sulfonylureas. The safety of sulfonylureas depends on their mode of metabolism and their half-life. Use of short-acting agents primarily metabolized by the liver is, in general, safer in dialysis patients. Acetohexamide, chlorpropamide, and tolazamide are excreted to a large extent in the urine. These drugs should not be used in dialysis patients because their half-lives will be greatly prolonged in the absence of renal function, possibly resulting in severe and prolonged hypoglycemia. The excretion of glyburide is 50% hepatic, and prolonged hypoglycemia may follow the use of this drug in dialysis patients. Metabolism of glipizide and tolbutamide is almost completely hepatic. Consequently, these drugs should be considered if an oral hypoglycemic agent is desired. Many drugs frequently used in dialysis patients either antagonize (phenytoin, nicotinic acid, diuretics) or enhance (sulfonamides, salicylates, warfarin, ethanol) the hypoglycemic action of sulfonylureas.

2. Metformin. Metformin, a biguanide, is associated with increased incidence of lactic acidosis in dialysis patients and should not used.

3. α-Glycosidase inhibitors. Acarbose inhibits α-glycosidase in the enteric mucosa and moderates postprandial hyperglycemia. Its side effects are primarily gastrointestinal. It may prove to be a useful adjunct to other diabetic medications in dialysis patients, but in the absence of clinical data cannot be recommended for use at this time. High-fiber diets have similar effects on postprandial hyperglycemia but may cause decreased absorption of vitamins and other nutrients.

4. Peroxisome proliferator-activated receptor (PPAR) agonists. PPAR-γ agonists include drugs such as rosiglitazone and pioglitazone. These drugs sensitize the target tissues to insulin, increase glucose uptake in muscle and adipose tissue, and decrease hepatic glucose production. They may also have beneficial anti-inflammatory, vascular, and metabolic (hypolipidemic) effects. Drugs that act on both PPAR-α receptors and PPAR-γ agonists, such as muraglitazar, are new agents being evaluated. Protective effects on renal function of PPAR-γ agonists have been reported, including reduction of proteinuria or urinary albumin excretion. Both pioglitazone and rosiglitazone have been used for adjunctive therapy in ESRD patients; addition of these drugs lowered HbA1c levels as well as blood pressure, and in one study, they increased high-density lipoprotein (HDL) cholesterol levels and reduced triglyceride concentrations (see Iglesias and Diez [2006] for a review). Rosiglitazone increased insulin sensitivity in CAPD patients.

PPARγ agonists are metabolized by the liver, and so the doses do not generally need to be reduced in renal failure, although the lowest possible dose should be used to start. They have been associated with weight gain, edema, and congestive heart failure in nonuremic patients; the mechanism is thought to be increased renal retention of sodium and water. For this reason, the glitazones are relatively contraindicated in patients with class 3 or 4 congestive heart failure. Postmarketing data on rosiglitazone have revealed an increased incidence of macular edema. Diabetics taking this class of drugs should immediately report any symptoms consistent with worsening macular edema (blurred or distorted vision, decreased color sensitivity, or decreased dark adaptation) (Kendall and Woolterton, 2006). Acute myopathy has been reported when glitazones were given in conjunction with fibrates. Troglitazone, the first of this class of drugs, was associated with a risk of severe hepatotoxicity. Isolated case reports of hepatotoxic reactions have been reported in patients receiving newer agents such as rosiglitazone, but causality has not been established.

5. Insulin secretagogues. Another class of drugs that may be useful in controlling blood glucose in diabetics with renal disease is the insulin secretagogues. Repaglinide and nateglinide are representative agents. They do have slightly prolonged half-lives in patients with renal failure, but initial doses have not usually been reduced (Devineni et al., 2003).

V. Hyperkalemia. Hyperkalemia occurs commonly in diabetic patients treated by maintenance hemodialysis. The causal factors include insulin deficiency and resistance, aldosterone deficiency, acidosis, hyperkalemic drugs, anuria, intracellular to extracellular fluid shifts attendant to hyperglycemia, and excesses in dietary potassium intake. Severe hyperkalemia is much less frequently found in patients on maintenance peritoneal dialysis. In a preliminary analysis of more than 6,000 serum samples obtained in 62 diabetic patients on chronic dialysis, we found serum potassium concentrations of >6 mmol/L in 0.6% of the samples in patients on peritoneal dialysis and in 5% of the samples in patients on hemodialysis.

VI. Hypertension and peripheral vascular disease

A. Control of hypertension. The incidence of hypertension is high in diabetic dialysis patients. Control of high blood pressure is very important for the prevention of cardiovascular sequelae and deterioration of vision. Most diabetics have volume-sensitive hypertension that can be controlled by appropriate sodium and fluid restriction and by removal of excess extracellular fluid by dialysis. If medications are needed, then several drugs can be used. Angiotensin-converting enzyme inhibitors or angiotensin receptor antagonists have the advantage of conferring cardioprotective effects but may lead to dangerous hyperkalemia, especially in nonoligoanuric patients. A vasodilator or calcium channel blocker can be used as an alternative first-choice agent. Many nephrologists prefer clonidine or labetalol, but these agents require more frequent dosing, which decreases compliance. Beta-blockers, which were avoided in diabetics because they interfere with the recognition of hypoglycemia by the patient (they block the epinephrine effect), can aggravate hyperkalemia by inhibiting β-2 adrenergically mediated muscle uptake of potassium (this should only occur with nonselective agents such as propranolol or higher doses of β-1 selective agents). Beta-blockers are used more frequently now, particularly in patients with ischemic cardiac disease. Loop diuretics in large doses may be beneficial in patients with residual renal function. If antihypertensive drugs are used, the smallest dose that can lead to the desired effect should be sought. It should also be kept in mind that dialysis hypotension may be aggravated by the use of antihypertensives; consequently, removal of excess fluid may become problematic.

B. Peripheral vascular disease. Diabetic patients on dialysis have a very high rate of amputation (O'Hare et al., 2003).

Frequent examination of the feet by a podiatrist is important in diabetic dialysis patients; with regular care focused on prevention of ulcer development, the risk of amputation can be minimized.

VII. Cerebrovascular disease. The incidence of stroke is higher in diabetic dialysis patients than in their nondiabetic counterparts. Although the use of aspirin has been shown to reduce the risk of stroke in nonuremic patients, the benefit of such therapy in diabetic dialysis patients is unknown, and the use of aspirin theoretically increases the risk of intraocular hemorrhage. The danger of intraocular bleeding also deters use of the coumarin anticoagulants in this population.

VIII. Eye problems in diabetics on dialysis. Ophthalmic complications of diabetes mellitus are the most prevalent eye disorders (other than myopia) noted in dialysis patients. Since diabetes was present in 45% of ESRD patients in the USRDS report of 2004, active collaboration with an ophthalmologist skilled in laser photocoagulation is vital to provide adequate care for such patients. In the United States, laser therapy for the retinal complications of diabetes was performed in 75% of ESRD diabetics by the time dialysis was initiated. Additional laser therapy and regular screening for glaucoma are vital components of comprehensive yet "routine" care for diabetic dialysis patients.

Diabetic patients on dialysis are subject to eye complications, which are common to all patients on dialysis. Conjunctivitis and keratitis are treated with ophthalmic preparations of antibiotic, antifungal, or antiviral agents in the usual doses. The dose of antibiotics given systematically should be adjusted for dialysis. Certain pathogens grow well in glucose-containing media and create a risk of severe eye infection in diabetics on dialysis.

Band keratopathy (corneal–conjunctival calcification) may afflict both diabetic and nondiabetic dialysis patients with elevated calcium–phosphorus product (>70, when both calcium and phosphorus concentrations are expressed in milligrams per deciliter). A "red-eye syndrome" due to irritation of the conjunctiva by calcium phosphate deposits may complicate band keratopathy. Superficial keratectomy or chelation of the calcium deposits with local application of ethylenediamine tetraacetic acid (EDTA) has been used to treat refractory cases.

Although few studies have addressed the point directly, heparinization during hemodialysis does not increase the risk of hemorrhagic complications due to diabetic retinopathy. One approach to assessing the heparin-induced risk of retinal hemorrhage is to compare the course of diabetic eye disease in individuals treated with peritoneal dialysis versus those undergoing hemodialysis. A prospective, uncontrolled study that evaluated visual changes in 112 diabetic patients, of whom 63% and 37% were treated with hemodialysis and peritoneal dialysis, respectively, found that the loss of vision was independent of the dialysis modality, glucose control, and type of diabetes. Provided that hypertension is effectively managed, there therefore does not appear to be an undue hazard imposed by heparin anticoagulation during hemodialysis to diabetic patients with retinopathy.

A.   Diabetic retinopathy. Retinopathy is present in essentially every patient with ESRD due to diabetic nephropathy. Indeed, because the correlation between diabetic retinopathy and diabetic nephropathy is so strong (nearly 100% coincidence), diabetes should be doubted as the cause of renal insufficiency in any patient with a normal retinal examination that includes fluorescein angiography.

Hypertension, which is also present in the majority of dialysis patients, accelerates progression of diabetic retinopathy, and may, by itself, cause retinal and vitreous hemorrhage. Vascular events secondary to hypertensive retinopathy (branch retinal vein occlusion from obstruction at the site of AV crossing) can cause sudden decreases in vision. Control of hypertension may prevent this complication, as well as the more rare central retinal vein and artery occlusion.

In the past, as many as one third of diabetic dialysis patients were legally blind at the time of initiation of dialytic therapy. Retinopathy is the most common cause of blindness in diabetics on dialysis; less common causes of blindness include macular edema, glaucoma, cataracts, and corneal disease. The early stage of background retinopathy, with leakage and occlusion of small retinal blood vessels, can cause visual loss if the macular area is involved. Slowing the progression of this stage requires careful control of blood pressure and blood glucose, and, in pre-ESRD patients without protein malnutrition, restriction of daily dietary protein intake to about 0.6 g/kg. Pegaptanib, a drug that acts against VEGF, and which has been shown to be beneficial in age-related wet macular degeneration, may be of benefit in diabetic retinopathy as well (Adamis, 2006).

Retinopathy progresses to a proliferative stage believed to be secondary to local hypoxia and characterized by intense proliferation of new blood vessels in the retina. These vessels, which are located in the surface layer of the retina, cause loss of vision through vitreous bleeding, macular distortion, or detachment. Discovery of proliferative retinopathy is an indication for laser treatment, which decreases the risk of detachment and the need for oxygen (by destroying nonessential parts of the retina). Vitreous hemorrhages from proliferative retinopathy obstruct the path of light and may lead to retinal detachment and blindness. Vitrectomy and other microsurgical techniques (removal of retinal membranes, reattachment of retina) can improve vision in one third to one half of patients.

Progression of retinopathy is associated with long duration of diabetes, poor blood pressure control, and female gender, but not with the use of heparin in hemodialysis. Good blood pressure control during the dialysis period is imperative. Systematic ophthalmologic examinations at frequent intervals combined with aggressive but judicious use of surgical techniques such as vitrectomy and scleral buckling to reattach a detached retina may restore vision in selected patients. Glaucoma and cataracts in dialysis patients are treated in the same way as in the general population. Proactive eye surveillance and intervention has proven effective in sustaining at least ambulatory vision in nearly all diabetic dialysis patients.

IX. Impotence. Impotence is common in diabetic dialysis patients. Autonomic neuropathy and peripheral vascular disease associated with diabetes are operative, as are the usual uremic causes. Management of impotence is discussed in Chapter 39.

X. Referral for transplantation. In diabetic patients in whom no contraindication to transplantation exists, renal transplantation is the preferred method of managing ESRD. In such patients, dialysis should be considered as a temporary measure only. Diabetic patients with severe preexisting cardiac disease may not benefit from transplantation because in this group transplantation is associated with a high mortality rate (Philipson et al., 1986).

XI. Bone disease. Among diabetics with ESRD, adynamic bone disease is common (see Chapter 35). This bone disease is characterized by a low bone formation rate. This low bone formation rate is believed to predispose diabetic patients to aluminum toxicity; diabetic patients on dialysis have been shown to accumulate bone aluminum at a faster rate than their nondiabetic counterparts (Andress et al., 1987). For this reason, every effort should be made to avoid use of aluminum-containing phosphate binders, especially in diabetics.

XII. Anemia. The response to erythropoietin is satisfactory for anemic diabetics treated with either hemodialysis or peritoneal dialysis.

XIII. Conclusion. The care of diabetic patients is a demanding task. It requires intense attention to multiple details. In addition to members of the dialysis team, representatives of other specialties (e.g., vascular surgery, podiatry, ophthalmology, neurology) are needed. The existence of a diabetic team, with all of the subspecialties available, working under the coordination of a nephrologist acting as a primary care physician and a nurse-specialist in diabetes, who should provide continuous patient teaching, is highly desirable to provide the best care for this demanding and increasing dialysis population.

SELECTED READINGS

Adamis AP, et al. Changes in retinal neovascularization after pegaptanib (Macugen) therapy in diabetic individuals. *Ophthalmology* 2006;113(1):23–28.

Al-Kudsi RR, et al. Extreme hyperglycemia in dialysis patients. *Clin Nephrol* 1982;17:228–231.

Amin K, et al. Intraperitoneal ondansetron hydrochloride for intractable nausea and vomiting due to diabetic gastroparesis in a patient on peritoneal dialysis. *Perit Dial Int* 2002;22:539–540.

Andress DL, et al. Early deposition of aluminum in bone in diabetic patients on hemodialysis. *N Engl J Med* 1987;316:292–296.

Aoki J, et al. Coronary revascularization improves long-term prognosis in diabetic and non-diabetic end-stage renal disease. *Circ J* 2002;66:595–599.

Arora SK, McFarlane SI. The case for low carbohydrate diets in diabetes management. *Nutr Metab (Lond)* 2005;2:16.

Beardsworth SF, et al. Intraperitoneal insulin: a protocol for administration during CAPD and review of published protocols. *Perit Dial Int* 1988;8:145.

Brownlee M. Advanced products of nonenzymatic glycosylation and the pathogenesis of diabetic complications. In: Porte D, Sherwin RS, eds. *Ellenberg and Rifkin's diabetes mellitus*, 5th ed. Stamford, CT: Appleton & Lange, 1997:229.

Cai W, et al. Association of advanced glycoxidation end products and inflammation markers with thrombosis of arteriovenous grafts in hemodialysis patients. *Am J Nephrol* 2006;26(2):181–185.

Cai W, et al. High levels of dietary advanced glycation end products transform low-density lipoprotein into a potent redox-sensitive mitogen-activated protein kinase stimulant in diabetic patients. *Circulation* 2004;110(3):285–291.

Czock D, et al. Pharmacokinetics and pharmacodynamics of lispro-insulin in hemodialysis patients with diabetes mellitus. *Int J Clin Pharmacol Ther* 2003;41:492–497.

Dasgupta MK. Management of patients with type 2 diabetes on peritoneal dialysis. *Adv Perit Dial* 2005;21:120–122.

Daugirdas JT, et al. Hyperosmolar coma: cellular dehydration and the serum sodium concentration. *Ann Intern Med* 1989;110:855–857.

Devineni D, et al. Pharmacokinetics of nateglinide in renally impaired diabetic patients. *J Clin Pharmacol* 2003;43:163–170.

Flynn CT. The Iowa Lutheran protocol. *Perit Dial Bull* 1981;1:100.

Goldberg T, et al. Advanced glycoxidation end products in commonly consumed foods. *J Am Diet Assoc* 2004;104(8):1287–1291.

Hatorp V. Clinical pharmacokinetics and pharmacodynamics of repaglinide [Review]. *Clin Pharmacokinet* 2002;41(7):471–483.

Ifudu O, et al. Interdialytic weight gain correlates with glycosylated hemoglobin in diabetic hemodialysis patients. *Am J Kidney Dis* 1994;23:686–691.

Iglesias P, Diez JJ. Peroxisome proliferator-activated receptor gamma agonists in renal disease. *Eur J Endocrinol* 2006;154(5):613–621.

Jackson MA, et al. Hemodialysis-induced hypoglycemia in diabetic patients. *Clin Nephrol* 2000;54:30–34.

Kendall C, Wooltorton E. Rosiglitazone (Avandia) and macular edema. *Can Med Assoc J* 2006;174(5):623.

Khanna R, et al. The Toronto Western Hospital protocol. *Perit Dial Bull* 1981;1:101.

Legrain M, Rottembourg J. The "Pitie-Salpetriere" protocol. *Perit Dial Bull* 1981;1:101.

Little R, et al. Can glycohemoglobin be used to assess glycemic control in patients with chronic renal failure? *Clin Chem* 2002;48:784–785.

Locatelli F, et al. Renal replacement therapy in patients with diabetes and end-stage renal disease. *J Am Soc Nephrol* 2004;Suppl. 1:S25–S29.

Lin CL, et al. Improvement of clinical outcomes by early nephrology referral in type II diabetics on hemodialysis. *Ren Fail* 2003;25:455–464.

Markel MS, Friedman EA. Care of the diabetic patient with end-stage renal disease. *Semin Nephrol* 1990;10:274.

Marshall J, et al. Glycemic control in diabetic CAPD patients assessed by continuous glucose monitoring system (CGMS). *Kidney Int* 2003;64:1480–1486.

Nakamoto H, et al. Effect of diabetes on peritoneal function assessed by peritoneal dialysis capacity test in patients undergoing CAPD. *Am J Kidney Dis* 2002;40:1045–1054.

Philipson JD, et al. Evaluation of cardiovascular risk for renal transplantation in diabetic patients. *Am J Med* 1986;81:630–634.

O'Hare AM, et al. Factors associated with future amputation among patients undergoing hemodialysis: results from the Dialysis Morbidity and Mortality Study Waves 3 and 4. *Am J Kidney Dis* 2003;41:162–170.

Quellhorst E. Insulin therapy during peritoneal dialysis: pros and cons of various forms of administration. *J Am Soc Nephrol* 2002;13(Suppl 1):S92–S96.

Phakdeekitcharoen B, Leelasa-nguan P. Effects of an ACE inhibitor or angiotensin receptor blocker on potassium in CAPD patients. *Am J Kidney Dis* 2004;44(4):738–746.

Popli S, et al. Asymptomatic, nonketotic, severe hyperglycemia with hyponatremia. *Arch Intern Med* 1990;150:1962–1964.

Schomig M, et al. The diabetic foot in the dialyzed patient. *J Am Soc Nephrol* 2000;11:1153–1159.

Thorp ML, et al. Three diabetic peritoneal dialysis patients receiving intraperitoneal insulin with dosage adjustment based on capillary glucose levels during peritoneal equilibrium tests. *Am J Kidney Dis* 2004;43:927–929.

Tzamaloukas AH, et al. Serum tonicity, extracellular volume and clinical manifestations in symptomatic dialysis-associated hyperglycemia treated only with insulin. *Int J Artif Organs* 2004;27:751–758.

Uribarri J, et al. Diet-derived advanced glycation end products are major contributors to the body's AGE pool and induce inflammation in healthy subjects [Review]. *Ann N Y Acad Sci* 2005;1043:461–466.

Uribarri J, et al. Restriction of dietary glycotoxins reduces excessive advanced glycation end products in renal failure patients. *J Am Soc Nephrol* 2003;14:728–731.

Wens R, et al. Overestimation of blood glucose measurements by auto-analyzer method in CAPD patients treated with icodextrin [Abstract]. *J Am Soc Nephrol* 1997;8:275a.

Windus DW, et al. Prosthetic fistula survival and complications in hemodialysis patients: effects of diabetes and age. *Am J Kidney Dis* 1992;19:448–452.

Yale JF. Oral antihyperglycemic agents and renal disease: new agents, new concepts [Review]. *J Am Soc Nephrol* 2005;16(Suppl 1):S7–10.

WEB REFERENCE

Diabetes and ESRD links: http://www.hdcn.com/ch/diabet/

Hypertension

Carmine Zoccali

Treatment of hypertension represents a major area of intervention for cardiovascular risk reduction in dialysis patients (stage 1–4 chronic kidney disease [CKD] patients are discussed in Chapter 1).

I. **Definition and measurement.** Studies in the general population have demonstrated that diastolic pressure is a better predictor than systolic pressure of coronary heart disease in the young. In the elderly the opposite is true (Franklin et al., 2001). Among dialysis patients, greater emphasis is now given to the systolic and pulsatile component of blood pressure (BP); in retrospective cohort studies, pulse pressure, which correlates with vascular calcification, stiffness, and pathologically increased pulse wave velocity, has been identified as the strongest predictor of cardiovascular events (Klassen et al., 2002). Studies of outcome versus BP in dialysis patients are confounded by the increased early mortality seen with low blood pressures, which are associated with severe heart failure (Stidley et al., 2006).

In patients without background cardiovascular complications, one can aim for BP targets suggested by the Seventh Report of the Joint National Committee on Prevention, Detection, Evaluation, and Treatment of High Blood Pressure (JNC7) for patients with CKD—namely, <130/80. As pointed out in Table 31-1, however, in older patients with atherosclerosis and stiff blood vessels as evidenced by high pulse pressures, such aggressive BP targets may be difficult to achieve practically and may not be safe (Ritz, 2006), and for them a systolic BP target of 140–150 is a reasonable goal.

Predialysis BP seems superior to postdialysis measurements as a measure of the pressure load on the heart (Zoccali et al., 2002a), and we recommend that this be the pressure to follow. Twenty-four-hour ambulatory monitoring is the most accurate estimation of BP load on the cardiovascular system and allows the study of night–day arterial pressure changes. Dialysis patients often fail to show the normal nocturnal drop in blood pressure, a phenomenon that may have prognostic implications (Amar et al., 2000). Ambulatory BP correlates better than clinic BP with the presence of left ventricular hypertrophy (LVH) (Agarwal et al., 2006b) and other outcomes (Tripepi et al., 2005). Home dialysis BP also can be measured reliably (Agarwal et al., 2006a).

II. **Pathophysiology**

A. **Extracellular volume expansion and sodium retention** is the main cause. Intensive and prolonged dialysis ultrafiltration treatments such as those given in daily dialysis or in long overnight dialysis are associated with good BP control in

Table 31-1. Indications for drug therapy of hypertension in dialysis patients

Definition

Hypertension: Predialysis systolic pressure >140 and/or
  diastolic pressure >90 mm Hg when the patient is believed
  to be at so-called "dry weight" (see text).

Drug therapy goals

Arterial pressure goals should be established individually,
  taking into account age, comorbid conditions, cardiac
  function, and neurologic status.
  In patients with raised systolic and diastolic pressure and
    few background cardiovascular complications, a reasonable
    predialysis BP goal is <130/80 mm Hg, that targeted by
    JNC7 for patients with chronic renal disease.
  In patients with isolated systolic hypertension and wide
    pulse pressure (usually elderly patients with
    atherosclerotic complications), excessive lowering of BP
    may be hazardous. For them a target predialysis systolic
    pressure of about 140–150 mm Hg is prudent.

BP, blood pressure.

most. Beyond causing hypertension, chronic volume overload
is associated with increased pulse wave velocity, which is an
indicator of arterial rigidity (Tycho Vuurmans et al., 2002),
and with left ventricular hypertrophy, which is strongly associated with mortality. Large interdialytic weight gains, though
confounded with better food intake and thus survival in uncontrolled analyses, are associated with shorter survival when
comorbidity is taken into account (Foley et al., 2002).

  B. Inappropriately high vascular tone. The renin–
angiotensin system is inappropriately activated in relation to
volume status, a problem that may be amplified in patients
with antecedent renovascular disease. Sympathetic overactivity, possibly triggered by afferent signals originated in dis-
eased kidneys, plays an important role (Converse et al., 1992).
Serum endothelin levels are elevated and correlate with degree of blood pressure elevation. In about one third of patients
treated with an erythropoiesis-stimulating agent (ESA), an
increase in arterial pressure >10 mm Hg occurs; the risk of
hypertension with ESA treatment is particularly high in patients with preexisting hypertension and/or when correction
of anemia is too rapid.

  Accumulation of endogenous inhibitors of nitric oxide like
asymmetric dimethyl-arginine (ADMA) is a strong predictor
of incident cardiovascular complications (Zoccali et al., 2001b).
ADMA impairs endothelium-dependent vasodilation, but its
role in hypertension remains undefined. Plasma concentrations of several vasodilatory peptides like atrial natriuretic
factor (ANF), calcitonin gene-related peptide (CGRP), and
adrenomedullin are markedly increased, but their role in the
disturbed regulation of vascular tone is unclear.

III.   Treatment
A.   Prevention
    1.   Sodium and fluid restriction. Most fluid ingestion is driven by salt ingestion, and nutritional recommendations are discussed in Chapter 28. Sodium restriction of 2 g per day (87 mmol) should not be onerous, and if the patient is open to a more stringent sodium restriction and caloric and protein intake seem adequate, then this should be encouraged. One should avoid becoming enamored with high-sodium dialysis solution strategies for controlling intradialytic symptoms; the amount of thirst and interdialytic fluid ingestion is closely related to the time-averaged sodium level present in the dialysis solution. Some patients naturally present with a lower predialysis sodium level, and for them, dialysis solution sodium level should be set close to the plasma level. Although most fluid intake is driven by sodium intake, not all is, and peculiar dietary beliefs or customs should be looked for when questioning the patient about fluid intake.

    2.   Longer and/or more frequent/longer dialysis sessions. In some patients, a three times per week dialysis schedule using 3- to 4-hour session lengths will be insufficient to maintain euvolemia. In such patients, the choices are to increase the dialysis session length, or to switch to a four times per week, or even six times per week, dialysis schedule (Fagugli et al., 2006). These are discussed in Chapter 14.

    3.   Residual renal function. This is key in helping to maintain euvolemia, and should be carefully protected by avoiding nephrotoxic agents and bouts of hypotension due to overaggressive fluid removal. Higher-dose loop diuretics sometimes help in maximizing urine output at higher levels of residual glomerular filtration rate.

B.   Correction of salt and fluid overload
    1.   Clinical assessment of dry weight. Ideally, dialysis treatment should bring the patients back to a normal extracellular volume. In clinical practice, the **"dry weight"** is defined as the level below which further fluid removal would produce hypotension, muscle cramps, nausea, and vomiting. However, the occurrence of such symptoms depends on how quickly fluid is removed, on the dialysis strategy used, on the predialysis volume status, and on concomitant drug treatment (many antihypertensive drugs impair the reflex cardiovascular adjustments to volume removal). Furthermore, edema may not be detectable until the interstitial volume has risen by about one third above normal (e.g., about 5 L).

    a.   Time delay in BP fall after correction of fluid overload. There may be a time delay between lowering extracellular fluid and a fall in blood pressure (Charra et al., 1998). For this reason, if BP does not fall initially after lowering the dry weight, this does not exclude hypervolemia as a cause of the hypertension.

    b.   Need for frequent reassessment. Dry weight and the nutritional status should be re-evaluated frequently, because loss of flesh weight due to malnutrition or to intercurrent illness can result in fluid overload at a previously determined level of "dry weight" at which the patient is no longer "dry."

2. **Technology**

   a. **Bioimpedance analysis (BIA).** When fluid removal becomes symptomatic and the patient remains hypertensive, the nephrologist is left with the problem of deciding whether or not the extracellular volume is still expanded. BIA is now often applied to answer this question. BIA measures resistance and reactance of the body to the passage of low-frequency (<10 kHz) and high-frequency alternating currents. These measurements are then converted into volumes by use of equations including reference coefficients for extracellular conductivity and tissue density; the latter is derived from isotope dilution measurements in nonuremic subjects. The assumption is generally made that the human body can be represented by a single cylinder. The validity of these assumptions in dialysis patients is uncertain, and "volumes" derived using BIA should be interpreted with caution. Nevertheless, a graphical approach may be useful, which compares the resistance/reactance relationship of the patient in question to that of the general population (Piccoli et al., 2004). Another approach is use of multifrequency BIA applied to the lower extremities during dialysis; the change in BIA during dialysis is followed in real time, and when the BIA is no longer changing, attainment of dry weight is inferred (Kuhlmann, 2005).

   b. **Other methods.** Continuous recording of hematocrit during dialysis (Crit-line Monitor) is considered a useful method by some, but relative blood volume reduction during dialysis does not reliably identify hypotension-prone versus resistant patients (Andrulli et al., 2002). Ultrasonography can be used to study the inferior vena cava diameter, and this might be the method of choice were it not so difficult to do routinely (Kayatas et al., 2006). Plasma ANF can be measured, but this is also highly dependent on left ventricular mass (Zoccali et al., 2001a), confounding its interpretation as a marker of volume status.

C. **Common clinical problems**

   1. **Excessive ultrafiltration.** Overzealous ultrafiltration may precipitate severe hypotension and disastrous cardiovascular consequences such as myocardial or cerebral infarction and mesenteric ischemia. Frequent intradialytic hypotensive episodes are associated with increased mortality, although it is not clear if this is an association or causal (Shoji et al., 2004). Hypotension may further damage the kidney and hasten the rate of decline of residual renal function. Methods of minimizing the risk of intradialytic hypotension are discussed in Chapter 10.

   2. **Postdialysis rise in blood pressure.** In about 14% of patients there is a paradoxic postdialysis rise in arterial pressure (Cheigh et al., 1993). This does not necessarily imply a state of relative dehydration, as in such cases evidence

of activation of the renin–angiotensin or sympathetic systems (which physiologically counterregulate volume deficiency) typically has been found.

3. Recurrent hypertension. If hypertension recurs in a patient after being well controlled by volume subtraction, a return to a state of volume excess is usually the cause.

D. Antihypertensive drug use

1. Calcium channel blockers. These drugs are the most frequently used for the treatment of volume-resistant hypertension in dialysis patients. A meta-analysis conducted in 2000 showed that calcium antagonists are more efficacious than beta-blockers in reducing the risk of stroke, but that they are less efficacious in reducing the risk of cardiac ischemia (Neal et al., 2000). In one large study of end-stage renal disease patients, the use of a calcium antagonist was associated with substantially lower risks of total (21%) and cardiovascular (26%) mortality (Kestenbaum et al., 2002).

　a. Side effects and dosing adjustments. Verapamil can cause cardiac conduction problems, bradycardia, and constipation. Calcium channel blockers should be used very cautiously in combination with β-adrenergic blockers, because congestive heart failure can be precipitated. Other side effects are ankle edema, headache, flushing, palpitations, and hypotension.

　　Long-acting preparations should be used. Calcium channel blockers are excreted primarily by the liver, their pharmacokinetic profile is unaltered in chronic renal failure and by dialysis (Table 31-2), and their dosage does not require any adjustment.

2. Sympatholytic drugs (e.g., methyldopa, clonidine, guanabenz). As noted above, there appears to be increased tonic sympathetic activity in dialysis patients, so use of central sympatholytic drugs, which inhibit sympathetic outflow by stimulating α-adrenoreceptors in the brain stem, is theoretically attractive. One side benefit of clonidine is its usefulness in the treatment of diarrhea due to autonomic neuropathy. Moreover, methyldopa and clonidine are relatively inexpensive—often an important consideration. Moxonidine added to other antihypertensive drugs was well tolerated in one study of patients with advanced renal failure and was comparable to nitrendipine in terms of efficacy (Vonend et al., 2003).

　a. Side effects and dosing adjustments. This class of drugs does have side effects. For clonidine these include sedation, dry mouth, depression, and postural hypotension. The last may be a particular problem in diabetic patients. Clonidine may cause rebound hypertension if it is abruptly withdrawn. Such side effects are substantially reduced with the transdermal formulation. Guanabenz and guanfacine are less likely to cause rebound hypertension but are more expensive. A large clinical trial of moxonidine in heart failure, MOXCON, was stopped because of excessive deaths in the moxonidine group, and therefore use of this drug in dialysis patients with heart failure is presently unwarranted. Methyldopa may cause hepatotoxicity or a positive direct or indirect Coombs test, interfering with cross-matching of blood.

Methyldopa, clonidine, and guanfacine are excreted substantially by the kidneys, and dosage reductions may be required. Methyldopa is removed by hemodialysis to a substantial extent. Guanabenz is metabolized by the liver and requires no dosage adjustment in renal failure.

3. **β-, α/β-, and α-Adrenergic blockers.** Beta-blockers counteract the cardiovascular effects of high sympathetic activity and lower plasma renin activity (PRA) and angiotensin II, which may all participate in causing high blood pressure in dialysis patients. Many show a documented cardioprotective effect in the setting of myocardial ischemia or infarction. Their use is associated with longer survival in the U.S. Renal Data System (USRDS) database (Foley et al., 2003).

High plasma noradrenaline associates with cardiovascular mortality in ESRD (Zoccali et al., 2002b). Carvedilol, an alpha/beta-blocker, reduces morbidity and mortality in patients with heart failure and in dialysis patients with systolic dysfunction (Cice et al., 2003).

a. **Side effects and dosing adjustments.** Alphablockers may cause postural hypotension. Prazosin has been associated with first-dose syncope, so the first dose must be administered at bedtime. β-Adrenergic blockers have a high incidence of side effects, such as drowsiness, lethargy, and depression. Beta-blockers need to be used cautiously in patients with a tendency toward pulmonary edema or asthma and in patients already being treated with some calcium channel blockers. Beta-blockers have an adverse effect on serum lipids; they also may have an adverse effect on cell potassium uptake, tending to increase the serum potassium level. They can mask the symptoms of hypoglycemia and augment insulin-induced hypoglycemia. All may cause bradycardia and interfere with reflex tachycardia following volume depletion.

Water-soluble beta-blockers such as atenolol and nadolol are primarily excreted by the kidney and require dosage reduction when treating renal failure patients. Atenolol and nadolol are removed substantially by hemodialysis, possibly contributing to paradoxic hypertension during dialysis.

4. **Angiotensin-converting enzyme (ACE) inhibitors and angiotensin II receptor blockers (ARBs).** These drugs generally are well tolerated by dialysis patients. The use of ACE inhibitors in dialysis patients is theoretically attractive. In dialysis patients, prekallikrein levels are low and ACE levels are high. The PRA level is overtly high in some dialysis patients and inadequately suppressed in volume-expanded patients. Angiotensin II in itself may contribute to LVH; in dialysis patients the ACE inhibitor perindopril partially reversed LVH, while the calcium antagonist nitrendipine had no such effect (London et al., 1994). ACE inhibitors, but not amlodipine, have been shown

Table 31-2. Antihypertensive drugs in dialysis patients: dosages and removal during dialysis

Drug	Tablet Size (mg)	Initial Dose in Dialysis Patients (mg)	Maintenance Dose Dialysis Patients (mg)	Removal During Hemodialysis
Ca antagonists				
Amlodipine	5	5 q24h	5 q24h	No
Diltiazem extended release	120, 180, 240, 300, 360	120 q24h	120–300 q24h	No
Felodipine	5, 10	5 q24h	5–10 q24h	No
Isradipine	5	5 q24h	5–10 q24h	No
Nicardipine (slow release)	30	30 b.i.d.	30–60 b.i.d.	No
Nifedipine XL	30, 60	30 q24h	30–60 q24h	No
Verapamil	40, 80, 120	40 b.i.d.	40–120 b.i.d.	No
ACE inhibitors				
Benazepril	5, 10, 20, 40	5	5–20 q24h	Yes (*)
Captopril	25, 50	12.5 q24h	25–50 q24h	Yes (*)
Enalapril	2.5, 5, 10, 20	2.5 q24h or q48h	2.5–10 q24h or q48h	Yes (*)
Fosinopril	10, 20	10 q24h	10–20 q24h	Yes (*)
Lisinopril	5, 10, 20, 40	2.5 q24h or q48h	2.5–10 q24h or q48h	Yes (*)
Perindopril	4	2 q.o.d.	2 q.o.d	Yes (*)
Quinapril	5, 10, 20, 40	2.5	10–20 q24h	No
Ramipril	1.25, 2.5, 5, 10	2.5–5 q24h	2.5–10 q24h	Yes (*)

Beta-blockers

Acebutolol	200, 400	200 q24h	200–300 q24h	Yes (*)
Atenolol	50, 100	25 q48h	25–50 q48h	Yes (*)
Carvedilol	5	5 q24h	5 q24h	Yes (*)
Metoprolol	50, 100	50 b.i.d.	50–100 b.i.d.	Yes (*)
Nadolol	20, 40, 80, 120, 160	40 q48h	40–120 q48h	Yes (*)
Pindolol	5, 10	5 b.i.d.	5–30 b.i.d.	Yes (*)
Propranolol	10, 40, 80	40 b.i.d.	40–80 b.i.d.	Yes (*)

Adrenergic modulators

Clonidine	0.1, 0.2, 0.3, TTS 0.2	0.1 b.i.d.	0.1–0.3 b.i.d., TTS weekly	No
Guanabenz	4, 8	4 b.i.d.	4–8 b.i.d.	No
Guanfacine	1, 2	1 q48h	1–2 q24h	No
Labetalol	100, 200, 300	200 b.i.d.	200–400 b.i.d.	No
Prazosin	1, 2, 5	1 b.i.d.	1–10 b.i.d.	No
Terazosin	1, 2, 5	1 b.i.d.	1–10 b.i.d.	No

continued

Table 31-2. *Continued.*

Drug	Tablet Size (mg)	Initial Dose in Dialysis Patients (mg)	Maintenance Dose Dialysis Patients (mg)	Removal During Hemodialysis
Vasodilators				
Hydralazine	10, 25, 50, 100	25 b.i.d.	50 b.i.d.	No
Minoxidil	2.5, 10	2.5 b.i.d.	2.5–10 b.i.d.	Yes (*)
Angiotensin II receptor blockers				
Candesartan	4, 8, 16, 32	4 q24h	8–31	No
Eprosartan	400, 600	400 q24h	400–600	No
Irbesartan	75, 150, 300	75–150 q24h	150–300	No
Losartan	50	50 q24h	50–100 q24h	No
Telmisartan	40, 80	40 q24h	20–80	No
Valsartan	80, 160	80 q24h	80–160	No

q24h, daily; b.i.d., two times per day; q48h, every other day; ACE, angiotensin-converting enzyme.
The dose of drugs that are removed by hemodialysis should be scheduled so that it is administered after dialysis (*). None of the drugs in the table undergoes substantial removal during continuous ambulatory peritoneal dialysis.

to reverse increased muscle sympathetic nerve activity associated with chronic renal failure (Ligtenberg et al., 1999). The Losrtan Intervention for Endpoint (LIFE) study in hypertensive diabetics with electrocardiogram evidence of LVH showed that losartan compared to atenolol resulted in a significant reduction of cardiovascular morbidity and mortality and more marked LVH reversal at similar BP levels (Lindholm et al., 2002), although another study found no benefit of ramipril on LVH in ESRD (Yu et al., 2006). Losartan and other ARBs have also been shown to be similarly effective in diabetics. Losartan and trandolapril improve arterial stiffness in ESRD (Ichihara et al., 2005). ACE inhibitors have been used with success in patients with congestive heart failure.

   a. Side effects and dosing adjustments. ACE inhibitors, by interfering with bradykinin breakdown, may be associated with an increased incidence of anaphylactoid reactions during dialysis. See Chapter 10.

   ACE inhibitors have been associated with hyperkalemia in patients with renal insufficiency, but often can be used in dialysis patients with minor adjustment to the potassium content of the diet if needed. Other side effects are cough, skin rash, alteration of taste, and, rarely, agranulocytosis or angioedema. Lower angioedema and cough risk are factors in favor of ARBs. Worsening of anemia and erythropoietin resistance is another purported side effect of ACE inhibitors, an effect that depends on the accumulation of N-acetyl-seryl-aspartyl-lysyl-proline, a physiologic inhibitor of hematopoiesis whose degradation depends on ACE (Le Meur et al., 2001). Because plasma half-life of many ACE inhibitors (or of their active metabolites) is prolonged in renal failure, reduction in dosage is often required.

   The efficacy of losartan and other drugs of this class in dialysis patients is comparable to that of ACE inhibitors. These drugs are extensively metabolized by the liver and do not require dose adjustment.

5. **Vasodilators** (e.g., hydralazine, minoxidil). These are third-line drugs. They usually require addition of a sympatholytic or beta-blocking drug because they tend to cause reflex tachycardia. Side effects of both drugs relate primarily to this reflex tachycardia and resulting palpitations, dizziness, and worsening of angina pectoris. Hydralazine is effective and inexpensive but can cause a lupus-like syndrome at dosages of more than 200 mg per day. Because of diminished renal excretion of its active metabolite(s), the maximum allowable dosage should be reduced in dialysis patients. Minoxidil has been associated with pericarditis and is generally avoided in women because of hypertrichosis. Minoxidil is usually reserved to treat resistant hypertension.

6. **Spironolactone.** Since publication of the Randomized Aldactone Evaluation Study (RALES) trial, there has been interest in whether blocking aldosterone in addition to angiotensin may have additive benefits. Risk of hyperkalemia with such dual blockade is theoretically increased. One

small study (Gross et al., 2005) suggested that addition of spironolactone to dialysis patients might result in further lowering of blood pressure, but this area needs to be studied further.

IV.   Hypertensive urgencies and emergencies

A.   Hypertensive urgency. The term hypertensive urgency is reserved for patients who are at significant risk of a serious morbid event within a matter of days if left untreated.

   1.   Treatment. The ideal rate of BP reduction in hypertensive urgencies is a balance between the risks of inadequate versus too-rapid lowering. In chronic hypertension the range of cerebral autoregulation is reset upward so that patients may be less able to compensate for a sudden fall in blood pressure, which may precipitate cerebral infarction and blindness. For this reason abrupt forms of therapy should be avoided. The short-acting formulation of nifedipine was used as a first-line drug for severe hypertension in the past but is no longer recommended, as there are now a number of reports documenting myocardial, cerebral, and retinal ischemia after its use. The long-acting preparation of nifedipine or other long-acting calcium antagonist, or clonidine, should be used instead as first-line therapy. If the patient is already on treatment with such drugs, a beta-blocker, an ACE inhibitor, or a combination thereof could be added. If oral therapy fails, parenteral drugs should be used (see below).

B.   Hypertensive emergencies are defined as increases in arterial pressure that, if sustained *for a few hours,* would cause irreversible organ damage. Hypertensive encephalopathy, hypertensive left ventricular failure, hypertension associated with unstable angina/myocardial infarction, hypertension with aortic dissection, and cerebral hemorrhage/brain infarction are such emergencies. Hypertensive emergencies should be treated with parenteral drugs. Nitroprusside administered by continuous IV infusion (0.3–0.8 mcg/kg per minute initially to a maximum of 8 mcg/kg per minute) is particularly useful in heart failure and dissecting aneurysm but requires careful monitoring because its toxic metabolite (thiocyanate) is retained in renal failure. Cyanide levels should be monitored every 48 hours and should not exceed 10 mg/dL. The symptoms of thiocyanate toxicity are nausea, vomiting, myoclonic movements, and seizures. In general, the infusion should not be prolonged for more than 48 hours. Both nitroprusside and its metabolites are readily removed by dialysis. Intravenous labetalol may also be considered in patients without heart failure, asthma, or heart block (2 mg/minute to a total of 2 mg/kg). Hydralazine 10–20 mg given slowly intravenously is a well-tried alternative, but this drug should be avoided in ischemic heart disease.

SELECTED READINGS

Amar J, et al. Nocturnal blood pressure and 24-hour pulse pressure are potent indicators of mortality in hemodialysis patients. *Kidney Int* 2000;57:2485–2491.

Andrulli S, et al. The role of blood volume reduction in the genesis of intradialytic hypotension. *Am J Kidney Dis* 2002;40:1244–1254.

Agarwal R, et al. Home blood pressure monitoring improves the diagnosis of hypertension in hemodialysis patients. *Kidney Int* 2006a;69(5):900–906.

Agarwal R, et al. Out-of-hemodialysis-unit blood pressure is a superior determinant of left ventricular hypertrophy. *Hypertension* 2006b;47(1):62–68.

Chan CT, et al. Regression of left ventricular hypertrophy after conversion to nocturnal hemodialysis. *Kidney Int* 2002;61:2235–2239.

Charra B, et al. Blood pressure control in dialysis patients: importance of the lag phenomenon. *Am J Kidney Dis* 1998;32:720–724.

Cheigh JS, et al. Mechanism of refractory hypertension in hemodialysis patients. *J Am Soc Nephrol* 1993;4:340.

Chen J, Gul A, Sarnak MJ. Management of intradialytic hypertension: the ongoing challenge. *Semin Dial* 2006;19(2):141–145.

Chobanian AV, et al. The seventh report of the Joint National Committee on Prevention, Detection, Evaluation, and Treatment of High Blood Pressure: the JNC 7 report. *JAMA* 2003;289:2560–2572.

Cice G, et al. Carvedilol increases two-year survival in dialysis patients with dilated cardiomyopathy: a prospective, placebo-controlled trial. *J Am Coll Cardiol* 2003;41:1438–1444.

Converse RL, et al. Sympathetic overactivity in patients with chronic renal failure. *N Engl J Med* 1992;327:1912–1918.

Dheenan S, et al. Preventing dialysis hypotension: a comparison of usual protective maneuvers. *Kidney Int* 2001;59:1175–1181.

Fagugli RM, et al. Effects of short daily hemodialysis and extended standard hemodialysis on blood pressure and cardiac hypertrophy: a comparative study. *J Nephrol* 2006;19(1):77–83.

Foley RN, et al. Blood pressure and long-term mortality in United States hemodialysis patients: USRDS Waves 3 and 4 Study. *Kidney Int* 2002;62:1784–1790.

Franklin SS, et al. Does the relation of blood pressure to coronary heart disease change with aging? The Framingham Study. *Circulation* 2001;103:1245–1249.

Gross E, et al. Effect of spironolactone on blood pressure and the renin-angiotensin-aldosterone system in oligo-anuric hemodialysis patients. *Am J Kidney Dis* 2005;46(1):94–101.

Ichihara A, et al. Low doses of losartan and trandolapril improve arterial stiffness in hemodialysis patients. *Am J Kidney Dis* 2005;45(5):866–874.

Kayatas M, et al. Comparison of the non-invasive methods estimating dry weight in hemodialysis patients. *Ren Fail* 2006;28(3):217–222.

Kestenbaum B, et al. Calcium channel blocker use and mortality among patients with end-stage renal disease. *Kidney Int* 2002,61:2157–2164.

Klassen PS, et al. Association between pulse pressure and mortality in patients undergoing maintenance hemodialysis. *JAMA* 2002;287:1548–1555.

Kuhlmann MK, et al. Bioimpedance, dry weight and blood pressure control: new methods and consequences. *Curr Opin Nephrol Hypertens* 2005;14(6):543–549.

Kuriyama S, et al. [Antihypertensive therapy for refractory morning hypertension in patients on peritoneal dialysis]. *Nippon Jinzo Gakkai Shi* 2005;47(1):38–45.

Le Meur Y, et al. Plasma levels and metabolism of AcSDKP in patients with chronic renal failure: relationship with erythropoietin requirements. *Am J Kidney Dis* 2001;38:510–517.

Ligtenberg G, et al. Reduction of sympathetic hyperactivity by enalapril in patients with chronic renal failure. *New Engl J Med* 1999;340:1321–1328.

Lindholm LH, et al. Cardiovascular morbidity and mortality in patients with diabetes in the Losartan Intervention For Endpoint reduction in hypertension study (LIFE): a randomised trial against atenolol. *Lancet* 2002;359:1004–1010.

Locatelli F, et al. Relevance of the conductivity kinetic model in the control of sodium pool. *Kidney Int Suppl* 2000;76:S89–95.

London GM, et al. Cardiac hypertrophy, aortic compliance, peripheral resistance, and wave reflection in end-stage renal disease. Comparative effects of ACE inhibition and calcium channel blockade. *Circulation* 1994;90:2786–2796.

Maggiore Q, et al. The effects of control of thermal balance on vascular stability in hemodialysis patients: results of the European randomized clinical trial. *Am J Kidney Dis* 2002,40(2):280–290.

Marshall M, et al. Associations of hemodialysis dose and session length with mortality risk in Australian and New Zealand patients. *Kidney Int* 2006;69:1229–1236.

Neal B, et al. Effects of ACE inhibitors, calcium antagonists, and other blood-pressure-lowering drugs: results of prospectively designed overviews of randomised trials. Blood Pressure Lowering Treatment Trialists' Collaboration. *Lancet* 2000,356:1955–1964.

Piccoli A, et al. Bioelectrical impedance vector distribution in peritoneal dialysis patients with different hydration status. *Kidney Int* 2004;65:1050–1063.

Ritz E. Lowering of blood pressure—the lower, the better? *J Am Soc Nephrol* 2006;17:2345–2352.

Santoro A, et al. Blood volume controlled hemodialysis in hypotension-prone patients: a randomized, multicenter controlled trial. *Kidney Int* 2002;62:1034–1045.

Saran R, et al. Longer treatment time and slower ultrafiltration in hemodialysis: associations with reduced mortality in the DOPPS. *Kidney Int* 2006;69:1222–1228.

Selby NM, et al. Automated peritoneal dialysis has significant effects on systemic hemodynamics. *Perit Dial Int* 2006;26(3):328–335.

Shoji T, et al. Hemodialysis-associated hypotension as an independent risk factor for two-year mortality in hemodialysis patients. *Kidney Int* 2004;66:1212–1220.

Stidley CA, et al. Changing relationship of blood pressure with mortality over time among hemodialysis patients. *J Am Soc Nephrol* 2006;17(2):513–512.

Tripepi G, et al. Prognostic value of 24-hour ambulatory blood pressure monitoring and of night/day ratio in nondiabetic, cardiovascular events-free hemodialysis patients. *Kidney Int* 2005;68:1294–1303.

Tycho Vuurmans JL, et al. Contribution of volume overload and angiotensin II to the increased pulse wave velocity of hemodialysis patients. *J Am Soc Nephrol* 2002;13:177–183.

Vonend O, et al. Moxonidine treatment of hypertensive patients with advanced renal failure. *J Hypertens* 2003;21:1709–1717.

Yu WC, et al. Effect of ramipril on left ventricular mass in normotensive hemodialysis patients. *Am J Kidney Dis* 2006;47(3):478–484.

Zoccali C, et al. Cardiac natriuretic peptides are related to left ventricular mass and function and predict mortality in dialysis patients. *J Am Soc Nephrol* 2001a;12:1508–1515.

Zoccali C, et al. Plasma concentration of asymmetrical dimethylarginine and mortality in patients with end-stage renal disease: a prospective study. *Lancet* 2001b;358:2113–2117.

Zoccali C, et al. Hypertension as a cardiovascular risk factor in end-stage renal failure. *Curr Hypertens Rep* 2002a;4:381–386.

Zoccali C, et al. Plasma norepinephrine predicts survival and incident cardiovascular events in patients with end-stage renal disease. *Circulation* 2002b;105:1354–1359.

Hematologic Abnormalities

Steven Fishbane

I. Anemia

A. Etiology. The anemia of chronic kidney disease (CKD) is primarily due to insufficient production of the glycoprotein hormone erythropoietin (EPO). Although EPO can be produced in many of the body's tissues, EPO required for erythropoiesis is generally produced by endothelial cells in proximity to the renal tubules. As excretory renal function is lost, there is a relative decline in the production of EPO that correlates with the declining glomerular filtration rate. The severity of the resulting anemia varies, but if untreated, then hematocrit values in end-stage renal disease (ESRD) of 18%–24% are typical. While the primacy of EPO deficiency is indisputable, other factors may play important contributory roles. Also, patients with ESRD may develop any of the other causes of anemia common in nonuremic subjects.

B. Consequences of anemia

1. Symptoms. The manifestations of anemia may be due both to the effects of decreased oxygen delivery to tissues and to the heart's compensatory changes. The most prominent symptoms of anemia are fatigue and dyspnea. Symptoms develop slowly and the patient may gradually constrict his or her activities in compensation. The patient's overall sense of well-being is diminished. Other symptoms may include difficulty concentrating, dizziness, sleep disorders, cold intolerance, and headaches. The heart responds to diminished oxygen-carrying capacity of blood by attempting to maintain systemic oxygen delivery with increased cardiac output and left ventricular hypertrophy. Patients may notice worsening dyspnea and palpitations at this stage. Other problems include deranged hemostatic function, impaired immune function, and diminished cognitive and sexual function. Exacerbations of angina, claudication, and transient ischemic attacks may also be observed.

2. Physical examination. The primary physical examination finding of anemia is pallor, which may be best detected on the palms of the hands, the nail beds, and the oral mucosa. A systolic ejection murmur due to increased cardiac flow may be heard over the precordium.

C. Treatment

1. Medications. There are two forms of recombinant human erythropoietin commercially available in the United States: Epoetin alfa (Epogen, Procrit) and darbepoetin alfa (Aranesp). At the time of this writing, a new drug application had been filed for continuous erythropoietin receptor activator (CERA), a pegylated form of erythropoietin with an extended serum half-life. In the past, the common terminology for this drug class was recombinant human erythropoietins. This is increasingly unsatisfactory because newer drugs are modified and increasingly divergent from the structure of native erythropoietin. Accordingly, a broader term is gaining favor, erythropoiesis-stimulating agents (ESAs). Epoetin alfa is a glycoprotein that is indistinguishable from native erythropoietin. It is manufactured by recombinant DNA technology and has a molecular weight of 30,400 d and a circulating half-life after intravenous administration of approximately 8.3 hours. Darbepoetin alfa is a synthetic analog of erythropoietin with increased carbohydrate content that increases the molecular weight by approximately 20% compared to native erythropoietin. As a result of the altered structure, the drug's pharmacokinetics are changed and the serum half-life is increased approximately threefold compared to epoetin alfa. Whether this results in the ability to extend the dosing interval compared to epoetin alfa is not clear.

2. **Benefits of anemia treatment**

   a. **Effect on outcomes.** Cross-sectional and retrospective studies have suggested that anemia in hemodialysis patients is associated with increased mortality, particularly when the hemoglobin concentration is <10 g/dL (100 g/L). Analyses of large administrative and clinical databases have shown that risk for mortality, hospitalization rate, and hospitalization days continue to decrease even at hemoglobin levels >11 g/dL (110 g/L) (Ma et al., 1999; Ofsthun et al., 2003). In contrast to these observational studies, interventional studies have not demonstrated reduced mortality with ESA treatment. Moreover, at least one study in hemodialysis patients with heart disease found increased mortality risk (nearly statistically significant) among patients treated with ESA to a target Hct of 42% (Besarab et al., 1998). More recently, a study of epoetin alfa in patients with CKD was terminated prematurely when patients randomized to a higher Hgb target (13.5 g/dL or 135 g/L) were found to experience adverse outcomes. Therefore, treatment to higher levels of Hgb may potentially be harmful.

   b. **Reduction in transfusion-related complications.** Prior to ESA therapy, up to 20% of patients on dialysis required frequent transfusions with attendant risk of immediate transfusion reactions, viral infection, iron overload, and immune sensitization. The rate of blood transfusion has been greatly reduced by the use of ESA therapy.

   c. **Improved quality of life and overall sense of well-being.** Various assessment tools, such as the Karnofsky score, SF-36 values, and Sickness Impact Profiles, have documented an improved quality-of-life and functional status in ESRD patients treated with ESA. Patients feel less fatigued, and their exercise capacity increases. There may be improvement as well in pruritus, sexual functioning, and leg cramps. The target level of hemoglobin for optimized quality-of-life is not completely known, but studies suggest that improvements may continue as hemoglobin is raised toward the normal range (Foley et al., 2000; Furuland, 2003; Parfrey et al., 2005).

d.   Regression of left ventricular hypertrophy (LVH). The left ventricle compensates for anemia and reduced oxygen delivery by undergoing hypertrophy, a maladaptive change that is independently associated with an increased risk of morbidity and death. Observational studies in patients with CKD demonstrate a strong relationship between anemia and risk for left ventricular hypertrophy (Levin et al., 1999). Smaller interventional studies have suggested that ESA treatment may induce LVH regression. However, larger randomized controlled trials have generally failed to demonstrate that treatment of anemia with ESA results in improvement in established LVH (Roger et al., 2004; Foley et al., 2000; Parfrey et al., 2005; Levin et al., 2005).

e.   Cognitive function. Cognitive function is improved after ESA therapy both at a physiologic level (evoked somatosensory potential latencies) and at a clinical level (tests of cognitive function). Patients may notice an improved ability to focus and concentrate.

f.   Improved hemostasis. ESRD patients in whom hemoglobin is <10 g/dL (100 g/L) often have increased bleeding time that responds to correction of anemia. With ESA therapy, serum fibrinogen and factor VIII concentrations increase and platelet aggregation is improved.

3.   Indications for ESA therapy and target hemoglobin. ESA therapy should be initiated in CKD patients when the hemoglobin falls below 11 g/dL (110 g/L). The optimal hemoglobin for a patient with ESRD is not known. The National Kidney Foundation's (NKF) Kidney Disease Outcome Quality Initiative (KDOQI) anemia guidelines (2006) recommend that hemoglobin for dialysis patients should be >11 g/dL (110 g/L). There always has been interest in the question of whether hemoglobin levels should be raised further, even to the normal range. Since this is a particularly expensive therapy, a strong supporting body of evidence would be required to demonstrate the benefit of higher hemoglobin targets. One study involved the randomization of over 1,200 hemodialysis patients with cardiac disease to a hematocrit level of 30% versus a "normal" 42%. The study was terminated prematurely due to a trend toward more adverse outcomes in the higher hematocrit group (Besarab et al., 1998). Similarly, in a recent randomized controlled study of 416 patients with different stages of chronic kidney disease, there was no reduction in risk for mortality with normalization of hemoglobin (Furuland et al., 2003). Therefore, raising the hemoglobin level toward the normal range cannot be recommended at this time.

4.   Route of administration

a.   Subcutaneous versus intravenous ESAs. The subcutaneous route improves the efficiency of therapy, resulting in a reduced dosing requirement for ESA for a given hemoglobin value (Kaufman et al., 1998). However, the vast majority of hemodialysis patients continue to be treated via the intravenous route. The primary reason is probably discomfort with subcutaneous injections, whereas reduced dosing requirements are a benefit that does not directly accrue to the patient. For patients on peritoneal dialysis, subcutaneous injections remain the dominant route of administration.

5. **Dosing**

   a. **Initial dose.** Treatment with ESA should ideally be initiated in the CKD period prior to ESRD. If treatment needs to be initiated for a patient already on dialysis, then reasonable starting doses of epoetin alfa for a hemodialysis patient would be 4,000–6,000 units three times per week, and for a peritoneal dialysis patient 8,000 units once per week. A typical dose of darbepoetin alfa would be approximately 25 mcg once weekly for a hemodialysis patient or 60 every 2 weeks for a patient on peritoneal dialysis. Selection of a specific dose requires clinical judgment as to how symptomatic the patient is and the starting level of hemoglobin. An excessively rapid rise in the hemoglobin should be avoided, as this may lead to an increased risk of worsening hypertension.

   b. **Initial response and plateau effect.** During the initiation phase of therapy, hemoglobin should be checked every 1–2 weeks, and the ESA dose adjusted as needed. It is very common during the initiation of treatment for a "plateauing" of effect to occur; either the hemoglobin stops increasing, or escalating doses of ESA are required to reach therapeutic targets. This period of blunted response is often due to the induction of iron deficiency. Once the target level of hemoglobin has been reached, the hemoglobin should be checked every 2–4 weeks. During this maintenance phase of therapy, the dose of ESA should be adjusted based on subsequent changes in hemoglobin (Fig. 32-1).

   The patient's responsiveness to ESA should be reassessed on a continuing basis. A certain proportion of patients will be highly responsive, with hemoglobin values consistently >11 g/dL (110 g/L), and an epoetin dose of <5,500 units three times per week. At the other end of the spectrum, many patients will be somewhat resistant to therapy, with a blunted erythropoietic response. These patients need to be fully evaluated for causes of ESA resistance. The remaining patients will demonstrate intermediate responsiveness. The hemoglobin of such patients will correlate with the ESA dose prescribed and will increase in response to an increase in dose. The responsiveness to ESA in all patients should be evaluated on an ongoing basis because the degree of responsiveness changes over time. In our experience, the development of resistance often signals the presence of iron deficiency or infection.

D. **Side effects of ESA therapy**

   1. **Worsening of hypertension.** This is a common problem during the partial correction of anemia with ESA therapy. In approximately 33% of patients, there will be

Continually reassess for the presence of ESA hyporesponsiveness, Hgb <11 g/dL or need for high ESA doses

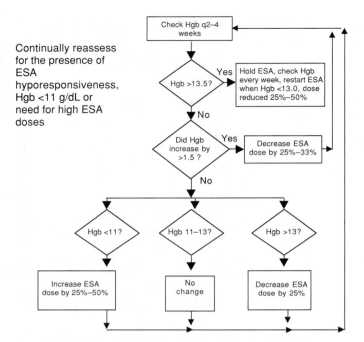

Figure 32-1. Flow chart for adjusting the erythropoiesis-stimulating agents (ESA) dose based on hematocrit (Hct) results.

a need to increase antihypertensive medication doses. However, it is rare for ESA to be withdrawn because of uncontrollable hypertension. Risk factors include preexisting hypertension, a rapid increase in hemoglobin, the presence of native kidneys, and severe anemia prior to treatment. The cause of the hypertensive effect is incompletely understood. Factors that may contribute include the partial reversal of hypoxic vasodilation as the hemoglobin rises, increased blood viscosity, a direct effect of ESA on the vasculature, and increased cardiac output. ESA induces a dose-dependent increase in the ratio of vasoconstrictive to vasodilatory prostanoids, increased vascular responsiveness to norepinephrine, and increased synthesis of endothelin-1 (Bode-Boger et al., 1996; Rodrigue et al., 2003). Various antihypertensives including long-acting calcium channel blockers are effective for treating hypertension associated with ESA.

2. Seizures. These may occur in a small number of patients during periods of rapidly increasing hemoglobin in association with hypertension. The risk of seizures is small using current ESA dosing protocols.

3. Graft clotting. The increase in blood viscosity with higher hemoglobin values on ESA could theoretically cause increased dialyzer and arteriovenous graft clotting. Studies to date have not consistently demonstrated an increased risk of thrombosis when the hemoglobin is raised to the 11–12 g/dL (110–120 g/L) range. The impact of higher hemoglobin levels is controversial. It should be clear that some patients may experience substantial hemoconcentration during or after the hemodialysis treatment, and effects on blood viscosity and risk for access thrombosis may be a particular concern in this setting.

4. Effect on *Kt*/*V*. Dialysis urea clearance may decrease slightly as the hemoglobin rises during ESA therapy, due to a diminished proportion of plasma to red cell volume, but with hemoglobin levels of <36%, the effect on urea clearance is of little clinical significance (see Chapter 3). The effect on creatinine clearance may be somewhat greater.

5. Phosphorus balance. Control of the serum phosphate concentration may become slightly more difficult during ESA therapy. An improvement in appetite and dietary intake of phosphate in combination with a reduction in dialyzer clearance of phosphate at the higher hemoglobin level may explain this phenomenon.

6. Hyperkalemia. This was occasionally seen in early studies of ESA. Subsequent clinical experience has not demonstrated any increase in the risk for hyperkalemia during ESA therapy.

E. Causes of decreased response to ESA therapy

1. Iron deficiency. The most important cause of a suboptimal response to ESA therapy is iron deficiency. Iron deficiency can be present at the outset of therapy, but more commonly, it develops during therapy, either due to rapid utilization of iron to support erythropoiesis or as the result of blood loss (Table 32-1).

a. Blood loss. Hemodialysis patients develop iron deficiency primarily because of chronic blood loss. Between retention of blood in the dialysis lines and filter, surgical blood loss, accidental bleeding from the access, blood sampling for laboratory testing, and occult gastrointestinal bleeding, iron losses may be substantial. Because of the overall burden of blood loss, it is very difficult to maintain iron stores in hemodialysis patients using oral iron supplements only. Losses in peritoneal dialysis patients are substantially less, and these patients often can be maintained on oral iron therapy.

b. Functional iron deficiency. In addition to a depleted iron supply, the demand for iron increases during ESA treatment, leading to a further strain on depleted iron stores. After the intravenous injection of ESA, there is an increase in the rate of erythropoiesis that leads to a greater immediate need for iron. In this setting, iron deficiency may occur even in the face of normal body iron stores. This phenomenon has been termed "functional iron deficiency" and may be noted clinically by low

Table 32-1.   Causes of iron deficiency in hemodialysis patients

- Depletion of iron stores
- Chronic blood loss
  1. Blood retention by the dialysis lines and filter
  2. Blood sampling for laboratory testing
  3. Accidents related to the vascular access
  4. Surgical blood loss
  5. Occult gastrointestinal bleeding
- Decreased dietary iron absorption
  1. Phosphate binders inhibit iron absorption
  2. Histamine-2 blockers, proton pump blockers, and functional achlorhydria impair iron absorption
  3. Uremic gut does not absorb iron optimally
- Increased iron demand
  1. Due to increased rate of erythropoiesis induced by erythropoiesis-stimulating agents
  2. Impaired release of iron from storage tissues (reticuloendothelial blockade)

transferrin saturation despite a normal or elevated serum ferritin concentration.

c.   Reticuloendothelial blockade. Iron deficiency may also be exacerbated in patients with ESRD by the presence of reticuloendothelial blockade. In this condition, which may be common in patients on dialysis, the presence of low-grade chronic inflammation may lead to impaired release of iron from its storage sites.

d.   Poor absorption of dietary iron. Iron deficiency among patients on dialysis may be exacerbated by poor absorption of dietary or medicinal iron. However, the subject is controversial and results from studies have been conflicting.

2.   Diagnosis

a.   Serum ferritin and transferrin saturation. The serum ferritin concentration and transferrin saturation percentage (TSAT) have been the two most widely used tests of iron status for dialysis patients. However, neither test is very accurate for the assessment of iron deficiency in this patient population; the tests provide only a rough estimate of iron status. Thus, patients should not be treated intensively with intravenous iron based only on the results of these indices. Instead, test results should be interpreted in the context of the patient's responsiveness to ESA therapy. The NKF's KDOQI anemia guidelines state that iron tests should be interpreted in the context of patients' clinical status, Hgb level, and ESA responsiveness. In our opinion, intensification of iron therapy should be considered at a serum ferritin of <200 ng/mL or transferrin saturation of <20% in patients who are reasonably

ESA responsive, and at a serum ferritin of <300 ng/mL or transferrin saturation <25% among patients with ESA resistance. Iron testing should usually be delayed for 1 week after treatment with intravenous iron.

b. **Reticulocyte hemoglobin content (CHr).** This test is a direct measure of iron availability at the level of the erythron (Brugnara, 2003). Several studies document a good level of diagnostic accuracy and cost effectiveness. In particular, it is a far more stable measure (less variability) than other tests of iron status (Fishbane et al., 2001). When the CHr value is <29–32 pg, patients are usually iron deficient and benefit from intravenous iron treatment.

c. **Other tests.** Other tests such as percentage of hypochromic red cells, zinc protoporphyrin, and soluble transferrin receptor levels have all been studied in patients with ESRD. All show at least some promise for aiding in iron management. However, at the time of this writing, none is yet widely available for clinical use in the United States.

3. **Iron treatment**

a. **General principles.** Iron therapy is an integral component of ESA treatment, particularly the regular use of parenteral iron in hemodialysis patients, resulting in higher hemoglobin levels and lower dose requirements for ESA. Intravenous iron may be administered on an episodic basis as needed when iron deficiency develops, or by the repeated administration of small doses to maintain iron balance.

A treatment flow chart is shown in Figure 32-2. In general, most patients on dialysis require iron supplementation as long as they are not iron overloaded.

b. **Oral iron.** Oral iron preparations are safe and relatively inexpensive. However, these supplements are associated with poor efficacy and troublesome side effects, such as constipation, dyspepsia, bloating, or diarrhea. Three randomized trials have compared oral iron to either placebo or no iron treatment in hemodialysis patients; none of the three was able to demonstrate any efficacy for oral iron. Therefore, oral iron should not be used for most hemodialysis patients.

For patients on peritoneal dialysis, oral iron is much more convenient than intravenous iron. Since these patients experience less chronic blood loss, oral iron may be sufficient to maintain iron stores. Intravenous iron therapy should be used in peritoneal dialysis patients only when marked resistance to ESA is present and the serum ferritin is <100 ng/mL and the TSAT is <20%.

(1) **Dosage and administration.** Oral iron usually is given as ferrous sulfate, fumarate, or gluconate, in a dosage of 200 mg of elemental iron per day. The timing of the iron dose is important; ideally, iron should be taken on an empty stomach to optimize efficacy.

The primary sites of iron absorption are the duodenum and proximal jejunum, and gastrointestinal

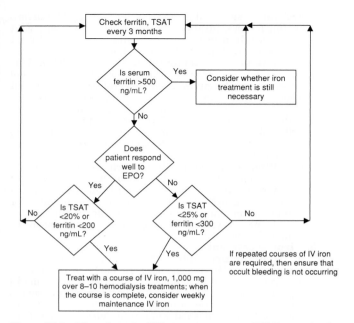

Figure 32-2.   Flow chart for IV iron management. TSAT, transferrin saturation percentage; EPO, erythropoietin.

symptoms are proportional to the amount of elemental iron presented to the duodenum at a single time; reduction of symptomatology may require changing the oral preparation, using pediatric dosages at more frequent intervals, or even taking the iron dosage with food. Others have suggested giving the medication during dialysis sessions (e.g., at the beginning and the end of the session) to help ensure patient compliance. Yet another strategy is to give oral iron only at bedtime. A common problem with oral iron is constipation, which can be partially managed, if necessary, with stool softeners or laxatives. Some iron preparations contain small doses of ascorbic acid to enhance iron absorption, but the advantage of the added vitamin is not established. Phosphorus binders, antacids, histamine-2 antagonists, and proton pump inhibitors may all inhibit the absorption of oral iron supplements.

Readily available delayed-release preparations of iron (e.g., Ferro-Gradumet, Slow Fe, Ferro Sequels) minimize the release of iron in the stomach and may cause less gastrointestinal irritation. Iron–polysaccharide complexes supply elemental iron rather than the iron salt (e.g., Niferex-150, Nu-Iron). Both delayed-release preparations and iron–polysaccharide complex–based tablets are substantially more expensive than the plain iron salts. It is not clear that any specific oral iron preparation causes fewer side effects than others. More recently, heme iron polypeptide has been evaluated as a potentially more effective and better tolerated form of oral iron. It is generally prescribed as a tablet containing 12 mg of elemental iron, with a dose of three tablets per day. At least one study has found the supplement to have excellent efficacy and tolerability (Nissenson et al., 2003).

c. Intravenous iron: General considerations. Three preparations are widely used: Iron dextran, ferric gluconate, and iron sucrose. Intravenous iron therapy has superior availability and efficacy when compared with oral iron therapy. In hemodialysis patients, achieving the target hemoglobin level associated with improved quality-of-life and reduced mortality and hospitalization risk is difficult to achieve without intravenous iron treatment. As a result, the NKF KDOQI anemia treatment guidelines note that most hemodialysis patients will require intravenous iron on regular basis. In contrast, intravenous therapy costs more, and its safety profile is less clear than that of oral iron. There are two commonly used intravenous iron dosing strategies. One is to treat established iron deficiency with a repletive 1,000-mg dose administered over 8–10 consecutive hemodialysis treatments. Alternatively, since iron deficiency occurs so frequently in hemodialysis patients, a weekly maintenance dose of 25–100 mg may be used. There is no significant evidence to suggest that one of these treatment strategies is more effective than the other. When intravenous iron is required for peritoneal dialysis patients, infusions of 250 mg of iron may be administered over 1–2 hours.

(1) Intravenous iron safety: Anaphylaxis. The best understood complication of intravenous iron treatment is the rare occurrence of anaphylactoid-type reactions. These are characterized by the abrupt occurrence of hypotension, dyspnea, flushing, and back pain. With iron dextran, the rate has been estimated as 0.7% of patients treated. Such reactions are less frequently observed, and are probably of milder intensity with the nondextran forms of iron. In the most rigorous study, which involved direct observation of patients after drug administration, the rate of serious reactions with single-dose exposure to ferric gluconate was 0.04%, a rate the authors considered to be less than expected with iron dextran (Michael et al., 2002). Iron sucrose, another nondextran form of iron, probably has a similar safety profile.

(2) Intravenous iron safety: Infection. Iron is a vital growth factor for micro-organisms, and intravenous iron treatment has the potential to make iron more readily available to these pathogens. In addition, in vitro studies suggest that iron treatment may interfere with phagocytic function of white blood cells. Early retrospective studies found higher serum ferritin levels in hemodialysis patients to be associated with increased risk of infection. In contrast, a large, prospective, multicenter study (Hoen et al., 1998, 2002) found no relation between serum ferritin or treatment with intravenous iron with the risk for bacteremia. The current literature on this subject remains inconclusive, but a prudent approach would be to avoid intravenous iron treatment during acute infectious episodes.

(3) **Intravenous iron safety: Oxidation.** Iron is a highly oxidative substance, and treatment with intravenous iron has the potential to overburden the body's native antioxidant systems. Oxidative damage to proteins such as albumin and fibrinogen has been demonstrated, although the clinical significance of such findings is not clear (Anraku et al., 2004). A potential harmful effect of vascular oxidation would be an acceleration of atherosclerotic processes. Support is found in the work of Drueke et al. (2002), who found increased carotid artery intima media thickness in relation to intravenous iron sucrose treatment and protein oxidation in hemodialysis patients. One study, which needs confirmation, suggested that vitamin E may attenuate oxidative stress associated with intravenous iron therapy (Roob et al., 2000).

d. **Intravenous iron drugs**

(1) **Intravenous iron dextran.** Because of the higher expected risk of anaphylaxis, iron dextran use should generally be reserved for patients who have a long history of prior safe use of the drug. Iron dextran is supplied as a sterile liquid, containing 50 mg of elemental iron per milliliter. In nonuremic patients, immediate allergic reactions to intravenous iron dextran have been reported. These usually occur within 5 minutes of injection but may be delayed by 45 minutes or more. Anaphylactic reactions can cause hypotension, syncope, purpura, wheezing, dyspnea, respiratory arrest, and cyanosis. For this reason, epinephrine and other means to treat anaphylaxis must be at hand when intravenous iron dextran is administered. Importantly, Walters and Van Wyck (2005) recently reported that almost all severe reactions occur with the test dose or first therapeutic dose. Milder immediate hypersensitivity reactions to iron dextran infusion include itching and urticaria. Delayed reactions can manifest as lymphadenopathy, myalgia, arthralgia, fever, and headache.

(2) **Sodium ferric gluconate.** Intravenous sodium ferric gluconate is a nondextran form of iron used in the United States since 1999 and in Europe for several decades. As discussed above, adverse reactions are less frequent and less severe than those seen with iron dextran. With single-dose exposure the rate of severe

reactions was 0.04%, and no severe reactions were observed with repeated administration of 13,151 doses to 1,321 patients (Michael et al., 2002, 2004). Intravenous sodium ferric gluconate may be administered to hemodialysis patients in the amount of 1,000 mg given in divided doses over eight consecutive treatments (i.e., 125 mg/dose).

(3) **Iron sucrose.** Intravenous iron sucrose was approved for use in the United States in 2000 and has been in use in Europe for many years. Like sodium ferric gluconate, the other widely used nondextran form of iron, reports generally indicate a good safety and efficacy profile. No serious adverse reactions occurred in 665 hemodialysis patients receiving 8,583 doses of the drug (Aronoff et al., 2004). The drug may be administered as iron replacement therapy, 100 mg for 10 consecutive doses, or as a weekly dose of 25–100 mg.

e. **Other causes of ESA resistance**

(1) **Hyperparathyroidism.** Hyperparathyroidism may be a cause of ESA resistance. The effect may be related most to the amount of marrow fibrosis, and it is unclear that the serum parathyroid hormone level (iPTH) is a good marker for resistance. Nonetheless, in the ESA-resistant patient who is found to have elevated iPTH levels, an intensification of the treatment of hyperparathyroidism is indicated. Among patients with severe hyperparathyroidism refractory to medical therapy, parathyroidectomy has been demonstrated to result in a significant improvement in erythropoiesis.

(2) **Inflammation and infection.** As with infection, inflammatory states lead to an increased resistance to ESA therapy. In patients on dialysis, inflammatory conditions may be occult with the cause obscure, or may be due to the bioincompatibility of the dialysis treatment itself. There is no perfect marker for occult inflammation, but C-reactive protein (CRP) is emerging as a valuable test for predicting ESA hyporesponsiveness caused by inflammation (Kalantar-Zadeh et al., 2003). A retained, nonfunctioning renal allograft can increase CRP levels and be a source of EPO resistance (Lopez-Gomez et al., 2004). The release of cytokines during infection leads to a diminished bone marrow response to ESA. A search for occult infection should be undertaken in patients with unexplained ESA resistance. If infection is present, higher doses of ESA may be effective by partially overcoming the temporary resistance. One occult site of infection is in old, nonfunctioning, arteriovenous accesses, where treatment of the infection may reverse ESA resistance (Nassar et al., 2002).

(3) **Inadequate dialysis.** An association between the adequacy of hemodialysis and responsiveness to ESA has been suggested (Ifudu et al., 1996), but this is not found universally, and in the HEMO trial, neither dose of dialysis nor assignment to use of a high-flux membrane affected ESA requirements or Hgb levels.

With more frequent dialysis, and especially with use of nocturnal dialysis, evidence for reduced ESA requirements is more convincing. With use of hemodiafiltration, some studies also suggest that less ESA is needed, but this is controversial. See Chapters 14 and 15.

(4)   Aluminum intoxication. Although problems with aluminum have become less common among dialysis patients, occasional problems may still occur, especially in patients who have been on dialysis for many years. The effect on erythropoiesis is a microcytic anemia associated with impaired iron utilization. Interestingly, intestinal aluminum absorption is significantly increased in patients with iron deficiency. A serum aluminum level provides a rough guide to aluminum status; if the results are suggestive, then either a deferoxamine stimulation test (see Chapter 43) or bone biopsy may be warranted.

(5)   Bleeding. An important cause of an apparent hyporesponsiveness to ESA is bleeding. Sometimes the bleeding may be occult, as in gastrointestinal blood loss. Often the bleeding may be obvious, as in patients undergoing surgery, menstruating women, or those with accidents involving the vascular access. It is vitally important to limit blood loss by any means possible. In addition, fecal occult blood testing should be performed every 3–6 months when unexplained ESA resistance is present.

(6)   Angiotensin-converting enzyme (ACE) inhibitors. ACE inhibitors may reduce EPO production in patients with chronic renal failure or following renal transplant. Among patients on dialysis, a reduction in ESA responsiveness has not been uniformly demonstrated in association with these agents.

(7)   Serum albumin. An association has been noted between hematocrit and serum albumin, suggesting a possible link between ESA responsiveness and either inflammation or nutritional state. However, there is no evidence of causality in this relationship or that an improvement in nutrition would necessarily lead to an improvement in ESA responsiveness.

(8)   Pure red cell aplasia. An outbreak of immune-mediated pure red cell aplasia has been reported, primarily in Europe, in association with ESA treatment. In the first 10 years of worldwide ESA availability, only three cases were noted among more than a million treated patients. Subsequently, the rate increased dramatically, with at least 184 cases reported between 1998 and 2003. The majority of cases have occurred in Europe, with epoetin alfa sold under the brand name of Eprex. A smaller number of cases have been reported with other forms of epoetin alfa or epoetin beta. The cause of the syndrome is now recognized as being the development of neutralizing antierythropoietin antibodies, usually after at least 6 months of drug exposure. While the cause is still under investigation, there is a strong association with the use of the stabilizer polysorbate. There is evidence that polysorbate caused leaching of organic compounds from uncoated rubber stoppers in prefilled syringes. Presumably these organic substances could interact with erythropoietin to elicit immunogenicity (Boven et al., 2005). In addition, almost all cases have been with subcutaneous administration of the drugs, leading in 2002 to health authorities to recommend against subcutaneous administration of epoetin alfa in Europe. Since then the number of cases has decreased substantially (Bennett et al., 2004, Rossert et al., 2004). Clinically, the syndrome is recognized by a continuous decrease in hemoglobin and the development of transfusion dependence, with a low reticulocyte count. Bone marrow shows a severe deficiency of red cell precursors and antierythropoietin antibodies are detected in plasma. Upon diagnosis, all ESA drugs must be discontinued, as there is universal cross-reaction with antierythropoietin antibodies. Many patients will respond successfully to treatment with steroids or other immunosuppressive medications.

(9) Other hematologic disease. Patients on dialysis are at risk for developing the same hematologic diseases as nonuremic subjects. Because of the emphasis on EPO deficiency, other hematologic diseases may go unrecognized. Among the potential causes are vitamin B_{12} or folic acid deficiency, hematologic malignancy, myelodysplastic syndromes, or hemolysis. Vitamin B_{12} and folic acid levels should be checked when unexplained ESA resistance is present. When an exhaustive evaluation for causes of resistance is unrevealing, hematology consultation and a bone marrow biopsy may be considered as a last step in the process to rule out unexpected hematologic disease. The percentage of hemodialysis patients with macrocytosis (mean corpuscular volume [MCV] >98 fl) has been reported to have increased between 1998 and 2004 in U.S. hemodialysis patients (Pollak and Lorch, 2005). Folate and vitamin B_{12} in selected patients with macrocytosis was normal. The generalizability of this observation and its clinical importance are not currently known.

F. Red blood cell transfusions. Transfusion of packed red cells should be used in severely anemic patients who are experiencing symptoms. Transfusion should never be utilized without a concurrent evaluation for causes of bleeding.

G. Carnitine. It has been suggested that carnitine may enhance responsiveness to ESA. A recent systematic review found that carnitine administration led to a reduction in overall epoetin requirements (Hurot et al., 2002). However, the process for selection of patients appropriate for this therapy remains unclear.

H. Ascorbic acid. Although the literature is mixed, several studies have found that intravenous ascorbic acid may improve epoetin responsiveness for patients on hemodialysis

(Attallah et al., 2006; Tarng et al., 1998; Keven et al., 2003). A typical regimen is intravenous vitamin C given three times weekly with the hemodialysis treatment. The effect may be mediated via improved iron availability to the erythroid marrow. Since vitamin C may lead to increases in oxalate production, appropriate caution must be used in patient selection and duration of therapy.

I. Nandrolone decanoate. Androgens have occasionally been used to increase Hgb level when ESAs are not available, or as an adjuvant to ESA treatment. However, a variety of adverse events have been noted, including priapism, liver dysfunction, and hepatocellular carcinoma. As a result, the NKF KDOQI anemia guidelines include an evidence-based guideline stating that androgens should not be used as an adjuvant to ESA therapy.

J. Nephrogenic fibrosing dermopathy. This relatively new complication of dialysis, first described in 1977, is of unknown cause. See Chapter 41 for a full description. A few reports have attempted to link this to high-dose EPO therapy (Swaminathan et al., 2005), although causality is far from established.

II. Hemolysis

A. General comments. Destruction of red blood cells, either intravascularly or extravascularly, may occasionally contribute to anemia in dialysis patients. Generally speaking, red cell survival appears to be shortened with chronic renal failure (approximately 30% compared to healthy subjects [Ly et al., 2004]). It is likely that this is due not to an inherent abnormality of the red cell, but to an effect of the uremic environment.

B. Diagnosis. Chronic hemolysis should be suspected when the patient develops high-grade ESA resistance in the presence of increased serum lactic dehydrogenase (LDH), unconjugated bilirubin, or a decrease in serum haptoglobin. The differential diagnosis of chronic hemolysis is broad, and includes all causes of hemolysis seen in nonuremic patients (Table 32-2) and several causes specific to patients treated with hemodialysis. Occasionally, hemolysis can be severe, associated with hypotension, back pain, and encephalopathy developing during the dialysis procedure.

C. Etiology. The most common correctible cause of hemolysis is due to some problem with the hemodialysis system. Faulty or kinked blood line tubing can do this. Chloramine in the dialysis solution, copper in the water supply, formaldehyde not rinsed out of the dialyzer after reprocessing, and use of a hypotonic or overheated dialysis solution are among the causes. Machine/dialysis solution–based issues are discussed in Chapters 4 and 5.

D. Treatment. If acute, severe hemolysis is suspected, then the dialysis treatment should be terminated immediately. Circulatory support should be provided as needed, and an electrocardiogram must be obtained to determine if hyperkalemic changes are present (which may be delayed) and to assess for acute cardiac ischemia. A blood sample should be obtained for determination of hemoglobin, hematocrit, and serum chemistries.

Table 32-2. Causes of hemolysis in dialysis patients

Related to the hemodialysis procedure
    Dialysis solution
        Contaminants
        Chloramine
        Copper, zinc
        Nitrates, nitrites
        Overheated
        Hypo-osmolar
    Reuse of sterilants (formaldehyde)
    Kinked or defective tubing—trauma to RBCs
    Needle trauma to RBCs
    Subclavian catheter (helmet cells, schistocytes)
Insufficient dialysis
Hypersplenism
Associated diseases
    Sickle cell anemia
    Other hemoglobinopathies
    Connective tissue diseases with vasculitis
Drug-induced
Hypophosphatemia

RBCs, red blood cells.

III. Disorders of hemostasis

A. Introduction. The formation of a blood clot in response to vascular injury is a complex and highly conserved process in mammalian species. Disorders of platelet quantity or function lead to bleeding in superficial sites, such as the skin and mucous membranes. Disorders of the coagulation system usually lead to bleeding into deeper structures, such as muscle and joints. Prior to the introduction of dialysis, bleeding tendencies were long recognized among uremic subjects. Dialysis partially reverses the abnormal hemostasis, but ecchymoses, excessive access bleeding, and occasional severe bleeding episodes still occur.

B. Pathophysiology. Many factors contribute to the deranged state of uremic hemostasis, with disorders in platelet function (thrombasthenia) being most important. Platelet aggregation is abnormal, probably due to reduced platelet granule adenosine phosphate and serotonin levels, and defective thromboxane A_2 production. Platelet function may also be hindered in uremic patients by increased endothelial nitric oxide production (Remuzzi et al., 1990). An adhesion receptor, the glycoprotein (GP) IIb–IIIa complex, plays an important role in controlling the formation of platelet thrombi. In uremic patients, the activation of the GP IIb–IIIa receptor is impaired, but activation is partially restored by dialysis. There has been a suggestion that abnormalities of von Willebrand factor (important for maintaining platelet adhesion in rapid blood flow) may contribute to disordered uremic hemostasis, but study results have been inconsistent. Finally, anemia itself probably contributes to uremic bleeding; abnormally prolonged bleeding time is significantly improved when the hematocrit is increased to >30%.

C. Assessment. Disordered hemostasis should be evaluated in terms of clinical manifestations and by testing of skin bleeding time. Patients with ecchymoses, excessive access bleeding, or any clinically significant bleeding episodes (including hemorrhagic pericarditis) should have platelet count, prothrombin time, partial thromboplastin time, and bleeding time tested. The bleeding time becomes abnormal when the platelet count is decreased, when platelet function is impaired, or if the vascular wall is damaged. The risk for hemorrhage increases when the bleeding time is elevated to more than 10 minutes.

D. Treatment. The management of dialysis patients experiencing bleeding requires (a) an estimate of the severity of blood loss, (b) hemodynamic stabilization, (c) transfusion with blood products as needed, (d) identification of the bleeding source, and (e) treatment of platelet dysfunction and other factors contributing to the bleeding diathesis. Intensive dialysis results in some improvement in bleeding tendency in two thirds of patients. The administration of cryoprecipitate (a plasma extract with high concentrations of von Willebrand factor) does not consistently result in improved platelet function. In one study only two of five treated patients had normalized bleeding time and a favorable outcome (Triulzi et al., 1990). Desmopressin (a synthetic analog of antidiuretic hormone) leads to increased release of von Willebrand factor multimers. A dose of 0.3 mcg/kg body weight may be administered diluted in 50 mL of saline intravenously over 30 minutes. In a well-designed study, this regimen led to a reduction in bleeding time in 1 hour, which lasted for 8 hours. Alternatively, a dose of 3.0 mcg/kg body weight may be injected subcutaneously. The drug has little vasoconstrictive effect and is only rarely associated with hyponatremia. Finally, repetitive intravenous infusions of conjugated estrogens may reduce bleeding time significantly. More practically, one oral dose of 25 mg conjugated estrogen (Premarin) normalizes bleeding time for up to 10 days. This effect is in contrast to the relatively short period of action of cryoprecipitate or desmopressin. We recommend the use of desmopressin empirically for dialysis patients with severe acute bleeding. In contrast, conjugated estrogens may be helpful in correcting an abnormal bleeding time prior to planned surgery or to treat chronic gastrointestinal bleeding in patients with telangiectasia. Estrogens alone, PO, IV, or transdermally (Sloand and Schiff, 1995) or estrogen–progesterone combinations have all been used (Boccardo et al., 2004). See the Web references for detailed dosing protocols.

SELECTED READINGS

Alarcon MC, et al. [Hormone therapy with estrogen patches for the treatment of recurrent digestive hemorrhages in uremic patients]. *Nefrologia* 2002;22(2):208–209.

Anraku M, et al. Intravenous iron administration induces oxidation of serum albumin in hemodialysis patients. *Kidney Int* 2004;66(2):841–848.

Aronoff G, et al. Iron sucrose in hemodialysis patients: safety of replacement and maintenance regimens. *Kidney Int* 2004;66(3): 1193–1198.

Attallah N, et al. Effect of intravenous ascorbic acid in hemodialysis patients with EPO-hyporesponsive anemia and hyperferritinemia. *Am J Kidney Dis* 2006;47(4):644–654.

Bennett CL, et al. Pure red-cell aplasia and epoetin therapy. *N Engl J Med* 2004;351(14):1403–1408.

Besarab A, et al. The effects of normal as compared with low hematocrit values in patients with cardiac disease who are receiving hemodialysis and epoetin. *N Engl J Med* 1998;339:584–590.

Boccardo P, et al. Platelet dysfunction in renal failure. *Semin Thromb Hemost* 2004;30(5):579–589.

Bode-Boger SM, et al. Recombinant human erythropoietin enhances vasoconstrictor tone via endothelin-1 and constrictor prostanoids. *Kidney Int* 1996;50:1255–1261.

Boven K, et al. Epoetin-associated pure red cell aplasia in patients with chronic kidney disease: solving the mystery. *Nephrol Dial Transplant* 2005;20(Suppl 3):iii33–40.

Brugnara C. Iron deficiency and erythropoiesis: new diagnostic approaches. *Clin Chem* 2003;49(10):1573–1578.

Drueke T, et al. Iron therapy, advanced oxidation protein products, and carotid artery intima-media thickness in end-stage renal disease. *Circulation* 2002;106(17):2212–2217.

Duffy R, et al. Multistate outbreak of hemolysis in hemodialysis patients traced to faulty blood tubing sets. *Kidney Int* 2000;57(4): 1668–1674.

Escolar G, Diaz-Ricart M, Cases A. Uremic platelet dysfunction: past and present [Review]. *Curr Hematol Rep* 2005;4(5):359–367.

Fishbane S, et al. A randomized trial of iron deficiency testing strategies in hemodialysis patients. *Kidney Int* 2001;60(6):2406–2411.

Foley RN, et al. Effect of hemoglobin levels in hemodialysis patients with asymptomatic cardiomyopathy. *Kidney Int* 2000;58:1325–1335.

Furuland H, et al. A randomized controlled trial of haemoglobin normalization with epoetin alfa in pre-dialysis and dialysis patients. *Nephrol Dial Transplant* 2003;18(2):353–361.

Gunnell J, et al. Acute-phase response predicts erythropoietin resistance in hemodialysis and peritoneal dialysis patients. *Am J Kidney Dis* 1999;33:63–72.

Hoen B. EPIBACDIAL: a multicenter prospective study of risk factors for bacteremia in chronic hemodialysis patients. *J Am Soc Nephrol* 1998;9(5):869–876.

Hoen B, et al. Intravenous iron administration does not significantly increase the risk of bacteremia in chronic hemodialysis patients. *Clin Nephrol* 2002;57(6):457–461.

Hurot JM, et al. Effects of L-carnitine supplementation in maintenance hemodialysis patients: a systematic review. *J Am Soc Nephrol* 2002;13:708–714.

Ifudu O, et al. The intensity of hemodialysis and the response to erythropoietin in patients with end-stage renal disease. *N Engl J Med* 1996;334:420–425.

Kalantar-Zadeh K, et al. Effect of malnutrition-inflammation complex syndrome on EPO hyporesponsiveness in maintenance hemodialysis patients. *Am J Kidney Dis* 2003;42(4):761–773.

Kaufman JS, et al. Subcutaneous compared with intravenous epoetin in patients receiving hemodialysis. Department of Veterans Affairs Cooperative Study Group on Erythropoietin in Hemodialysis Patients. *N Engl J Med* 1998;339:578–583.

Keven K, et al. Randomized, crossover study of the effect of vitamin C on EPO response in hemodialysis patients. *Am J Kidney Dis* 2003;41(6):1233–1239.

Levin A, et al. Canadian randomized trial of hemoglobin maintenance to prevent or delay left ventricular mass growth in patients with CKD. *Am J Kidney Dis* 2005;46(5):799–811.

Levin A, et al. Left ventricular mass index increase in early renal disease: impact of decline in hemoglobin. *Am J Kidney Dis* 1999; 34(1):125–134.

Lopez-Gomez JM, et al. Presence of a failed kidney transplant in patients who are on hemodialysis is associated with chronic inflammatory state and erythropoietin resistance. *J Am Soc Nephrol* 2004;15(9):2494–2501.

Ly J, et al. Red blood cell survival in chronic renal failure. *Am J Kidney Dis* 2004;44(4):715–719.

Ma JZ, Ebben J, Collins AJ. Hematocrit level and associated mortality in hemodialysis patients [Abstract]. *J Am Soc Nephrol* 1999;10:610–619.

Macdougall IC, et al. Pharmacokinetics of novel erythropoiesis stimulating protein (NESP) compared with epoietin alfa in dialysis patients. *J Am Soc Nephrol* 1999;10:2392–2395.

Michael B, et al. Sodium ferric gluconate complex in haemodialysis patients: a prospective evaluation of long-term safety. *Nephrol Dial Transplant* 2004;19(6):1576–1580.

Michael B, et al. Sodium ferric gluconate complex in hemodialysis patients: adverse reactions compared to placebo and iron dextran. *Kidney Int* 2002;61(5):1830–1839.

Nassar GM, et al. Occult infection of old nonfunctioning arteriovenous grafts: a novel cause of erythropoietin resistance and chronic inflammation in hemodialysis patients. *Kidney Int Suppl* 2002;(80):49–54.

National Kidney Foundation—KDOQI. II. Clinical practice guidelines and clinical practice recommendations for anemia in chronic kidney disease in adults. *Am J Kidney Dis* 2006;47(5 Suppl 3):S16–85.

Nissenson AR, et al. Clinical evaluation of heme iron polypeptide: sustaining a response to rHuEPO in hemodialysis patients. *Am J Kidney Dis* 2003;42(2):325–330.

Noris M, Remuzzi G. Uremic bleeding: closing the circle after 30 years of controversies? *Blood*. 1999;94:2569–2574.

Ofsthun N, et al. The effects of higher hemoglobin levels on mortality and hospitalization in hemodialysis patients. *Kidney Int* 2003;63(5):1908–1914.

Parfrey PS, et al. Double-blind comparison of full and partial anemia correction in incident hemodialysis patients without symptomatic heart disease. *J Am Soc Nephrol* 2005;16(7):2180–2189.

Pollak VE, Lorch JA. Macrocytosis in chronic hemodialysis (HD) patients [Abstract]. *J Am Soc Nephrol* 2005;16:477A.

Remuzzi G, et al. Role of endothelium derived nitric oxide in the bleeding tendency of uremia. *J Clin Invest* 1990;86:1768–1771.

Rodrigue MF, et al. Relationship between eicosanoids and endothelin-1 in the pathogenesis of erythropoietin-induced hypertension in uremic rats. *J Cardiovasc Pharmacol* 2003;41(3):388–395.

Roger S, et al. Effects of early and late intervention with epoetin alpha on left ventricular mass among patients with chronic kidney disease (stage 3 or 4): results of a randomized clinical trial. *J Am Soc Nephrol* 2004;15(1):148–156.

Roob JM, et al. Vitamin E attenuates oxidative stress induced by intravenous iron in patients on hemodialysis. *J Am Soc Nephrol* 2000;11:539–549.

Rossert J, et al. Anti-erythropoietin antibodies and pure red cell aplasia. *J Am Soc Nephrol* 2004;15(2):398–406.

Sloand JA, Schiff MJ. Beneficial effect of low-dose transdermal estrogen on bleeding time and clinical bleeding in uremia. *Am J Kidney Dis* 1995;26:22–26.

Spinowitz BS, et al. The safety and efficacy of ferumoxytol therapy in anemic chronic kidney disease patients. *Kidney Int* 2005;68:1801–1806.

Swaminathan S, et al. Nephrogenic fibrosing dermopathy is linked to high dose erythropoietin therapy [Abstract]. *J Am Soc Nephrol* 2005;16:480A.

Tarng DC, Huang TP. A parallel, comparative study of intravenous iron versus intravenous ascorbic acid for erythropoietin-hyporesponsive anaemia in hemodialysis patients with iron overload. *Nephrol Dial Transplant* 1998;13:2867–2872.

Teruel JL, et al. Androgen versus erythropoietin for the treatment of anemia in hemodialyzed patients: a prospective study. *J Am Soc Nephrol* 1996;7:140–144.

Triulzi DJ, Blumberg N. Variability in response to cryoprecipitate treatment for hemostatic defects in uremia. *Yale J Biol Med* 1990;63(1):1–7.

Van Wyck DB, et al. Safety and efficacy of iron sucrose in patients sensitive to iron dextran: North American Clinical Trial. *Am J Kidney Dis* 2000;36:88–97.

Walters BA, Van Wyck DB. Benchmarking iron dextran sensitivity: reactions requiring resuscitative medication in incident and prevalent patients. *Nephrol Dial Transplant* 2005;20(7):1438–1442.

Xia H, et al. Hematocrit levels and hospitalization risks in hemodialysis patients. *J Am Soc Nephrol* 1999;10:1309–1316.

WEB REFERENCES

Anemia management protocols, links, and updates: http://www.hdcn.com/ch/rbc

NKF KDOQI guidelines for anemia: http://www.kidney.org

Infections

David J. Leehey, Joan P. Cannon,
and Joseph R. Lentino

I. **Derangement of immune function in uremia**
   A. **Etiology.** In dialysis patients there is impairment of several aspects of lymphocyte and granulocyte function. Unidentified uremic toxins are thought to be responsible; malnutrition or vitamin D deficiency can sometimes be contributory factors.
   B. **Clinical implications**
      1. **Increased susceptibility to infection**
         a. **Frequency of bacterial infections.** Bacterial infections occur more often in dialysis patients than in their nonuremic counterparts; the increase is probably related more to frequent violation of normal skin and mucosal barriers than to immune system dysfunction.
         b. **Severity of bacterial infections.** Bacterial infections in dialysis patients appear to progress more quickly and to resolve less promptly than in nonuremic patients. However, formal documentation of this clinical impression is lacking. Whereas dialysis patients should not be considered as immunocompromised hosts in the same fashion as transplant recipients, initiation of antimicrobial therapy should be considered sooner and at a lower level of documentation of bacterial infection than in nonuremic patients.
         c. **Role of hemodialysis membrane or peritoneal dialysis solution**. Some of the immune defects previously attributed to uremia may be due, in part, to periodic exposure of the blood to certain dialysis membranes or to lack of removal of putative inhibitors of immune function by low-flux membranes. However, in the HEMO study, infection-related deaths were not reduced by utilization of biocompatible, high-flux dialyzers (Allon et al., 2004). In peritoneal dialysis patients, peritoneal neutrophil function is depressed due to removal of opsonins (immunoglobulin and complement) in the dialysate and to regular exposure to low pH, high osmolality, and glucose degradation products present in some dialysis solutions.

II. **Derangement of temperature control in uremia**
   A. **Baseline hypothermia in uremic patients.** In 50% of hemodialysis patients, the predialysis body temperature is subnormal. The reason for this is unknown.
   B. **Reduced pyrexic response associated with infections.** Uremia per se does not appear to affect the temperature response to pyrogens. In addition, the degree of interleukin-1 (IL-1) production by stimulated uremic monocytes is normal. However, because of baseline hypothermia, and possibly

because of frequently coexisting malnutrition, severe infections in some dialysis patients may not be associated with fever.

III. Bacterial infections in dialysis patients
A. Related to the access site
1. Hemodialysis patients.
Prevention, diagnosis, and treatment of vascular access infections are described in Chapters 6 (venous access) and 7 (fistulas and grafts). Several additional clinical points are emphasized here.

a. Bacteremia versus pyrogen reaction. The dialysis patient with bacteremia generally presents with chills and fever and may appear quite toxic. On occasion, however, symptoms and signs of infection are remarkably few or absent. Although redness, tenderness, or exudate at the access site may help to incriminate it as the source of the infection, in many cases an infected access site can appear normal. Delayed treatment of sepsis in dialysis patients is an important cause of morbidity and mortality.

(1) Pyrogen reaction. Low-grade fever during hemodialysis may be related to pyrogens present in the dialysis solution rather than to actual infection. The time course of fever may be somewhat helpful in making the distinction between pyrogen reaction and infection: Patients with pyrogen-related fever are afebrile prior to dialysis but become febrile during dialysis; fever resolves spontaneously after cessation of dialysis. Patients with access site–related bacteremia often are febrile prior to institution of dialysis and, in the absence of treatment, fever persists during and after dialysis. There is one exception to the rule: Fever and chills that occur shortly after catheter manipulation (for instance, commencement or cessation of dialysis) suggests catheter-associated bacteremia. Use of high-flux dialysis (especially in conjunction with bicarbonate dialysate) and dialyzer reuse are associated with an increased incidence of pyrogenic reactions. Blood cultures should always be obtained in any febrile hemodialysis patient, even when a pyrogen reaction is the suspected cause of the fever.

(2) Contamination of hemodialysis machines or solutions. Occasionally bacteremia may result from contamination of hemodialysis machines. These are generally Gram-negative and occasionally fungal infections. Outbreaks of such infections have been caused by inadequate disinfection of water treatment or distribution systems or reprocessed dialyzers. Contamination of the waste drain ports of the hemodialysis machine has also been described.

b. Prophylactic antimicrobial administration

(1) Prophylaxis prior to an invasive procedure likely to result in bacteremia. Although there is no definite evidence in the literature, it is our policy to administer antimicrobial prophylaxis to hemodialysis patients prior to invasive procedures associated with a substantial risk of bacteremia because of the abnormal vascular communication present. These include dental procedures (especially extractions); gastrointestinal procedures such as esophageal stricture dilation, sclerotherapy for esophageal varices, and endoscopic retrograde cholangiography with biliary obstruction (not necessary for routine endoscopy with or without biopsy); and genitourinary procedures including cystoscopy, urethral dilation, and transurethral prostate resection. The recommended antimicrobial is amoxicillin 2.0 g 1 hour before the procedure (or ampicillin 2.0 g IM or IV 30 minutes before the procedure). In penicillin-allergic patients, either clindamycin 600 mg PO or IV (dental or esophageal procedures) or vancomycin 1.0 g IV (other gastrointestinal and genitourinary procedures) can be substituted.

(2) Long-term, continuous prophylaxis. The skin and nasal carriage rate of *Staphylococcus aureus* in hemodialysis patients is about 50%. Prophylactic antimicrobial therapy with rifampin has been shown to be effective in decreasing infections due to this organism in such patients (Yu et al., 1986). Intranasal mupirocin ointment is also effective in eradicating the carrier state and in uncontrolled studies has decreased the incidence of staphylococcal infection. Decision analysis suggests that weekly use of this agent in all patients without screening will decrease infection rates and is cost effective (Bloom et al., 1996). However, controlled trials in support of this contention need to be performed. A major concern is the development of mupirocin resistance with chronic use. We believe that nasal mupirocin is best reserved for patients with repetitive infections and nasal *S. aureus* carriage.

c. Vancomycin-resistant   Gram-positive   infections. Concern about an increasing prevalence of vancomycin-resistant enterococci (VRE) in hospitalized patients has resulted in recommendations that vancomycin use be restricted in dialysis patients. Because of the relatively high incidence of staphylococcal organisms resistant to antistaphylococcal penicillins and cephalosporins, it is currently our policy to utilize vancomycin as initial therapy of life-threatening suspected *S. aureus* infections (e.g., catheter-related bacteremia). If sensitivity results warrant, vancomycin can be discontinued in several days and prolonged treatment with an alternative antibiotic can then be employed. Certain cephalosporins (e.g., cefazolin) have a very prolonged half-life in end-stage renal disease (ESRD) patients and can be dosed conveniently postdialysis.

2. Peritoneal dialysis patients. See Chapter 24.

a. Antimicrobial prophylaxis. In the absence of other indications for prophylaxis, we do not routinely administer antibiotics prior to invasive procedures unless a vascular access is present. Long-term, continuous prophylaxis is discussed in Chapter 24.

B.   Unrelated to the access site

1.   Urinary tract infection. In dialysis patients the incidence of urinary tract infection is high, especially in patients with polycystic kidney disease. In patients with a neurogenic bladder (e.g., diabetic patients), pyocystis (pus in the defunctionalized bladder) may be an unsuspected source of infection. See Chapter 39 for a full discussion of these topics.

2.   Pneumonia. Pneumonia is an important cause of mortality in this population; the possibility of Gram-negative infection should be considered in patients dialyzed in a hospital setting. Dialysis patients may have unusual pulmonary infiltrates due to pulmonary calcification (now uncommon), which can resemble those due to pneumonia. Pleural effusions commonly are exudative in character due to uremia-associated inflammation, even in the absence of infection.

3.   Intra-abdominal infections. Diverticulosis and diverticulitis occur commonly in dialysis patients and especially in those with polycystic kidney disease. Strangulated hernia is also frequently encountered. In peritoneal dialysis patients, the differentiation between dialysis-associated peritonitis and peritonitis due to a disease process involving the abdominal viscera can be difficult (see Chapters 24 and 38). Acalculous cholecystitis has been reported. Intestinal infarction can occur as a complication of hypotension occurring during a dialysis session or between dialyses; bowel infarction should always be suspected in a dialysis patient with unexplained, refractory septic shock.

4.   Tuberculosis. The incidence of tuberculosis has been estimated to be as much as tenfold higher among hemodialysis patients than among the general population. Tuberculosis in hemodialysis patients is frequently extrapulmonary; disseminated disease may occur in the absence of chest x-ray abnormalities. Difficulty in making the diagnosis is increased because delayed skin hypersensitivity to tuberculin reagent is often absent or diminished due to cutaneous anergy. A number of subtle, atypical presentations of tuberculosis can be encountered; for instance, patients may present with ascites and intermittent fever only, or with hepatomegaly, weight loss, and anorexia. The diagnosis of tuberculosis in extrapulmonary cases is usually made by demonstrating typical caseating granulomas on pleural or hepatic biopsy or by recovery of tubercle bacilli from culture of biopsy material. When the index of suspicion for tuberculosis is high, presumptive therapy with antitubercular agents is sometimes warranted. Mortality in dialysis patients with tuberculosis has been reported to be as high as 40%.

5.   Listeriosis. Listeriosis, an unusual infection in the nonimmunocompromised host, has been reported to occur in hemodialysis patients suffering from iron overload.

6.   *Salmonella* septicemia. In dialysis patients severe *Salmonella* septicemia has been noted to occur; in nonuremic patients *Salmonella* enteritis rarely progresses to sepsis.

7. ***Yersinia* septicemia.** This infection has been reported in dialysis patients receiving deferoxamine chelation therapy.

8. **Mucormycosis.** This sometimes fatal infection is seen with unusual frequency in patients being treated with deferoxamine (see Chapter 43).

9. ***Helicobacter pylori*.** Although patients with ESRD frequently have upper gastrointestinal (GI) complications, the prevalence of this infection appears to be the same in ESRD patients as in patients with normal renal function. Therapy is similar to that for nonuremic patients (see Chapter 38).

IV. **Viral infections**

A. **Hepatitis A.** The incidence of hepatitis A in dialysis patients is no greater than in the general population, given that transmission is usually by the fecal–oral route. The disease pursues the usual clinical course in dialysis patients. Chronic hepatitis after hepatitis A infection is believed to occur rarely, if at all.

B. **Hepatitis B**

1. **Epidemiology**

   a. **Hemodialysis patients.** The incidence of infection with hepatitis B virus (HBV) is now quite low (Finelli et al., 2005). The low incidence is due to screening of the blood supply for evidence of this infection and to low transfusion requirements due to the availability of erythropoietin. However, recent outbreaks of hepatitis B in several hemodialysis units have occurred. Although hepatitis B vaccine should be administered to all susceptible hemodialysis patients, <60% of patients in the United States are vaccinated (Tokars et al., 2002). Of note, only 50%–60% of vaccinated hemodialysis patients develop a protective antibody response.

   b. **Peritoneal dialysis patients.** This group is at very low risk of acquiring hepatitis B infection. Nevertheless, hepatitis B can be transmitted through exposure to peritoneal effluent.

2. **Clinical presentation.** Hepatitis B infection is largely asymptomatic in dialysis patients. Commonly, malaise is the only complaint. The occurrence of visible jaundice is rare. The only manifestation of infection may be an unexplained, mild (two- to threefold) elevation in the serum aspartate (AST) or alanine aminotransferase (ALT) level, or even a move from a lower to a higher level within the normal range. The serum bilirubin and alkaline phosphatase concentrations may remain normal or be elevated only slightly.

3. **Chronic hepatitis B infection.** Hepatitis B infection in dialysis patients often runs a protracted course and in 50% of cases progresses to a chronic, Hb_sAg-positive state. Development of clinically important persistent (or active) hepatitis is not nearly as common. Patients with high serum ferritin levels appear to be at increased risk for developing

persistent hepatitis. Interferon, lamivudine, or adefovir can be utilized for the treatment of chronic hepatitis B. The dosing for lamivudine and adefovir are 100 mg PO daily and 10 mg PO daily, respectively.

4. Routine screening. Hemodialysis patients should be screened periodically (usually every 3–6 months) for the presence of hepatitis B infection by determination of serum alanine and aspartate aminotransferase and HbsAg values.

5. Prevention

a. Restricting the possibility of exposure to the virus. Epidemiologic principles can be utilized to decrease the risk of hepatitis B infection, both among patients and among dialysis staff. Table 33-1 lists the required precautions. Some centers recommend that patients with hepatitis B antigenemia be treated with either home hemodialysis or home peritoneal dialysis in order to decrease the chance of transmission to other patients and staff.

b. Vaccination. See Section V below.

c. Hepatitis B immune globulin. This should be given after any exposure to the body fluids of a person known to be infected with the hepatitis B virus.

C. Hepatitis C. The prevalence of antibodies to hepatitis C virus (anti-HCV) in dialysis patients is higher than in healthy populations. Recent data indicate that 8%–10% of dialysis patients in the United States have anti-HCV. Worldwide, there is considerable variability in the prevalence of anti-HCV, ranging from 1%–63%. However, there is also great variability in HCV testing practices in dialysis centers (Meyers et al., 2003). The high incidence and prevalence of HCV infection among dialysis patients can be attributed to several risk factors including number of blood transfusions, duration of dialysis, mode of dialysis (lower risk in peritoneal dialysis patients), and a history of previous organ transplantation or intravenous drug abuse. Infection rates among dialysis patients in the United States have not changed appreciably since tests for anti-HCV were first developed in the early 1990s. At the present time, there is no evidence that sharing of dialysis machines, type of dialysis membrane used, and dialyzer reprocessing are risk factors. Therefore, the Centers for Disease Control and Prevention (CDC) does not recommend dedicated machines, isolation of patients, or prohibition of reuse in hemodialysis patients with anti-HCV. However, observations suggest both a higher incidence of new cases of hepatitis C in units with a higher prevalence of HCV infection and a decreased incidence of HCV in units that implement infection control measures; therefore, in dialysis units with a high prevalence of infection, isolation of HCV-positive patients, use of dedicated machines, and restriction on dialyzer reuse for patients infected with HCV may be warranted.

The prevalence of anti-HCV among dialysis staff is similar to that of the general population (0%–6%). Immune globulin and/or α-interferon for postexposure prophylaxis of hepatitis C in health care workers is not recommended.

Table 33-1. Infection control practices in the hemodialysis unit

1. General precautions for staff and patients
   a. Surveillance for hepatitis B surface antigen (HB$_s$Ag) and antibody (HB$_s$Ab) every 3–6 months
   b. Isolation of HB$_s$Ag-positive patients (not necessary for human immunodeficiency virus [HIV]- and hepatitis C virus [HCV]-infected patients)
   c. Cleansing of dialysis machines and blood/body fluid contaminated areas with 1% sodium hypochlorite (bleach) solution
   d. Dialyzer reuse prohibited for HIV- and HBV-positive patients (acceptable for patients with anti-HCV)
   e. Universal precautions (see below)
   f. Protocol for exposure to blood/body fluids (see below)
2. Universal precautions
   a. Staff must wear fluid-impermeable garments
   b. Gloves are to be used whenever there is potential for exposure to blood or body fluids
   c. Gloves must be changed and hands washed between patients
   d. Protective eyewear and face shields are worn when there is potential for splashing of blood (e.g., initiation and discontinuation of dialysis, changing the blood circuit)
   e. No recapping of contaminated needles; prompt disposal in appropriate container
   f. No eating or drinking in dialysis unit
3. Exposure to blood
   a. Testing for HB$_s$Ag and HB$_s$Ab at time of incident and 6 weeks later
   b. Testing for HIV (employee consent required) at time of incident and 6 weeks and 6 months later
   c. If HB$_s$Ag status of source patient is positive or unknown, administer hepatitis B immune globulin
   d. Test source patient for HIV (inform patient; consent may not be required)

The natural history of hepatitis C in dialysis patients is difficult to ascertain since there have been no large studies in which liver biopsy has been performed in this population. The association between liver enzymes (e.g., ALT) and histologic severity is poor. Multivariate analyses have shown an increased risk for death in hepatitis C–infected patients, with excess mortality predominantly due to cirrhosis and liver cancer.

Treatment options are suboptimal. α-Interferon results in decreased transaminase levels and improved liver histology in most patients, with a sustained response in about 40% of patients, a response rate at least comparable to that seen in patients without renal disease. However, the incidence of side effects is substantial. Common side effects are myalgias, headache, fatigue, and depression, but more serious adverse effects, including bone marrow suppression, pancreatitis, cardiac failure, and lymphoma, have been reported. Therefore, the benefit-to-risk ratio in the dialysis population is unclear. It is of note that a large prospective trial of interferon α-2b in ESRD patients was terminated early due to the high rate of adverse effects (Degos et al., 2001). There is little information on the use of peginterferon or interferon–ribavirin combination therapy. In one trial of six patients, this combination was used; reduced doses of 50 or 135 mcg per week of pegylated interferon α-2b or α-2a, respectively, plus reduced doses of ribavirin were used with encouraging results (Bruchfeld et al., 2006). Ribavirin is normally renally excreted and causes dose-related hemolysis; therefore, it must be used with extreme caution and at a reduced dose in dialysis patients. Treatment for hepatitis C should at present be considered only for patients with significant liver disease with a reasonable likelihood of prolonged survival, especially in patients in whom transplantation is planned.

D. Cytomegalovirus and mononucleosis. These viral infections can mimic hepatitis due to B or C virus but occur uncommonly in dialysis patients.

E. Influenza. Dialysis patients are at increased risk for developing complications during influenza infection and should be vaccinated (see below). Use of antiviral agents for influenza prevention and treatment is discussed below (VI A 11)

F. Human immunodeficiency virus (HIV)

1. Incidence and prevalence. The rate of HIV infection in hemodialysis patients is elevated but only slightly above that in the general population. The incidence of HIV infection in the U.S. ESRD program is stable. Both incidence and prevalence are much higher in large urban areas serving minorities.

2. Clinical manifestations. Dialysis patients who are HIV positive may be asymptomatic or may present with the full-blown acquired immunodeficiency syndrome (AIDS). HIV-related renal disease may be an important cause of renal failure in some patients. Since the availability of highly active antiretroviral therapy (HAART) in 1996, the prognosis of HIV-infected patients has markedly improved and many patients who are HIV positive without other clinical manifestations can live for many years on dialysis.

3. Routine screening. There exists much controversy as to whether hemodialysis patients without clinical evidence of AIDS should be routinely screened for HIV positivity. The recommendation from the CDC is that routine screening not be performed. However, some dialysis units (especially those serving high-risk populations) are screening for HIV. Issues of confidentiality must be balanced against the risk to other patients and dialysis staff.

4. Dialysis in patients who are HIV positive. The CDC recommendation is that the choice between hemodialysis and peritoneal dialysis should not be affected by the finding of HIV positivity. However, home dialysis will lessen any possible risk to other patients and to dialysis staff. The peritoneal effluent of HIV-positive patients should be considered infectious and handled appropriately. If hemodialysis is elected, the CDC guidelines maintain that only the usual body fluid precautions attendant to routine dialysis need be followed. The CDC does not recommend that a special dialysis machine be set aside for HIV-positive patients, and dialyzer reuse in HIV-positive patients is not forbidden.

A number of dialysis units see the CDC recommendations as too liberal and are treating HIV-positive patients in the same manner as patients who are Hb_sAg positive (see Table 33-1). At the time of this writing, no HIV infection has been known to occur in a dialysis staff member in relationship to dialysis of an HIV-positive patient. However, health care workers have developed HIV infection after skin or mucous membrane contact with HIV-infected blood, underscoring the importance of universal precautions while performing dialysis.

V. Vaccination. In dialysis patients the antibody response to a number of commonly used vaccines is suboptimal. Nevertheless, vaccination against pneumococcus, influenza, and hepatitis is believed to be indicated for almost all dialysis patients. Table 33-2 lists the recommended frequency of administration of commonly used vaccines. For all vaccines other than hepatitis B, the dosage is identical to that used in the general population.

A. Vaccination against hepatitis B. All dialysis patients except those who are Hb_sAg or Hb_sAb (antibody) positive should receive the hepatitis B vaccine. To increase the chances of successful vaccination, the dosage of hepatitis B vaccine in dialysis patients should be twice the normal amount. A series of four IM injections of 40 mcg Hb_sAg should be given into the deltoid muscles at intervals of 0, 1, 2, and 6 months to complete the primary immunization series. Injection into the gluteal muscle is not recommended because gluteal injection

Table 33-2. Immunizations recommended for dialysis patients

Vaccine	Frequency of Administration
Influenza A and B	Annually
Tetanus, diphtheria	Booster every 10 years
Pneumococcus	Revaccination dependent on antibody response
Hepatitis B	For initial vaccination schedule give a total of four double doses with each injection split between the left and right deltoid muscles
	Requirement for revaccination not yet known

has been associated with failure to develop antibody or with loss of antibody 6 months to 1 year following immunization (in nonuremic as well as in uremic patients).

Overall, the percentage of successful vaccination against hepatitis B in dialysis patients is less than in the general population, and rates as low as 50%–60% have been reported. Some patients may not have responded because of gluteal vaccine administration or because of failure to complete the vaccination regimen. The usefulness of adjuvant vaccines and vaccines given intradermally continues to be studied.

VI. Antimicrobial usage in dialysis patients. Table 33-3 lists dosing guidelines for most commonly used antimicrobial, antifungal, and antiviral agents.

A. Comments pertaining to selected drug groups

1. Penicillins. Most penicillins are normally excreted by the kidney to a substantial extent (40%–80%) and are removed to a moderate degree by both hemodialysis and peritoneal dialysis. Therefore, both dosage reduction and posthemodialysis supplementation are generally recommended. From a practical standpoint, postdialysis supplementation is probably unnecessary; however, dosing should be timed so that a dose is given immediately after dialysis. Two exceptions to this general rule are nafcillin and oxacillin; because these drugs are substantially excreted by both the liver and kidney, dosage reduction is not necessary unless liver function is also impaired. Because of the high therapeutic index of penicillins, monitoring of serum levels is generally not necessary.

Clavulanate is a β-lactamase inhibitor that slows bacterial breakdown of penicillins. Clavulanate is popularly combined with amoxicillin or ticarcillin. The half-life of clavulanate increases from 0.75 to about 5.0 hours with renal failure, but clavulanate is dialyzable. The dosing recommendations for the parent antimicrobial in Table 33-3 will usually apply as well to the antimicrobial–clavulanate combination.

2. Cephalosporins. Most cephalosporins are excreted by the kidney to a large extent (e.g., 30%–96%) and dosage reduction is almost always necessary for dialysis patients. Most are removed to some extent by dialysis. Some of the long-acting cephalosporins (e.g., cefazolin, ceftazidime, ceftizoxime) can be administered thrice weekly (e.g., after each hemodialysis session in patients being dialyzed three times a week).

3. Carbapenem/monobactams. Cilastatin is an inhibitor of the renal dipeptidase enzyme that normally breaks down imipenem. Cilastatin half-life is prolonged from 1 hour to about 15 hours in renal failure, but cilastatin is dialyzable. Imipenem is available only with cilastatin and only in a 1:1 dosage ratio between the two compounds. The recommendations in Table 33-3 pertaining to imipenem apply to the imipenem–cilastatin combination.

Ertapenem is the newest addition to the carbapenem family. Ertapenem has a broad spectrum of activity, covering the Gram-positives, Gram-negatives, and anaerobes. Unlike

Table 33-3.   Systemic antibiotic, antiviral, and antifungal drug dosages for an adult dialysis patient

Drug	Usual Nonuremic Dose^a	Half-life Non-Uremic Patient (hours)	Half-life Dialysis Patient (hours)	Dialysis Patient Dosage (% of Non-Uremic Dose)	Usual Dialysis Patient Dosage	Post-HD Supplement	Dosage for CAPD
Antibiotics							
Penicillins							
Amoxicillin PO	500 mg q8h	1.5	10–15	50–75	500 mg q12h	DAD	Same^b
Ampicillin IV	0.5–2.0 g q4–6h	1.0	10–15	50	0.5–1 g q12h	DAD	Same
Ampicillin/sulbactam IV	1.5 g q6h	1.1	See ampicillin		1.5 g q12h	DAD	Same
Bacampicillin PO	400–800 mg q8–12h		4–20	50	400–800 mg q12–24h	No	
Cloxacillin IV/IM	250–500 mg q4–6h	0.5–1	1–3	100	250–500 mg q4–6h	No	Same
Cloxacillin PO	250–500 mg q6h	0.5–1	1–3	100	250–500 mg q6h	No	Same
Dicloxacillin PO	0.25 g q6h	0.7	1.3	100	0.25 g q6h	No	Same
Flucloxacillin IV/IM	250 mg–1 g q6h	0.75–1.5		100	250 mg–1 g q6h	No	Same
Flucloxacillin PO	250 mg q6h	0.75–1.5		100	250 mg q6h	No	Same
Nafcillin IV	0.5–1.0 g q4–6h	0.5	1.2	100	0.5–1.0 g q4–6h	No	Same
Oxacillin IV	0.5–1.0 g q4–6h	0.4	1.0	100	0.5–1.0 g q4–6h	No	Same

Penicillin G IV/IM	0.3–5.0 mU q4–6h	0.5	10	25–50	1.5 mU q12h	DAD	Same
Penicillin V PO	250 mg q6h	1.0	4.0	50	250 mg q12h	250 mg	Same
Piperacillin IV	3–4 g q4–6h	1.2	4.2	50	2–3 g q8h	DAD	Same
Piperacillin/tazobactam IV	3.375 g q4–6h	1.5	See piperacillin / 15	25	2.25 g q8h	0.75 g	Same
Ticarcillin IV	3 g q4–6h				2 g q12h	2 g	Same[c]
Ticarcillin/clavulanate IV	3.1 g q6h	See ticarcillin			3.1 g q12h	3.1 g	Same
Cephalosporins							
Cefaclor PO	0.25–0.5 g PO q8h	0.75	2.8	33	250 mg q12h	250 mg	Same
Cefadroxil PO	0.5–1 g q12h	1.4	22	25–50	0.5–1 g q24–48h	0.5–1 g	Same
Cefamandole IV/IM	0.5–2 g q4–6h	1.0	11	25	0.5 g q8–12h	500 mg	Same
Cefazolin IV/IM	0.5–1.5 g q8h	1.8	35	10–25	1 g q48h	500 mg[c]	500 mg q24h
Cefdinir PO	600 mg q.d. or 300 mg q12h	1.7	?	?	300 mg q24h	DAD	?
Cefditoren PO	400 mg q12h or 100–200 mg t.i.d.	1.3–2.0	?	?	no data		
Cefepime IV	1–2 g q8–12h	2.0	13.5	25	0.25–1 g q24h	DAD	Same
Cefixime PO	200 mg q12h	3.6	13	50	200 mg q24h	200 mg	Same
Cefonicid IV	1.0–2.0 g q24h	4.4	17–56	10	250 mg q72h	No	Same
Cefoperazone IV	2 g q12h	2.1	2.9	100	2 g q12h	1 g	Same
Ceforanide IV/IM	0.5–1 g q12h	3.5–2.5	25	?	0.5–1 g q24–48h	0.5–1 g	?
Cefotaxime IV	1–2 g q6h	1.0	2.6	50	1 g q24h	1 g	Same

continued

Table 33-3. *Continued.*

Drug	Usual Nonuremic Dose[a]	Half-life Non-Uremic Patient (hours)	Half-life Dialysis Patient (hours)	Dialysis Patient Dosage (% of Non-Uremic Dose)	Usual Dialysis Patient Dosage	Post-HD Supplement	Dosage for CAPD
Cefotetan IV/IM	1–2 g q12h	3.0	14–35	25	1–2 g q48h	500 mg[d]	1 g q24h
Cefoxitin IV/IM	1–2 g q4–6h	0.7	18	15	0.5–1.0 g q24h	750 mg	Same
Cefpirome IV	1–2 g q12h	2.0	9.4	25	1 g LD, then 250–500 mg q12	250–500 mg	1 g LD, then 250–500 mg q12
Cefpodoxime PO	100–400 mg q12h	2–3	9.8	25	100–400 mg t.i.w.	DAD	100–400 mg q24h
Cefprozil PO	500 mg q24h, or 250–500 mg q12h, or 250 mg t.i.d.	1–2	6.0	25	250 mg (on dialysis days)	DAD	?
Ceftazidime IV/IM	0.5–2.0 g q8–12h	1.6	18–34	15	500–750 mg q48h	500 mg[d]	500 mg q24h
Ceftibuten PO	400 mg q24h	1.5–2.5	18–29	25–50	400 mg q24h	DAD	?
Ceftizoxime IV/IM	1–2 g q8–12h	1.4	30	10–25	1 g (on dialysis days)	DAD	1 g q24h
Ceftriaxone IV	1–2 g q12–24h	8.0	15	50–100	1 g q24h	DAD	750 mg q12h
Cefuroxime IV	0.75–1.5 g q8h	1.7	17	33	0.75 g q24h	DAD	0.75–1.5 g q24h

Cefuroxime PO	250–500 mg q12h	1.7	17	33	250–500 mg q24h	DAD	250–500 q12h
Cephalexin PO	0.25–1.0 g q6h	0.9	30	25	500 mg q12h	DAD	Same
Cephalothin IV	0.5–2.0 g q4–6h	0.7	12	50	1 g q12h	DAD	Same
Cephradine PO	0.5 g q6h	1.3	12	25	250 mg q12h	DAD	Same
Moxalactam IV	1–2 g q8h	2.3	21	25	1 g q24h	1 g	1 g q36–48h

Carbapenems/monobactams

Aztreonam IV	0.5–2.0 g q6–8h	1.7	6	25–50	125–500 mg q6–8h	DAD	Same
Ertapenem IV/IM	1 g q24h	4.0	14	50	500 mg q24h	DAD	?
Imipenem IV/IM	0.5–1.0 g q6–8h	1.0	3.7	50	250–500 mg q12h	DAD	Same
Meropenem IV	0.5–2 g q8h	1.0	20	25	500 mg q24h	DAD	?

Fluoroquinolones

Ciprofloxacin IV	400 mg q8–12h	4.0	5.8	50	200–400 mg q24h	?	?
Ciprofloxacin PO	250–750 mg q12h	4.0	5.8	50	250–500 mg q24h	No	Same
Levofloxacin IV/PO	500 mg q24h	7.0	35	25	250 mg q48h	No	Same
Lomefloxacin PO	400 mg q24h	8	45	50	400 mg × 1d 200 mg q24h	No	Same
Moxifloxacin IV/PO	400 mg q24h	9–16	9–16	100	400 mg q24h	No	Same

continued

Table 33-3. *Continued.*

Drug	Usual Nonuremic Dose[a]	Half-life (hours) Non-Uremic Patient	Half-life (hours) Dialysis Patient	Dialysis Patient Dosage (% of Non-Uremic Dose)	Usual Dialysis Patient Dosage	Post-HD Supplement	Dosage for CAPD
Nalidixic acid PO	1 g q6h	Avoid in renal failure					
Norfloxacin PO	400 mg q12h	3–4		?	400 mg q24h	DAD	?
Ofloxacin IV/PO	200–400 mg q12h	7.0	8.34	25	100–200 mg q24h	DAD	Same
Oxolinic acid PO	750 mg q12h	4.0	4.0	100	750 mg q12h	No	Same
Pefloxacin IV/PO	400 mg q12h	7–14	35	50	200 mg q12h	No	?
Pipemidic acid PO	400 mg q12h	2.1–4.6	5.7–16	?	Data are lacking	?	?
Sparfloxacin PO	400 mg LD, then 200 mg q24h	20	35	50	200 mg q48h	?	?
Trovafloxacin[e] IV/PO	100–300 mg q24h	9–12	9–12	100	100–300 mg q24h	No	Same
Aminoglycosides							
Amikacin IV	5–7.5 mg/kg q8–12h	3.1	86	10	See text	See text	See text
Gentamicin IV	1.5 mg/kg q8h	3.1	60	10	See text	See text	See text
Neomycin PO	6.6 mg/kg q6h	Avoid in renal failure					
Netilmicin IV	1.3–2.2 mg/kg q8h	2.7	40	10	See text	See text	See text
Streptomycin IM	500 mg q12h	2.5	70	15	No data	See text	See text
Tobramycin IV	1.5 mg/kg q8h	3.1	70	10	See text	See text	See text

Macrolides and ketolides

Macrolides and ketolides							
Azithromycin IV/PO	500 mg q24h × 1 day 250 mg q24h × 4 days	41	?	100	500 mg q24h × 1 day 250 mg q24h × 4 days	DAD	Same
Clarithromycin PO	250–500 mg q12h	3–7	?	50	250 mg q24h	DAD	Same
Dirithromycin PO	500 mg q24h	8.0	?	100	500 mg q24h	No	Same
Erythromycin IV	500 mg–1 g q6h	1.6	4.5	100(?)	See text	No	Same
Erythromycin PO	250–500 mg q6–12h	1.6	4.5	100(?)	See text	No	Same
Roxithromycin PO	150 mg q12h or 300 mg q24h	12	?	?	150 mg q24 or 300 mg q48h	No	Same
Telithromycin PO	800 mg PO q24h	10–13	14.64	?	Dose adjustment not yet established		
Glycopeptides							
Teicoplanin IV/IM	12 mg/kg LD, then 3–6 mg/kg q24h	90–157	149–163	50	6 mg/kg q3 days	No	Same
Vancomycin IV	1 g q12h	5.6	200	<10	1 g q 7–10 days	See text	See text
Tetracyclines							
Chlortetracycline PO	250–500 mg q6h	5.5	Avoid in renal failure	?	reduce dose	?	?
Demeclocycline PO	150 mg q6h or 300 mg q12h	Avoid in renal failure					
Doxycycline IV/PO	100 mg q24h	18	21	100	100 mg q24h	No	Same

continued

Table 33-3. *Continued.*

Drug	Usual Nonuremic Dose[a]	Half-life Non-Uremic Patient (hours)	Dialysis Patient	Dialysis Patient Dosage (% of Non-Uremic Dose)	Usual Dialysis Patient Dosage	Post-HD Supplement	Dosage for CAPD
Minocycline IV/PO	200 mg LD, 100 mg q12h	11–22	?	100	100 mg PO q12h	No	Same
Methacycline PO	300 mg q12h or 150 mg q6h	Avoid in renal failure					
Oxytetracycline PO	250–500 mg q6h	8.5–9.6	?	?	250–500 mg q24h	DAD	?
Tetracycline PO	250–500 mg q6h	8–10	100	?	250–500 mg q24h	No	?
Nitroimidazoles							
Metronidazole IV/PO	500 mg q6–8h	8.5	8.5	100[f]	500 mg q6–8h	DAD	250 mg q6–8h
Ornidazole IV/PO	500 mg q12h	11–14	11–14	100	500 mg q12h	DAD	?
Tinidazole IV	800 mg q24h or 400 mg q12h	11.1–14.7	11.1–14.7	100	800 mg q24h or 400 mg q12h	200–400 mg	?
Tinidazole PO	1 g q24h or 500 mg q12h	11.1–14.7	11.1–14.7	100	1 g q24h or 500 mg q12h	250–500 mg	?
Diaminopyrimidines							
Pyrimethamine PO	25–50 mg q24h	80–96		100	25–50 mg q24h	No	?
Trimethoprim (T)/sulfamethoxazole(S) IV/PO	See text	11 (T) 35 (S)	26 (T) 50 (S)	50	See text	See text	See text

Antituberculars

Drug							
Ethambutol PO	15 mg/kg q24h	3.1	9.0	60	15 mg/kg q48h	DAD	Same
Isoniazid IV/PO	300 mg q24h	1.4	2.3 (fast acetylators) 10.7 (slow acetylators)	66–100[g]	300 mg q24h	DAD	Same
Pyrazinamide PO	15–30 mg/kg/day	5.2	Avoid in renal failure				
Rifabutin PO	300 mg q24h	45	ND	100	300 mg q24h	?	?
Rifampin IV/PO	600 mg q24h	3.5	4.0	100	600 mg q24h	No	Same
Rifapentine PO	600 mg 2×/wk	13.2	?	?	?	?	?

Miscellaneous antibiotics

Drug							
Chloramphenicol IV	1 g q6h	4.0	4.0	100	1 g q6h	No	Same
Clindamycin PO	150–450 mg qid	4.0	4.0	100	150–450 mg q.i.d.	No	Same
Clindamycin IV	600–900 mg q8h	2.7	4.0	100	600–900 mg q8h	No	Same
Dapsone PO	50–100 mg q24h	10–50	?	100	50–100 mg q24h	?	?
Daptomycin IV	4 mg/kg q24h	7–11	30	50	4 mg/kg q48h	DAD	Same
Fusidic acid IV	>50 kg: 500 mg q8h <50 kg: 6–7 mg/kg q8h	5–6	?	100	>50 kg: 500 mg q8h <50 kg: 6–7 mg/kg q8h	No	?

continued

Table 33-3. *Continued.*

Drug	Usual Nonuremic Dose[a]	Half-life Non-Uremic Patient (hours)	Half-life Dialysis Patient (hours)	Dialysis Patient Dosage (% of Non-Uremic Dose)	Usual Dialysis Patient Dosage	Post-HD Supplement	Dosage for CAPD
Fusidic acid PO	500 mg–1 g q8h	5–6	?	100	500 mg–1 g q8h	No	?
Linezolid IV/PO	600 mg q12h	5.0	?	100	600 mg q12h	DAD	?
Methenamine PO	1 g q6h (mandelate) 1 g q12h (hippurate)	Avoid in renal failure					
Nitrofurantoin PO	0.5–1.0 g q6h	Avoid in renal failure					
Quinupristin/ Dalfopristin IV	7.5 mg/kg q8–12h	1.3–1.5	?	100	7.5 mg/kg q8–12h	No	Same
Spectinomycin IM	2 g once	1.7	24	100	2 g once	No	Same
Antivirals							
Acyclovir IV	5–10 mg/kg q8h	3.0	19.5	15–20	2.5–5 mg/kg q24h	2.5 mg/kg	Same
Acyclovir PO	0.2–0.8 g 5×/day	3.0	19.5	15–20	0.2–0.8 g q24h	0.4 g	Same
Adefovir PO	10 mg q24h	7.5	?	?	10 mg q7d	DAD	?
Amantadine PO	100 mg q12h	24	500	<10	100 mg q wk[h]	No	Same

				Contraindicated with creatinine clearance ≤55 mL/minute			
Cidofovir IV	5 mg/kg weekly to every other week						
Famciclovir PO	125–500 mg q8–12h	2.3	13	25	125–250 mg q48h	?	?
Foscarnet IV	60 mg/kg q8h × 3 wk, then 90–120 mg/kg q24h	3.0	?	See text	See text	?	?
Ganciclovir IV	5 mg/kg/day	2.7	29	25	1.25 mg/kg	DAD	?
Ganciclovir PO	1 g t.i.d.	2.7	29	25	500 mg t.i.w.	DAD	?
Oseltamivir PO	75 mg b.i.d.		No data				
Ribavirin PO	200 mg q8h	30–60	?	50	200 mg q12h	No	Same
Rimantadine PO	100 mg q12h	24–33	44	50	100 mg q24h	No	Same
Valacyclovir PO	0.5–1 q q 8–12h	3.0	14	16	500 mg q24h	DAD	Same
Valganciclovir PO	900 mg q12–24h			Avoid in patients receiving hemodialysis			
Antiretrovirals							
Abacavir PO	300 mg q12h	1.5	?	100	300 mg q12h	?	?
Atazanavir PO	300–400 mg q24h	7.0	?	?	300–400 mg q24h	?	?
Delavirdine PO	400 mg q8h	4.0	?	100	400 mg q8h	?	?
Didanosine EC PO	250–400 mg q24h	1.3–1.5	3.1–3.6	25–50	125 mg q24h	No	Same

continued

Table 33-3. *Continued.*

Drug	Usual Nonuremic Dose[a]	Half-life Non-Uremic Patient	Half-life Dialysis Patient (hours)	Dialysis Patient Dosage (% of Non-Uremic Dose)	Usual Dialysis Patient Dosage	Post-HD Supplement	Dosage for CAPD
Efavirenz PO	600 mg q.h.s.	40–55	?	100	600 mg q.h.s.	?	?
Enfuvirtide SC	90 mg q12h			100	90 mg q12h	?	?
Emtricitabine PO	200 mg q24h	10	?	?	200 mg q96h	DAD	?
Fosamprenavir PO	1,400 mg q24h	7.7	?	?	1,400 mg q24h		?
Indinavir PO	800 mg q8h	1.8	?	100	800 mg q8h	?	?
Lamivudine PO	150 mg q12h or 300 mg q24h	6	19	10	150 mg LD, then 25 mg q24h	No	Same
Lopinavir/ritonavir PO (1 tablet = 200 mg lopinavir and 50 mg ritonavir)	2 tablets q12h	4.4–6.1		100	2 tablets q12h	No	?
Nelfinavir PO	1250 mg q12h	4	?	100	1250 mg q12h	?	?
Nevirapine PO	200 mg q12h	25–30	?	100	200 mg q12h	?	?
Ritonavir PO	600 mg q12h	3.5	?	100	600 mg q12h	?	?

Drug	Dose				Adjusted dose		
Saquinavir	1000 mg b.i.d. with 100 mg ritonavir b.i.d.	7–13	?	100	1000 mg b.i.d. with 100 mg ritonavir b.i.d.	?	?
Stavudine PO	20–40 mg q12h, depending on wt	1.2	8	12	>60 kg: 20 mg q24h; <60 kg: 15 mg q24h	?	?
Tenofovir PO	300 mg PO q24h	4–8	?	?	300 mg weekly	DAD	?
Zalcitabine PO	0.75 mg q8h	2	8.5	50	Insufficient data	No	Same
Zidovudine PO	300 mg b.i.d.	1.0	1.4	See text	100 mg q8h	No	Same
Antifungals							
Amphotericin B deoxycholate IV	0.5–1.5 mg/kg q24h	24	24	100	0.5–1.5 mg/kg q24h	No	Same
Amphotericin B lipid complex (Abelcet®)IV	2.5–5 mg/kg q24h	24	?	100	2.5–5 mg/kg q24h	No	Same
Amphotericin B liposome (AmBisome®)IV	3–5 mg/kg q24h	174	?	100	3–5 mg/kg q24h	No	Same
Caspofungin IV	70 mg LD, 50 mg q24h	9–11	?	100	70 mg LD, 50 mg q24h	No	?
Fluconazole IV/PO	100–800 mg q24h	30	?	100	50–400 mg q24h	DAD	Same
Flucytosine PO	1.5 g q6h	4.2	100	10–25	0.5–1.0 g q48h	DAD	0.5–1.0 gm q24h

continued

Table 33-3. *Continued.*

Drug	Usual Nonuremic Dose[a]	Half-life Non-Uremic Patient (hours)	Half-life Dialysis Patient	Dialysis Patient Dosage (% of Non-Uremic Dose)	Usual Dialysis Patient Dosage	Post-HD Supplement	Dosage for CAPD
Griseofulvin PO	0.5–1 g q24h (microsize) 330–750 mg q24h (ultramicrosize)	9–22	?	100	0.5–1 g q24h (microsize) 330–750 mg q24h (ultra-microsize)	?	
Itraconazole IV	200 mg q12h, × 4 doses, then 200 mg q24h	21	25	100	Do not use with a CrCl <30 mL/ minute		
Itraconazole PO	200 mg q12h	21	25	100	200 mg q12h	No	Same
Ketoconazole PO	200 mg q12–24h	8.0	8.0	100	200 mg q12–24h	No	Same
Micafungin IV	50 or 150 mg q24h	14–17	?	?	50 or 150 mg q24h	No	Same
Terbinafine PO	250 mg q24h, 125 mg q12h	Not recommended in patients with creatinine clearance ≤50 mL/minute					

			Not recommended in patients with creatinine clearance ≤50 mL/minute		
Voriconazole IV	6 mg/kg q12h LD, 4 mg/kg q12h	6		≥40 kg: 200 mg q12h <40 kg: 100 mg q12h	No	Same
Voriconazole PO	≥40 kg: 200 mg q12h <40 kg: 100 mg q12h	100		≥40 kg: 200 mg q12h <40 kg: 100 mg q12h	No	Same

DAD, no post-HD supplement required, but on hemodialysis days schedule the usual dialysis patient dose after the dialysis session; HD, hemodialysis; CAPD, continuous ambulatory peritoneal dialysis; IM, intramuscular; IV, intravenous; LD, loading dose; PD, peritoneal dialysis (primarily CAPD; PO, oral; SC, subcutaneous; q24h, daily; q.h.s., at bedtime; t.i.d., three time/day; b.i.d., two times/day; t.i.w., three times/week.

[a]Usual doses recommended for treatment of moderate to severe infections.

[b]Give usual dialysis patient dose.

[c]Some recommend increasing the dose during PD to 3 g q12h.

[d]Prolonged half-life allows dosing thrice weekly post-HD.

[e]Trovafloxacin use limited due to serious liver toxicity leading to liver transplantation and/or death.

[f]Some authors recommend a reduction in dosage.

[g]No dosage reduction needed in patients known to be fast acetylators.

[h]Long-term administration best avoided unless blood levels are followed.

Sources: Data from *Goodman and Gilman's the physiological basis of therapeutics*, 11th ed, Brunton LL, et al. (eds), McGraw-Hill, New York, NY, 2006; *Physicians' desk reference 2006*, Thomson Healthcare, Montvale, NJ, 2006; Gilbert DN, et al., *The Sanford guide to antimicrobial therapy 2006*, 36th ed. Antimicrobial Therapy Inc., Sperryville, VT, 2006; Lacy CF, *Lexi Comp's drug information handbook*, 14th ed, Lexi-Comp, Inc., Hudson, OH, 2006; Brater DC, *Manual of drug use in clinical medicine*, 7th ed, Improved Therapeutics, Indianapolis, IN, 1996; *Antibiotics and chemotherapy*, 8th ed, Finch RG (ed) Churchill Livingstone, London, 2003; Rodriguez RA, McNicoll IR, *Dosing of antiretroviral drugs in renal insufficiency and hemodialysis* (updated July 2006), AETC National Resource Center, http://www.aids-ed.org/aidsetc?page=et-03-00-02.

imipenem/cilastatin, ertapenem lacks coverage against *Pseudomonas* and *Acinetobacter*. Ertapenem has the advantage of once-daily dosing. The dose should be reduced by 50% in patients with renal dysfunction.

Aztreonam is a monobactam antibiotic. It has Gram-negative coverage only (including coverage of *Pseudomonas*). Due to the cost of aztreonam, this antibiotic is typically reserved for patients who have a history of rash to both penicillins and cephalosporins, or patients who have an immediate-type allergy (i.e., anaphylaxis) to the penicillins. For patients receiving dialysis, 25% of the normal dose should be given at the regular interval (q6–8h).

4. Fluoroquinolones. Moxifloxacin is the newest fluoroquinolone. This fluoroquinolone has better coverage against Gram-positive pathogens (particularly *Streptococcus pneumoniae*) versus the older fluoroquinolones. The majority of the fluoroquinolones can be administered both orally and intravenously. Moxifloxacin, oxolinic acid, and trovafloxacin are the only antibiotics in this class that do not require dosage adjustment. The use of trovafloxacin is extremely limited as serious liver toxicity leading to transplantation and/or death has been reported.

5. Aminoglycosides. Aminoglycosides should be administered carefully in dialysis patients. The percentage of renal excretion is normally >90%, and a substantial increase in dosing interval is necessary. Drug removal by dialysis is important, requiring a postdialysis supplement or addition of aminoglycoside to peritoneal dialysis solutions. The therapeutic index of these agents is low, with the major risk (in dialysis patients) being otovestibulotoxicity. Loss of clinically important residual renal function may also occur.

a. Gentamicin and tobramycin

(1) Hemodialysis patients. The usual loading dose (1.5–2.0 mg/kg) is given; subsequently, 1.0 mg/kg is infused after each hemodialysis session. Although removal of gentamicin and tobramycin is primarily renal, extrarenal excretion of up to 20–30 mg per day has been reported in dialysis patients. Furthermore, many dialysis patients have some residual renal function, accounting for some renal drug removal. The postdialysis dose will have to replace drug lost during hemodialysis and drug removed due to nonrenal and residual renal excretion; thus, the amount of postdialysis dose may vary considerably from the suggested 1.0 mg/kg amount and should be adjusted based upon the plasma drug levels achieved (see below).

(2) Peritoneal dialysis patients. The easiest strategy for treating nonperitoneal infections in continuous ambulatory peritoneal dialysis (CAPD) and continuous cycling peritoneal dialysis (CCPD) patients is to give the usual loading dose IV and then to add 6 mg/L to the peritoneal dialysis solution. Although the strategy is simple, its efficacy and safety have not been evaluated. An alternative strategy for patients receiving CAPD or CCPD would be to give the usual loading dose followed

by parenteral (IV or IM) or intraperitoneal administration of additional small doses based on serum drug
levels.

b. **Amikacin.** The strategy for amikacin is identical to
that for dosing gentamicin or tobramycin; however, the
loading dose should be 5.0–7.5 mg/kg. In hemodialysis patients, the posthemodialysis supplement should be in the
range of 4.0 to 5.0 mg/kg. In peritoneal dialysis patients,
the recommended amount of amikacin to add to the peritoneal dialysis solution was formerly 18–25 mg/L. Now
there has been a trend to use lower doses of amikacin
(e.g., for peritonitis; see Chapter 24).

c. **Netilmicin.** For netilmicin, the loading dose is 2
mg/kg, with a posthemodialysis supplement of 1–2 mg/kg.
For patients receiving peritoneal dialysis, the strategy is
similar to that described for gentamicin and tobramycin,
above.

d. **Streptomycin.** One-half of the normal (nonuremic)
dosage should be administered after hemodialysis. In
CAPD patients, 20 mg/L should be added to the dialysis
solution.

e. **Monitoring of serum aminoglycoside levels.**
Serum drug levels should be monitored in all dialysis patients receiving aminoglycosides, except perhaps
those being treated with intraperitoneal (IP) aminoglycosides for peritonitis. Monitoring of serum aminoglycoside
levels is especially important in cases of serious infection where maximal efficacy is of paramount importance
and during prolonged use where otovestibular toxicity is
common.

(1) **Peak aminoglycoside levels.** The volume of distribution for aminoglycosides in dialysis patients is
similar to that of nonuremic patients; therefore, peak
serum levels should be similar to those in nonuremic
patients given a similar dosage with a similar trough
(predose) serum concentration. Ideally, peak levels
should be drawn 60 minutes after a dose.

(2) **Trough aminoglycoside levels.** In nonuremic
patients, the dosing interval of the aminoglycosides
is adjusted based on the trough (predose) level, as
trough levels >2 mcg/mL (gentamicin, tobramycin,
netilmicin) or 10 mcg/mL (amikacin) are associated
with toxicity. In dialysis patients, the altered pharmacokinetics of aminoglycosides may lead to difficulties in
dosing. For example, when gentamicin is given postdialysis, the magnitude of a subsequent predialysis
level will depend on the frequency of dialysis, as well
as on the amount administered and the gentamicin
half-life. With daily or even every-other-day dialysis, therapeutic peak levels of approximately 4.0–6.0
mcg/mL may be associated with predialysis levels of
>2.0 mcg/mL. Thus, predialysis levels >2.0 mcg/mL
may need to be accepted if therapeutic peak levels are
desired. Whether predialysis levels of >2.0 mcg/mL in
a dialysis setting predisposes to otovestibulotoxicity is

unknown. This may be an important consideration with prolonged (>7–10 days) therapy.

Prolonged aminoglycoside therapy in peritoneal dialysis patients using IP maintenance dosages will result in random serum aminoglycoside levels of >2 mcg/mL (for gentamicin, tobramycin, netilmicin) or >8 mcg/mL for amikacin. For example, the addition of 6 mg/L of gentamicin into the dialysate may result in a steady-state serum level of 3–6 mcg/mL, which may result in otovestibulotoxicity. Recommendations include administering IP aminoglycoside once daily only or decreasing the concentration of IP aminoglycoside when prolonged therapy is indicated (see Chapter 24).

(3) When the minimum inhibitory concentration (MIC) is known. When the organism is known and the aminoglycoside MIC has been determined, the strategy should be to achieve a peak serum drug level at least four times greater than the MIC value. Of course, one cannot exceed maximum safe peak drug levels; however, in some instances the MIC may be quite low, allowing a reduction in aminoglycoside dosage and serum drug levels without compromising treatment efficacy.

6.   Macrolides and ketolides. Erythromycin (12% renal excretion in nonuremic patients) requires no dosage adjustment in the presence of renal insufficiency. The use of erythromycin has been largely supplanted by newer macrolides (e.g., azithromycin and clarithromycin), which have a more favorable side effect profile and fewer drug–drug interactions. As with erythromycin, the newer agents also do not require dosage adjustment in renal insufficiency.

The ketolides are a new class of antibiotics, similar to the macrolides. To date, telithromycin is the first and only agent on the market in the United States. The difference between these two classes is that ketolides have greater affinity for the ribosomal binding site than macrolides. Compared to the macrolides, the ketolides have additional activity against multiresistant *Streptococcus pneumoniae, S. aureus* (methicillin- and erythromycin-susceptible isolates only), *Haemophilus influenzae, Moraxella catarrhalis, Chlamydia pneumoniae,* and *Mycoplasma pneumoniae.* The ketolides are currently used for the treatment of respiratory infections. Dose adjustment for renal dysfunction has yet to be established, but as only 13% of telithromycin is excreted by the kidney, substantial dose reduction would not be expected (Shi et al., 2005).

7.   Glycopeptides. Vancomycin is an extremely useful agent for the treatment of severe Gram-positive infections in dialysis patients. As vancomycin is excreted by the kidneys, dosing intervals can be substantially increased in patients with renal failure. In the past, doses could be administered every 7–10 days in patients with no renal excretory function since drug removal is negligible when conventional dialyzers are employed. However, now that high-flux membranes are commonly used, substantial extracorporeal removal of vancomycin during dialysis can be expected.

Measurement of serum drug levels is necessary to ensure adequate bactericidal levels and to avoid ototoxicity. Target peak and trough plasma concentrations are 30–40 mcg/mL and 5–10 mcg/mL, respectively. In hospitalized patients with life-threatening infection, we recommend administration of a 20 mg/kg initial dose with measurement of the peak serum level (30 minutes after the completion of the administration of the dose); additional serum values are then obtained daily during the first week of therapy in order to guide subsequent dosing. In less ill patients who are managed in the outpatient hemodialysis center, it is probably most convenient to administer vancomycin (e.g., 500 mg) after each hemodialysis session. A recent publication gives a sample algorithm (Pai et al., 2004). Vancomycin is removed to only a minimal extent by peritoneal dialysis and dosing is similar to that for hemodialysis patients.

8. Tetracyclines. Use of tetracyclines is generally avoided in patients with renal insufficiency because of the antianabolic effect of these drugs; the use of tetracyclines can lead to an increase in the plasma urea nitrogen level and to worsening acidosis. When a tetracycline is needed, doxycycline is often utilized. Although doxycycline also has antianabolic effects, the percentage of renal excretion for doxycycline (normally 40%) is lower than that for tetracycline (60%); no dosage adjustment for doxycycline is necessary in dialysis patients. Doxycycline is poorly removed by dialysis; hence, the timing of the doxycycline dose relative to a dialysis treatment is not important. Minocycline and chlortetracycline are minimally excreted by the kidney and can be given in the usual dosages.

9. Diaminopyrimidines. Trimethoprim may raise serum creatinine values in patients with renal impairment due to interference with tubular secretion of creatinine; this is not accompanied by a reduction in the true glomerular filtration rate (as measured by the clearance of inulin). Trimethoprim is normally 80%–90% excreted by the kidney. Renal excretion of sulfamethoxazole is normally 20%–30%. Trimethoprim and sulfamethoxazole are removed well by hemodialysis but poorly by peritoneal dialysis.

For treatment of urinary tract infections, one single-strength tablet containing 80 mg of trimethoprim and 400 mg of sulfamethoxazole should be given twice daily. When giving high-dose IV trimethoprim/sulfamethoxazole (e.g., for treatment of *Pneumocystis carinii* pneumonia) in dialysis patients, 50% of the usual dose (the latter being 20 mg/kg per day based on the trimethoprim component) is given; the incidence of leukopenia may be increased when treating dialysis patients, and careful monitoring is essential. For hemodialysis patients a large postdialysis supplement (e.g., 50% of the maintenance dosage) may be necessary to offset drug removal during dialysis.

10. Antituberculars. Rifampin is a drug of increasing importance in dialysis patients, primarily because of its application to the treatment of *S. aureus* skin exit site infections. Renal excretion of rifampin in nonuremic patients is only 7%; dosage does not need to be adjusted in dialysis patients. The percentage of renal excretion of isoniazid will vary depending on whether the patient acetylates the drug slowly (renal excretion = 30%) or rapidly (renal excretion = 7%). Isoniazid is removed well by dialysis. The dosage does not usually need to be adjusted in dialysis patients because decreased renal excretion is balanced by removal during dialysis. However, some authors recommend a small dosage reduction (e.g., 200 mg per day rather than 300 mg per day), because accumulation of isoniazid may occur at the 300 mg per day dosage in patients who are "slow acetylators."

Ethambutol is largely excreted by the kidney in nonuremic patients. In dialyzed patients, an increase in the dosing interval is required (see Table 33-3).

11.   Antivirals. Amantadine, used for the prophylaxis and treatment of the influenza A virus, should be used with great caution in hemodialysis patients as excretion of amantadine is almost exclusively renal. Because of its large volume of distribution, amantadine is removed very slowly by either hemodialysis or peritoneal dialysis.

A better alternative to amantadine is rimantadine, since this drug is metabolized by the liver with <25% typically excreted unchanged by the kidney. Dosage is 100 mg daily for 5–7 days in dialysis patients and can be used for treatment (if given within 48 hours of onset of symptoms) or prophylaxis. The drug is not removed by hemodialysis.

Oseltamivir, a relatively new antiviral, targets both influenza A and B. However, there are no data available for the dosing in patients with a creatinine clearance (CrCl) of <10 mL per minute. Normally an active metabolite produced in the liver is excreted via glomerular filtration and tubular secretion by the kidney—a process that can be blocked by probenecid (Hill et al., 2002); therefore, one would assume that substantial dose reduction would be necessary in dialysis patients.

Acyclovir, famciclovir, and valacyclovir are all used to treat herpes simplex and varicella-zoster infections. Published literature and clinical experience suggest that commonly recommended dosages of oral acyclovir for the treatment of herpes zoster in dialysis patients (e.g., 800 mg q12h) are too high and may cause neurotoxicity, especially in CAPD patients (Davenport et al., 1992). The dosages recommended in Table 33-3 are safe in our experience. Both famciclovir and valacyclovir also require dosage reduction.

Several antiviral agents are currently employed for the treatment of cytomegalovirus (CMV) infections and CMV prevention in transplanted patients (cidofovir, foscarnet, ganciclovir, valganciclovir). Cidofovir is utilized at a dosage of 5 mg/kg per week for 2 weeks and then maintained at 5 mg/kg every 2 weeks for CMV disease in patients with normal renal function, but is contraindicated in patients with a CrCl ≤55 mL per minute. Little information about dosing in ESRD patients is available for foscarnet. The prolonged half-life of this drug dictates a reduction in dose interval and total dosage. Foscarnet given at a dosage of 60 mg/kg three times per week after hemodialysis appears to be safe (MacGregor et al., 1991). The dosage of ganciclovir requires reduction by approximately 75%. Since hemodialysis results in substantial (50%) decreases in serum drug levels, doses should be administered after dialysis. Valganciclovir is an oral form of ganciclovir with much higher oral bioavailability than oral ganciclovir. The manufacturer recommends that valganciclovir be avoided in patients receiving hemodialysis. Patients should be closely observed for bone marrow toxicity while on any of these four antivirals.

12. Antiretrovirals. The nucleoside/nucleotide reverse transcriptase inhibitors (NRTIs) were the first class of antiretrovirals available for clinical use. Zidovudine (azidothymidine or AZT), the first NRTI to be approved for the treatment of HIV/AIDS, has now been used for over a decade in patients with ESRD. It is predominantly hepatically metabolized to the inactive glucuronide metabolite GZDV with only about 20% excreted unchanged by the kidneys. However, in renal failure, alteration in elimination possibly due to GZDV accumulation necessitates dosage reduction (generally a 50% reduction) in order to avoid toxicity. We have observed that a 100 mg t.i.d. dosage can cause severe granulocytopenia in ESRD patients. There is no significant removal of the drug or its metabolite by either hemodialysis or peritoneal dialysis. Other nucleoside reverse transcriptase inhibitors (didanosine, emtricitabine, lamivudine, tenofovir, zalcitabine) also require dosage adjustments in renal failure (see Table 33-3). Abacavir is the only NRTI that does not require dosage adjustment. Although there are inadequate data regarding dosage adjustment for zalcitabine, this NRTI is used infrequently. Tenofovir, a relatively new NRTI, has been reported to cause nephrotoxicity, which could be important in patients with residual renal function.

All of the protease inhibitors (PIs)—fosamprenavir, indinavir, nelfinavir, ritonavir, and saquinavir, with the exception of atazanavir—do not require dosage adjustment in renal failure. Atazanavir is the newest agent of the PI class. To date, there are no data available on dosage adjustment of atazanavir in renal dysfunction. There are numerous drug–drug interactions with PIs due to metabolism of these drugs by the hepatic cytochrome P450 isoenzyme system.

The nonnucleoside reverse transcriptase inhibitors (NNRTIs) nevirapine, delavirdine, and efavirenz are a heterogenous group with respect to renal clearance (see Table 33-3).

Enfuvirtide belongs to a new class of antiretrovirals (a fusion inhibitor). This drug is reserved only for patients who require salvage therapy and are resistant to all classes of antiretrovirals. The use of this antiretroviral is limited by the need for subcutaneous injections and the substantial cost (around $20,000 annually). Currently, there are insufficient data in patients with CrCl <35 mL per minute.

13. Antifungals. The use of amphotericin B deoxycholate (conventional amphotericin B), although the gold standard for the treatment of fungal infections, has always been limited because of its nephrotoxicity potential. Two lipid-based amphotericin B formulations are Food and Drug Administration approved (Abelcet and AmBisome) with significantly less nephrotoxicity versus amphotericin B deoxycholate. Nephrotoxicity may be a consideration with prolonged use of amphotericin B in patients with residual renal function.

The systemic azole antifungals include fluconazole, itraconazole, ketoconazole, and, most recently, voriconazole. Fluconazole is typically utilized for the treatment of *Candida albicans* infections. Fluconazole was a useful antifungal for the treatment of *Candida glabrata*; however, resistance of *C. glabrata* to fluconazole is increasing. Voriconazole has a broader spectrum of activity versus fluconazole, with activity against *Aspergillus*, *Fusarium* spp., *Scedosporium* spp., and *Candida* spp. The only azole antifungal that requires dosage adjustment in renal dysfunction is fluconazole; some will decrease the dose by one half in patients with renal dysfunction while others will extend the interval to q48h while keeping the dose the same. The latter may be more appropriate due to fluconazole's dose dependence (e.g., the higher the dose, the higher the serum concentration will be above the MIC of the organism). While oral itraconazole and voriconazole are not dose adjusted with renal dysfunction, the IV form of both drugs cannot be given if a patient's CrCl is <30 mL per minute and 50 mL per minute, respectively. This is due to the accumulation of the vehicle used in the IV formulation. Although itraconazole, ketoconazole, and voriconazole do not require dosage adjustment in renal dysfunction, these antifungals are metabolized hepatically and have numerous drug–drug interactions. A patient's medication profile should be reviewed carefully before prescribing these agents, particularly voriconazole, as several medications are contraindicated if given with voriconazole concomitantly.

Caspofungin and micafungin are antifungal agents in a class of antifungals called the echinocandins. This class of antifungals works on the fungal cell wall compared to the amphotericin formulations and the azole antifungals, which act on the fungal cytoplasmic membranes. Caspofungin has a broad spectrum of activity, with in vitro activity against *Aspergillus* species and *Candida* species (including *Candida glabrata* and *Candida krusei*). Caspofungin is available in the intravenous form only. The dose of caspofungin (70 mg loading dose, followed by 50 mg daily) does not need to be adjusted in patients with renal dysfunction. However, in patients with moderate hepatic insufficiency (Child-Pugh score 7–9), the maintenance dose should be reduced to 35 mg daily. Side effects and adverse effects associated with caspofungin are generally minimal. Caspofungin should be used cautiously in patients who are receiving cyclosporine, due to the potential of abnormal liver function tests.

Micafungin has in vitro activity against the *Candida* species. This antifungal was recently approved for the treatment of esophageal candidiasis as well as prophylaxis of *Candida* infections in patients undergoing hematopoietic stem cell transplantation. The recommended dosage for these two indications is 150 mg and 50 mg daily, respectively. There is no dosage adjustment for renal or hepatic insufficiency. Similar to caspofungin, this antifungal is only available intravenously.

B. Postdialysis supplements. Recommended posthemodialysis supplements are listed in Table 33-3. These should be given in addition to the maintenance dosages listed. The posthemodialysis supplements recommended here are geared for a conventional, 4-hour hemodialysis treatment only. In other instances, the amount of drug removed by hemodialysis is not substantial enough to necessitate a posthemodialysis supplement, but timing of dosing so that a dose is given after dialysis is recommended. In general, peritoneal dialysis patients can be treated with usual hemodialysis patient doses. Drug dosing during continuous renal replacement therapy has recently been reviewed elsewhere (Joy et al., 1998).

SELECTED READINGS

Allon M. Dialysis-catheter related bacteremia: treatment and prophylaxis. *Am J Kidney Dis* 2004;44:779–791.

Ballantine L. Tuberculosis screening in a dialysis program. *Nephrol Nurs J* 2000;27(5):489–499; quiz 500–501.

Bloom S, et al. Clinical and economic effects of mupirocin calcium on preventing Staph. aureus infection in hemodialysis patients. *Am J Kidney Dis* 1996;27:687–694.

Bruchfeld A, et al. Pegylated interferon and ribavirin treatment for hepatitis C in haemodialysis patients. *J Viral Hepat* 2006;13(5): 316–321.

Davenport A, et al. Neurotoxicity of acyclovir in patients with end-stage renal disease treated with continuous ambulatory peritoneal dialysis. *Am J Kidney Dis* 1992;20:647.

Degos F, et al. The tolerance and efficacy of interferon-alpha in haemodialysis patients with HCV infection: a multicentre, prospective study. *Nephrol Dial Transplant* 2001;16:1017–1023.

Deray G, et al. Pharmacokinetics of 3'-azide-3 deoxy-thymidine (AZT) in a patient undergoing hemodialysis. *Therapie* 1989;44:405.

Dinits-Pensy M, et al. The use of vaccines in adult patients with renal disease. *Am J Kidney Dis* 2005;46:997–1011.

Finelli L, et al. National surveillance of dialysis-associated diseases in the United States, 2002. *Semin Dial* 2005;18(1):52–61.

Hill G, et al. The anti-influenza drug oseltamivir exhibits low potential to induce pharmacokinetic drug interactions via renal secretion-correlation of in vivo and in vitro studies. *Drug Metab Dispos* 2002;30(1):13–19.

Jaber BL. Bacterial infections in hemodialysis patients: pathogenesis and prevention. *Kidney Int* 2005;67:2508–2519.

Joy MS, et al. A primer on continuous renal replacement therapy in critically ill patients. *Ann Pharmacother* 1998;32:362–375.

Lok CE, et al. Hemodialysis infection prevention with Polysporin ointment. *J Am Soc Nephrol* 2003;14:169–179.

MacGregor RR, et al. Successful foscarnet therapy for cytomegalovirus retinitis in an AIDS patient undergoing hemodialysis: rationale for empiric dosing and plasma level monitoring. *J Infect Dis* 1991;164:785.

Marr KA, et al. Catheter-related bacteremia and outcome of attempted catheter salvage in patients undergoing hemodialysis. *Ann Intern Med* 1997;127:275–280.

Masuko K, et al. Infection with hepatitis GB virus C in patients on maintenance hemodialysis. *N Engl J Med* 1996;334:1485–1490.

Messing B, et al. Antibiotic-lock technique: a new approach to optimal therapy for catheter-related sepsis in home-parenteral nutrition patients. *J Parenter Enter Nutr* 1988;12:185–189.

Meyers CM, et al. Hepatitis C and renal disease: an update. *Am J Kidney Dis* 2003;42:631–657.

Pai AB, Pai MP. Vancomycin dosing in high flux hemodialysis: a limited-sampling algorithm. *Am J Health Syst Pharm* 2004; 61:1812–1816.

Pollard TA, et al. Vancomycin redistribution: dosing recommendations following high-flux hemodialysis. *Kidney Int* 1994;45:232–237.

Rodby RA, Trenholme GM. Vaccination of the dialysis patient. *Semin Dial* 1991;4:102.

Shi J, Montay G, Bhargava VO. Clinical pharmacokinetics of telithromycin, the first ketolide antibacterial [Review]. *Clin Pharmacokinet* 2005;44(9):915–934.

Tokars JI, et al. National surveillance of hemodialysis associated diseases in the United States, 2000. *Semin Dial* 2002;15:162–171.

Tong NKC, et al. Immunogenicity and safety of an adjuvanted hepatitis B vaccine in pre-hemodialysis and hemodialysis patients. *Kidney Int* 2005;68:2298–2303.

Van Geelen JA, et al. Immune response to hepatitis B vaccine in hemodialysis patients. *Nephron* 1987;45:216.

Vidal L, et al. Systematic comparison of four sources of drug information regarding adjustment of dose for renal function. *Br J Med* 2005;331:263.

Yu VL, et al. *Staphylococcus aureus* nasal carriage and infection in patients on hemodialysis: efficacy of antibiotic prophylaxis. *N Engl J Med* 1986;315:91–96.

Zampieron A, et al. European study on epidemiology and management of hepatitis C virus (HCV) infection in the haemodialysis population. Part 3: prevalence and incidence. *EDTNA ERCA J* 2006;32(1):42–44.

Endocrine Disturbances

Michael J. Flanigan and Victoria S. Lim

Chronic kidney disease alters endocrine and metabolic function in subtle, often complex ways. Consequently, interpreting standard endocrine function tests and diagnosing endocrine deficiency or excess can be difficult. Much of the information obtained has been based on hemodialysis patients; peritoneal dialysis and transplant patient data on endocrine function are less available. Some of the endocrine disturbances with the greatest clinical impact are highlighted below.

I. Insulin

A. Pathophysiology. The most prominent and perhaps important endocrine/metabolic defect in uremia is the "metabolic syndrome." This complex of abundant circulating free fatty acids, elevated fasting insulin, postreceptor insulin resistance, hypertriglyceridemia, depressed high-density lipoprotein (HDL) cholesterol, excess adiponectin, and hypertension is ubiquitous as the glomerular filtration rate (GFR) falls below 50 mL per minute and is associated with an increased likelihood of manifest diabetes, renal failure, and cardiovascular disease. Insulin and adipokine clearances by renal and extrarenal mechanisms are reduced, pancreatic β-cell response to hyperglycemia is blunted, and pulsatile insulin release erratic. Postreceptor insulin resistance, blunted β-cell responsiveness, and hyperlipidemia are partially corrected by hemodialysis as well as by control of hyperparathyroidism and vitamin D therapy.

B. Clinical issues. In nondiabetic uremic patients, impaired renal metabolism of peptide hormones results in altered clearance kinetics of insulin, glucagon, and adipokines. These changes in peripheral metabolism are associated with peripheral hormone resistance and excessive circulating free fatty acids and triglycerides, a diabetic glucose tolerance curve, and a normal fasting blood glucose because of elevated plasma insulin levels. Hyperinsulinemia stimulates very low-density lipoprotein synthesis, and insulin resistance impairs lipoprotein lipase activity and increases serum triglycerides. Peritoneal dialysis and transplant patients may have markedly increased insulin requirements due to the use of glucose as the osmotic agent and immunosuppressive therapy, respectively. Issues regarding diabetic dialysis patients are discussed in Chapter 30.

II. Norepinephrine and epinephrine

A. Pathophysiology. Resting plasma catecholamine levels are generally elevated in patients with chronic renal failure. Increased synthesis appears an unlikely cause because both tyrosine hydroxylase and dopamine β-hydroxylase (DBH), the catecholamine-synthesizing enzymes, are reduced. De-

creased renal excretion is well documented. Reduced catechol-
O-methyltransferase activity impairs degradation of both norepinephrine and epinephrine. Decreased neuronal uptake as a
potential cause is suggested by catecholamine depletion in the
adrenergic nerve terminals of uremic subjects' salivary glands.

B. Clinical issues. Elevated circulating catecholamines
(noradrenaline) are associated with increased mortality
(Zoccali et al., 2002).

    1. Pheochromocytoma. Urinary catecholamine quan-
tification obviously is not useful. Because plasma norepinephrine levels may be moderately elevated in dialysis
patients, the diagnosis of pheochromocytoma based primarily on plasma catecholamine values is less useful unless levels are extremely high. The utility of plasma metanephrine,
normetanephrine, and the clonidine suppression test in this
setting have not been evaluated. Other appropriate diagnostic tests might include computed tomography (CT) and/or
magnetic resonance imaging (MRI) of the adrenal glands
and abdomen.

III. Cortisol

A. Pathophysiology. Plasma cortisol half-life is prolonged
in patients with renal insufficiency, and basal as well as integrated 24-hour plasma cortisol levels are not infrequently
elevated in dialysis patients. Plasma-free cortisol is increased
to a greater extent than total cortisol, suggesting decreased
binding to cortisol-binding globulin. Increased plasma cortisol
levels may be offset, to some degree, by tissue resistance to
glucocorticoid hormone action.

    Additionally, hemodialysis patients have reduced 11β-
hydroxysteroid dehydrogenase type 2 activity (11β-HSD2 is
a cortical collecting duct enzyme that interconverts cortisol
and cortisone). This results in an abnormal accumulation of
cortisol (compound F) and cortisone (compound E), metabolites with pronounced increases in plasma tetrahydrocortisol
(THF), 5α-tetrahydrocortisol (5α-THF) and tetrahydrocorti-
sone (THE), and insufficient dialysis removal. The clinical relevance of these high concentrations of plasma THF, 5α-THF,
and THE is unknown. Elevated plasma cortisol levels may
sometimes be a spurious finding because some commercially
available antisera cross-react with steroid metabolites that
accumulate in dialysis patients. For this reason, unexpectedly
high cortisol levels should be rechecked with alternative assay
procedures.

    1. Suppression and stimulation tests. In dialysis pa-
tients, plasma cortisol increases appropriately with adrenocorticotropic hormone (ACTH) stimulation. The suppressive
effect of dexamethasone is demonstrable but blunted. The
conventional 1-mg oral dose does not fully suppress cortisol secretion, but an 8-mg oral dose or a 1-mg intravenous
dose will suppress plasma cortisol levels to about 2 mcg/dL
(20 mcg/L). In nonuremic patients with Cushing syndrome,
plasma cortisol remains ≥10 mcg/dL (100 mcg/L) even after
intravenous administration of 1 mg of dexamethasone. The
blunted suppression of plasma cortisol by oral dexamethasone may represent abnormal pituitary–adrenal feedback

or be a consequence of decreased absorption or accelerated catabolism of dexamethasone.

B. Clinical issues. Dialysis patients do not ordinarily present with signs or symptoms of Cushing syndrome. If Cushing syndrome is suspected, cortisol suppression should be evaluated using 1 mg of intravenous dexamethasone. A primary hypoadrenocorticism diagnosis in dialysis patients is based on a low basal plasma cortisol and a poor ACTH response.

IV. Thyroid function

A. Pathophysiology. Serum total thyroxine (TT_4) is either normal or reduced in hemodialysis patients. The free thyroxine index (FT_4I), an indirect estimate of free T_4 derived from the product of TT_4 and the triiodothyronine (T_3) uptake ratio, usually changes in the same direction as TT_4, but to a lesser degree. The free fraction of T_4, measured by equilibrium dialysis, is increased and calculated levels of free T_4 are usually normal. Serum thyroxine binding globulin (TBG) levels are normal. The discrepancy between the T_3 uptake ratio and TBG binding capacity measurement suggests a displacement of T_4 from its binding sites by uremic toxins, inhibitors, or drugs.

Serum total T_3 is frequently low among dialysis patients, but normalizes with correction of systemic acidosis; free T_3 index and free T_3 levels are likewise reduced during acidosis. A low free T_3 level also is associated with elevated markers of inflammation such as interleukin (IL)-6 (Zoccali et al., 2005). Serum levels of total reverse T_3 are normal, while free reverse T_3 levels are elevated.

Serum thyroid-stimulating hormone (TSH) is normal, and the TSH response to thyrotropin-releasing hormone (TRH) is either normal or blunted.

In patients undergoing peritoneal dialysis, significant amounts of TBG, T_4, and T_3 are lost in the peritoneal effluent. Despite this, serum TBG remains normal. Serum levels of TT_4 and TT_3 are either normal or reduced, but TSH is normal or minimally elevated.

B. Clinical issues. Serum free T_4 increases transiently after hemodialysis, an effect attributed to heparin, which competes with T_4 for its binding sites either directly or through increased levels of free fatty acids. Long-term hemodialysis is associated with a decrease in the serum levels of the TT_4 and FT_4 index, but the serum TT_3 remains either unchanged or modestly increased.

Most dialysis patients are euthyroid. A diagnosis of hypothyroidism should not be made solely on the basis of low circulating T_4 and T_3 levels, but requires documentation of a substantial TSH elevation (TSH levels >5 mIU/L but <20 mIU/L may occur in 20% of uremic patients but are more likely indicative of nonthyroidal illness than true hypothyroidism). Inappropriate thyroid hormone supplementation will result in excessive protein nitrogen wasting as low thyroid hormone in this situation is a protective adaptation for nitrogen conservation. Clinically asymptomatic multinodular goiter is common in continuous ambulatory peritoneal dialysis (CAPD), hemodialysis, and transplant patients (as high as 50% in endemic areas), and the incidence of goiter appears to be proportional to the size of the anion gap.

V. Testicular function

A. Pathophysiology

1. Gonadal function. Total and free serum testosterone levels are reduced in uremia. Decreased Leydig cell testosterone production is believed to be the cause. The germinal epithelium is also adversely affected: Seminal fluid volume is small, and both sperm numbers and motility are decreased.

2. Pituitary function. Pituitary function does not appear to be abnormal: Plasma luteinizing hormone (LH) is either normal or slightly elevated. Plasma follicle-stimulating hormone (FSH) is normal. Plasma levels of both gonadotropins increase appropriately following administration of gonadotropin-releasing hormone or clomiphene (a nonsteroidal antiestrogen that stimulates gonadotropin secretion by blockade of estrogen-mediated negative feedback on the hypothalamus), suggesting intact pituitary function. Similarly, testosterone administration suppresses plasma LH appropriately.

3. Hypothalamic function. The evidence supporting hypothalamic dysfunction is substantial and includes sustained elevation of plasma FSH following restoration of renal function with transplantation and decreased LH pulsatile frequency. Children with renal failure have reduced gonadotropin pulsatility for their stage of pubertal maturation.

4. Hyperprolactinemia. Serum prolactin levels are elevated in about 30% of dialysis patients; the magnitude of elevation is mild, about three to six times the levels found in control subjects. Extreme hyperprolactinemia (>100 ng/mL) suggests a concomitant pituitary disease and requires investigation. Increased serum prolactin levels are due to a combination of decreased metabolic clearance and increased pituitary secretion. The latter may be augmented by medication, such as methyldopa, metoclopramide, and phenothiazine, which further inhibit the dopamine-stimulated pituitary expression of neuronal nitric oxide synthase.

Hyperprolactinemia in dialysis patients is rather resistant to inhibition by L-dopa or dopamine, but bromocriptine often can normalize the serum prolactin levels.

B. Clinical issues. Decreased libido, impotence, and infertility are widely prevalent among dialysis patients. One should initially consider nonendocrine causes of impotence, including vascular insufficiency, anemia, fatigue, depression, and autonomic neuropathy. Diagnosis and treatment are discussed in Chapter 39.

VI. Ovarian function

A. Pathophysiology. In most female adult dialysis patients plasma estradiol levels are normal, suggesting relatively intact ovarian function. Estrogen normally exerts a negative feedback on pituitary gonadotropin secretion. In uremic patients, this negative feedback relation is intact as evidenced by increased plasma LH and FSH values following clomiphene administration and during menopause. However, the positive feedback effect of estrogen on the hypothalamus, responsible for the midcycle LH and FSH surge, is lost. The latter was demonstrated by failure of LH and FSH to increase following exogenous estrogen administration.

B.   Clinical issues. About half of the women on hemodialysis are amenorrheic. In women who continue to menstruate, the menses are irregular and generally anovulatory. However, metromenorrhagia may also occur, increasing the transfusion requirement. Although infertility is common, conception can take place, especially in well-dialyzed and well-nourished patients. Thus, contraception is advised in women who do not wish to become pregnant. See Chapter 40.

VII.   Growth hormone

A.   Pathophysiology. Renal failure patients have elevated fasting growth hormone (GH) levels. GH is not suppressible following glucose infusion and increases in an exaggerated fashion after arginine infusion. The high serum level is due to a combination of decreased degradation and increased secretion.

GH induces skeletal growth indirectly by inducing hepatic synthesis of insulin-like growth factors I and II (IGF-I and IGF-II), which stimulate growth of the epiphyseal cartilage. In chronic renal failure patients, circulating IGF activity, measured by bioassay, is reduced despite elevated levels by radioimmunoassay. This is explained by the presence of reduced intact but elevated serum levels of insulin-like growth factor binding proteins (IGFBP) in uremic plasma. Measurement of serum IGF-I and IGF-II by radioimmunoassay showed levels ranging from low to higher than normal, while ultrafiltration analysis suggests depressed IGF availability.

B.   Clinical issues. Statural growth is impaired in children with renal insufficiency; height age is usually more retarded than bone age. Delayed bone age and sexual maturation are beneficial because the opportunity for statural growth is prolonged. Attempts to induce growth include adequate dialysis, increased nutritional intake, renal osteodystrophy management, correction of metabolic acidosis, and recombinant human growth hormone (rhGH) administration.

As a result of rhGH treatment, children with renal failure exhibit a rise in growth velocity and an increase in body weight and midarm muscle circumference, suggesting a net anabolic effect. This salutary effect is achieved without adverse effects on glucose tolerance or creatinine clearance. More importantly, the accelerated growth does not hasten bone age maturation, thus preserving growth potential. Among adult dialysis patients with protein-energy malnutrition, rhGH therapy can favorably affect protein anabolism and bone turnover.

VIII.   Parathyroid hormone (PTH)

A.   Pathophysiology

1.   Baseline PTH levels. Plasma concentrations of PTH are elevated in dialysis patients due primarily to increased secretion caused by (a) vitamin D deficiency, (b) a reduction in serum ionized calcium, and (c) an elevation in serum phosphorus value. Hypocalcemia in uremia is due to a combination of the following: (a) phosphate retention and hyperphosphatemia, (b) reduced intestinal calcium absorption, and (c) skeletal resistance to PTH.

Hyperphosphatemia causes a reduction in plasma ionized calcium levels both by reducing residual renal 1,25-dihydroxyvitamin D_3 production and direct complexing with ionized calcium. Factors b and c are, in part, a result of reduced serum $1,25(OH)_2D_3$ activity.

In uremia, $1,25(OH)_2D_3$ deficiency results in a higher set point (i.e., a greater than normal level of serum calcium is needed to suppress PTH secretion) for the negative feedback between serum calcium and PTH secretion.

2.   PTH assays. Serum PTH levels are assay dependent. Almost all PTH assays cross-react with retained PTH degradation products, which are normally metabolized by the kidneys. Interpretation of the various PTH assays is discussed in Chapter 35.

B.   Clinical issues. The principal bone lesion of secondary hyperparathyroidism is osteitis fibrosa cystica. Extraskeletal manifestations of disordered calcium/phosphorus metabolism include the following: (a) calcium deposition in the media of various arteries, sometimes resulting in ischemic necrotizing skin lesions; (b) periarthritis and myopathy; (c) pruritus; and (d) anemia and bone marrow fibrosis.

Hypothesized associations between hyperparathyroidism and cardiovascular disease, impotence, neuropathy, encephalopathy, and impaired immune response are not firmly established.

Diagnosis of parathyroid-associated bone disease, and prevention and treatment of hyperparathyroidism, including when to recommend parathyroidectomy, are discussed in Chapter 35.

IX.   Vitamin D_3

A.   Pathophysiology. Vitamin D_3 is hydroxylated at the 25-position in the liver and at the 1-position in the kidney. The 1,25-dihydroxy form of D_3 is biologically the most active form. In dialysis patients, plasma concentrations of $1,25(OH)_2D_3$ are almost universally depressed, and 25%–50% of patients also demonstrate low 25-hydroxy D_3 levels. The primary reason for the depressed 1,25-dihydroxy D_3 is reduced hydroxylation by the kidney, while depressed 25-hydroxy D_3 levels are likely related to dietary restriction and lack of sun exposure. Reduced 1-hydroxylation may result from either intrinsic renal damage or hyperphosphatemia. The physiologic consequence of a low 1,25-dihydroxyvitamin D_3 is decreased intestinal calcium and phosphorus absorption, reduced skeletal sensitivity to PTH, and inhibition of synthesis and release of pre-pro-PTH in response to calcium receptor protein stimulation.

B.   Clinical issues. The dihydroxy form of vitamin D_3 is now available for the treatment of secondary hyperparathyroidism; it may be administered either orally or intravenously. It effectively suppresses PTH, but hypercalcemia is a common complication. Several vitamin D analogs (22-oxacalcitriol, 19-nor-$1\alpha,25(OH)_2D_2$, and 1α-$(OH)D_2$) are also available for clinical use and appear to have selectively greater affinity for parathyroid rather than intestinal and bone vitamin D receptors. The administration and complications of vitamin D treatment are discussed in Chapter 35.

SELECTED READINGS

Charlesworth JA, et al. Insulin resistance and postprandial triglyceride levels in primary renal disease. *Metab Clin Exper* 2005;54: 821–828.

DeFronzo RA, et al. Glucose intolerance in uremia: quantification of pancreatic beta cell sensitivity to glucose and tissue sensitivity to insulin. *J Clin Invest* 1978;62:425–435.

Fine RN. Growth hormone and the kidney: the use of recombinant human growth hormone (rhGH) in growth-retarded children with chronic renal insufficiency. *J Am Soc Neprhol* 1991;1:1136–1145.

Handelsman DJ. Hypothalamic—pituitary gonadal dysfunction in renal failure, dialysis and renal transplantation. *Endocr Rev* 1985;6:151–182.

Kutlay S, et al. Thyroid disorders in hemodialysis patients in an iodine-deficient community. *Artif Organs* 2005;29(4):329–332.

Lim VS, et al. Ovarian function in chronic renal failure: evidence suggesting hypothalamic anovulation. *Ann Intern Med* 1980;93: 21–27.

Lim VS, et al. Protective adaptation of low serum triiodothyronine in patients with chronic renal failure. *Kidney Int* 1985;28:541–549.

Lim VS. Renal failure and thyroid function. *Int J Artif Organs* 1986;9:385–386.

Lim VS, et al. Thyroid dysfunction in chronic renal failure: a study of the pituitary—thyroid axis and peripheral turnover kinetics of thyroxine and triiodothyronine. *J Clin Invest* 1977;60:522–534.

Malyszko J, et al. Adiponectin, leptin and thyroid hormones in patients with chronic renal failure and on renal replacement therapy: are they related? *Nephrol Dial Transplant* 2006;21(1):145–152.

Nolan GE, et al. Spurious overestimation of plasma cortisol in patients with chronic renal failure. *J Clin Endocrinol Metab* 1981;52:1242–1245.

Phillips LS, Kopple JD. Circulating somatomedin activity and sulfate levels in adults with normal and impaired kidney function. *Metabolism* 1981;30:1091–1095.

Pupim LB, et al. Recombinant human growth hormone improves muscle amino acid uptake and whole-body protein metabolism in chronic hemodialysis patients. *Am J Clin Nutr* 2005;82(6):1235–1243.

Rigalleau V, Gin H. Carbohydrate metabolism in uraemia [Review]. *Curr Opin Clin Nutr Metab Care* 2005;8(4):463–469.

Ritz E, Bommer J. Discussion: zinc metabolism. *Contrib Nephrol* 1984;38:126.

Robey C, et al. Effects of chronic peritoneal dialysis on thyroid function tests. *Am J Kidney Dis* 1989;13:99–103.

Rosman PM, et al. Pituitary—adrenocortical function in chronic renal failure: blunted suppression and early escape of plasma cortisol levels after intravenous dexamethasone. *J Clin Endocrinol Metab* 1982;54:528–533.

Schaefer RM, et al. Improved sexual function in hemodialysis patients on recombinant erythropoietin: a possible role for prolactin. *Clin Nephrol* 1989;31:1–5.

Schaefer F, et al. Pulsatile gonadotropin secretion in pubertal children with chronic renal failure. *Acta Endocrinol* 1989;120:14–19.

Talbot JA, et al. Pulsatile bioactive luteinizing hormone secretion in men with chronic renal failure and following renal transplantation. *Nephron* 1990;56:66–72.

Wiederkehr MR, Kalogiros J, Krapf R. Correction of metabolic acidosis improves thyroid and growth hormone axes in haemodialysis patients. *Nephrol Dial Transplant* 2004;19:1190–1197.

Zoccali C, et al. Low triiodothyronine: a new facet of inflammation in end-stage renal disease. *J Am Soc Nephrol* 2005;16(9):2789–2795.

Zoccali C, et al. Plasma norepinephrine predicts survival and incident cardiovascular events in patients with end-stage renal disease. *Circulation* 2002;105(11):1354–1359.

WEB REFERENCES

HDCN calcium-phosphorus-PTH channel: http://www.hdcn.com/ch/calphos/

Bone Disease

Daniel W. Coyne, Steven C. Cheng, and James A. Delmez

I. Pathophysiology. Bone disease in dialysis patients is primarily due to the effects of secondary hyperparathyroidism. Hyperparathyroidism appears in many patients when the glomerular filtration rate (GFR) is in the range of 50 to 70 mL per minute. The causes of hyperparathyroidism include hypocalcemia, diminished circulating calcitriol levels, and phosphate retention. Low levels of calcitriol are due to reduced 1-hydroxylation of 25-hydroxyvitamin D_3 in the kidney. Additionally, low levels of vitamin D stores (assessed by measurement of 25-hydroxyvitamin D) are prevalent in the chronic kidney disease (CKD) population. Calcitriol inhibits parathyroid hormone (PTH) synthesis at the pre-pro-PTH messenger RNA (mRNA) level by acting on calcitriol receptors in parathyroid cells. In uremia, the calcitriol receptor density on parathyroid cells is reduced, making the cells less sensitive to this feedback inhibition. There is decreased sensitivity of the gland to calcium suppression, perhaps due to decreased expression of calcium receptors on parathyroid cells. Also, hyperphosphatemia stimulates PTH secretion by a direct effect on the parathyroid gland. Eventually, chronically low calcium levels, lack of calcitriol inhibition, and hyperphosphatemia cause the parathyroid glands to increase to many times their original size through hyperplasia. High PTH levels and likely inadequate production of other substances, such as bone morphogenic protein–7, result in progressive renal osteodystrophy.

Bone resistance to PTH action develops in dialysis patients and results in the need for higher PTH levels to effect normal bone turnover. Osteitis fibrosa (high bone turnover) develops in dialysis patients when PTH levels are chronically and markedly elevated, while PTH levels maintained in the normal range result in adynamic bone (low bone turnover). In dialysis patients, PTH levels that are moderately elevated (two to four times the normal range) frequently lead to a near normal bone histology.

II. Laboratory findings and target recommendations

A. PTH assays. Parathyroid hormone is an 84 amino acid peptide (PTH[1–84]) that activates a signaling cascade via the PTH1 receptor present on a variety of tissues. The N-terminal portion of the peptide is essential for binding and receptor activation, while large portions of the C-terminal are not. Fragments of PTH are rapidly cleared by the kidney and accumulate in renal failure. Most fragments cannot activate the PTH1 receptor due to loss of portions of the N-terminus; however, these fragments were usually detected by single antibody radioimmunoassays (RIAs) employed in the 1980s. The intact

PTH (iPTH) assay is a two-antibody immunometric assay (a capture antibody for the midregion and a detection antibody that binds near the N-terminus), which greatly diminishes interference of PTH fragments and initially was thought to identify PTH(1–84) alone.

However, one major fragment, PTH(7–84), is identified by this assay and accounts for about 48% of the PTH measured in dialysis patients. Recently a second-generation immunometric assay was developed, which employs a detection antibody that binds at or very near the first amino acid (Salusky et al., 2003). The new assay, referred to as biPTH, biointact PTH, or whole PTH, binds exclusively PTH(1–84). The biPTH results are approximately 55% of the corresponding iPTH values. Widespread use of biPTH has thus far been limited by the availability and technical demands of this assay.

Some investigators have suggested that the ratio of PTH(1–84) to the PTH(7–84) fragment may have diagnostic significance (Monier-Faugere et al., 2001). This ratio equals the [biPTH/(iPTH – biPTH)]. Ratios >1 or 1.5 have been found in some studies to be associated with high bone turnover, while low ratios are associated with adynamic bone. Other studies have found no diagnostic value in the ratio (Coen et al., 2002). There are insufficient data to support use of the ratio for diagnostic decisions at this time.

The present recommendations for target PTH in dialysis patients set by the National Kidney Foundation (NKF) are to maintain iPTH levels of 150–300 pg/mL (16–32 pmol/L), which is approximately a biPTH of 80–160 pg/mL (around 9–18 pmol/L). For proper management, physicians should know which assay is being employed in their dialysis center and hospital, and whether historical PTH values were done with the older iPTH or newer biPTH assay.

B.   Calcium. The normal range for serum calcium is 8.4–10.2 mg/dL (2.1–2.6 mmol/L), and the NKF Kidney Disease Outcome Quality Initiative (KDOQI) bone guidelines recommend a target predialysis corrected calcium within this normal range, and preferably ≤9.5 mg/dL (2.4 mmol/L). Serum calcium circulates in a free (ionized) and a protein-bound state. Total calcium reported on standard lab tests reflects both of these circulating forms. Protein-bound calcium is proportional to the concentration of albumin, which accounts for most protein binding of calcium. On average, total calcium falls by 0.8 mg/dL for every 1.0 g/dL decrease in albumin (0.2 mmol/L for every 10 g/L decrease in albumin). Consequently, in hypoalbuminemia the total calcium reported from the laboratory should be corrected by using the equation:

Corrected calcium (mg/dL)

= total calcium + (0.8 × (4.0 − albumin [in g/dL])

Corrected calcium (mmol/L)

= total calcium + (0.02 × (40 − albumin [in g/L])

In most new dialysis patients, corrected and ionized calcium concentrations are usually slightly low or in the low-normal range. In chronic dialysis patients, corrected calcium reflects the calcium exposure (via calcium-based binders and concentration of calcium in the dialysate), the level of PTH, and the effect of therapies to treat hyperparathyroidism.

Hypercalcemia is usually due to excessive use of calcium-based binders and use of active vitamin D agents, which increase calcium absorption. Patients with low PTH appear to have the highest range of serum calcium, which may reflect adynamic bone disease and poor ability of bone to buffer calcium. Advanced hyperparathyroidism associated with a large mass of autonomous parathyroid tissue can rarely result in hypercalcemia in the absence of oral calcium administration or the use of active vitamin D. This is referred to as tertiary hyperparathyroidism.

Low levels of total uncorrected calcium are often due to a low serum albumin. Low corrected calcium may be due to poor gastrointestinal absorption of calcium due to vitamin D deficiency, severe hyperphosphatemia, or use of the calcimimetic agent cinacalcet.

C. **Phosphorus.** The normal range for serum phosphorus is 2.7–4.6 mg/dL (0.9–1.5 mmol/L) in patients with normal renal function and stage 3 and 4 CKD. In dialysis patients, the KDOQI bone guidelines recommend target predialysis phosphorus of 3.5–5.5 mg/dL (1.1–1.8 mmol/L), slightly higher than the normal range, while the European Best Practice Guidelines recommend targeting the normal range.

Hyperphosphatemia can be due to gut absorption of phosphorus due to excessive dietary phosphorus intake, or inadequate use or noncompliance with phosphorus binders. Hyperphosphatemia can also result from missed dialysis treatments, excessive resorption of bone due to severe hyperparathyroidism, or use of active vitamin D agents, which increase gut absorption of phosphorus and increase bone resorption. Although PTH and phosphorus levels correlate, serum phosphorus values are a poor guide to the severity of the hyperparathyroidism.

Hypophosphatemia can be due to poor intake of dietary phosphorus, excessive use of binders, or a blood draw that occurred just following dialysis. Patients with persistent predialysis hypophosphatemia while off binders usually also have low protein intake, and should be counseled to increase dietary protein and phosphorus intake. Use of phosphorus supplements (K Phos Neutral, consisting of 8 mmol phosphorus, 13 mmol sodium, and 1.1 mmol potassium, starting at one tablet daily) is indicated if the serum phosphorus remains below 3.0 mg/dL (1.0 mmol/L).

D. **Alkaline phosphatase.** Alkaline phosphatase is frequently elevated in dialysis patients, usually due to osteitis fibrosa from hyperparathyroidism. However, alkaline phosphatase originates from sources in addition to bone, the most important being liver, intestine, and kidney. Bone-specific alkaline phosphatase is a readily obtainable test that reflects bone formation, and should be measured when the source of a high serum alkaline phosphatase is in doubt. Both total and bone-specific alkaline phosphatase are usually elevated in hyperparathyroidism and fall during successful treatment of this disorder. While there is reasonable correlation between PTH levels and these tests, this is rarely useful in the management of hyperparathyroidism.

E. **Vitamin D.** 25-OH vitamin D is synthesized by the liver and reflects vitamin stores. These are frequently low in dialysis patients. Several factors likely account for the high incidence of deficiency, including poor sun exposure in ill patients, restriction of vitamin D–fortified dairy products for purposes of phosphorus control, and the high prevalence of black patients who are frequently lactose intolerant and whose dark pigmentation reduces effective vitamin D formation upon ultraviolet light exposure. The lowest serum 25-vitamin D levels are typically found in black patients and in winter, but low values are found at all times of the year independent of race.

Treatment of vitamin D deficiency is appropriate despite the loss of adequate 1-α-hydroxylase activity in the kidney, as other tissues possess this enzyme to produce calcitriol for autocrine and paracrine actions. In fact, 1-α-hydroxylase activity has been demonstrated in the parathyroid gland itself (Ritter et al., 2005). Treatment should replete and then maintain adequate stores. Vitamin D stores are assessed by measuring 25-OH vitamin D in the blood. Levels >30 ng/mL (>75 nmol/L) are desirable. A 25-OH vitamin D level of 15–29 ng/mL (~40–75 nmol/L) should be treated with a single ergocalciferol (vitamin D_2) 50,000-IU capsule monthly; levels of 5–14 ng/mL (13–39 nmol/L) should be treated with one capsule weekly for a month, then monthly; and levels <5 ng/mL (<13 nmol/L) should be treated with 1 capsule weekly for 12 weeks, then monthly. Recommended daily intake for vitamin D in nonuremic persons is 200–400 IU per day, with at least 800 IU per day recommended for populations at risk of deficiency and during the winter. In CKD patients, 800–2,000 IU per day are likely sufficient and safe. In the United States vitamin D deficiency is treated with ergocalciferol, as cholecalciferol (vitamin D_3) is available only as a dietary supplement, and amounts are not regulated or standardized. Cholecalciferol is also added to a number of calcium supplements that are widely marketed.

III. **Bone biopsy and bone histology**

A. **Overview and indications.** Bone normally undergoes a coordinated turnover with osteoblast cells producing new bone matrix proteins (osteoid), which undergo mineralization, coupled with the activity of osteoclasts, which cause bone resorption. In most dialysis patients, the underlying bone pathology can be judged based on PTH levels. However, in those patients with unexplained bone pain, spontaneous fractures, or progressive bone loss, a bone biopsy provides an accurate diagnosis of the underlying bone lesion. It can also be helpful to rule out aluminum-related bone disease. Finally, some investigators recommend bone biopsies prior to parathyroidectomy to ensure the presence of osteitis fibrosa and absence of aluminum accumulation.

The pathologic classification of renal osteodystrophy is based both on the static and dynamic histologic parameters obtained by transiliac bone biopsy. Fluorescent labels, tetracycline, and demeclocycline are deposited along the lines of mineralization. Administration of such a label for 1–3 days followed 1–2 weeks later by the repeat administration of label allows for the determination of the rate of bone mineralization. With high bone turnover, for example, the distance between the two labels would be increased. Aluminum deposition is detected by staining the sample with acid solochrome azurin.

B. Osteitis fibrosa. This form of renal osteodystrophy occurs when PTH is persistently high. Although representing a spectrum of severity, it is characterized by accelerated formation and resorption of bone due to an increased number and activity of osteoblasts and osteoclasts and increased marrow fibrosis. The severity of osteitis fibrosa is roughly proportional to the degree and duration of PTH elevation. Mild osteitis fibrosa is probably preferable to adynamic bone (see below) in that bone strength is greater and there is less alteration in mineral metabolism. When more severe, bone is laid down so rapidly that it is not properly mineralized. In such cases, the amount of unmineralized bone (osteoid) is increased. The alignment of the collagen is irregular instead of the usually lamellar pattern. This "woven" bone may become mineralized as amorphous calcium phosphorus rather than hydroxyapatite. The resulting bone is more prone to fracture. The most prominent symptoms of severe osteitis fibrosa are bone and joint discomfort. Metastatic calcification with periarticular calcium deposits may lead to acute joint inflammation or pain and stiffness.

Radiologic findings usually are absent in mild disease but always are present in severe hyperparathyroidism. As such, plain x-rays of bone are not generally recommended for the assessment of bone disease in dialysis patients. Hand films most reliably demonstrate changes of hyperparathyroidism. The characteristic finding is bone loss (resorption) in the subperiosteal area, best seen on the radial side of the second and third phalanges. Associated erosion of the tuft of the distal phalanx also may be visible and, when severe, may lead to blunting of the fingertip. The latter changes are pathognomonic of present or past osteitis fibrosa. Evidence of bone resorption also may be seen elsewhere in the skeleton, including the skull, giving it a "salt-and-pepper" appearance, and in the long bones, particularly the lesser trochanter of the femur.

Disorganized, accelerated bone formation is associated with osteitis fibrosa and may be visible radiologically as osteosclerosis. Bone scanning using technetium radiopharmaceuticals will show increased skeletal uptake of isotope. The bone:soft tissue ratio of isotope uptake will be increased. However, bone scans generally add little to the diagnostic evaluation of osteitis fibrosa.

C. Adynamic bone. Adynamic bone disease is characterized by reduced osteoblast and osteoclast number and low or absent bone formation rate as measured by tetracycline labeling. The osteoid thickness is normal or reduced, distinguishing it from osteomalacia. Associated laboratory findings may include an iPTH <100 pg/mL (11 pmol/L) or biPTH <80 pg/mL (~9 pmol/L), low serum bone-specific alkaline phosphatase, and occasionally a slightly elevated serum ionized calcium level. Vertebral and peripheral bone densities tend to be normal or low.

The causes of adynamic bone histology are unknown, but persistently low (for dialysis patients) PTH levels play a major causal role. Susceptible populations include the elderly, women, diabetics, and those of Caucasian race. It is more common in peritoneal dialysis patients, as is a low PTH. Use of a dialysis solution calcium concentration of >2.5 mEq/L (1.25 mM) may increase the prevalence of adynamic bone and cause PTH oversuppression. Aluminum is now a rare cause of adynamic bone disease.

Initially thought to be asymptomatic and not requiring treatment, adynamic bone is now known to be associated with a higher fracture rate than osteitis fibrosa, hypercalcemia (likely due to impaired ability of the bone to buffer serum calcium), and vascular and other soft tissue calcification. Symptoms, such as pain from nontraumatic fractures, are usually absent until the disease is advanced.

D.   Osteomalacia. Like adynamic bone disease, osteomalacia represents a state of low bone turnover. It differs, however, because of the presence of large amounts of unmineralized osteoid. In nonuremic patients vitamin D deficiency is the most common cause of osteomalacia and in dialysis patients with low bone mass and frequent fractures it should be in the differential diagnosis as well (see Section II E). In the not-too-distant past, osteomalacia was often associated with aluminum overload, as aluminum prevents bone mineralization and suppresses PTH secretion. With recognition of its toxicity, aluminum is now rarely used as a long-term phosphorus binder and properly treated dialysate is free of aluminum. Consequently, the incidence of aluminum-induced osteomalacia has decreased substantially. An unusual cause of osteomalacia is iron overload.

E.   Mixed lesions. Some patients display histologic evidence of both osteitis fibrosa and osteomalacia on bone biopsy. Such patients frequently have high PTH levels and impaired bone formation and mineralization. In the past such mixed lesions often were found in patients with concomitant aluminum intoxication.

F.   Osteoporosis. The age of patients beginning dialysis continues to increase. Many have pre-existing osteoporosis documented with bone densitometry. Medical interventions used routinely for osteoporosis include bisphosphonates, selective or nonselective estrogens, teriparatide (Forteo) if the PTH is persistently low, and vitamin D. None of these treatments has demonstrated efficacy or safety in the hemodialysis population.

IV.   Management of PTH and bone disease

A.   PTH. The target range in dialysis patients for iPTH is 150–300 pg/mL (16–32 pmol/L), and 80–160 pg/mL for biPTH (around 9–18 pmol/L). Renal osteodystrophy is usually managed indirectly by control of PTH within this target range.

This is the best indirect method of bone disease management presently available.

Chronically low PTH results in adynamic bone disease in most patients, while PTH levels above the target range are likely to result in osteitis fibrosa (high bone turnover). The severity of osteitis fibrosa is also proportional to the duration and severity of hyperparathyroidism. However, the clinician should remember that PTH in a given range does not always correlate with the bone disease present in the individual patient. Adynamic bone disease has been found in patients with PTH values above the target range, osteitis fibrosa is not uncommon in patients with PTH levels maintained in the target range (although its severity is usually mild), and osteomalacia due to vitamin D deficiency has little correlation to PTH. Clinical events (e.g., fractures, hypercalcemia) that do not correlate with the results of repeated PTH measures warrant further evaluation.

B. Calcium

1. **Target.** The KDOQI bone guidelines recommend maintaining the predialysis corrected calcium between 8.4 and 10.2 mg/dL (2.1 and 2.6 mmol/L), with ideal values <9.5 mg/dL (2.4 mmol/L) based on association data. More recent and more sophisticated fixed and time-dependent analyses that adjust for use of vitamin D indicate corrected calcium values from 9.0 to 10.0 mg/dL (2.25–2.50 mmol/L) are associated with the lowest mortality (Kalantar Zadeh et al., 2006).

2. **Hemodialysis** solution dialysate calcium should be 2.5 mEq/L (1.25 mM) in most patients. This will usually maintain a neutral calcium balance. Cautious use of a 2.0 mEq/L (1.0 mM) calcium bath or lower can be used to control chronically high serum calcium or to stimulate PTH secretion in a patient with a chronically low PTH.

3. **Peritoneal dialysis** fluid calcium concentration should be 2.5 mEq/L (1.25 mM) in most patients. A 3.5 mEq/L (1.75 mM) dialysis solution is available, but should be reserved for patients with chronically low corrected calcium. The higher calcium concentration, especially when used in conjunction with calcium-based phosphorus binders, creates a chronically positive calcium balance in most patients, suppresses PTH, and may contribute to vascular calcification.

4. **Oral calcium as phosphorus binder and supplement.** Oral calcium (such as calcium carbonate or calcium acetate) should be given with meals when used as a dietary phosphorus binder and on an empty stomach (such as bedtime) when the goal is to provide additional calcium for absorption.

C. Phosphorus

1. **Target and rationale.** In hemodialysis and peritoneal dialysis patients, the target range for phosphorus is 3.5–5.5 mg/dL (1.13–1.78 mmol/L). Control of phosphorus ensures maintenance of a safe Ca × P product. High serum phosphorus has been associated with increased cardiovascular events and higher mortality. Control of phosphorus

Table 35-1.   Foods especially high in phosphorus

Dairy products (milk, yogurt, cheese)
Many soft drinks (particularly colas)
Some fruit juices, punches, coolers[a]
Liver, meat
"Enhanced meats" (to which phosphorus-containing chemicals have
  been added)[a]
Beans
Nuts
Whole grain breads and cereals, cereal bars[a]

[a]Food tables giving details of phosphorus content for various breakfast drinks as well as cereals have been published in three papers by Murphy-Gutekunst and Barnes in the *J Ren Nutr* 2005;15(2, 3, and 4). Links to the tables are provided at http://www.hdcn.com/ch/calphos/.

lowers serum PTH and likely inhibits parathyroid gland hyperplasia. High phosphorus levels also lower ionized calcium contributing to higher PTH secretion.

2.   Dietary intake. Restriction of phosphorus in the diet to 800–1,200 mg/day (26–39 mmol) is the keystone of control of serum phosphorus. Continuing patient education by a knowledgeable dietitian is the best method to establish and maintain proper dietary habits in a dialysis patient. See Table 35-1 for foods high in phosphorus. Phosphorus is present in many sources other than dairy products. Phosphorus additives to foods now can contribute as much as 1,000 mg/day (32 mmol/day) of phosphorus to the average diet. As absorption of these additives is almost 100% versus about 60% for phosphorus in grains, meat, and dairy; avoidance of additive-containing foods is paramount. It is well known that colas (Coke, Pepsi, Dr. Pepper) contain substantial amounts of phosphorus (about 40–60 mg [1.3–1.9 mmol] per 12-oz [350 mL] serving). Less well known is the fact that certain fruit punches and drinks and "coolers" can contain twice this amount. Breakfast cereals and cereal bars contain from 30 to 200 mg (1.0–6.5 mmol) of phosphorus per three-quarter cup (180 mL) serving. These often are supplemented with calcium, and more often than not, calcium phosphate is what is being added. A third source of phosphorus in the diet is the growing use of "enhanced meats," where a variety of phosphorus-containing compounds are injected into meats for use as flavor enhancers and tenderizers. Phosphorus content of foods is not required to be listed on food labels, and so many of these products are best avoided unless their phosphorus content can be obtained from the manufacturer (see Table 35-1 for a link to the appropriate reference tables). Boiling of (regular) meat greatly reduces its phosphorus content (about 50%) while having only a small (–15%) effect on its protein content (Cupisti et al., 2006).

3.   Removal of phosphorus by dialysis. Hemodialysis typically removes about 800 mg (26 mmol) of phosphorus per treatment, but this depends to some extent on predialysis serum levels. A predictive model for phosphate removal based on initial serum level and dialysis treatment parameters has been developed (Gotch et al., 2003). High-flux dialyzers and dialyzers with larger surface areas can increase phosphorus clearance to a limited degree, and hemodiafiltration results in a further (~15%–20%) increase in phosphorus removal (Lornoy, 2006). Increasing the time on dialysis is of significant but limited benefit because serum phosphorus level falls quickly during dialysis due to slow equilibration of phosphorus from tissues to blood resulting in reduced phosphorus gradient across the dialyzer in the latter part of the treatment. Therefore, short daily dialysis increases phosphorus removal, but 3-hour sessions are required six times per week to clinically impact phosphorus removal (see Chapter 14). Nocturnal dialysis given six times per week provides the greatest phosphorus removal by allowing steady clearance while tissues slowly release phosphorus into the blood. Most nocturnal dialysis patients require addition of phosphate to the dialysate to prevent hypophosphatemia. Peritoneal dialysis removes approximately 300 mg (9.7 mmol) per day of phosphorus with four exchanges of 2 L per day. The high prescribed dietary protein intake usually requires the use of binders to control phosphorus levels.

4.   Phosphorus binders. Phosphorus binders play an important role in phosphorus control in conjunction with dietary restriction. These agents bind phosphorus in the gut to prevent absorption. As such, they should be given with meals at doses proportional to the phosphorus content of meals. Combination therapies may be necessary to establish aggressive phosphorus control without exposing patients to excessive calcium supplementation and the subsequent risks of hypercalcemia. See Table 35-2 for a summary of phosphorus-binding agents.

   a.   Calcium-containing phosphorus binders. These agents are generally used as the initial management of hyperphosphatemia based on a profile of effective phosphorus binding and calcium supplementation. However, dose titration is limited by current KDOQI recommendations that elemental calcium supplementation should not exceed 1.5 g (37 mmol) per day. In addition, dialysis solution calcium concentration should be kept at 2.5 mEq/L (1.25 mM) to accommodate the added oral calcium load. The coadministration of calcium and active vitamin D preparations predispose patients to hypercalcemia and warrant close monitoring.

      (1)   Calcium carbonate is available in a variety of preparations and dose sizes including TUMS (200 mg [5.0 mmol] of elemental calcium per tab), Caltrate (240 mg [6.0 mmol] of elemental calcium per tab), and OsCal 500 (500 mg [12.5 mmol] of elemental calcium per tab). A reasonable starting dose is one to two tablets with each meal. However, the use of more than 1.5 g [37 mmol] of elemental calcium per day exposes patients to excessive calcium loading and the risk of hypercalcemia. This agent has the benefit of easy accessibility and low cost.

Table 35-2. Commonly used phosphate binders

Product	Trade Names	Dose (mg) per Tablet	Elemental Calcium per Tablet	Maximum Dose per Day	Comments
Calcium carbonate	(Generic, multiple names)	Multiple doses	40% elemental calcium	1.5 g of elemental calcium per day	Administered with meals as binder; on empty stomach as supplement
	TUMS	500 mg	200 mg (5.0 mmol)	As above (seven tablets)	
	TUMS EX	750 mg	300 mg (7.5 mmol)	As above (five tablets)	
	TUMS Ultra	1,000 mg	400 mg (10 mmol)	As above (three tablets)	
	TUMS 500	1,250 mg	500 mg (12.5 mmol)	As above (three tablets)	
	Os-Cal 500	1,250 mg	500 mg (12.5 mmol)	As above (three tablets)	
	Os-Cal+D	1,250 mg	500 mg (12.5 mmol)	As above (three tablets)	200 IU of vitamin D per tab
	Caltrate	600 mg	240 mg (6.0 mmol)	As above (six tablets)	
Calcium acetate	PhosLo	667 mg	169 mg (4.2 mmol)	As above (nine tablets)	More expensive than calcium carbonate Prescription medication
Magnesium carbonate	MagneBind	200: 200 mg $MgCO_3$ with 400 mg $CaCO_3$	160 mg (4.0 mmol)	Dose limited by serum Mg levels and diarrhea	85 mg (3.5 mmol) of elemental magnesium per tablet; dialysate magnesium concentrations should be adjusted
Magnesium carbonate	MagneBind	300: 300 mg $MgCO_3$ with 250 mg $CaCO_3$	100 mg (2.5 mmol)	Dose limited by serum Mg levels and diarrhea	85 mg (3.5 mmol) of elemental magnesium per tablet; dialysate magnesium concentrations should be adjusted
Lanthanum carbonate	Fosrenol	250-mg and 500-mg tablets	N/A	1,250 mg t.i.d.; higher doses have not been tested long term given up to a maximum average daily dose of 13 g daily in ESRD patients; dose may be limited by side effect of GI discomfort	Significantly more expensive than other products; must be chewed
Sevelamer hydrochloride	Renagel	400-mg and 800-mg tablets	N/A		Significantly more expensive than other products

t.i.d., three times per day; GI, gastrointestinal.

(2) Calcium acetate (PhosLo) is available in 667-mg tablets (169 mg [4.2 mmol] of elemental calcium), and the recommended initial dose is two tablets with each meal. Upward titration may be necessary to establish adequate phosphate control. Studies have shown that calcium acetate is, per gram, twice as potent as calcium carbonate. However, after the difference in dosage is taken into account, overall efficacy of the two drugs appears to be similar. Furthermore, because calcium carbonate is 40% calcium and calcium acetate is 25% calcium, the number of tablets that must be ingested daily is similar for the two drugs.

b. Sevelamer hydrochloride (Renagel) is a nonaluminum, non–calcium-based phosphorus binder that traps phosphorus in the bowel through ion exchange and hydrogen binding. The drug is available in 400- and 800-mg tablets and should be started at 800–1,600 mg three times per day with meals. It can be titrated upward to attain necessary phosphate control, though this may require a significant pill load and financial burden for the patient. The absence of an absorbable cation makes this agent extremely useful for those predisposed to hypercalcemia and those already at the limit of calcium supplementation. It is most effective at a pH between 5 and 7 (Chertow et al., 1999). In addition, sevelamer has the benefit of low-density lipoprotein (LDL) reduction through bile salt binding. The main side effect of sevelamer is gastrointestinal (GI) discomfort. Occasionally hypocalcemia or a mild metabolic acidosis occurs. A higher calcium bath or calcium supplementation can be utilized if patients develop hypocalcemia.

c. Lanthanum carbonate (Fosrenol) has good phosphate-binding properties and a low level of absorption. It is available in 250-, 500-, 750-, and 1,000-mg chewable tablets. A reasonable starting dose is 500 mg three times per day with upward titration as needed, not exceeding doses of 1,250 mg orally three times per day. Thus far, there has been no evidence of toxic accumulation or adverse effects on bone metabolism (D'Haese et al., 2003). Its main side effects are related to GI discomfort. In addition, the chewable preparation may be convenient for patients with a large swallowed pill load, but difficult for patients with poor dentition. Like sevelamer hydrochloride, lanthanum carbonate is particularly useful in individuals at risk for hypercalcemia. However, both products are notably more expensive than other available phosphate binders.

d. Aluminum-based binders were the primary therapy for hyperphosphatemia until the mid-1980s, when the accumulation of aluminum to toxic levels was found to result in hematologic, neurologic, and bone complications. As a general rule, these agents should no longer be used chronically. Usage of aluminum-based therapies for short periods may be necessary to reduce severely elevated phosphorus and calcium × phosphorus products in patients with severe hyperparathyroidism and/or concurrent hypercalcemia. Coingestion of citrate (Shohl solution, calcium citrate, fruit juices, Alka-Seltzer) greatly enhances aluminum absorption and can lead to acute aluminum neurotoxicity.

e. Magnesium binders have been used as phosphorus-reducing agents primarily in combination with calcium binders. Magnesium carbonate is available in preparation with calcium carbonate (Magnebind) in a 200-mg tablet (with 400 mg of calcium carbonate) and a 300-mg tablet (with 250 mg of calcium carbonate). The suggested starting dose is one to three tablets per meal, with dose titration limited by oral calcium load (1.5 g per day) and serum magnesium levels. In a study of 15 hemodialysis patients, magnesium carbonate, in conjunction with dialysis solution magnesium concentrations of 0.6 mg/dL (0.25 mM), allowed a reduction in calcium carbonate dose without compromising control of the serum phosphorus (Delmez et al., 1996). In addition, higher doses of calcitriol could be used without causing hypercalcemia. Despite a mean dose of 465 mg (19 mmol) per day of elemental magnesium during the trial, serum levels did not change, nor did diarrhea develop.

f. Nicotinamide (niacinamide) is widely available as a vitamin supplement in a variety of preparations. It has recently been shown to lower serum phosphate in animal models by inhibiting the sodium-dependent phosphate co-transporter present in the renal tubule and small intestine of rats. A study of 65 hemodialysis patients showed that nicotinamide decreased serum phosphorus and iPTH without an increase in serum calcium (Takahashi, 2004). The starting dose of nicotinamide is 500 mg daily with dose titration by 250 mg as needed to obtain control of the serum phosphorus. In addition, this agent reduced LDL levels and raised high-density lipoprotein (HDL) levels during this trial. Its main adverse effect was GI discomfort. Further clinical trials are necessary to confirm these results. Mild thrombocytopenia (Rottembourg et al., 2005) has recently been reported as a complication of nicotinamide use for this purpose.

g. Combination therapies. Combined treatment with different types of phosphate binders may be advantageous and cost effective. These regimens should be individually tailored to each patient. Combinations should take into account the patient's medication preferences, side effect tolerance, and financial considerations. Total daily exposure to elemental calcium, magnesium, or lanthanum should also factor into the choice of agents used. For example, the combination of calcium-based and non–calcium-based agents may provide target phosphorus control and calcium supplementation without risking excess exposure to calcium. Studies have not yet been done to establish the efficacy of such regimens.

V. Management of low PTH below the target range (an iPTH <150 pg/mL [16 pmol/L] or biPTH <80 pg/mL [~9 pmol/L]) is necessary to treat or prevent adynamic bone disease. The goal should be to increase the PTH into the target range.

A. Dialysis solution. Usually the hemodialysis solution calcium concentration should not exceed 2.5 mEq/L (1.25 mM) in these patients. Rarely, use of a higher dialysis solution calcium is necessary to maintain a corrected calcium in a safe range (generally >7.5 mg/dL [>1.9 mmol/L]). The low serum calcium in these patients is a potent stimulus to PTH secretion and gland hyperplasia, and therefore should generally be tolerated in this low PTH state. Use of dialysis solution calcium of 1.0–2.0 mEq/L (0.5–1.0 mM) for 3–6 months has been shown to stimulate PTH secretion by inducing repetitive intradialytic hypocalcemia. However, this treatment should be used with caution as intradialytic hypocalcemia can cause hypotension. In peritoneal dialysis patients with adynamic bone disease and low PTH levels, use of a 1.0 mM (2.0 mEq/L) calcium dialysis solution improved bone formation rate markedly and increased serum PTH values (Haris et al., 2006).

B. Calcium and phosphorus control. In this group of patients the serum calcium should be maintained in the low-normal range (8.4–9.5 mg/dL) or even below this range to stimulate PTH secretion.

   1. Low serum phosphorus levels inhibit PTH secretion and parathyroid gland hyperplasia. In patients with low PTH, predialysis serum phosphorus should be kept within the target range, and phosphorus binders should be reduced or eliminated to minimize the risk of hypophosphatemia. A mild elevation in serum phosphorus between 4.5 and 5.5 mg/dL (1.5 and 1.8 mmol/L) may be reasonable to stimulate PTH secretion.

   2. Calcium-based phosphorus binders should be avoided as the calcium absorbed further suppresses PTH.

      a. Vitamin D and calcimimetics. Use of active vitamin D should almost always be avoided in this population as it will further suppress PTH and inhibit parathyroid gland hyperplasia. Rarely, small doses of any form of active vitamin D are required to increase intestinal calcium absorption. The minimum dose needed to return corrected calcium to a safe range should be used. Supplementation of vitamin D (ergocalciferol, vitamin D_2 or cholecalciferol, vitamin D_3) is not contraindicated and may help prevent development of osteomalacia. Calcimimetics have no role in the management of low PTH.

      b. Miscellaneous therapies.

         (1) Bisphosphonates. While these agents can increase bone density in osteoporosis, they have not been adequately tested and shown to be efficacious in dialysis patients. Bisphosphonates decrease bone resorption by inhibiting osteoclasts. This reduction in bone turnover may be deleterious in dialysis patients, creating a form of adynamic bone disease. Generally, these agents should not be used in dialysis patients.

         (2) Teriparatide. A synthetic form of PTH(1–34), this polypeptide induces a marked increase in bone density in osteoporotic patients when administered as a daily subcutaneous injection. It has not been tested in dialysis patients, but may be of value in the treatment of adynamic bone disease, as PTH levels are usually low in this disorder. Further studies are needed to define its role in the low bone turnover disease in dialysis patients.

VI.   Management of PTH in target range. The PTH target range for dialysis patients is an iPTH of 150–300 pg/mL (16–32 pmol/L) or a biPTH of 80–160 pg/mL (around 9–18 pmol/L). This range is most likely to maintain bone turnover in a normal range.

A.   Dialysis solution. Virtually all these dialysis patients should be maintained on a 2.5 mEq/L (1.25 mM) calcium bath. Use of a lower calcium bath is likely to stimulate further PTH secretion and parathyroid hyperplasia, and use of a higher calcium bath is likely to suppress PTH and lead to chronic calcium overload in most patients.

B.   Calcium and phosphorus control. To maintain optimal PTH control, these patients should have corrected calcium maintained in the 8.4–10.2 mg/dL (2.1–2.6 mmol/L) range, and serum phosphorus between 3.5 and 5.5 mg/dL (1.1–1.8 mmol/L).

C.   Vitamin D and calcimimetics. Initiation of active vitamin D or calcimimetics is usually unnecessary when serum PTH is in the target range. Rarely, small doses of active vitamin D are required to increase intestinal calcium absorption and normalize serum calcium. Supplementation of vitamin D (ergocalciferol, vitamin D_2 or cholecalciferol, vitamin D_3) is not contraindicated and may help prevent development of osteomalacia.

VII.   Management of high PTH

A.   Dialysis solution. Most patients should be maintained on a 2.0–2.5 mEq/L (1.0–1.25 mM) calcium bath. A lower calcium bath can be used to treat or prevent hypercalcemia associated with use of active vitamin D; however, this intradialytic hypocalcemia will stimulate PTH secretion and may enhance gland hyperplasia. Use of a higher calcium bath will suppress PTH but chronically increase the calcium burden, and therefore is rarely a wise option. In patients receiving six times per week nocturnal dialysis, a 3.0 mEq/L dialysis solution (1.5 mM) is often used to prevent overstimulation of PTH secretion (see Chapter 14).

B.   Calcium and phosphorus control. The corrected calcium should be maintained in the 8.4–10.2 mg/dL (2.1–2.6 mmol/L) range, and serum phosphorus between 3.5 and 5.5 mg per dL (1.1 and 1.8 mmol/L). Although high serum calcium will lower PTH, it is inefficient and likely contributes to vascular and tissue calcification. Hyperphosphatemia increases PTH secretion and control of serum phosphorus will lower PTH.

C.   Active Vitamin D and D analogs suppress serum PTH in a dose-dependent fashion (Malluche et al., 2002). The higher the pretreatment PTH, the larger the dose required to suppress PTH into the target range. The medications are usually

Table 35-3. Characteristics of commonly used vitamin D analogs

Medication	Trade Name	Route	Dosing Information	Comments
Calcitriol	Rocaltrol	PO	Starting dose: 0.25 mcg daily or 0.5 mcg three times per week Dose range: 0.25–2 mcg daily Available in 0.25- and 0.5-mcg tablets	Monitor calcium and phosphorus at least monthly
	Calcijex	IV	0.02 mcg/kg (or 1–2 mcg) given three times weekly	
Doxercalciferol	Hectorol	PO	Titrate by 0.5–1 mcg every 2–4 weeks Starting dose: 2.5–5.0 mcg three times per week Titrate by 2.5 mcg every 8 weeks Available in 2.5-mcg tablets	A vitamin D prohormone that is metabolized in the liver to active 1,25(OH)$_2$ vitamin D$_2$ Oral administration in dialysis patients is more hypercalcemic and hyperphosphatemic than IV administration
	Hectorol	IV	Starting dose: 2.5–5.0 mcg three times per week Titrate by 1–2 mcg every 8 weeks	
Paricalcitol	Zemplar	PO	Dosing: 1–2 mcg daily or 2–4 mcg on a thrice-weekly regimen Titrate by 1-mcg increments on the daily schedule, or by 2 mcg on the thrice-weekly schedule	The oral form caused minimal alterations in calcium and phosphorus, comparable to placebo
	Zemplar	IV	0.04–0.1 mcg/kg or give dose in mcg equal to biPTH/40 or iPTH/80 three times per week Titrate by 30%–50% at 4-week intervals	The IV preparation can also be administered on a once-weekly regimen based on the cumulative weekly dose

given intravenously during each dialysis, but can be given orally, usually two to three times a week (Table 35-3).

1. **Calcitriol (Calcijex, Rocaltrol)** or $1,25(OH)_2D_3$ is a synthetic form of the natural compound, and is usually started at $1-2$ μg IV with each dialysis.

2. **Paricalcitol (Zemplar)** or 19-Nor-$1,25(OH)_2D_2$ is a vitamin D analog that has less hypercalcemic and hyperphosphatemic actions in animal studies. In humans, the evidence of superiority over calcitriol is more limited. A double blind trial versus placebo in CKD stage 3 and 4 patients showed potent PTH suppression with changes in serum calcium and phosphorus similar to placebo (Coyne et al., 2006). A large historical cohort study found improved survival in dialysis patients receiving paricalcitol compared to calcitriol (Teng et al., 2003). The initial dose in mcg per dialysis treatment can be estimated by dividing the pretreatment iPTH by 80 or biPTH by 40. Others have found that a starting dose of iPTH divided by 120 is equally effective and may require fewer dosing adjustments to prevent oversuppression of iPTH (Mitsopolous et al., 2006). An oral formulation of paricalcitol is also available for patients with CKD or patients on peritoneal dialysis who do not have regular intravenous access. A starting dose of 1 mcg daily or 2 mcg three times a week should be administered to patients with an iPTH ≤500 pg/mL (52 pmol/L). An initial dose of 2 mcg daily or 4 mcg three times a week should be started in patients with an iPTH >500 pg/mL (52 pmol/L).

3. **Doxercalciferol (Hectorol)** or $1\alpha(OH)D_2$ is a vitamin D prohormone that is metabolized by the liver to active $1,25(OH)_2D_2$. Initial dosing is 2.5–5.0 mcg intravenously or orally each dialysis treatment.

4. **Dose adjustments** of active vitamin D products for PTH control are based on subsequent PTH determinations, which should be performed monthly initially to establish control, then reassessed quarterly. If hypercalcemia (corrected calcium >10.2 mg/dL [>2.6 mmol/L]) develops, the dose should be decreased by 30%–50%, or held until the hypercalcemia resolves and then restarted at a lower dose (Fig. 35-1).

D. Calcimimetics bind to the calcium-sensing receptor on the parathyroid gland, making it more responsive to the ambient ionized calcium and resulting in suppression of PTH (Goodman et al., 2000). Unlike active vitamin D products, calcimimetics result in a decrease in serum calcium and phosphorus. Cinacalcet (Sensipar), the only calcimimetic presently available, is a pill available in 30, 60, and 90 mg. Maximal PTH suppression of 60%–80% occurs 2–4 hours after each dose, and 30%–50% suppression at 24 hours is observed in about two thirds of patients. Serum PTH should be measured 12–24 hours after a dose. The initial dose of cinacalcet should be 30 mg daily regardless of serum PTH, and should not be initiated if the corrected calcium is <8.4 mg/dL (<2.1 mmol/L). The dose should be increased by 30-mg increments up to a maximum of 180 mg per day, based on monthly or quarterly PTH results, provided the corrected calcium is >7.8 mg/dL (>2.0 mmol/L). A fall in serum calcium accompanies PTH

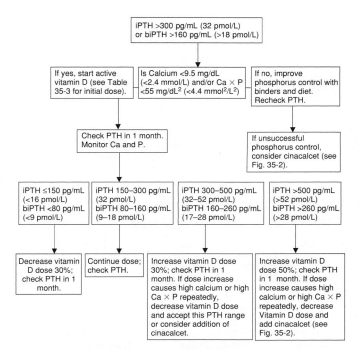

Figure 35-1. Guideline for vitamin D dosing in secondary hyperparathyroidism. iPTH, intact parathyroid hormone; biPTH, biointact parathyroid hormone.

suppression, and hypocalcemia of <7.5 mg/dL (<1.9 mmol/L) occurs in about 5% of patients. Hypocalcemia is rarely symptomatic, and can be managed by the addition of 500 to 1,000 mg of elemental calcium on an empty stomach, an increase or addition of active vitamin D, or an increase in dialysis solution calcium to 3.0–3.5 mEq/L (1.5–1.75 mM). The other major side effects of cinacalcet are nausea and vomiting, which occur in up to 30% of patients but can be minimized by taking the medication with a meal, and rash (Fig. 35-2).

E. Parathyroidectomy. Despite aggressive efforts to control PTH levels, surgical parathyroidectomy continues to be necessary in those patients with severe hyperparathyroidism. Parathyroidectomy rates were higher among patients who were younger, female, nondiabetic, and receiving peritoneal dialysis, and those with a longer duration of dialysis (Foley et al., 2005).

1. Indications. Failure of high-dosage intravenous active vitamin D and calcimimetic therapy to improve findings of hyperparathyroidism suggests the presence of large, poorly suppressible glands that require removal.

The indications for parathyroidectomy are listed in Table 35-4. When parathyroidectomy is being contemplated for

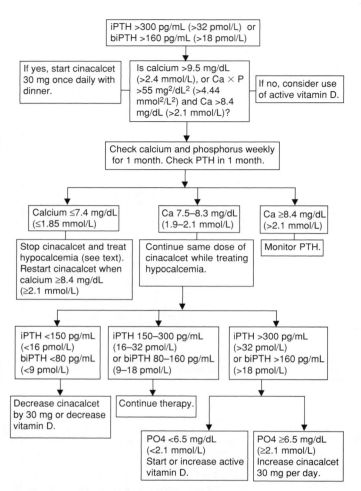

Figure 35-2.   Guideline for cinacalcet dosing in secondary hyperparathyroidism. iPTH, intact parathyroid hormone; biPTH, biointact parathyroid hormone.

the treatment of refractory osteitis fibrosa or hypercalcemia, very high PTH levels would be expected, and it is important to document a high serum PTH level (e.g., iPTH usually >1,000 pg/mL [~100 pmol/L] or biPTH usually >500 pg/mL [~50 pmol/L]) before contemplating surgery. A lower serum PTH level should be suppressible with calcimimetics or calcitriol. Also, lower serum PTH levels or normal bone-specific alkaline phosphatase should prompt one to question the diagnosis. Bone biopsy should show marked osteitis fibrosa

Table 35-4. Indications for parathyroidectomy

- Severe progressive symptomatic osteitis fibrosa (skeletal pain and/or fractures) despite adequate medical management, including serum phosphorus control and calcitriol therapy
- Very high levels of PTH plus any of the following:
  - Persistent hypercalcemia if other causes have been excluded
  - Severe intractable pruritus
  - Persistent severe soft tissue calcification despite attempts to control the serum phosphorus level
  - Idiopathic disseminated skin necrosis (calciphylaxis)
  - Incapacitating arthritis, periarthritis, and spontaneous tendon ruptures

with many osteoclasts, increased tetracycline labeling, and minimal aluminum staining.

2. Relative contraindications. Accumulation of aluminum on the bone mineralizing surface increases markedly after parathyroidectomy and suggests that parathyroidectomy should not be done in patients who are aluminum loaded. If there is a history of long-term aluminum exposure, a bone biopsy should be performed prior to parathyroidectomy to exclude significant aluminum accumulation.

3. Surgical strategy. Parathyroid surgery is a complex endeavor and requires the services of a surgeon with experience in this procedure. Aberrantly located glands, and three, five, or even six rather than the usual four glands, may be present. An attempt may be made to localize the glands preoperatively using 10-MHz ultrasonographic scanning or thallium–technetium scanning, but this is usually not necessary.

Traditionally, the operation of choice was subtotal parathyroidectomy: Total resection of three glands and 75% of the fourth. The alternative approach has been total parathyroidectomy, with autotransplantation of some parathyroid tissue into the forearm or, more recently, subcutaneously in the presternal area (Kinnaert et al., 2000). Both procedures entail some disadvantages, including the risks of permanent hypoparathyroidism and recurrence (or lack of resolution) of bone disease or hypercalcemia. Recurrence and failure to improve are troublesome problems; often it is uncertain whether the cause is hyperfunction of residual or transplanted parathyroid tissue or the unsuspected presence of an additional gland that was overlooked at the time of surgery. Total parathyroidectomy without implantation is sometimes performed in severe cases to minimize the risk of recurrence. However, this is not routinely done due to the potential risk of inducing persistent hypoparathyroidism.

4. Chemical ablation. Percutaneous injection of ethanol or calcitriol into the parathyroid glands of patients with severe secondary hyperparathyroidism has been used to cause regression of the glands and moderate parathyroid hormone secretion. It is performed using ultrasound or color Doppler flow mapping and may be considered in those who are poor surgical risks and in centers with the appropriate expertise (Kakuta et al., 1999). The risk of recurrent laryngeal nerve palsy has been reported to be low.

5. Postoperative hypocalcemia. Within several hours of parathyroidectomy, but especially during the first postoperative days, profound hypocalcemia can develop, the extent of which depends on the degree of osteitis fibrosa, which can be predicted by the extent of preoperative serum alkaline phosphatase elevation and bone histology. In addition to oral calcium supplements (2–4 g [50–100 mmol] per day), large dosages of intravenous calcium (0.5–5.0 g per day) and oral or intravenous calcitriol (2–6 mcg per day) may be required to maintain serum calcium levels in an acceptable range (Dawborn et al., 1983). Some advocate starting calcitriol and oral calcium therapy a few days before the procedure even in hypercalcemic patients.

VIII. Miscellaneous disorders and management issues
A. Calcific uremic arteriolopathy (CUA), previously known as "calciphylaxis," is an unusual disorder seen predominately in dialysis patients. Early signs and symptoms include livedo reticularis and painful red nodules, which progress to ulcerative and necrotic lesions. Risk factors include female gender, obesity, and Caucasian race. Exposure to the uremic milieu may be responsible for altering vascular smooth muscle cells and increasing the expression of factors involved in ectopic mineralization, such as osteopontin and core-binding factor alpha (Moe and Chen, 2003). Further mineralization from elevated calcium and phosphorus levels ultimately results in arteriolar calcification, occlusion, and tissue ischemia. A high index of suspicion is necessary to identify the disease as early as possible. The differential diagnosis includes vasculitis, Coumadin (warfarin)-associated skin necrosis, cryoglobulinemia, calcinosis cutis, and panniculitis. Bone scan has been reported to identify calcium deposition in 97% with early, plaque–only, CUA (Fine and Zacharias, 2002). Skin biopsy shows characteristic arteriolar calcifications in the medial layer.

Once the diagnosis is made, calcium-containing supplements and vitamin D analogs should be discontinued, and non–calcium-based phosphate binders should be titrated for aggressive phosphorus control. Parathyroidectomy is recommended for those with CUA and elevated iPTH (>500 pg/mL or >50 pmol/L), though hyperparathyroidism is not required for CUA and patients may in fact have low to normal iPTH levels (Bleyer et al., 1998). Coumadin (warfarin), which inhibits the calcium-regulatory matrix gla-protein, should be discontinued. Sodium thiosulfate, at a dose of 25 g IV three times per week, has been reported in a small number of patients to decrease pain and plaque size, presumably due to the high solubility of calcium-thiosulfate salts (Cicone et al., 2004). Pamidronate has also been cited in a single case report to exhibit rapid clinical improvements (Monney et al., 2004). Wound care is critically important in ulcerative lesions and surgical debridement and antibiotics may be necessary.

Hyperbaric oxygen (Basile et al., 2002) and low-dose tissue plasminogen activator (Sewell et al., 2004) have been reported to promote wound healing in single case studies.

B. Aluminum toxicity. Aluminum toxicity is rarely seen today due to the development of nonaluminum phosphorus binders and the improvement in water purity. Among those still exposed to aluminum-based compounds, greater risk for accumulation occurs in diabetics, the iron deficient, children, and those with exposure to citrate (which increases aluminum absorption). Aluminum bone disease results in diffuse bone pain or fractures with low iPTH, hypercalcemia, and normal alkaline phosphatase. See Chapter 43.

SELECTED READINGS

Asmus HG, et al. Two year comparison of sevelamer and calcium carbonate effects on cardiovascular calcification and bone density. *Nephrol Dial Transplant* 2005;20:1653–1661.

Basile C, et al. Hyperbaric oxygen therapy for calcific uremic arteriolopathy: a case series. *J Nephrol* 2002;15(6):676–680.

Bleyer AJ, et al. A case control study of proximal calciphylaxis. *Am J Kidney Dis* 1998;32:376–383.

Block GA, et al. Mineral metabolism, mortality, and morbidity in maintenance hemodialysis. *J Am Soc Nephrol* 2004;15:2208–2218.

Chertow GM, et al. Cinacalcet hydrochloride (Sensipar) in hemodialysis patients with active vitamin D derivatives with controlled PTH and elevated calcium × phosphate. *Clin J Am Soc Nephrol* 2006;1:305–312.

Chertow GM, et al. Long-term effects of sevelamer hydrochloride on the calcium × phosphate product and lipid profile of haemodialysis patients. *Nephrol Dial Transplant* 1999;14:2907–2914.

Cicone JS, et al. Successful treatment of calciphylaxis with intravenous sodium thiosulfate. *Am J Kidney Dis* 2004;43(6):1104–1108.

Clinical algorithms on renal osteodystrophy. *Nephrol Dial Transplant* 2000;15 (Suppl 5):40–57.

Coen G, et al. PTH 1-84 and PTH "7-84" in the noninvasive diagnosis of renal bone disease. *Am J Kidney Dis* 2002;40(2):348–354.

Coyne DW, et al. Paricalcitol capsule for the treatment of secondary hyperparathyroidism in stages 3 and 4 CKD. *Am J Kidney Dis* 2006;47:263–276.

Cupisti A, et al. Effect of boiling on dietary phosphate and nitrogen intake. *J Renal Nutr* 2006;16(1):36–40.

Dawborn JK, et al. Parathyroidectomy in chronic renal failure. *Nephron* 1983;33:100–105.

Delmez JA, et al. Calcium acetate as a phosphorus binder in hemodialysis patients. *J Am Soc Nephrol* 1992;3:96–102.

Delmez JA, et al. Magnesium carbonate as a phosphorus binder: a prospective, controlled, crossover study. *Kidney Int* 1996;49:163–167.

D'Haese PC et al. A multicenter study of the effects of lanthanum carbonate (Fogrenol) and calcium carbonate on renal bone disease in dialysis patients. *Kidney Int Suppl* 2003;85:S73–S78.

Fine A, Zacharias J. Calciphylaxis is usually non-ulcerating: risk factors, outcome and therapy. *Kidney Int* 2002;61:2210–2217.

Floege J. When man turns to stone: extraosseous calcification in uremic patients. *Kidney Int* 2004;65:2447–2462.

Foley RN, et al. The fall and rise of parathyroidectomy in U.S. hemodialysis patients, 1992 to 2002. *J Am Soc Nephrol* 2005;16: 210–218.

Goldsmith D, Ritz E, Covic A. Vascular calcification: a stiff challenge for the nephrologists. *Kidney Int* 2004;66:1315–1333.

Goodman WG, et al. A calcimimetic agent lowers plasma parathyroid hormone levels in patients with secondary hyperparathyroidism. *Kidney Int* 2000;58:436–445.

Gotch FA, et al. A kinetic model of inorganic phosphorus mass balance in hemodialysis therapy. *Blood Purif* 2003;21:51–57.

Hampl H, et al. Long-term results of total parathyroidectomy without autotransplantation in patients with and without renal failure. *Miner Electrolyte Metab* 1999;25:161–170.

Haris A, et al., Reversal of adynamic bone disease by lowering of dialysate calcium. *Kidney Int* 2006;70:931–937.

Henley C, et al. 1,25-dihydroxyvitamin D3 but not cinacalcet HCl (Sensipar/Mimpara) treatment mediates aortic calcification in a rat model. *Nephrol Dial Transplant* 2005;20:1370–1377.

Hutchison AJ, et al. Long-term efficacy and tolerability of lanthanum carbonate: results from a 3-year study. *Nephron Clin Practice* 2006;102:c61–c71.

Kakuta T, et al. Prognosis of parathyroid function after successful percutaneous ethanol injection therapy guided by color Doppler flow mapping in chronic dialysis patients. *Am J Kidney Dis* 1999;33:1091–1099.

Kalantar-Zadeh K, et al. Survival predictability of time-varying indicators of bone disease in maintenance hemodialysis patients. *Kidney Int* 2006;70(4):771–780.

Kim HW, et al. Calcitriol regresses cardiac hypertrophy and QT dispersion in secondary hyperparathyroidism on hemodialysis. *Nephron Clin Practice* 2006;102:c21–c29.

Kinnaert P, et al. Long-term results of subcutaneous parathyroid grafts in uremic patients. *Arch Surg* 2000;135(2):186–190.

LaClair RE, et al. Prevalence of calcidiol deficiency in CKD: a cross-sectional study across latitudes in the United States. *Am J Kidney Dis* 2006;45:1026–1033.

Lehmann G, et al. Specific measurement of PTH (1-84) in various forms of renal osteodystrophy (ROD) as assessed by bone histomorphometry. *Kidney Int* 2005;68(3):1206–1214.

London GM, et al. Arterial calcification and bone histomorphometry in end-stage renal disease. *J Am Soc Nephrol* 2004;15:1943–1951.

Lornoy W, et al. Impact of convective flow on phosphorus removal in maintenance hemodialysis patients. *J Ren Nutr* 2006;16(1): 47–53.

Malluche HH, Mawad H, Koszewski NJ. Update on vitamin D and its newer analogues: actions and rationale for treatment in chronic renal failure. *Kidney Int* 2002;62:367–374.

Manns B, et al. A systematic review of sevelamer in ESRD and an analysis of its potential economic impact in Canada and the United States. *Kidney Int* 2004;6:1239–1247.

Mistopoulos E, et al. Initial dosing of paricalcitol based on PTH levels in hemodialysis patients with secondary hyperparathyroidism. *Am J Kidney Dis* 2006;48(1):114–121.

Moe SM, Chen NX. Calciphylaxis and vascular calcification: a continuum of extra-skeletal osteogenesis. *Pediat Nephrol* 2003;18:969–975.

Monier-Faugere MC, et al. Improved assessment of bone turnover by the PTH-(1-84)/large C-PTH fragments ratio in ESRD patients. *Kidney Int* 2001;60(4):1460–1468.

Monney P, et al. Rapid improvement of calciphylaxis after intravenous pamidronate therapy in a patient with chronic renal failure. *Nephrol Dial Transplant* 2004;19(8):2130–2132.

Murphy-Gutekunst L. Hidden phosphorus in popular beverages: part 1. *J Ren Nutr* 2005;15(2):e1–e6. Available at: http://www.jrnjournal.org. Accessed 9/19/06.

Murphy-Gutekunst L, Uribarri J. Hidden phosphorus-enhanced meats: part 3. *J Ren Nutr* 2005;15(4):e1–e4. Available at: http://www.jrnjournal.org. Accessed 9/19/06.

Navarro JF, et al. Relationship between serum magnesium and parathyroid hormone levels in hemodialysis patients. *Am J Kidney Dis* 1999;34:43–48.

Qunibi WY, et al. Treatment of hyperphosphatemia in hemodialysis patients: the Calcium Acetate Renagel Evaluation (CARE study). *Kidney Int* 2004;65:1914–1926.

Ritter CS, et al. 25-Hydroxyvitamin D3 suppresses PTH synthesis and secretion by cultured bovine parathyroid cells: potential role for intracrine 1,25-dihydroxyvitamin D3 [Abstract]. *J Am Soc Nephrol* 2005(Oct); Renal Week SA-PO889.

Rottembourg JB, Launay-Vacher V, Massard J. Thrombocytopenia induced by nicotinamide in hemodialysis patients. *Kidney Int* 2005;68(6):2911–2912.

Salusky IB, et al. Similar predictive value of one turnover using first- and second-generation immunometric PTH assays in pediatric patients treated with peritoneal dialysis. *Kidney Int* 2003;63:1801–1808.

Scranton R, et al. Statin use and fracture risk: study of a U.S. veterans population. *Ann Intern Med* 2005;165:2007–2012.

Sewell LD, et al. Low-dose tissue plasminogen activator for calciphylaxis. *Arch Dermatol* 2004;140(9):1045–1048.

Spalding, EM, Chamney PW, Farrington K. Phosphate kinetics during hemodialysis: evidence for biphasic regulation. *Kidney Int* 2002;61:655–667.

Sprague SM, et al. Paricalcitol versus calcitriol in the treatment of secondary hyperparathyroidism. *Kidney Int* 2003;63:1483–1490.

Takahashi Y. Nicotinamide suppresses hyperphosphatemia in hemodialysis patients. *Kidney Int* 2004;65:1099–1104.

Teng M, et al. Survival of patients undergoing hemodialysis with paricalcitol or calcitriol therapy. *N Engl J Med* 2003;349:446–456.

Ubara Y, et al. Histomorphogenic features of bone in patients with primary and secondary hypoparathyroidism. *Kidney Int* 2003;63:1809–1816.

WEB REFERENCES

HDCN calcium:phosphorus:PTH:bone disease channel: http://www.hdcn.com/ch/calphos/

NKF KDOQI guidelines: http://www.kidney.org/

Dialysis in Infants and Children

Susan R. Mendley

Choices in dialysis treatment for infants and children are wide and include the full range of therapies utilized in adult patients. Theoretical considerations of clearance, kinetic modeling, and adequacy of dialysis apply equally in pediatric dialysis, although they are less well studied in this population than in adults. There are important technical considerations in performing dialysis on patients whose weights may vary by as much as 50-fold. Furthermore, there are indications for and complications of the dialysis procedure that are unique to children. Finally, chronic care of children receiving dialysis is complex and requires attention to growth and development, age-specific nutritional interventions, consequences of metabolic disturbances, and psychosocial adjustment to achieve the goal of complete rehabilitation.

I. Acute dialysis

A. Indications. The indications for acute dialysis in an infant, child, or adolescent are similar to those in adults and include:

1. Oliguric acute renal failure where optimal nutritional and medical support will require fluid and/or electrolyte removal

2. Volume overload with congestive heart failure, pulmonary edema, or severe hypertension not manageable with diuretics or conservative measures

3. Hyperkalemia with electrocardiographic abnormalities

4. Metabolic acidosis that cannot be safely corrected with sodium bicarbonate administration because of risk of sodium or volume overload

5. Symptoms of uremic encephalopathy, with particular attention to seizures

6. Uremic pericarditis

7. Tumor lysis syndrome or severe hyperuricemia complicating chemotherapy for malignancy

8. Progressively rising blood urea nitrogen (BUN) level in a situation where imminent recovery is not anticipated and uremic consequences are likely. The BUN level where concern arises will vary with the age of the child; 35–50 mg/dL (12–18 mmol/L) is potentially dangerous in an infant, whereas 150 mg/dL (54 mmol/L) in an adolescent may necessitate initiation of dialysis.

9. Inborn error of metabolism with severe organic acidemia or hyperammonemia

10. Toxic ingestion. Guidelines for extracorporeal therapy for poisoning are found in Chapter 17.

B. Choice of acute dialysis modality

1. **Acute peritoneal dialysis** is most often used in this age group and has several advantages. It does not require sophisticated equipment or technical expertise. One can avoid the need for vascular access, blood priming, and anticoagulation; hemodynamic instability is uncommon. Continuous peritoneal dialysis provides efficient clearance in small children. However, severe hyperammonemia, hyperphosphatemia, or hyperkalemia often requires more rapid correction; in such situations, hemodialysis (sometimes in combination with continuous hemo[dia]filtration) may be more appropriate. Furthermore, volume removal by ultrafiltration in peritoneal dialysis is often unpredictable and may not be rapid enough in some patients with congestive heart failure or pulmonary edema. Dialysate leakage with risk of peritonitis may limit acute peritoneal dialysis.

There are no guidelines as to what constitutes adequate peritoneal dialysis in acute renal failure (ARF), and one attempts maximum possible clearance to compensate for catabolic stress, utilizing continuous exchanges. The initial prescription may include hourly exchanges; more frequent exchanges can be performed, although a greater fraction of total time is then spent in filling and draining, rather than in solute exchange. An automated cycler facilitates this process, limiting nursing effort and repeated opening of the catheter. Most cyclers can deliver exchange volumes small enough for infants and young children. When a cycler is unavailable or when fill volumes <200 mL are desirable, a modification can be made by hanging a large dialysis solution bag attached to a buretrol device (in-line sterile graduated cylinder) connected to the patient's peritoneal dialysis catheter either by a stopcock or a Y set. A drainage line is attached to the other limb of the Y or the stopcock. One periodically measures the desired volume into the buretrol and infuses it into the patient. The effluent dialysate is drained via the other limb of the Y set and measured, and the process is repeated without opening the system. The Gesco DialyNate system (Utah Medical Products Ltd., Midvale, UT) has been used to perform closed circuit, low-volume, manual continuous peritoneal dialysis in infants and very small children.

Exchange volumes are targeted at 40 mL/kg or greater, but immediately after catheter placement, it is prudent to limit volumes to half or three fourths of this volume to avoid leakage, which predisposes to peritonitis. Hourly exchanges usually result in obligate ultrafiltration even when 1.5% dextrose concentration is used, so that parenteral or enteral fluid intake is needed to avoid volume depletion and prolongation of ARF.

2. **Acute hemodialysis** is performed when peritoneal dialysis is contraindicated because of an intra-abdominal process (including recent abdominal surgery, diaphragmatic hernia, omphalocele, or gastroschisis) or respiratory limitation.

Acute hemodialysis in infants and small children requires experience and technical expertise, as well as size-appropriate dialyzers, blood lines, and vascular catheters. Very small patients may require blood priming of the hemodialysis circuit. Small patient size allows efficient and rapid solute clearance where appropriate (i.e., ammonia) but must be approached with caution where overly rapid osmolar shifts could precipitate seizures (reportedly more common in children than in adults). Dialyzers are available in a wide range of sizes for neonates through older adolescents (Table 36-1); however, the choices for very small dialyzers are limited.

3. Continuous therapies. Continuous hemofiltration (C-HF) or continuous hemodiafiltration (C-HDF) has been utilized in pediatric patients, ranging from preterm infants to older adolescents. The physiologic principles are unchanged from those in adults (see Chapter 13); because of small patient size, clearance can be extremely efficient, replacing a large fraction of endogenous renal function. In particular, continuous therapies permit better phosphorus clearance than intermittent hemodialysis or peritoneal dialysis and are thus frequently employed in the tumor lysis syndrome in children with Burkitt lymphoma or acute lymphoblastic leukemia.

Maintaining vascular access with adequate flow in small vessels can be problematic (Table 36-2) and is often the limiting factor. We have found pump-driven venovenous C-HF (CVVH) to perform more reliably and to maintain circuit patency longer, although others have reported equal success with arteriovenous C-HF (CAVH). As in acute hemodialysis, the entire circuit volume must be considered and a blood prime used if it is >10% of the patient's blood volume. The electrolyte concentrations and pH of the blood prime are far from normal values and many infants will experience hemodynamic instability at initiation of therapy. Zero balance ultrafiltration has been proposed to bring the concentrations in the blood prime close to physiologic values, which might avoid instability at initiation (Hackbarth et al., 2005). Cooling of the blood circuit is a concern in infants; a blood warmer may be used inline, although it increases the circuit volume. Hemofilters appropriate for pediatric use are listed in Table 36-3. Ultrafiltration is controlled by volumetric pump or automated weighing to avoid errors in replacement fluid, which, if compounded over days of therapy, could be dramatic in a small, anuric patient. The Baxter BM11/BM14, the Gambro, Prisma, the Braun Biopact, and the Fresenius 200 BH have been used in pediatric patients. Although the reported precision of the pumps in most systems is merely ± 10%, clinical experience suggests that the delivered volumes are considerably closer to target. Several studies have demonstrated the success of these devices in critically ill infants and children. Ultrafiltration rates in infants and small children may be as low as 5–30 mL per hour without replacement fluid (slow continuous ultrafiltration, SCUF) or as high as 100–600 mL per hour with replacement fluid (C-HF); larger children can tolerate ultrafiltration and replacement rates near those of adults. Commercially available bicarbonate-based dialysis solution or replacement solution (Normocarb, PrismaSate, Accusol, Hemosol BO) is the safest choice; errors in local preparation of solutions in hospital pharmacies are well recognized and are no longer necessary now that standardized solutions are available. Lactate-based replacement solutions can present an excessive lactate load to a small patient and are best avoided in children. Successful circuit anticoagulation has been reported with both heparin and citrate. Since the citrate infusion rate is scaled to circuit blood flow, which is relatively large in infants and small children, citrate accumulation may occur after prolonged therapy resulting in "citrate lock" or persistently low ionized calcium levels despite calcium infusion. The combination of fixed concentration bicarbonate-containing replacement fluid and citrate anticoagulation may result in metabolic alkalosis after several days of therapy. In reported series, infants are more often anticoagulated with heparin. Doses for systemic heparin anticoagulation in infants are larger than those reported for adults and monitoring the system by activated clotting times (ACTs) is recommended. Circuit life is significantly shorter in pediatric patients run without anticoagulation.

II.   Chronic dialysis
A.   Indications. Optimal management of chronic renal failure (CRF) avoids some of the historical indications for initiation of dialysis. Anemia, acidosis, hyperparathyroidism, and growth delay can usually be managed medically, so nephrologists must be attuned to subtle indications of uremia, that is, diminished energy (less vigorous play), resumption of napping, anorexia (with absence of expected weight gain), and inattentiveness at school or failure to attain expected developmental milestones, in order to recognize the appropriate time to begin dialysis. The National Kidney Foundation's (NKF) Kidney Disease Outcome Quality Initiative (KDOQI) (2006 update) guidelines recommend that dialysis initiation in children be considered when glomerular filtration rate (GFR) falls below 14–15 mL per minute per 1.73 m^2; dialysis is recommended (peritoneal dialysis guidelines) when GFR falls below 8. Measurements and estimates of residual GFR in small children are problematic; clearly the clinical status of the child is the most important parameter in making therapeutic decisions. Medically unresponsive volume overload, poor nutritional status, hypertension, hyperphosphatemia, hyperkalemia, acidosis, growth failure, or symptomatic uremia would prompt initiation of dialysis. Chronic dialysis is usually an interim measure to allow time to prepare for kidney transplantation.
B.   Choice of chronic dialysis modality
    1.   Chronic peritoneal dialysis is often the therapy of choice for pediatric patients. Transperitoneal solute exchange in children appears to be as efficient as in adults. Since peritoneal surface area is correlated with body surface area, small children have a relatively large surface for solute exchange compared with adults, which makes peritoneal

Table 36-1. Characteristics of low-volume dialyzers suitable for pediatric use

Dialyzer	Priming Volume (mL)	Surface Area (m^2)	Urea Clearance (Q_B 200 or as Specified)	B_{12} Clearance (at Highest Tested Q_B)	K_0A	Membrane	Manufacturer
100 HG	18	0.2	76 $Q_B = 100$ 92 $Q_B = 150$ 106 $Q_B = 200$	17	170	Hemophan	Gambro/Hospal
Polyflux 6H	52	0.6	50 $Q_B = 50$ 97 $Q_B = 100$ 136 $Q_B = 150$ 167 $Q_B = 200$	90	465 $Q_B = 200$	Polyflux (Polyarylethersulfone, Polyvinylpyrrolidone, Polyamide)	Gambro
CA50, CA70, CA90, CA-HP90	35, 45, 60, 60	0.5, 0.7, 0.9, 0.9	128 (147 $Q_B = 300$), 153 (175 $Q_B = 300$), 166 (199 $Q_B = 300$), 213 ($Q_B = 300$)	27, 36, 45, 59	243, 333, 435, 512	Cellulose acetate	Baxter
F3, F4, F5, F40	28, 42, 63, 42	0.4, 0.7, 1.0, 0.7	125, 155 (183 $Q_B = 300$), 170 (206 $Q_B = 300$), 165 (200 $Q_B = 300$)	20, 34, 47, 86	231, 364, 472, 440	Polysulfone	Fresenius
Filtryzer $B_1$0.6, $B_1$0.8, $B_2$0.5, $B_3$0.5, $B_3$0.8	46, 55, 35, 35, 49	0.6, 0.8, 0.5, 0.5, 0.8	139, 152, 123, 137, 163	49, 56, 35, 45, 61	266, 330, 205, 265, 404	PMMA	Toray

						Material	Manufacturer
AM SD 300, AM SD 400 M	30, 49		187, 206 ($Q_B = 300$)	29, 41	371, 457	Cuprammonium rayon	Asahi
PAN03, PAN06	33, 63	0.3, 0.6	136, 178 ($Q_B = 300$)	53, 85	171, 258	PAN	Asahi
Filtral 6	48	0.6	136	45	273	AN69	Hospal
MF5, MF15, MF50	72	1.0	170, 172, 175	45, 59, 90	493, —, 514	Polysulfone	Meditech
BioF 10	55	1.0	172	57	514	Cellulose	Meditech
MO 08, MO 10	49, 56	0.8, 1.0	166, 171	42, 47	474, 525	Hemophan	Meditech
NP08, NP10	49, 58	0.8, 1.0	165, 169	41, 45	465, 504	Cuprophane	Meditech
ME-08H, ME-10H	46, 55	0.8, 1.0	160, 170	39, 46	408, 494	Cellulose	Kawasumi

AN69, acrylonitrile and sodium methallyl sulfonate; PAN, polyacrylonitrile; PMMA, polymethylmethacrylate.

Table 36-2.   Catheters for use in pediatric extracorporeal renal replacement therapy

Patient Size	Catheter Size	Access Location
Neonate	UVC—5.0 F	Umbilicus
	UAC—3.5, 5.0 F	Umbilicus
	or 5.0 F single lumen	Femoral vein(s)
	or 6.5, 7.0 F dual lumen	Femoral vein(s)
3–15 kg	6.5, 7.0 F dual lumen	Femoral/subclavian vein
16–30 kg	7.0, 9.0 F dual lumen	Femoral/internal jugular/subclavian
>30 kg	9.0, 11.5 F dual lumen	Femoral/internal jugular/subclavian

UVC, umbilical vein catheter; UAC, umbilical artery catheter.

dialysis an effective modality. Peritoneal equilibration testing (PET) shows that young children are more likely to fall in the category of high or high-average transport, although this observation may be the result of large surface area for transport rather than a difference in peritoneal membrane characteristics. Enhanced glucose absorption will result in relatively rapid attainment of osmotic equilibrium between dialysate and plasma, limiting ultrafiltration on long dwells. For this reason, automated forms of peritoneal dialysis utilizing short dwells are most commonly used in children.

Peritoneal dialysis offers additional benefits as a chronic dialysis modality. It is technically simple and avoids the need for chronic vascular access (which is particularly difficult in infants and small children). Blood pressure and volume status may be better controlled with peritoneal dialysis than with hemodialysis. Less time is spent in the hospital and in the dialysis unit, with more time spent at school and engaged in other age-appropriate activities. Parents often feel they have greater control over their child's care when they perform peritoneal dialysis.

a.   Limitations to peritoneal dialysis. Previous abdominal surgery may result in intra-abdominal adhesions that make peritoneal dialysis impossible, particularly repair of complex urogenital anomalies, which are often a cause of end-stage renal disease (ESRD) in children. The presence of a ventriculoperitoneal shunt is a relative contraindication to peritoneal dialysis because of the concern for ascending infection to the central nervous system; however, there are reports of successful peritoneal dialysis in this situation. The presence of a ureterostomy, pyelostomy, or loop ileostomy is not an absolute contraindication to performance of peritoneal dialysis, although the risk of exit site infection and peritonitis with urinary organisms is increased.

Table 36-3. Hemofilters Appropriate for Pediatric Use

Hemofilter	Priming Volume (mL)	Surface Area (m^2)	Ultrafiltration Rate (mL per minute, $Q_B = 100$)	Membrane	Manufacturer
Minifilter Plus	15	0.07	1–8	Polysulfone	Baxter
RenafloII HF 400, 700	28, 53	0.3, 0.7	20–35, 35–45	Polysulfone	Minntech
Miniflow 10, Multiflow 60	3.5, 48	0.04, 0.6	4.2 ($Q_B = 20$), 38	AN69	Hospal
PAN-03, -06	33, 63	0.3, 0.6	15–28, 28–43	PAN	Asahi
PRISMA M10, M60 set	50, 84	0.04, 0.6	4.2 ($Q_B = 20$), 38	AN69	Gambro

AN69, acrylonitrile and sodium methallyl sulfonate; PAN, polyacrylonitrile.

b. Transplantation in peritoneal dialysis patients. Peritoneal dialysis is continued up to the time of renal transplantation without increased risk of infection. The peritoneal dialysis catheter is often removed at the time of living-donor transplantation (assuming immediate graft function), but sometimes it is left in place if a cadaver transplantation is performed. The catheter is removed electively once graft function is stable; delay in catheter removal has been associated with posttransplantation peritonitis in the dry abdomen.

c. Complications of peritoneal dialysis. The complications of pediatric peritoneal dialysis include those already described in adults (see Chapters 24–26). Peritoneal dialysis presents particular problems for children and families. Months or years of a demanding regimen may result in "burnout" or caregiver fatigue, which exacerbates underlying family conflicts; nonadherence to therapy becomes common, particularly among adolescents. The presence of a peritoneal dialysis catheter may adversely affect body image. Children have a higher rate of peritonitis than adults, which further complicates therapy. Eradication of nasal *Staphylococcus aureus* carriage leads to decreased exit site infection and peritonitis in adults; studies in children showed no benefit. Congenital defects in the diaphragm may result in communication between the pleural and peritoneal spaces. In some cases, a change to automated peritoneal dialysis (APD) with empty periods may permit continuation of peritoneal dialysis. Some children become obese from excessive glucose absorption from dialysate; this presents additional problems for body image as well as adversely affecting blood lipid levels and an already increased risk of cardiovascular disease. Chronic hypoalbuminemia develops in some patients, particularly with repeated peritonitis; its long-term consequences for growth in stature and lean body mass are unknown.

C. Apparatus for acute and chronic peritoneal dialysis

1. Lactate-based peritoneal dialysis solutions are available in a range of bag sizes appropriate for small patients who perform chronic ambulatory peritoneal dialysis and automated (cycler) peritoneal dialysis. Calcium concentrations of 1.25 mM and 1.75 mM are used depending on the required dose of calcium-based phosphorus binder. Standard dextrose concentrations (1.5%, 2.5%, and 4.25%) are utilized depending on the need for ultrafiltration. Enhanced glucose absorption in small children occasionally warrants higher glucose concentration to maintain ultrafiltration, although short-dwell dialysis is usually preferred in that situation. Amino acid–containing peritoneal dialysis solution is tolerated in children, although there remains a greater reliance on supplemental nasogastric feeding in infants and young children. Icodextrin-containing solutions have been used in children in whom adequate ultrafiltration was otherwise not achievable. Neutral pH solutions of pure bicarbonate or a bicarbonate/lactate combination have been shown to be safe in children and offer a potential benefit of protection of peritoneal membrane integrity. The long-term impact of new solutions on acid–base and nutritional status is still unclear and their role in chronic care of pediatric peritoneal dialysis patients is still to be determined.

2. Peritoneal dialysis catheters are available in neonatal and pediatric sizes of almost any configuration used in adults, including Tenckhoff (curled and straight), swan-neck, and Toronto-Western, usually with a choice of one or two cuffs. Most commonly placed in children is a one-cuff, curled Tenckhoff catheter with a straight tunnel and a laterally oriented exit site; North American Pediatric Renal Transplant Cooperative Study data suggest a benefit to double-cuffed catheters and downward-oriented exit sites in decreasing peritonitis rates.

   a. Implantation. Chronic catheters are almost invariably implanted surgically in pediatric patients under general anesthesia. Laparoscopic placement is feasible and safe with experienced surgeons. Several technical points have been alleged to be important:

   (1) Sealing the peritoneum around the catheter (to prevent leakage) by use of a pursestring suture, which is also affixed to the cuff. The exit site should be directed caudally, as shown in Figure 36-1, to facilitate drainage and to minimize the risk of exit site infection.

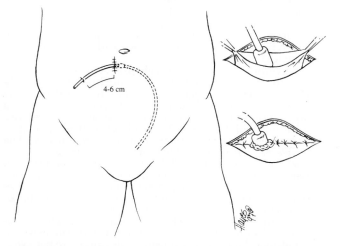

Figure 36-1. One method of implanting a peritoneal catheter in children. The pursestring suture used to seal the peritoneum includes the catheter cuff. A second pursestring suture (not shown) may also be used as described in the text to seal the posterior rectus sheath. (Modified from Alexander SR, et al. *Clinical parameters in continuous ambulatory peritoneal dialysis for infants and children. CAPD update.* **New York: Masson, 1981.)**

(2) Use of a second pursestring suture to seal the posterior rectus sheath opening and fix the posterior rectus sheath to the upper part of the cuff (to prevent leakage and displacement; this is not shown in Fig. 36-1).

(3) Performance of a partial omentectomy (to prevent obstruction)

(4) Intraoperative search for and closure of associated hernial defects, especially a patent tunica vaginalis

We try to allow 2 weeks for healing of the abdomen before using the catheter. It can be used immediately for acute peritoneal dialysis or unanticipated clinical deterioration in chronic renal failure, but one risks early leakage. Small exchange volumes and performance of APD in the supine position may help avoid dialysate leakage.

b. Acute "temporary" catheters can be placed after prefilling the abdomen with dialysate as in adults (see Chapter 20 for description of the technique in adults). Older acute PD catheters were much stiffer than chronic catheters, conferring a greater risk of bowel injury. Newer, more flexible acute PD catheters have been developed and some have reported success with their use with a low leakage and infection rate. Most centers utilize a surgically implanted chronic PD catheter for acute peritoneal dialysis, placing it at bedside in the intensive care unit in the most unstable patients.

3. APD cyclers have facilitated peritoneal dialysis in young patients, and all available cyclers permit sufficiently small exchange volumes to be used even in infants. Pediatric cycler tubing is available for some models of cyclers; it helps reduce dialysis inefficiency due to dead space in the tubing, which is an important consideration with very small dwell volumes (<200 mL).

D. Chronic peritoneal dialysis prescription

1. Continuous ambulatory peritoneal dialysis (CAPD). The technique for performing CAPD in the pediatric patient is similar to that in adults. Fill volumes are determined by patient comfort, but most children can tolerate 40 mL/kg or 800–1,000 mL/m^2 without discomfort or leakage once their catheter exit site is well healed. The NKF's KDOQI-recommended target fill volumes of 1,000–1,200 mL/m^2 (maximum 1,400 mL/m^2) are appropriate to reach clearance targets, although this may require assessment of intraperitoneal pressure. The choice of glucose concentration depends on ultrafiltration needs (fluid intake minus urine output and insensible losses).

a. Kinetic modeling of CAPD as Kt/V-urea and creatinine clearance has been performed in children; however, outcome data to define adequate clearance are not available. The NKF KDOQI (2006 update) recommendation for adequate CAPD in children is a weekly Kt/V-urea of 1.8 per week; if residual renal function contributes to this clearance, it should be measured regularly. Collections of effluent dialysate and residual urine output (in continent patients with normal bladder function) are used to ensure that target clearance values are being achieved and that loss of kidney function is not compromising the adequacy of therapy. Patients unable to perform urine collections should be assumed to have no residual GFR to avoid inadvertent underdialysis. Many patients can achieve acceptable clearance and ultrafiltration with four exchanges per day; some will require more. The risk of noncompliance with the dialysis prescription and missing exchanges increases as the task of dialysis becomes more burdensome and intrudes on usual family activities.

2. **APD** is well suited for chronic peritoneal dialysis in children, accommodating their efficient solute exchange and higher risk of peritonitis. APD can be performed without a daytime dwell (nightly intermittent peritoneal dialysis, NIPD), with a daytime dwell (continuous cycling peritoneal dialysis, CCPD), or with a daytime dwell and midday exchange if solute clearance or fluid removal necessitate. The daytime dwell is recommended to improve middle molecule clearance in those patients without residual renal function. NIPD may allow improved nutritional intake and decrease the risk of hernia formation, but clearance will likely be adequate only in patients with high or high-average transport as measured by PET or those with residual renal function. The day dwell of CCPD may allow one to shorten nightly treatments (desirable in older children) or improve clearance for low and low-average transporters; yet high transporters usually absorb most of their long dwell if it is left in all day. The initial prescription is guided by transport characteristics determined by PET, typically ranging from four to eight exchanges per night with dwell times of 45 minutes to 2 hours.

   a. **Kinetic modeling.** Although kinetic modeling of peritoneal dialysis delivery has been performed in children treated by CCPD and NIPD, outcome data to define adequate clearance are not available. Target clearance (peritoneal and renal) is the same as for CAPD, a weekly Kt/V-urea of 1.8. Dialysate and urine collections are performed to assess the actual delivered dialysis dose at a given prescription. Collections are repeated whenever the prescription is changed and at regular intervals to assess changes in residual renal function and peritoneal transport function. In practice, young children with PET-defined high or high-average permeability peritoneal membranes can almost always exceed these values, particularly if there is residual renal function. Older children with low-average permeability peritoneal membranes and without residual renal function often require a midday exchange to achieve acceptable clearances.

3. **Tidal dialysis** is used in children; it can enhance clearance in patients with borderline values for Kt/V who might otherwise need to change modalities. Children with abdominal pain at the end of a drain may be more comfortable if left with fluid in the abdomen at all times.

E. **Chronic hemodialysis.** Chronic hemodialysis is the appropriate modality for children and families not capable of providing reliable home care. Furthermore, large adolescents with low-permeability peritoneal membranes may not achieve adequate clearance on peritoneal dialysis without a burdensome exchange schedule, and such adolescents are appropriate candidates for hemodialysis. Because hemodialysis treatments take children out of usual activities (school and play), a hemodialysis unit must provide intensive nursing, tutoring, play therapy, age-appropriate toys, and occupational and physical therapy during dialysis treatments.

   1. Hemodialysis equipment

     a. Vascular access. Vascular access remains a major limitation to successful hemodialysis in small children. Placing and maintaining permanent accesses in small vessels requires experienced and dedicated surgeons and radiologists. Vascular catheters can be placed by interventional radiologists or surgeons depending on the best experience available in an institution. A conservative strategy for permanent access is critical because of the lifelong need for renal replacement therapy. Some young adults leave pediatric dialysis units after many years of hemodialysis treatments (with interval failed renal transplants), and one must ensure they have not depleted all options for long-term vascular access.

       (1) Catheters (Table 36-2). Available double-lumen hemodialysis catheters range from 7 F to 12 F in lengths appropriate for small children through older adolescents. Both temporary and permanent catheters are available, and precurved models for internal jugular cannulation are available in larger sizes. The catheter tip should be radiologically positioned in the junction of the superior vena cava and right atrium.

       In small infants and neonates, single-lumen catheters may be more appropriate considering vessel size. In neonates, a catheter can be inserted into the vena cava through the umbilical vessel if the vessel is still patent. Most of these catheters can be left in place for several weeks.

       (2) Fistulas and grafts. In older children, creation of an arteriovenous fistula between the radial artery and cephalic vein in the nondominant arm with an end-to-side anastomosis is a common mode of vascular access. When blood vessel size is too small for constructing an adequate fistula, a polytetrafluoroethylene (GoreTex or Impra) graft can be placed between an extremity artery and vein. Children with myelomeningocele may prefer a graft placed in the thigh because of absent sensation. Lower extremity grafts allow unimpeded play or schoolwork during dialysis treatments but risk leg edema and hypertrophy.

       (3) Blood flows. Desired blood flow rate is targeted to urea clearance specifications for a chosen dialyzer. In a patient with advanced uremia, an initial urea clearance of 3 mL per minute per kg is prudent to avoid symptomatic disequilibrium; higher urea removal rates are usually tolerated after the first few treatments.

Smaller blood vessels cause higher venous resistance than in adults, which eventually limits flow, typically in the range of 50–150 mL per minute in small children and 200–350 mL per minute in older children. Small catheters often limit flow to 25–100 mL per minute because of limited arterial inflow.

b. Dialyzers. A limited listing of dialyzers that may be appropriate for small patients is provided (Table 36-1).

c. Blood lines. Appropriately sized blood lines allow control of circuit volume. If the volume of the entire extracorporeal circuit exceeds 10% of the patient's blood volume (>8 mL/kg), a warmed blood (or albumin) prime is usually given to ensure hemodynamic stability. Blood lines are available in a range of sizes: Neonatal (~20 mL), infant (~40 mL), and pediatric (~70 mL). It is important that the blood pump be properly calibrated for the chosen blood lines. Neonatal lines are not compatible with some currently available volumetric dialysis machines.

d. Dialysis solution. Bicarbonate dialysis solution is standard for pediatric hemodialysis; it provides better hemodynamic stability and fewer intradialytic symptoms. Patients with small muscle mass will be unable to metabolize a large acetate load quickly.

e. Dialysis machines. Dialysis machines that provide volumetric ultrafiltration control are required. Small errors in ultrafiltration volume (of a few hundred milliliters) may cause symptomatic hypotension or chronic volume overload. Blood flows must be accurate within the range of 30–300 mL per minute and the blood pump calibrated to different size lines.

2. Hemodialysis prescription. A cautious approach to avoiding disequilibrium involves use of a target urea clearance of 3 mL per minute per kg, which is calculated from the specifications of the chosen dialyzer and the blood flow attainable through the patient's access. Early treatments may be programmed even more slowly if the patient is very uremic; repeated short treatments are usually advisable during initiation of hemodialysis when the BUN is extremely elevated. Once a stable, chronic dialysis prescription is attained, more efficient urea clearance is usually well tolerated and fluid removal is more often a cause of intradialytic symptoms. With conditioning and distraction, most children can tolerate hemodialysis sessions lasting 3–4 hours.

a. Anticoagulation. The strategy for heparin administration to infants and children is similar to that for adults. Clotting is infrequent when the ACT is prolonged to approximately 150% of the population baseline value. A "low-dose" heparin protocol would be used to prolong the clotting time to 125% of the population baseline value. The initial loading dosage is usually 10–20 units/kg, with higher dosages being used for infants and children weighing <15 kg. The initial maintenance heparin infusion rate (for the first 20–30 minutes) can be set at 0.3–0.5 units/kg per minute, with further adjustments based on changes in the ACT. Low molecular weight heparin has been used in children receiving chronic hemodialysis. Heparin-induced thrombocytopenia occurs in children and anticoagulation has been successful with danaparoid, hirudin, and argatroban, although published reports are few.

In older children, heparin-free dialysis can be performed successfully. Different dialyzer membrane types have not been systematically compared with regard to clotting. Clotting will be more likely in smaller children, in whom the blood flow rate is usually low relative to the size of the dialyzer. Intermittent saline flushes of the dialysis circuit will result in excessive volume administration in small children unless removal of excess fluid by ultrafiltration is carried out simultaneously.

b. Kinetic modeling of hemodialysis. Formal three-point urea kinetic modeling of hemodialysis has been performed in children, and results are useful in assessing the efficiency of the dialysis treatment as well as dietary protein intake (as a function of urea generation rate) during the interdialytic period. Recommended dietary protein intake in children is greater than that in adults, and the long-term effects of inadequate intake on growth and neurologic development are of even greater concern. The technical aspects of kinetic modeling are discussed in Chapter 3 and are applied similarly in children. The slow-flow technique for blood sampling is important for accurate measurement and the duration of slow flow is determined by the volume of the blood line from the needle or catheter to the sampling port. Pediatric blood lines can be adequately cleared by a slow-flow rate (60 mL per minute) for 17 seconds; we predict infant lines will require 12 seconds at a slow-flow rate of 20 mL per minute. The greater reliance on catheters in pediatric dialysis raises concern that recirculation will diminish treatment efficiency.

c. Adequacy of hemodialysis. When small patients receive efficient clearance (i.e., relatively high K/V), there is a greater amount of postdialysis urea rebound with reequilibration of urea from either the intracellular space or relatively underperfused tissues. Thus, single-pool modeling overestimates dose of dialysis and urea generation rate. The NKF KDOQI 2006 recommendation in adults is for a minimum delivered dialysis dose of a single-pool $Kt/V = 1.2$. The guidelines recommend using single-pool Kt/V to guide therapy, but to increase the minimum dose for smaller patients, including children. A minimum spKt/V value of 1.4–1.5 would seem to be appropriate for children, and in pratice such a minimum value is easily achievable. Equilibrated Kt/V is recommended by the European Best Practice Guidelines, and this can be derived from single-pool Kt/V and the rate of dialysis using either the rate equation described in Chapter 3, or the Tattersall equation described in Appendix A, Table A-4. Yet another approach is to extrapolate from a post-dialysis sample taken 15 minutes after dialysis (Goldstein et al., 1999). Whether spKt/V or equilibrated

Kt/V is used to target dose, it is prudent to err on the side of providing more therapy when treating this vulnerable population. Residual renal function can significantly impact the hemodialysis prescription, especially in very small patients. Regular measurements are needed to ensure overall treatment adequacy as the GFR falls. If patients are unable to perform urine collections, they should be assumed to have no residual GFR to avoid inadvertent underdialysis.

  d. Complications
  (1) Disequilibrium and seizures. Infants and small children develop seizures as a manifestation of the disequilibrium syndrome more commonly than adults. For this reason, the blood flow rate and session length are usually limited for the first few treatments. Overly rapid urea removal is generally avoided by choosing an appropriately sized dialyzer to provide 3 mL per minute per kg urea clearance for the initial treatments; often, blood flows are limited by the caliber of the dialysis access. Other measures sometimes utilized to help prevent disequilibrium syndrome include keeping the dialysate sodium at or slightly above the plasma level and the prophylactic infusion of mannitol (0.5–1.0 g/kg body weight) during the hemodialysis session.
  (2) Hypotension. Intradialytic hypotension and cramping with fluid removal >5% of body weight are common, yet interdialytic weight gains can be large in anuric children on largely liquid diets and in noncompliant adolescents, resulting in sustained interdialytic hypertension. Volume removal must be closely monitored because blood pressure is normally lower in children than in adults and there is a narrower margin to hypotension. Infants and very young children are prone to precipitous falls in blood pressure with no warning and no ability to communicate distress. Isolated ultrafiltration or lower dialysate temperature may make fluid removal more tolerable. If hypoalbuminemia is present, intravenous albumin infusion (0.5–1.5 g/kg) will increase oncotic pressure and may permit ultrafiltration. Repeated treatments may be the only way to remove fluid safely, and many children require more than three treatments per week for fluid and blood pressure management.
  (3) Hypothermia with isolated ultrafiltration. If warmed dialysis solution is not circulated, then the extracorporeal blood circuit will function as a radiator, cooling the blood and the child. Core body temperature should be monitored throughout dialysis, especially during isolated ultrafiltration.
III. Care of the pediatric ESRD patient
A. Nutrition. Comprehensive nutritional management is important for the achievement of growth and physical development through ESRD. The recommended energy intakes for pediatric dialysis patients depend on their ages and should be

the same as the recommended dietary allowances (RDAs) for their nonuremic counterparts. For infants, the RDA for energy is approximately 100 kcal/kg per day. Such high intakes may require supplementation, either orally or by gavage feeding, which can be performed at night concomitant with CCPD. Attempts to provide calories well in excess of the RDA to further enhance growth are usually not effective and induce obesity. However, failure of expected weight gain is an indication for increased energy intake. In older children, the recommended energy intake ranges from 40 to 70 kcal/kg per day, depending on age and activity level.

Protein requirements for children depend on their age and are greater than adult RDA. The recommended dietary protein intake (DPI) for pediatric hemodialysis patients is 0.4 g/kg per day above their RDA for age. The recommended DPI for peritoneal dialysis patients is greater to compensate for anticipated peritoneal losses, which are more significant in infants and toddlers; such very young pediatric peritoneal dialysis patients should consume 0.7–0.8 g/kg per day above their RDA with close monitoring of the adequacy of protein stores. There is limited experience with the use of amino acid–containing peritoneal dialysis fluids, although individual patients have been treated for up to a year.

Supplementation of water-soluble vitamins is routine practice for children treated with chronic peritoneal dialysis or hemodialysis. Fat-soluble vitamins should not be supplemented as clearance of vitamin A metabolites are impaired, risking hypervitaminosis A; an appropriate multivitamin must be selected.

It is difficult to impose fluid, sodium, phosphate, and potassium restrictions on pediatric patients; however, such restrictions may be unnecessary when peritoneal dialysis is the treatment modality. For hemodialysis patients, restrictions depend on the amount of residual urinary output, but always require individual dietary guidance to achieve stringent fluid, sodium, and potassium intake. Infants pose a particular challenge; daily fluid intake in an anuric infant on hemodialysis should be limited to 400–500 mL/m^2, and formula should be concentrated and appropriately supplemented to achieve nutritional goals. However, polyuric infants will require supplemental fluid and sodium to maintain volume status and permit growth.

Enteral feeding supplements designed for adults should be used cautiously in young children. Fortunately specialized infant formulas low in phosphorus and potassium are available; commercially available phosphorus-depleted milk (Dairy Delicious, Delicious Milk Company, Inc., New York, NY) can also be used.

B. Hypertension. Hypertension is a particular concern given the accelerated rate of cardiovascular disease in children with chronic renal failure. Attention is directed to the maintenance of normal volume status and age-appropriate blood pressure. High blood pressure in children undergoing peritoneal dialysis is usually the result of incorrect dialysate glucose concentrations chosen at home coupled with excessive sodium and fluid intake; it is usually managed with dietary counseling, parent education, and close monitoring of weight and blood pressure at home. In hemodialysis patients, hypertension is the result of inadequate fluid removal during dialysis and nonadherence to sodium and fluid restrictions. In patients who continue to remain hypertensive despite increased dialysis time, lowered dialysate temperature or isolated ultrafiltration may make volume removal more tolerable. Dietary and psychological counseling for the patient and family are advisable in cases of repeated nonadherence as this may reflect more serious difficulties in coping with the chronic disease process. If modifications in the dialysis prescription are not adequate for blood pressure control, antihypertensive medications are indicated. All antihypertensive agents typically prescribed for adults have been used successfully in pediatric dialysis patients, and doses should be titrated to age-appropriate blood pressure targets and reassessed frequently.

C. Anemia. Children undergoing hemodialysis tend to be anemic more often than adults and have a lower hemoglobin at the initiation of dialysis. Children respond quite well to erythropoietin; the indications, route of administration, and potential complications are similar for children and adults. Dosage per kilogram is often higher in very young children (150–300 units/kg per week) than in adults. Iron deficiency and repeated episodes of peritonitis adversely affect the erythropoietin response, and nonadherence to home therapy is occasionally a problem. Iron supplementation, either intravenous or oral, is usually necessary in pediatric ESRD patients; blood loss in the hemodialysis circuit is an important cause of iron deficiency in very small patients, especially when more than three treatments per week are prescribed. Androgen therapy, while rarely used in adults, is contraindicated in prepubertal children because it will lead to premature closure of epiphyses.

D. Growth. Few longitudinal studies describing growth in pediatric patients undergoing CAPD or APD have been undertaken. Initial data comparing growth with CAPD or APD to that obtained with hemodialysis seemed to favor the peritoneal dialysis approach; however, definitive controlled studies have not been performed. In children undergoing CAPD or APD, improvement in growth has been linked to a reduction in the degree of secondary hyperparathyroidism. Others have attributed better growth with CAPD or APD to improved nutritional intake, but, as noted above, increasing energy intake much above the RDA will not usually be of benefit.

    1. Recombinant human growth hormone (rhGH) therapy. There is evidence that rhGH treatment increases growth rate in children receiving chronic dialysis, although not as effectively as in children with chronic renal insufficiency. The usual dosage is 0.05 mg/kg per day or 30 IU/m^2 per week as a nightly subcutaneous injection, although other dosing strategies have been used. Slipped capital femoral epiphyses and worsening of metabolic bone disease may occur with rhGH; secondary hyperparathyroidism should be controlled prior to initiation of therapy. Use of rhGH after renal transplantation is some-what controversial; early reports raised concern about an increase in renal transplant rejection rates, although most centers find it an important adjunct to steroid minimization or withdrawal protocols.

2.   Acidosis. Metabolic acidosis is common in children with ESRD and is more problematic in those receiving hemodialysis than those treated with peritoneal dialysis. Chronic acidosis may impair growth by affecting bone mineralization through the growth hormone/insulin-like growth factor-1 axis, as well as exerting a catabolic effect on lean body mass. Some pediatric patients benefit from oral sodium bicarbonate or sodium citrate therapy or higher dialysate bicarbonate concentrations to maintain a serum bicarbonate concentration ≥22 mmol/L.

3.   Renal osteodystrophy. Renal osteodystrophy can be largely prevented or treated in pediatric patients undergoing CAPD or CCPD by assiduous attention to the serum calcium, phosphorus, bicarbonate, intact parathyroid hormone, and alkaline phosphatase levels. The serum alkaline phosphatase levels vary with age, and normal age-related values should be consulted whenever test results are being interpreted. Active vitamin D (as calcitriol or analogs) is used to treat hyperparathyroidism and associated bone disease. Hyperphosphatemia should be controlled by dietary manipulation and by oral administration of phosphate binders to an age-appropriate serum phosphorus level. Phosphorus restriction is particularly difficult to achieve in infants and children because of the higher recommended protein intakes, and we rely on low-phosphorus infant formula and phosphorus-depleted milk. Phosphorus intake should be restricted to 100–275 mg (3.2–8.9 mmol) per day in infants and to 500–1250 mg (16–40 mmol) per day in children and adolescents, with greater restriction in patients with hyperphosphatemia or hyperparathyroidism. Calcium carbonate and calcium acetate have long been used as phosphate binders, and remain the mainstays of treatment in infants and young children. Older children and adolescents are treated with calcium-containing binders or sevelamer, the latter being used because of the recognition of early cardiac calcification in adolescents and young adults with ESRD. Sevelamer is not currently available in liquid formulation for young children. The use of aluminum-containing phosphate binders should be avoided in infants and young children with chronic renal failure because of bone and neurotoxicity. There are no data on the use of lanthanum in children.

SELECTED READINGS

Coleman J, et al. Gastrostomy buttons for nutritional support on chronic dialysis. *Nephrol Dial Transplant* 1998;13:2041–2046.

Coppo R, et al. Providing the right stuff: feeding children with chronic renal failure. *J Nephrol* 1998;11:171–176.

Daugirdas JT. Simplified equations for monitoring Kt/V, PCRn, eKt/V, and ePCRn. *Adv Ren Replace Ther* 1995;2:295–304.

Edefonti A, et al. A prospective multicentre study of the nutritional status in children on chronic peritoneal dialysis. *Nephrol Dial Transplant* 2006;21:1946–1951.

Furth SL, et al. Peritoneal dialysis catheter infections and peritonitis in children: a report of the North American Pediatric Renal Transplant Cooperative Study. *Pediatr Nephrol* 2000;15:179–82.

Goldstein SL, et al. Evaluation and prediction of urea rebound and equilibrated *Kt/V* in the pediatric hemodialysis population. *Am J Kidney Dis* 1999;34(1):49–54.

Goldstein SL, et al. Pediatric patients with multi-organ dysfunction syndrome receiving continuous renal replacement therapy. *Kidney Int* 2005;67:653–658.

Goldstein SL, et al. Quality of life for children with chronic kidney disease. *Semin Nephrol* 2006;26(2):114–117.

Gorman G, et al. Clinical outcomes and dialysis adequacy in adolescent hemodialysis patients. *Am J Kidney Dis* 2006;47(2):285–293.

Hackbarth RM, et al. Zero balance ultrafiltration (Z-BUF) in blood-primed CRRT circuits achieves electrolyte and acid-base homeostasis prior to patient connection. *Pediatr Nephrol* 2005;20:1328–1333.

Mian AN, Mendley SR. Acute dialysis in children. In: Henrich WL ed. *Principles and practice of dialysis,* 3rd ed. Philadelphia: Lippincott Williams & Wilkins, 2004F;617–628.

Monagle P, et al. Antithrombotic therapy in children: the Seventh ACCP Conference on antithrombotic and thrombolytic therapy. *Chest* 2004;126(Suppl 3):645S–687S.

NKF. KDOQI clinical practice guidelines for bone metabolism and disease in children with chronic kidney disease. *Am J Kidney Dis* 2005;46(Suppl 1):S1–S121.

NKF. KDOQI clinical practice guidelines for hemodialysis adequacy, update 2006. Guideline 8. Pediatric hemodialysis prescription and adequacy. *Am J Kidney Dis* 2006;48(Suppl 1):S45–47.

NKF. KDOQI clinical practice guidelines for peritoneal dialysis adequacy, update 2006. Guideline 6. Pediatric peritoneal dialysis. *Am J Kidney Dis* 2006;48(Suppl 1):S127–129.

Schaefer F, et al. Peritoneal transport properties and dialysis dose affect growth and nutritional status in children on chronic peritoneal dialysis. Mid-European Pediatric PD Study Group. *J Am Soc Nephrol* 1999;10:1786–1792.

Smye SW, et al. Paediatric haemodialysis: estimation of treatment efficiency in the presence of urea rebound. *Clin Phys Physiol Meas* 1992;13:51–62.

Symons JM, et al. Continuous renal replacement therapy in children up to 10 kg. *Am J Kidney Dis* 2003;41:984–989.

Warady B, et al. *Pediatric dialysis.* Dordrecht: Kluwer Academic, 2004.

WEB REFERENCES

ESRD in children. Links and guidelines: http://www.hdcn.com/crf/kids

North American Pediatric Renal Transplant Cooperative Study annual report and bibliography: http://spitfire.emmes.com/study/ped/studydoc.htm

KDOQI clinical practice guidelines: http://www.kidney.org/

Pediatric continuous renal replacement therapy: http:// www.pcrrt.com/

Cardiovascular Disease

Daniel E. Weiner, Anthony J. Nicholls,
and Mark J. Sarnak

In end-stage renal disease (ESRD) patients, mortality due to cardiovascular disease (CVD) is 10–30 times higher than in the general population. This is likely due to an increased prevalence of diabetes, hypertension, and left ventricular hypertrophy as well as nontraditional risk factors such as chronic volume overload, hyperphosphatemia, anemia, oxidant stress, and other aspects of the uremic milieu (Table 37-1). In this chapter we focus on epidemiology and management of traditional and nontraditional CVD risk factors and on ischemic heart disease, heart failure, pericardial effusion, valvular disease, and arrhythmia.

I. Traditional risk factors

A. **Blood pressure.** See Chapter 31.

B. **Diabetes.** Diabetics are at higher risk for acute coronary syndromes and have worse outcomes following coronary interventions than nondiabetics. Additionally, there is increased prevalence of heart failure. Poor blood glucose control (as assessed by glycosylated hemoglobin levels) is associated with increased mortality in dialysis patients. See Chapter 30.

C. **Smoking.** Smoking is associated with progression in early-stage CKD patients, and may well adversely impact residual renal function in dialysis patients, although data here are scant. Smoking strongly associates with incident heart failure, incident peripheral vascular disease, and all-cause mortality in the U.S. Renal Data System (USRDS). Former smokers had similar risk as lifelong nonsmokers, suggesting a benefit of smoking cessation and a role for directed intervention.

D. **Dyslipidemia.** Dyslipidemia is very common in dialysis patients. Based on the National Kidney Foundation's (NKF) Kidney Disease Outcome Quality Initiative (KDOQI) recommendations, over 60% of dialysis patients have lipid abnormalities sufficient to require therapy.

    1. **Cholesterol.** In dialysis, the relationship of total or low-density lipoprotein (LDL) cholesterol to mortality is U-shaped; patients with LDL cholesterol levels above 100 mg/dL (2.6 mmol/L) are most likely at increased risk for adverse cardiovascular outcomes, but low levels, probably indicating malnutrition, also are associated with higher mortality rates. Despite frequently reduced levels of total and LDL cholesterol, atherogenic lipoprotein remnants and lipoprotein (a) are generally increased and high-density lipoprotein (HDL) cholesterol levels are generally reduced, likely contributing to CVD risk.

    2. **Hypertriglyceridemia.** Nearly one third of dialysis patients have hypertriglyceridemia, defined by levels above

Table 37-1. Traditional and nontraditional cardiovascular risk factors

Traditional Risk Factors	Nontraditional Factors
Older Age	Extracellular fluid volume overload
Male gender	Abnormal calcium/phosphate
Hypertension	metabolism
Diabetes	Vitamin D deficiency
Smoking	Anemia
Dyslipidemia	Oxidant stress
Left ventricular hypertrophy	Inflammation
Physical inactivity	Homocysteine
Menopause	Malnutrition
Family history of	Albuminuria
cardiovascular disease	Thrombogenic factors
	Sleep disturbances
	Altered nitric oxide/endothelin
	balance
	Marinobufagenin
	Uremic toxins

Reproduced and modified with permission from Sarnak MJ, et al. Kidney disease as a risk factor for development of cardiovascular disease: a statement from the American Heart Association Councils on Kidney in Cardiovascular Disease, High Blood Pressure Research, Clinical Cardiology, and Epidemiology and Prevention. *Circulation* 2003;108:2154–2169.

200 mg/dL (2.26 mmol/L), with levels occasionally up to 600 mg/dL (6.8 mmol/L). The predominant underlying cause is a deficiency of lipoprotein lipase, resulting in reduced lipolysis of triglyceride (TG)-rich very low-density lipoproteins (VLDLs) and yielding high quantities of atherogenic remnant lipoproteins. Enrichment of LDL particles with triglycerides also suggests partial deficiency of hepatic lipase. These basic defects may be enhanced by β-adrenergic blockers, high-carbohydrate diets, absorption of glucose from peritoneal dialysate, the use of heparin, and decreased hepatic blood flow from cardiac insufficiency.

3. **Measurement.** If possible, dialysis patients should be evaluated with a fasting (although perhaps recommended we know not practical) serum lipid panel that includes total and HDL cholesterol as well as triglycerides.

   a. **LDL cholesterol** is commonly computed by subtracting the serum triglyceride level divided either by 5 (when TGs are measured in mg/dL) or by 2.19 (when TGs are measured in mmol/L) as well as the HDL cholesterol level from the total cholesterol. This use of the Friedewald equation is reliable in dialysis patients.

   b. **Atherogenic, remnant lipoproteins and non-HDL cholesterol.** In persons without elevated triglyceride levels (TG <200 mg/dL [2.26 mmol/L]), levels of atherogenic remnant lipoproteins correlate well with the calculated LDL cholesterol. When 200 <TG <500 mg/dL

(2.26 <TG <5.64 mmol/L), levels of atherogenic remnant lipoproteins correlate well with VLDL levels—these can be estimated as total minus HDL cholesterol and form the basis of the treatment recommendation targeting non-HDL cholesterol (bottom row, Table 37-1).

   c. Frequency and technique. Measurements generally should be repeated yearly, but also several months after a therapeutic intervention. Serum for measurement of triglyceride levels should be obtained prior to heparin administration (heparin stimulates the action of lipoprotein lipase) and, if possible, after an overnight fast. In peritoneal dialysis patients, the presence of glucose in the abdomen prior to blood sampling does not result in a true fasting determination; however, for practical reasons, dialysis is not stopped prior to testing.

  4. Treatment (Fig. 37-1)

   a. Target lipid levels. Because dialysis patients are in the highest risk group for CVD events, current KDOQI guidelines recommend that dyslipidemia should be more aggressively treated than in the general population, with an LDL cholesterol target level below 100 mg/dL (2.6 mmol/L). Even lower LDL targets (70 mg/dL or 1.8 mmol/L) have been advocated in diabetic patients during the earlier stages of CKD based on extrapolation from results in nonuremic individuals (Molitch, 2006). However, there is no direct trial evidence to support these lower LDL targets in diabetic patients with any stage of CKD. Treatment of very high TG levels (>500 mg/dL [>5.7 mmol/L]) is recommended to protect against TG-induced pancreatitis. KDOQI also recommends medical therapy

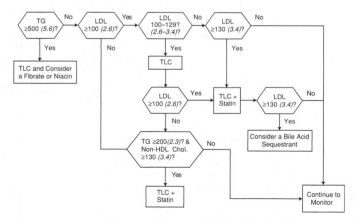

Figure 37-1. Treatment of dyslipidemias in adults. TG, triglyceride; LDL, low-density lipoprotein; TLC, therapeutic lifestyle changes; HDL, high-density lipoprotein. Units are mg/dL (*mmol/L*). (Modified with permission from National Kidney Foundation. K/DOQI clinical practice guidelines for managing dyslipidemias in chronic kidney disease. *Am J Kidney Dis* 2003;41(4 suppl 3): S1–S92.

for high levels of non-HDL cholesterol when serum TGs are elevated, as a proxy for high levels of atherogenic remnant lipoproteins (Table 37-2).

b. Therapeutic lifestyle changes. As in the general population, first-line therapy for most patients is dietary and lifestyle modification. Dietary prescriptions are best accomplished with guidance from a nutritionist with experience in management of kidney disease patients. Recommendations listed in Chapter 28 should generally be followed. These include consumption of a diet containing about 25%–35% of total calories as fat; of this, about 20% should be monounsaturated, 10% polyunsaturated, and <7% saturated fat. In patients with hypertriglyceridemia, mild restriction of total carbohydrate intake and limitation of the use of refined carbohydrate are indicated. Additionally, alcohol ingestion should be strongly discouraged. Despite the risk of malnutrition in many dialysis patients, there may be a minority where overall calorie restriction is indicated to achieve ideal body weight, especially among those receiving peritoneal dialysis. Due to beneficial effects on volume overload, sodium restriction in peritoneal dialysis patients may reduce the use of higher dialysis solution glucose concentrations; this would yield less glucose absorption and decrease the stimulus for hypertriglyceridemia (see Chapter 26). If possible, physical training and regular exercise are recommended as they result in reduced serum triglyceride concentrations and an improved sense of well-being.

c. Drug therapy. If therapeutic lifestyle changes are unsuccessful in controlling dyslipidemia, drug therapy is then recommended. Suggested first- and second-line drug therapies are listed in Table 37-2.

(1) Statins. When therapeutic lifestyle changes fail to adequately lower either LDL cholesterol or non-HDL cholesterol levels in the setting of normal or moderately elevated TGs, statins are the first drug of choice. Statins are not indicated for initial therapy of very high TG levels alone; here fibrates and/or nicotinic acid are recommended. While associated with lower mortality in observational studies (Seliger, 2002), statin use has not been shown to mitigate CVD risk in one large randomized, controlled trial (RCT) performed in diabetic dialysis patients (4D trial, Wanner et al., 2005). Thus, recommendations for use of statins predate the results of the 4D trial and are based on extrapolation of beneficial results in the general population. Confirmatory RCTs in the dialysis population are ongoing.

Table 37-3 reviews therapeutic options for dyslipidemia. Dosages of most statins should be reduced in dialysis patients. While statins generally are safe in the dialysis population, a number of medications increase blood levels of statins via cometabolism by hepatic cytochrome P450 enzymes; these include cyclosporine, macrolide antibiotics, azole antifungal agents, calcium channel blockers, fibrates, and nicotinic acid. Potential

Table 37-2. Treatment recommendations for dyslipidemia in dialysis patients

Dyslipidemia	Treatment Goal	Initial Regimen	Increased Regimen	Alternative Regimen
TG $\geq$500 mg/dL ($\geq$5.6 mmol/L)	TG <500 mg/dL (<5.6 mmol/L)	TLC	TLC + fibrate or niacin	Fibrate or niacin
LDL 100–129 mg/dL (2.6–3.4 mmol/L)	LDL <100 mg/dL (<2.6 mmol/L)	TLC	TLC + low-dose statin	Bile acid seq or niacin
LDL $\geq$130 mg/dL ($\geq$3.4 mmol/L)	LDL <100 mg/dL (<2.6 mmol/L)	TLC + low-dose statin	TLC + max. dose statin	Bile acid seq or niacin
TG $\geq$200 mg/dL ($\geq$2.3 mmol/L) and non-HDL $\geq$130 mg/dL ($\geq$3.4 mmol/L)	Non-HDL <130 mg/dL (<3.4 mmol/L)	TLC + low-dose statin	TLC + max. dose statin	Fibrate or niacin

TG, triglyceride; TLC, therapeutic lifestyle changes; LDL, low-density lipoprotein cholesterol; HDL, high-density lipoprotein cholesterol. Adapted from National Kidney Foundation. Kidney Disease Outcomes Quality Initiative. *Am J Kidney Dis* 2003;41(4 Suppl 3):S40.

Table 37-3. Lipid-lowering medication dose adjustments for reduced GFR

Therapeutic Agent	GFR (mL per minute per 1.73 m²)			Notes
	60–90	15–59	<15	
Statins[a]				
Atorvastatin	No	No	No	None
Fluvastatin	No	→ to 50%	→ to 50%	Decrease dosage by half at GFR <30
Lovastatin	No	→ to 50%	→ to 50%	Decrease dosage by half at GFR <30
Pravastatin	No	No	No	Starting dose of 10 mg per day recommended for GFR <60
Rosuvastatin	No	→	→	Decrease to a maximum of 10 mg per day at GFR <30; recommended starting dose is 5 mg per day
Simvastatin	No	No	?	If GFR <10, start at 5 mg per day and use doses above 10 mg daily with caution
Bile acid seq				
Cholestyramine	No	No	No	Not absorbed
Colestipol	No	No	No	Not absorbed
Colesevelam	No	No	No	Not absorbed
Fibrates[a]				
Bezafibrate	No	→ to 25%	See note	If GFR <15, avoid unless on dialysis; max. dose of 200 mg three times per week in dialysis patients
Ciprofibrate	No	?	Avoid	Dose 100 mg every other day at reduced GFR; may increase serum creatinine[b]
Clofibrate	→ to 50%	→ to 25%	Avoid	May increase serum creatinine[b]
Fenofibrate	→ to 50%	→ to 25%	Avoid	May increase serum creatinine[b]
Gemfibrozil	No	No	No	Likely no effect on serum creatinine
Miscellaneous				
Ezetimibe	No	No	No	None
Nicotinic Acid	No	No	→ to 50%	May worsen glycemic control and cause orthostasis, hyperuricemia, and flushing

GFR, glomerular filtration rate.

[a]Because of increased risk of myositis and rhabdomyolysis, statin therapy in conjunction with a fibrate should be avoided in patients with chronic kidney disease.

[b]The increase in levels of serum creatinine seen with most fibrates has not been appreciated with gemfibrozil.

Weiner DE, Sarnak MJ. Managing dyslipidemia in chronic kidney disease. *J Gen Intern Med* 2004;19:1045–1052.

drug–drug interactions should be assessed in each patient. Statins may cause myopathy, and the risk of myopathy is increased in CKD and with concurrent use of fibrates. It is prudent to check the serum creatinine phosphokinase (CPK) level at initiation of therapy in order to guide safety monitoring of these medications and to question the patient in detail about muscle-related complaints during the course of therapy.

(2) Alternatives to statins. Alternatives include bile acid sequestrants (including the phosphate binder sevelamer), nicotinic acid, ezetimibe, and fibrates. Notably, **bile acid sequestrants** can interfere with absorption of other medications. They should not be used when TGs are >400 mg/dL (>4.5 mmol/L), and are relatively contraindicated when TGs are >200 mg/dL (>2.3 mmol/L) since they may increase triglycerides in some patients. Doses do not need to be reduced in dialysis patients (Table 37-3). Dose ranges (g per day) would be 4–16 for cholestyramine, 5–20 for colestipol, and 2.6–3.8 for colesevelam (Kasiske, 2004). **Sevelamer** also has bile acid sequestrant effects and lowers both total and LDL cholesterol; sevelamer is a good choice when phosphate binding is also indicated with the caveat that it may worsen metabolic acidosis. While not as effective for LDL lowering, **nicotinic acid** has the greatest favorable effects on HDL cholesterol levels of available drug therapies. The dosage of nicotinic acid should be reduced by about 50% in ESRD, given its substantial renal excretion. The potential of nicotinic acid as a phosphate binder has been touted, but a recent case report documented transient thrombocytopenia when used in conjunction with sevelamer in hemodialysis (see Chapter 35). Other adverse effects can include hyperglycemia and hepatotoxicity in individuals with underlying liver disease or with high medication doses. Flushing may be attenuated with concurrent aspirin use or longer-acting preparations. Nicotinic acid is more often used as a first-line therapy when severe hypertriglyceridemia (>500 mg/dL [5.8 mmol/L]) needs to be treated to protect against pancreatitis, or when therapeutic lifestyle changes fail to control levels of "remnant" lipoproteins and a statin is contraindicated. **Ezetimibe** is a drug that inhibits cholesterol absorption. There are few data available on its use in kidney failure. **Fibrates** include gemfibrozil, bezafibrate, ciprofibrate, clofibrate, and fenofibrate. Of these, gemfibrozil may be the best choice, as it does not require dose reduction in CKD. Gemfibrozil is used primarily to treat severe hypertriglyceridemia or significantly increased remnant lipoprotein levels as reflected by elevated non-HDL cholesterol (Table 37-1). Fibrates both cause myopathy and increase the blood levels of statins; therefore, concurrent fibrate and statin use in individuals with CKD is contraindicated. Fibrates have only a small effect on LDL and should not be used for lowering LDL in normotriglyceridemic patients.

(3) Drug combinations. Drug combinations to further lower LDL cholesterol should seldom be necessary in the dialysis population. Perhaps the safest combination would be a statin plus a bile acid sequestrant. There are no data on combined use of a statin with nicotinic acid in dialysis patients.

E. Left ventricular hypertrophy

1. Epidemiology. Left ventricular hypertrophy (LVH) is very common in both predialysis (20%–40%) and dialysis (50%–75%) patients. Most LVH is initially concentric, representing a uniform increase in wall thickness secondary to pressure overload from hypertension, stiffened blood vessels, or aortic valve stenosis. Anemia and volume overload resulting from chronic inability to effectively remove ingested sodium and fluid may each result in eccentric hypertrophy. The endpoint is often a dilated cardiomyopathy with eventual reduction in systolic function. Such end-stage patients typically have low blood pressure and may be responsible for the J-shaped (or U-shaped) relationship observed between blood pressure and mortality in dialysis patients. LVH in dialysis patients is an independent risk factor for adverse CVD outcomes and all-cause mortality.

2. Prevention and management. Some data suggest that with modification of risk factors, including anemia and systolic blood pressure, strict management of volume, and use of angiotensin-converting enzyme (ACE) inhibitor and angiotensin receptor blocker therapy, regression of LVH may occur in dialysis patients. Studies have documented regression of LVH with more frequent dialysis, such as six times per week short daily dialysis given 18 hours per week (Ayus, 2005), or six times per week nocturnal dialysis (Chan, 2002). Disordered mineral metabolism has also been associated with LVH, with identified risk factors including elevated calcium-phosphate product, elevated serum parathyroid hormone (PTH), and markedly reduced serum PTH levels. Other data suggest that vitamin D deficiency may be further implicated in cardiovascular disease beyond its complex effects on mineral metabolism: vitamin D influences the regulation of inflammation, myocardial cell hypertrophy and proliferation, and the regulation of the renin-angiotensin system.

II. Nontraditional risk factors. These are listed in Table 37-1. In-depth discussion of some of these is beyond the scope of the *Handbook,* but we briefly summarize the most pertinent issues. Volume control is discussed in Chapters 10 and 31.

A. Calcium, phosphorus, PTH, and vitamin D. Mineral metabolism is discussed in Chapter 35. Disorders of calcium and phosphorus metabolism can affect the cardiovascular system in several ways. Both elevated PTH and reduced vitamin D levels may directly affect the myocardium, promoting hypertrophy. Hyperphosphatemia, as well as calcium flowing into a system where bone buffering is impaired, plus other factors in the uremic milieu including loss of calcification inhibitors, can combine to promote vascular calcification. Vascular calcification occurs at both the arterial media and the intima, with medial calcification generally more pronounced among dialysis patients. Medial calcification is associated with stiffer blood vessels, as evidenced by increased pulse wave velocity. This increases cardiac afterload and promotes LVH. Furthermore, during the cardiac cycle, the systolic pressure wave normally reflects back onto the heart during early diastole, promoting coronary filling. With stiffened arteries and increased pulse wave velocity, this reflected wave returns to the heart prematurely—during late systole. This results in loss of the coronary filling effect and increased afterload as the heart has to pump against the reflected pressure wave from the previous contraction.

Vascular calcification may be diagnosed in several ways. Plain radiographs are specific but insensitive. Electron beam and spiral computed tomography are sensitive and specific but expensive and associated with significant radiation exposure on repeated use. Ultrasound, most commonly of the carotid arteries, is relatively inexpensive and noninvasive but requires a trained operator and may lack precision to closely track changes over time. Use of such tests needs to be justified by their impact on clinical decision making. At the present time there is no reliable method of reversing cardiac calcification, although some studies have suggested that use of sevelamer may slow progression. Whether this possible effect is due to avoidance of calcium loading or to the lipid-lowering effects of sevelamer is not known. Other data suggest that with six times per week nocturnal dialysis, where phosphorus balance becomes negative, vascular calcification may be slowed. A reasonable (albeit not evidence based) strategy might be to limit use of calcium-containing phosphorus binders if possible in patients in whom extensive vascular calcification has been documented. In all patients, total calcium intake from all sources should be limited to 2 g per day (50 mmol) according to current KDOQI guidelines.

B. Anemia. Anemia is common in CKD patients, especially at dialysis initiation, and the extent of desirable correction is a matter of some debate. Anemia correlates with the extent of LVH, and correction of anemia in one small study of patients with heart failure was associated with improved functional status. However, at the present time, correction of anemia to hemoglobin levels above 12 g/dL (120 g/L) has not been associated with a cardiovascular or survival benefit. Maintenance of hemoglobin levels above 11 g/dL (110 g/L) is currently recommended and may prevent further progression of LVH.

C. Sleep. Sleep abnormalities, discussed in Chapter 42, are highly prevalent in dialysis patients and are associated with coronary artery disease. Nocturnal hypoxemia associated with sleep apnea predicts CVD events and may represent a potentially modifiable risk factor.

D. Homocysteine
   1. Epidemiology. Hyperhomocysteinemia is much more common in dialysis patients than in the general population.

Homocysteine is typically measured in the plasma and normal levels range between 5 and 12 mcmol/L. In the general population, hyperhomocysteinemia is an independent risk factor for adverse CVD outcomes and is commonly associated with deficiencies in folate and vitamins B_6 and B_{12}. B-vitamin and folate supplementation effectively reduce homocysteine levels in the general population and recent extensive folate supplementation in foods has lowered the overall prevalence of hyperhomocysteinemia in the nondialysis population. Homocysteine levels increase dramatically as kidney function declines, with as many as 80% of dialysis patients classified as having hyperhomocysteinemia. In dialysis patients, some but not all studies suggest that hyperhomocysteinemia is independently associated with CVD mortality. Nutritional status confounds these analyses, since better nourished patients tend to have higher homocysteine levels.

2. Treatment. In the general population, several large RCTs have been unable to show a beneficial effect on CVD outcomes by lowering levels of homocysteine with aggressive vitamin supplementation. In dialysis patients, high levels of homocysteine are often resistant to folate and B-vitamin administration; however, high-dose supplementation, especially with pharmacologic doses of folate or the more active form, folinic acid, as well as vitamin B_{12}, often results in improvement but not normalization of homocysteine levels. Use of hemodiafiltration and six times per week nocturnal dialysis also has been associated with lower homocysteine levels. RCTs of homocysteine lowering in the dialysis population are ongoing; at this time there are insufficient data to recommend aggressive therapy of hyperhomocysteinemia.

E. Oxidant stress and inflammation. Numerous factors in the dialysis patient increase oxidant stress. These include inflammation (as marked by elevated C-reactive protein), malnutrition (by reducing antioxidant defenses), uremic toxins, and, potentially, the dialysis procedure itself. Many protective mechanisms are impaired, including reduced plasma protein-associated free thiols such as glutathione. This may magnify the impact of oxidant stress in the dialysis population. At this time, specific treatment strategies to reduce inflammation or oxidant stress are neither widely used nor adequately supported by RCTs. Therapies with various antioxidants, including vitamin E (especially γ-tocopherol), vitamin C, α-lipoic acid, and acetylcysteine, are among promising treatment options.

III. Ischemic heart disease

A. Overview. Acute myocardial infarction (AMI) is common in the ESRD population. Outcomes for patients with AMI are poor, with 50% 1-year mortality. Both atherosclerosis and arteriosclerosis contribute to pathogenesis; arteriosclerosis may cause LVH with increased myocardial oxygen demand and altered coronary perfusion with subsequent subendocardial ischemia. Small vessel coronary artery disease also plays a role: In one study, up to 50% of nondiabetic dialysis patients

with symptoms of myocardial ischemia did not have significant large-caliber coronary artery disease, implicating isolated
small vessel disease as a cause of ischemia.

B. Diagnosis. Routine screening is not currently recommended. There are no preoperative screening guidelines specific to dialysis patients, and it is reasonable to use general
population guidelines, recognizing that the extent of comorbid conditions prevalent in the dialysis population is likely
to place them into the highest cardiovascular risk group. Because many dialysis patients are unable to achieve adequate
exercise levels for valid stress tests, pharmacologic stress tests
should be used in this population. Furthermore, because of the
high incidence of baseline electrocardiogram abnormalities, either nuclear or echocardiographic imaging should be utilized
in stress testing. The utility of cardiac markers to diagnose
AMI in dialysis patients is reviewed in Chapter 29.

C. Prevention. Aspirin, beta-blockers, ACE inhibitors, and
nitrate preparations are all appropriate for primary therapy
of AMI and are likely appropriate for secondary prevention,
although data on aspirin for secondary prevention of coronary artery disease remain inadequate to date. Observational
studies suggest that medical therapies including aspirin, beta-
blockers, and ACE inhibitors may be underutilized in dialysis
patients.

D. Treatment

    1. Management of angina pectoris. The pharmacologic
approach to angina in dialysis patients is similar to that
in the general population. The progressive introduction of
sublingual nitrates, oral long-acting nitrates, beta-blockers,
and calcium channel blockers is appropriate. The usual
dosages of sublingual and oral nitrates can be given to dialysis patients.

    2. Angina during the hemodialysis session. For
patients whose angina manifests primarily during the
hemodialysis session, a number of therapeutic options are
available. Nasal oxygen should be given routinely. If the
anginal episode is associated with hypotension, then initial
treatment should include raising the blood pressure by
elevating the feet and by cautiously administering saline.
Sublingual nitroglycerin can be given as soon as the blood
pressure has increased to a clinically acceptable value.
Consideration should be given to reducing the blood flow
rate and stopping ultrafiltration until the anginal episode
subsides. Predialysis administration of 2% nitroglycerin
ointment may be of benefit when applied 1 hour prior to
a hemodialysis session, assuming that the blood pressure
will tolerate this intervention. Predialysis administration
of beta-blockers and oral nitrates may be of benefit but
must be done cautiously because the risk of hypotension
during the dialysis session may be increased. Calcium
channel blockers could be of use in situations where
beta-blockade is contraindicated or inadequate; however,
given the negative cardiac inotropy associated with this
class and the high prevalence of systolic dysfunction in
dialysis patients, calcium channel blockers, particularly the

nondihydropyridines (diltiazem and verapamil), should be used with caution.

3. Revascularization. Coronary artery bypass grafting and angioplasty with stenting are each of benefit as compared to medical management of operable coronary lesions. As with most procedures, those done on an emergent basis are associated with worse outcomes. Thrombolytics and glycoprotein IIb/IIIa antagonists are likely beneficial, particularly when interventional cardiology is unavailable, but may be associated with a higher risk of bleeding complications. Historically, the results of percutaneous transluminal coronary angioplasty in dialysis patients have been disappointing, with high rates of restenosis at 6 months, but this information was denied from studies done before use of newer coronary stent technologies. Pre- and postoperative management of dialysis patients undergoing cardiac surgery is similar to that for any other major operation, and older retrospective data have shown that bypass surgery is a viable option for dialysis patients.

IV. Cardiomyopathy and heart failure

A. Pathophysiology. Heart failure is highly prevalent in the dialysis population and is associated with many traditional and nontraditional CVD risk factors. Although there is no universally accepted definition, heart failure is generally characterized by volume overload, pulmonary edema, and dyspnea. Heart failure may occur as a result of left ventricular dysfunction (systolic dysfunction) or diastolic dysfunction, in which the left ventricle has a normal ejection fraction but impaired filling. Diastolic dysfunction is often associated with left ventricular hypertrophy and systemic hypertension, both of which are extremely common in dialysis patients. Systolic dysfunction frequently is a result of ischemic disease and dilated cardiomyopathy. Although, for obvious reasons, dialysis patients are particularly vulnerable to fluid overload, pulmonary edema even in the setting of marked fluid overload may represent cardiac dysfunction. Additionally, frequent pulmonary edema with minimal intradialytic weight gain may be an important clue of cardiac dysfunction. A further clue may be dialysis-related hypotension, as dysfunctional hearts likely have reduced capacity for adaptation to intravascular volume loss.

Although the diagnosis of heart failure is clinical, echocardiography is invaluable for diagnosing systolic and diastolic dysfunction. Echocardiography may also suggest the cause of disease, identifying wall motion abnormalities that may indicate ischemia and infarcts, LVH that may predispose to diastolic dysfunction, and valvular disease with its effects on cardiac morphology. KDOQI guidelines recommend obtaining echocardiograms at dialysis initiation after dry weight is established and every 3 years thereafter; these recommendations are opinion based.

B. Treatment. Chronic therapy for heart failure in dialysis patients has not been adequately studied; therefore, most recommendations are either extrapolated from the general population or based on smaller trials. Restriction of sodium intake is of great importance, since, with most three times per week dialysis schedules, the ability to remove excess fluid is limited. Maintaining a balance between pulmonary edema on the one hand and symptomatic hypotension on the other may be extremely difficult in some dialysis patients. In these patients, moving to a four times per week or even more frequent schedule or nocturnal dialysis may reduce the risk of hospitalization for heart failure.

    1. **Traditional drug therapy**

        a. **ACE inhibitors** are beneficial in nonuremic patients with chronic heart failure and are likely beneficial in dialysis patients. If there is a contraindication for ACE inhibitors, it seems reasonable to extrapolate from data in the general population and substitute angiotensin receptor blockers.

        b. **Beta-blockers,** another mainstay of heart failure therapy in the general population, may be of benefit in the dialysis population. Carvedilol, well studied for heart failure in the general population, reduced mortality in dialysis patients with left ventricular dysfunction. Carvedilol dosing is the same as in the general population; however, several of the beta-blockers (e.g., atenolol) do accumulate in renal failure and should either not be used or be used in markedly reduced dosage (see Table 31-2). In general, non–kidney-metabolized beta-blockers can be safely titrated to heart rate and blood pressure.

        c. **Aldosterone-blocking agents,** including spironolactone and eplerenone, have proven beneficial in the general population with heart failure and, given the known effects of aldosterone on arterial stiffness and cardiac remodeling, could be beneficial in the dialysis population. However, use of these agents has not been adequately studied in the dialysis population for safety or efficacy.

        d. **Cardiac glycosides,** namely digoxin, are frequently used in heart failure in the general population where it has been shown that they improve morbidity but not mortality. Digoxin, when used in dialysis patients, should be utilized judiciously with careful attention to dosage and drug levels. Maintenance dosing should begin at low doses (0.0625 mg or 0.125 mg) every other day. A loading dose generally should not be used. Care should be taken in complex drug regimens as many other medications affect digoxin levels.

        e. **Aspirin.** While there is strong evidence for the benefits of aspirin for secondary prevention in individuals with intact kidney function and ischemic cardiomyopathy, there have been conflicting reports of worse heart failure outcomes associated with aspirin use in patients with chronic kidney disease. This may relate to attenuation of the beneficial effects of ACE inhibitors due to aspirin-mediated inhibition of kinin-mediated prostaglandin synthesis. Very limited observational data in dialysis patients have shown that aspirin use may increase the incidence of new and recurrent heart failure episodes.

2. Role of arteriovenous (AV) fistulas and grafts. Although forearm fistulas occasionally lead to a high output state (MacRae et al., 2006), this problem is more often encountered with upper arm brachial fistulas, and close attention to the size of the AV fistula is essential during surgical construction. Bradycardia during fistula or graft occlusion (by finger pressure) suggests that the AV shunt is importantly and pathologically contributing to an increased cardiac output (Branham sign). The test is specific, but absence of bradycardia on fistula or graft occlusion by no means exonerates the AV communication as a cause of the heart failure.

3. Carnitine. Predominantly anecdotal evidence has suggested cardiovascular benefits with L-carnitine therapy at recommended intravenous doses of 20 mg/kg of total body weight following the dialysis procedure. Indications for carnitine therapy include anemia with extremely high erythropoietin requirements, intradialytic hypotension, and muscle weakness. L-carnitine may also be indicated for treatment of symptomatic cardiomyopathy with a documented impaired ejection fraction that has not responded adequately to standard medical therapy. Carnitine should be discontinued if there is no improvement within 9–12 months.

V. Pericardial disease. Pericardial disease most commonly manifests as acute uremic or dialysis-associated pericarditis, although chronic constrictive pericarditis may also be seen. Most estimates of the clinical incidence of pericardial disease in prevalent dialysis patients are <20%.

A. Uremic pericarditis. Uremic pericarditis describes patients who develop clinical manifestations of pericarditis prior to or within 8 weeks of initiation of renal replacement therapy. In the current era, uremic pericarditis is rare but remains an indication for and responds extremely well to initiation of renal replacement therapy.

B. Dialysis-associated pericarditis. Dialysis-associated pericarditis is a syndrome that occurs after a patient is stabilized on dialysis and is much more common than uremic pericarditis. The cause of dialysis pericarditis remains unknown but may be at least in part dependent on inadequate dialysis and volume overload. However, other causative factors are likely present, given that intensification of dialysis frequently does not result in resolution.

1. Clinical manifestations and diagnosis. The most common symptom of pericarditis is chest pain, generally pleuritic in nature and exacerbated by reclining and reduced with leaning forward. Pericarditis may be accompanied by nonspecific symptoms including fever, chills, malaise, dyspnea, and cough, with respiratory symptoms potentially reflecting a pericardial effusion. Physical examination may reveal a pericardial friction rub. When hemodynamically significant, pericardial disease accompanied by an effusion may be characterized by hypotension, particularly during hemodialysis. Jugular venous distension, elevated pulsus paradoxus, and distant heart sounds may also be present. Chest radiograph may reveal an enlarged cardiac silhouette that may be difficult to distinguish from LVH. Dialysis-related pericarditis often does not manifest with the classical electrocardiogram finding of diffuse ST segment elevation because there may only be minimal inflammation of the epicardium. Echocardiography is useful in identifying pericardial effusions, but effusions may be absent in patients who have adhesive, noneffusive pericarditis.

2. Treatment

   a. Monitoring. Small (<100 mL), asymptomatic pericardial effusions are fairly common in dialysis patients and require no acute intervention. Larger effusions present a risk for tamponade and need to be monitored closely using serial echocardiograms. Hemodynamic and even echocardiographic signs of impending tamponade are not always reliable.

   b. Intensification of hemodialysis is the mainstay of therapy but is only effective approximately 50% of the time. This may be accomplished by increasing dialysis frequency to 5–7 days per week with careful attention to electrolytes, volume, and nutrition. Supplemental potassium often must be added to the dialysate to avoid hypokalemia; the dialysate bicarbonate level should be reduced to avoid alkalosis; and, in some cases, phosphate supplementation may be required. Heparin during dialysis has traditionally been avoided out of concern for hemorrhagic tamponade.

   c. Adjuvant medical therapies, including oral and parenteral glucocorticoids and nonsteroidal anti-inflammatory medications, have generally not been effective and are not indicated.

   d. Surgical drainage. Failure to recognize the need for timely surgical drainage of large pericardial effusions may have dire consequences for the patient as the onset of tamponade may be rapid and without premonitory signs. Hence, regular echocardiographic monitoring of the size of an effusion is vital. Drainage of the pericardial effusion, preferably by subxiphoid pericardiostomy, should be strongly considered whenever the effusion size is estimated by echocardiography to exceed 250 mL (posterior echo-free space >1 cm), even when hemodynamic compromise is absent. Drainage is mandatory when overt tamponade appears.

   (1) Subxiphoid pericardiostomy is likely the surgical drainage procedure of choice (i.e., insertion typically under local anesthesia of a large-bore tube into the pericardial space). The tube is left in place to closed drainage for several days until drainage ceases. Case series have indicated considerable success with this approach. Instillation of locally acting steroids has not been proven necessary and increases the risk of infection.

   (2) Pericardiocentesis with echocardiographic or fluoroscopic guidance and extended catheter drainage is performed in many centers for drainage of uremic pericardial effusions. There are no data comparing this approach with subxiphoid pericardiostomy, although anecdotal reports favor subxiphoid pericardiostomy in patients with relative hemodynamic stability. Importantly, unguided pericardiocentesis is extremely dangerous and only indicated as an emergent therapy for patients with life-threatening tamponade when no other options exist. Hemorrhagic effusions are poorly evacuable through the needle, and the risk of coronary artery or cardiac puncture and arrhythmia is substantial.

(3) **Anterior pericardiectomy** has been favored by some, but general anesthesia and thoracotomy are unnecessary risks given the uniformly successful response to drainage by subxiphoid pericardiostomy.

C. **Constrictive pericarditis.** Constrictive pericarditis can appear as an unusual complication of dialysis-associated pericarditis or as the first manifestation of pericardial disease. Constrictive pericarditis may also masquerade as congestive cardiac failure; the best means of differentiation is by right heart catheterization. Even then, the diagnosis may be in doubt and can be proven only by a favorable response to total pericardiectomy.

D. **Purulent pericarditis.** Occasionally, patients are found to have purulent pericarditis as a complication of septicemia, often as a result of access site infection. These patients often require anterior pericardiectomy in addition to antimicrobial therapy.

VI. **Valvular disease**

A. **Endocarditis.** Infective endocarditis is a relatively common complication of hemodialysis. Venous hemodialysis catheters are prone to infection and endocarditis is a frequent complication of catheter-related bacteremia. The majority of cases are due to Gram-positive organisms (*Staphylococcus aureus*, *S. epidermidis*, and *Enterococcus*). The mitral valve is the most commonly affected, followed by the aortic valve. The presence of underlying valvular disease including calcification may increase the risk. Prevention is focused on avoiding use of venous catheters as much as possible, as well as prolonged antimicrobial therapy for staphylococcal bacteremia when it occurs. In many patients, acute bacterial endocarditis will complicate an already recognized episode of *S. aureus* bacteremia, and the latter infection should be treated as a presumed endocarditis unless transesophageal echocardiography confirms the absence of a valvular infection.

1. **Symptoms and signs.** Dialysis patients with endocarditis usually have fever. Murmurs, leukocytosis, and septic emboli may also be present; however, the clinical evaluation of murmurs may prove difficult because cardiac murmurs are common in the ordinary dialysis population owing to anemia, valvular calcification, and the presence of AV fistulas. Because a substantial percentage of dialysis patients are normally hypothermic, the body temperature with infection may be elevated to only slightly above the normal range or not at all. Often the only clinical

manifestation of endocarditis may be orthostatic dizziness in a patient with positive blood cultures, occasionally accompanied by mild neurologic manifestations that may be misinterpreted as being due to the disequilibrium syndrome or to uremia.

2. Diagnosis is chiefly dependent on positive blood cultures and clinical suspicion. Transthoracic and in particular transesophageal echocardiography may be critical to making the diagnosis.

3. Treatment of endocarditis in hemodialysis patients will usually be directed at Gram-positive organisms and regimens tailored to bacterial sensitivities. In general, empiric therapy in individuals with fever and a dialysis catheter will be initiated with vancomycin, both because of the high incidence of methicillin-resistant *S. aureus* and the ease of administration. Some practitioners will add empiric Gram-negative coverage with an aminoglycoside, third-generation cephalosporin, or fluoroquinolone. In the presence of methicillin-sensitive *S. aureus*, antistaphylococcal penicillins like nafcillin or first-generation cephalosporins like cefazolin are preferable. In cases of severe *S. aureus* infection, other agents may be added for synergy including aminoglycosides and rifampin. Notably, care must be taken with aminoglycoside use due to the incidence of ototoxicity. Newer antistaphylococcal agents have been developed but use should be judicious and aided by input from an infectious disease specialist to avoid development of widespread resistance. In all cases, there should be a high degree of suspicion for line and access infections and a low threshold for removal of central venous catheters. Therapy should be continued for at least 4–6 weeks. Such prolonged antimicrobial therapy should help avoid the complication of valvular sequestration of infection in most patients with bacteremia diagnosed at an early stage.

4. Valve replacement. ESRD is not a contraindication to valve surgery. Indications for surgery are the same as in the general population: Progressive valvular destruction, progressive heart failure, recurrent embolization, and failure to respond to appropriate antibiotic therapy.

VII. Valvular calcification and stenosis

A. Mitral annular calcification. Mitral annular calcification may occur in as many as 50% of patients on dialysis and is also common in the elderly general population. It is recognized on echocardiography as a uniform echodense rigid band located near the base of the posterior mitral leaflet and may progressively involve the posterior leaflet. Complications include conduction abnormalities, embolic phenomena, mitral valve disease, and increased risk of endocarditis. There are no proven preventive or treatment strategies.

B. Aortic calcification and stenosis. Aortic valve calcification occurs in 25%–55% of dialysis patients. It occurs more frequently in patients with elevated parathyroid hormone, calcium, and/or phosphorus levels. Increased patient age and dialysis vintage are also risk factors. Calcification may result in progressive immobilization of the aortic leaflets, eventually restricting flow. Functional aortic stenosis exists when the valve leaflets thicken to the extent that a pressure gradient develops across the aortic valve.

1. Symptoms and signs. Angina, congestive heart failure, and syncope are the cardinal symptoms of critical aortic stenosis. Frequent episodes of intradialytic hypotension may be a clue as the heart has difficulty in adapting to conditions of reduced filling. The classical systolic murmur that radiates to the carotid arteries may be present; this typically begins after S1 and ceases prior to S2; additionally, S2 may be fixed or paradoxically split. However, it is often difficult to differentiate the murmur of aortic stenosis from that heard in aortic sclerosis or from benign flow murmurs.

2. Diagnosis is by echocardiography and cardiac catheterization.

3. Valve replacement is the therapy of choice. Timing depends on perceived risks versus anticipated benefits. Studies from the USRDS have not demonstrated any difference in survival based on the use of tissue versus nontissue bioprosthetic valves. The mortality rate for valve replacement (with or without concurrent coronary artery bypass surgery) is relatively high for dialysis patients; however, in most cases the prognosis is worse if clinically indicated surgery is not performed or if emergent surgery rather than elective surgery is performed.

VIII. Arrhythmias, cardiac arrest, and sudden cardiac death

A. Risk factors. Many comorbid conditions that are highly prevalent in dialysis patients are also associated with arrhythmias. These include LVH, chamber enlargement, valve abnormalities, and ischemic heart disease. Additionally, serum levels of cations that can affect cardiac conduction, including potassium, calcium, hydrogen, and magnesium, are often abnormal and undergo rapid fluctuation during hemodialysis.

B. Cardiac arrest and acute arrhythmias. According to the 2001 USRDS, cardiac arrest of unknown cause and identified arrhythmias account for 60% of cardiac deaths in dialysis patients. Thirty-day survival after cardiac arrest is only 32% and 1-year survival 15%. Potential strategies to reduce the risk of fatal cardiac risk include careful attention to fluid and electrolyte shifts. Risk of arrhythmias and cardiac arrest are increased in patients being dialyzed using a dialysate potassium level of <2.0 mM; these low potassium solutions should not be used unless the benefits outweigh the risks. For acute arrhythmias that occur during dialysis, the dialysis session should be terminated and blood returned cautiously. Urgent cardioversion per the American Heart Association's Advanced Cardiovascular Life Support (ACLS) guidelines is indicated for all patients who are unstable. Amiodarone, currently the first-line pharmacologic intervention for ventricular tachycardia in the general population, is dosed identically in dialysis patients. Airway management and cardiac monitoring are essential. Administration of procainamide and other class Ia antiarrhythmics should be undertaken with caution as they may cause QT prolongation and torsades de pointes in dialysis patients.

C. Chronic arrhythmias

1. **Atrial fibrillation** remains the most common arrhythmia in both the general and dialysis population and often occurs in patients with structural heart disease and in particular left atrial enlargement.

a. **Drug therapy.** When restoration of sinus rhythm cannot be maintained, rate control becomes the focus of therapy. Several medications have traditionally been used for rate control in atrial fibrillation, including digoxin, beta-blockers, nondihydropyridine calcium channel blockers, and amiodarone. Beta-blockers or nondihydropyridine calcium channel blockers such as diltiazem are good choices for rate control in patients with intact systolic function but may be contraindicated in subjects with reduced cardiac function due to their negative inotropic effects. In these subjects, there clearly is a tradeoff, as chronic control of tachycardia may offset any drug-related decrease in cardiac inotropy by changing the Frank-Starling relationship. Although a less effective agent for rate control, digoxin is frequently used in patients with reduced systolic function. Paradoxically, digoxin use is also associated with a high risk of arrhythmias. When digoxin is used in dialysis patients, extreme care must be taken to minimize electrolyte shifts and, in particular, hypokalemia. These patients should generally be on a 3.0-mM potassium bath. Less alkaline dialysate may also be necessary to prevent potassium shifts. In patients with reduced ejection fraction in whom digoxin does not adequately control heart rate or in whom electrolyte abnormalities remain difficult to manage, amiodarone may be the drug of choice. Importantly, due to drug interactions among warfarin, amiodarone, and digoxin, combinations of these drugs should be used with extreme caution if at all in dialysis patients.

b. **Anticoagulation.** The risks and benefits of warfarin therapy should be considered on an individual basis in all dialysis patients with chronic and paroxysmal atrial fibrillation. Unfortunately, there are no consistent data regarding anticoagulation for atrial fibrillation in the dialysis population. Of note, warfarin is associated with an increased risk of vascular calcification in the general population and in individuals with CKD; this is likely due to warfarin-induced decreased activity of mineralization inhibitor matrix Gla protein. There may also be an association between calciphylaxis and warfarin use; however, as of publication, these data have only been published in abstract form.

2. **Ventricular arrhythmias and ectopy** are common in the dialysis population. There are no data indicating that cardiac management of patients prone to arrhythmia should be any different than in the general population. When indicated, dialysis patients may benefit from implantable defibrillators. Amiodarone therapy is generally well tolerated and dosing is identical to that in the general population.

SUGGESTED READINGS

Achinger SG, Ayus JC. The role of vitamin D in left ventricular hypertrophy and cardiac function. *Kidney Int* 2005;67(S95): s37–s42.

Ayus JC, et al. Effects of short daily versus conventional hemodialysis on left ventricular hypertrophy and inflammatory markers: a prospective, controlled study. *J Am Soc Nephrol* 2005;16:2778–2788.

Becit N, et al. Subxiphoid pericardiostomy in the management of pericardial effusions: case series analysis of 368 patients. *Heart* 2005;91:785–790.

Berger AK, Duval S, Krumholz HM. Aspirin, beta-blocker, and angiotensin-converting enzyme inhibitor therapy in patients with end-stage renal disease and an acute myocardial infarction. *J Am Coll Cardiol* 2003;42:201–208.

Block GA. Effects of sevelamer and calcium on coronary artery calcification in patients new to hemodialysis. *Kidney Int* 2005;68: 1815–1824.

Bonaa KH, et al. Homocysteine lowering and cardiovascular events after acute myocardial infarction. *N Engl J Med* 2006;354: 1578–1588.

Chan CT, et al. Regression of left ventricular hypertrophy after conversion to nocturnal hemodialysis. *Kidney Int* 2002;61:2235–2239.

Cho BC, et al. Clinical and echocardiographic characteristics of pericardial effusion in patients who underwent echocardiographically guided pericardiocentesis: Yonsei Cardiovascular Center experience, 1993–2003. *Yonsei Med J* 2004;45:462–468.

Clarke R, Lewington S, Landray M. Homocysteine, renal function, and risk of cardiovascular disease. *Kidney Int Suppl* 2003;63(84): S131–133.

Covic A, Gusbeth-Tatomir P, Goldsmith DJ. Is it time for spironolactone therapy in dialysis patients?. *Nephrol Dial Transplant* 2006;21:854–858.

Daugirdas JT, et al. Subxiphoid pericardiostomy for hemodialysis-associated pericardial effusion. *Arch Intern Med* 1986;146:1113–1115.

deFilippi C, et al. Cardiac troponin T and C-reactive protein for predicting prognosis, coronary atherosclerosis, and cardiomyopathy in patients undergoing long-term hemodialysis. *JAMA* 2003;290: 353–359.

Gibney EM, et al. Cardiovascular medication use after coronary bypass surgery in patients with renal dysfunction: a National Veterans Administration study. *Kidney Int* 2005;68:826–832.

Hegarty J, et al. Calcific uraemic arteriolopathy causing skin necrosis: the UK National Epidemiological Survey [Abstract]. *J Am Soc Nephrol* 2005;16:SA-PO785.

Herzog CA. Cardiac arrest in dialysis patients: approaches to alter an abysmal outcome. *Kidney Int Suppl* 2003;63 (S84):S197–200.

Kalantar-Zadeh K, et al. Reverse epidemiology of cardiovascular risk factors in maintenance dialysis patients. *Kidney Int* 2003;63: 793–808.

Kasiske B, et al. Clinical practice guidelines for managing dyslipidemias in kidney transplant patients. *Am J Transplantation* 2004: 4(Suppl 7):13–53.

Kennedy DJ, et al. Uremic cardiomyopathy—an endogenous digitalis intoxication? Central role for the cardiotonic steroid marinobufa-genin in the pathogenesis of uremic cardiomyopathy. *Hypertension* 2006;47:488–495.

Kim HW, et al. Calcitriol regresses cardiac hypertrophy and QT dispersion in secondary hyperparathyroidism on hemodialysis. *Nephron Clin Practice* 2006;102:c21–c29.

London GM, et al. Arterial structure and function in end-stage renal disease. *Nephrol Dial Transplant* 2002;17:1713–1724.

Longenecker JC, et al. Traditional cardiovascular disease risk factors in dialysis patients compared with the general population: the CHOICE Study. *J Am Soc Nephrol* 2002;13:1918–1927.

MacRae JM, et al. The cardiovascular effects of arteriovenous fistulas in chronic kidney disease: a cause for concern? *Semin Dial* 2006;19:349–448.

Mallamaci F, et al. Hyperhomocysteinemia predicts cardiovascular outcomes in hemodialysis patients. *Kidney Int* 2002;61:609–614.

Middleton RJ, Parfrey PS, Foley RN. Left ventricular hypertrophy in the renal patient. *J Am Soc Nephrol* 2001;12:1079–1084.

Molitch ME. Management of dyslipidemias in patients with diabetes and chronic kidney disease. *Clin J Am Soc Nephrol* 2006;1:1090–1099.

National Kidney Foundation. KDOQI clinical practice guidelines for cardiovascular disease in dialysis patients. *Am J Kidney Dis* 2005;45(4 Suppl 3):s1–s153.

Pilkey RM, et al. Lifetime warfarin exposure is associated with aortic valve calcification in hemodialysis patients. *J Am Soc Nephrol* 2005;16:729A.

Sarnak MJ, et al. Kidney disease as a risk factor for development of cardiovascular disease: a statement from the American Heart Association Councils on Kidney in Cardiovascular Disease, High Blood Pressure Research, Clinical Cardiology, and Epidemiology and Prevention. *Circulation* 2003;108:2154–2169.

Schleithoff S, et al. Vitamin D supplementation improves cytokine profiles in patients with congestive heart failure: a double-blind, randomized, placebo-controlled trial *Am J Clin Nutr* 2006;83:754–759.

Seliger SL, et al. HMG-CoA reductase inhibitors are associated with reduced mortality in ESRD patients. *Kidney Int* 2002;61:297–304.

Spittle MA, et al. Oxidative stress and inflammation in hemodialysis patients. *Am J Kidney Dis* 2001;38:1408–1413.

Wanner C, et al. Atorvastatin in patients with type 2 diabetes mellitus undergoing hemodialysis. *N Engl J Med* 2005;353:238–248.

Weiner DE, Sarnak MJ. Managing dyslipidemia in chronic kidney disease. *J Gen Intern Med* 2004;19:1045–1052.

Yuen D, et al. The natural history of coronary calcification progression in a cohort of nocturnal haemodialysis patients. *Nephrol Dial Transplant* 2006;21:1407–1412.

WEB REFERENCES

HDCN cardiovascular disease channel: http://www.hdcn.com/ch/highbp/

Digestive Tract

Susie Q. Lew and Juan P. Bosch

I. Common gastrointestinal (GI) symptoms

A. Anorexia. Anorexia is a nonspecific symptom that is a manifestation of uremia but may be due to any number of other causes. Covert infection should always be suspected if anorexia suddenly manifests or worsens.

B. Nausea and vomiting. Prior to the initiation of dialysis, patients may complain of nausea and vomiting. These symptoms usually disappear with dialysis and removal of uremic toxins but may recur if dialysis becomes inadequate. Nausea and vomiting are not uncommon during a dialysis session, and then are thought to be due either to a mild form of disequilibrium syndrome or are associated with hypotension (see Chapter 10). If either uremia or the dialysis session is not likely to be at fault, then a thorough evaluation for possible cerebral or GI causes is indicated.

C. Dyspepsia. Dyspepsia is persistent or recurrent abdominal discomfort centered in the upper abdomen (epigastrium). "Indigestion" is a common patient-used synonym. Symptoms may include epigastric pain or discomfort, bloating, belching, eructations, and flatulence. Dyspepsia may be due to a true GI pathologic process, such as peptic ulcer, gastroesophageal reflux, gastritis, duodenitis, or, in diabetic patients, gastroparesis. Alternatively, dyspepsia may be related to medications that dialysis patients are required to take, such as phosphate binders or iron supplements. Evaluation for an organic lesion is warranted if the history and physical examination are suggestive. Prokinetic agents, histamine-2 receptor antagonists, and proton pump inhibitors are the most widely used medications in management (Table 38-1). Antacids should be used sparingly and those containing aluminum or magnesium are best avoided.

D. Constipation. Constipation is not an uncommon complaint among dialysis patients. The causes are multifactorial. Patients' fluid intake is limited. Dietary restriction of high-potassium-containing fruits and vegetables decreases fiber intake. Calcium-containing phosphate binders and iron supplements cause constipation. Patient inactivity and underlying medical conditions may contribute. Narcotic analgesics such as codeine and meperidine can cause it. All of these factors operate on a background prolongation of colonic transit time in these patients (Wu et al., 2004).

Constipation may result in obstipation with obstruction, fecal impaction, and even bowel perforation. Long term it may contribute to diverticular disease as well as hemorrhoids. In patients treated with peritoneal dialysis, decreased bowel motility can cause dialysate outflow obstruction.

Table 38-1.   Doses of histamine-2 blockers and proton pump inhibitors in ESRD

Name	Dose
Histamine-2 blockers	
Cimetidine (Tagamet)	400–800 mg PO q24h
Ranitidine (Zantac)[a]	150 mg PO q24h
Famotidine (Pepcid)	20–40 mg PO q.h.s.
Nizatidine (Axid)[a]	150–300 mg PO q48h
Proton pump inhibitors	
Esomeprazole (Nexium)	20–40 mg PO q24h
Omeprazole (Prilosec)	20–40 mg PO q24h
Lansoprazole (Prevacid)	15–30 mg PO q24h
Pantoprazole (Protonix)	40 mg PO q24h
Rabeprazole (AcipHex)	20 mg PO q24h

[a]Clearance is mainly renal.
ESRD, end-stage renal disease; PO, by mouth; q24h, daily; q.h.s., at bedtime; q48h, every other day.

Increasing the fiber content of the diet usually helps. If constipation persists, the following agents may be used: Emollient: Docusate sodium (Colace) 100 mg PO q24h to t.i.d. PRN (as needed), casanthranol and docusate sodium (Peri-Colace) one to two capsules or one to two tablespoons PO q.h.s. (every evening at bedtime) PRN; Stimulant: Bisacodyl (Dulcolax) one to three tablets PO q24h PRN; and Hyperosmotic: Lactulose (Chronulac) 30 mL PO q.h.s., polyethylene glycol (Miralax) one teaspoon in water PO q24h Soap suds, mineral oil, and tap water enemas or bisacodyl or glycerin suppositories once daily may be used for more immediate results.

Sodium polystyrene sulfonate resin plus sorbitol (Kayexalate) has been associated with intestinal necrosis in end-stage renal disease (ESRD) patients, either given by enema or by the oral route (Dardik et al., 2000). It is not clear if the sorbitol component alone is equally dangerous. Whereas the combination is still widely used to treat hyperkalemia, use of sorbitol to treat constipation, when there are alternatives available, may not be wise.

Medicinal fiber in the form of psyllium (Metamucil) also should be avoided. Both sodium and potassium are present in the preparation, and a large volume of liquid is required in preparation. Laxatives containing magnesium, citrate, or phosphate should be avoided (e.g., milk of magnesium, magnesium citrate, and Fleet's products containing phosphate). Magnesium is poorly handled by patients with ESRD. Hypermagnesemia can result in development of neurologic disorders or in dangerous bradycardia with arrhythmias. Citrate, in general, should be avoided in patients with ESRD because it increases absorption of aluminum from the GI tract. **Severe hyperphosphatemia, dangerous**

hypocalcemia, coma, rectal necrosis, and vascular cal-cification have all been reported in ESRD patients after use of phosphate-containing enemas.

E. Diarrhea. An episode of diarrhea on an occasional ba-sis is not uncommon and may be related to bowel irritability associated with dietary intake or to a viral GI disorder.

Diarrhea following a period of constipation may signal fe-cal impaction. Treatment is then focused on alleviating the constipation.

An acute episode of bloody diarrhea associated with abdom-inal pain, fever and signs of sepsis, and hypotension may suggest ischemic bowel disorder or bowel infarction. Diar-rhea associated with fever suggests an infectious cause. Blood and stool specimen for culture and sensitivity are required. *Clostridium difficile* enteritis may occur after prolonged an-timicrobial therapy. Oral vancomycin 125–500 mg PO q.i.d. or metronidazole 500 mg PO t.i.d. is used in the treatment of *C. difficile* enteritis.

Persistent diarrhea requires a workup similar to that in patients without ESRD. Autonomic neuropathy should be suspected in patients with diabetes mellitus. Endoscopy is required to diagnose inflammatory bowel disorders. Malab-sorption is suspected if food fibers or fat are found in the stool. Dietary adjustment or digestive enzyme replacement may help or correct malabsorption.

In noninfectious diarrhea, attapulgite (Kaopectate), lop-eramide hydrochloride (Imodium), or diphenoxylate hy-drochloride and atropine sulfate (Lomotil) may be used for temporary relief.

The use of probiotics to repopulate the gut with bene-ficial bacteria, especially after a course of antibiotics, has not been evaluated specifically in chronic kidney disease (CKD) patients. *Bifidobacterium infantis* has been beneficial in nonuremic patients with diarrhea due to irritable bowel syndrome as well as in patients with inflammatory bowel disease.

F. Hiccups. Diaphragmatic irritation, hyponatremia, or other metabolic derangements, such as uremia, may result in intractable hiccups. Those due to uremia can be corrected with dialysis.

G. Other GI symptoms. Dysgeusia, a metallic taste in the mouth, and a peculiar odor to the breath are often noted by ure-mic patients. **Uremic stomatitis** is a peculiar oral inflamma-tion that some patients manifest. **Parotitis and sicca syn-drome** are commonly present, thus limiting compliance with fluid restriction. Vitamin B_{12} deficiency might then be looked for (Andres et al., 2006). Such oral and gustatory complications may contribute to decreased nutritional intake.

II. Upper GI diseases

A. Gastritis, duodenitis, and peptic ulcer disease. The prevalence of ulcer disease and *Helicobacter pylori* gastritis is not significantly different from the general population. How-ever, upper endoscopy of stable dialysis patients reveals ab-normalities in up to 83% of cases. Gastritis, duodenitis, and mucosal erosions are most commonly seen. *H. pylori* is present in almost all cases of nonerosive chronic active gastritis and in some cases of chronic gastritis without the active component.

B. Upper GI bleeding. Causes for upper GI bleeding in patients with chronic renal failure in one study were as follows: angiodysplasia of the stomach or duodenum (24%), erosive gastritis (18%), duodenal ulcer (17%), erosive esophagitis (17%), gastric ulcer (12%), Mallory-Weiss (8%), and erosive duodenitis (3%). It is possible that angiodysplastic lesions in both the upper and lower tract in these patients are no more common than in the general population. However, they may be discovered more frequently because angiodysplastic lesions in patients with chronic renal failure are more likely to bleed than such lesions in patients without renal failure. Uremic platelet dysfunction may play a contributory role.

Recently, a so-called "watermelon stomach" has been described (Stefanidis et al., 2006) characterized by gastric antral vascular ectasia. Treatment is by endoscopic bipolar electrocoagulation.

  1. Diagnosis. Esophagogastroduodenoscopy (EGD) is more likely to provide an accurate diagnosis than a single-contrast barium meal radiograph in patients with upper GI bleeding.

  2. Management

  a. Treatment for *H. pylori* includes one to three antibiotics given in combination with a proton pump inhibitor. For dosing of these agents in renal failure, see Table 38-1. Use of bismuth-based regimens should be avoided because of accumulation of bismuth due to impaired renal excretion (Gladziwa and Koltz, 1994).

  b. Treatment of upper GI bleeding is the same as for nonuremic patients. It consists of nasogastric aspiration, transfusion, and the administration of acid secretion inhibition with proton pump inhibitors or histamine-2 blockers. Proton pump inhibitors can be used in the usual dose. Histamine-2 blockers are partially excreted renally, and their usual dosage should be reduced by at least 50% in chronic renal failure.

  Antacids containing aluminum and magnesium hydroxide should be avoided in dialysis patients because of risk of aluminum toxicity and hypermagnesemia. Sucralfate (Carafate) is a sulfated polysaccharide, sucrose octasulfate, complexed with aluminum hydroxide. Sucralfate should not be used in dialysis patients because of the risk of intestinal aluminum absorption (Robertson et al., 1989).

  Risk factors for ulcer formation (nonsteroidal antiinflammatory drug or aspirin ingestion, smoking) should be eliminated if possible.

C. Gastric retention. Gastric retention is uncommon in nondiabetic dialysis patients but does occur, and its correction results in improved nutritional status (Ross and Koo, 1998). Patients on continuous ambulatory peritoneal dialysis may complain of symptoms of gastric retention when dialysate is present in the abdomen; symptoms are relieved with draining of the dialysate.

Gastroparesis is frequently encountered in patients with diabetes mellitus, and is associated with autonomic neuropathy. Diagnosis can be made with an isotopic gastric emptying study. Prokinetic drugs block dopaminergic receptors in the upper alimentary tract, stimulating motility of the esophagus, stomach, and upper small intestine. Prokinetic agents include domperidone and metoclopramide. In nonuremic patients, both are equally efficacious, but central nervous system side effects may be less with domperidone (Patterson et al., 1999). There is little information about the pharmacokinetics of domperidone in renal failure patients (Lauritsen et al., 1990). Metoclopramide is renally excreted to a large extent, and the usual dose of 10–15 mg q.i.d. needs to be reduced by 50% in patients with minimal renal function. Metoclopramide is normally given 30 minutes before meals and at bedtime. Cisapride, which in some hands was a more efficacious drug than either domperidone or metoclopramide, is no longer sold in the United States because of the regular occurrence of QT interval prolongation, worsened by coadministration of many other common drugs, and occasional occurrence of fatal arrhythmia.

D. Gallbladder disease. Chronic cholecystitis and cholelithiasis are common in dialysis patients. In one study, gallstone disease was detected in 33% of the dialysis population, of whom 82% were asymptomatic. The stones were radiolucent in 88% of cases. In patients with polycystic kidney disease, dilation of the common bile duct is common (Ishikawa et al., 1996). Symptomatic patients can be treated with laparoscopic cholecystectomy or traditional cholecystectomy. Asymptomatic patients usually undergo cholecystectomy if they are renal transplant candidates.

III. Lower GI disease

A. Diverticulosis and diverticulitis. Right-sided diverticular disease is more common in the dialysis population than in the general population. Constipation due to dietary restriction of fluid, fruits, and vegetables and due to the use of phosphate binders may predispose dialysis patients to diverticular disease. Colonic diverticula are increased among those suffering from polycystic kidney disease. Complications of diverticulosis include diverticulitis and colonic perforation. Diverticulitis is a relative contraindication for peritoneal dialysis. In renal transplant candidates with recurrent diverticulitis, segmental resection of the lesions prior to transplantation may lower the risk of perforation associated with high-dose steroid therapy once immunosuppression has been initiated.

B. Spontaneous colonic perforation. Spontaneous colonic perforation may be seen in patients with increased risk, such as those with diverticular disease, amyloidosis, constipation, posttransplantation immunosuppressive treatment, and infections. Spontaneous perforation may occur in the absence of an obvious cause or risk factor. A vasculitic pathogenesis has been proposed. When a patient receiving dialysis presents with abdominal pain, consider impending or actual colonic perforation. If perforation occurs, the mortality rate is extremely high.

C.   Discrete colonic ulceration. A patient with ESRD who is receiving hemodialysis and who presents with symptoms similar to those of appendicitis or carcinoma of the colon, or even with rectal bleeding, may have discrete, nonspecific single ulcers of the cecum or ascending colon. The pathogenesis of such lesions is unknown. Treatment is oriented toward symptoms.

D.   Intestinal necrosis. Necrosis of the small and large intestines has been reported in renal failure patients receiving oral or rectal sodium polystyrene sulfonate in sorbitol. Whether the culprit is the exchange resin or sorbitol is unknown.

E.   Colon cancer. The official clinical practice guidelines for detection in the general population should apply.

F.   Angiodysplasia. Angiodysplasias are acquired lesions of the GI tract affecting submucosal and mucosal blood vessels. These lesions, multiple and small (measuring <5 mm), usually are located in the cecum and right colon. The diagnosis is best made by angiography or endoscopy. Angiodysplasia can cause acute and chronic blood loss in ESRD patients and presents predominantly in patients over the age of 50. In addition to correcting platelet dysfunction and decreasing the dose of heparin used during dialysis treatments, conservative therapy with low-dose estrogens (i.e., oral conjugated estrogen therapy, 0.3–0.625 mg per day) has been shown to stop the bleeding, whereas bowel resection did not help because of the presence of multiple lesions. Electrocautery can be used to stop an actively bleeding lesion seen during colonoscopy.

G.   Ischemic bowel disease. The combination of atherosclerosis involving the intestinal vasculature and prolonged episodes of hypotension, especially during and after hemodialysis treatments, predisposes patients to ischemic bowel disease and bowel infarction. Some patients present with abdominal pain, hypotension, and bloody diarrhea, whereas others present with signs and symptoms of sepsis without an obvious cause. Arteriography may be required to make the diagnosis.

H.   Peritonitis. See Chapter 24.

I.   Hernia. See Chapter 25.

IV.   Ascites

A.   Hemodialysis-associated ascites. The diagnosis is one of exclusion and is made only when evidence for alternative causative factors such as congestive heart failure, cirrhosis of the liver, lupus, or abdominal malignancy have been excluded. The pathogenesis might be multifactorial: Increased capillary hydrostatic pressure caused by volume overload and a decrease of oncotic pressure by hypoalbuminemia, in the face of abnormally high peritoneal permeability and reduced lymphatic drainage of the ascitic fluid.

Treatment is first to ensure that adequate dialysis is being given. Fluid overload needs to be corrected by sodium restriction and adequate fluid removal during dialysis (including use of isolated ultrafiltration, although the need for this is controversial). Patients should be encouraged to eat well in order to maintain adequate nutritional status. Ascitic fluid can be difficult to remove by dialysis because of continued patient noncompliance with sodium and fluid restriction. Also, increased intra-abdominal pressure caused by the ascites can interfere with cardiac function and venous return, causing intradialytic hypotension. Finally, over time, the ascitic fluid can develop a high oncotic pressure. (Protein concentration tends to be low initially, but then may increase.)

Other methods for the removal of dialysis-associated ascites include placing the patient on peritoneal dialysis or performing a renal transplantation.

Chylous ascites associated with acute pancreatitis has been seen; the peritoneal fluid is typically milky white, so the diagnosis is difficult to miss.

V. Liver disease
A. Hepatitis. See Chapter 33.
B. Hemosiderosis. Hemosiderosis (iron overload) is now rarely seen in dialysis patients compared with the pre-erythropoietin era when blood transfusion, and therefore iron loading, was given to maintain hematocrit. If hemosiderosis is detected, it is better to use erythropoietin to consume iron rather than to use iron-chelating agents. The chelating agent deferoxamine has been associated with cerebral, pulmonary, and intestinal mucormycosis.

VI. Pancreatitis. Acute pancreatitis occurs at a rate of 0.03 per patient year in peritoneal dialysis patients and 0.01 per patient year in hemodialysis patients. Acute pancreatitis follows organ transplantation in 2%–9% of patients. About half of these attacks occur beyond the sixth postoperative month (Padilla et al., 1994). Acute pancreatitis is suspected when a patient complains of left upper quadrant pain with elevated serum amylase and lipase levels. The serum amylase level is often elevated in dialysis patients without pancreatitis. However, the level rarely exceeds two to three times the upper limit of normal. The use of laboratory tests to diagnose pancreatitis is discussed in Chapter 29.

The usual causes for pancreatitis should be considered. Treatment is the same as for nonuremic patients. Supportive care of acute pancreatitis consists of analgesia for pain control, restoration and maintenance of intravascular volume, and frequent monitoring of physical findings and vital signs. To minimize pancreatic secretions, patients should be given nothing by mouth. Nasogastric suction is indicated for symptomatic relief of vomiting, severe nausea, and developing or complete paralytic ileus. Once the pain has subsided, small feedings of a diet high in carbohydrate but low in protein and fat are begun, with increments to regular food several days later as tolerated but avoiding large meals. The use of histamine-2 blockers is controversial.

VII. Bowel preparation for surgery, radiography, or colonoscopy. Electrolyte solutions containing ethylene glycol polymers (i.e., Colyte, GoLYTELY, or NuLYTELY) may be used in bowel preparation procedures. Because of the osmotic properties of the polyethylene glycol, little if any of the administered solution is absorbed. The solution is promptly evacuated by rectum, thus cleansing the bowel. Other effective preparations include castor oil, extract of senna fruit, or bisacodyl tablets or suppositories. Dosage for these need not be adjusted for renal function.

SELECTED READINGS

Al-Mueilo SH. Gastroduodenal lesions and *Helicobacter pylori* infection in hemodialysis patients. *Saudi Med J* 2004;25(8):1010–1014.

Andres E, et al. Primary Sjögren's syndrome and vitamin B12 deficiency: preliminary results in 80 patients. *Am J Med*. 2006;119(6): e9–10.

Badalamenti S, et al. High prevalence of silent gallstone disease in dialysis patients. *Nephron* 1994:66(2)225–227.

Bender JS, et al. Acute abdomen in the hemodialysis patient population. *Surgery* 1995;117(5):494–497.

Bruno MJ, et al. Acute pancreatitis in peritoneal dialysis and haemodialysis: risk, clinical course, outcome, and possible aetiology. *Gut* 2000;46:385–389.

Dardik A, et al. Acute abdomen with colonic necrosis induced by Kayexalate-sorbitol. *South Med J* 2000;93(5):511–513.

Fabbian F, et al. Esophagogastroduodenoscopy in chronic hemodialysis patients: 2-year clinical experience in a renal unit. *Clin Nephrol* 2002;58(1):54–59.

Gladziwa U, Koltz U. Pharmacokinetic optimisation of the treatment of peptic ulcer in patients with renal failure. *Clin Phamacokinet* 1994;27(5):393–408.

Huang JJ, et al. Diagnostic efficacy of (13)C-urea breath test for Helicobacter pylori infection in hemodialysis patients. *Am J Kidney Dis* 2000;36(1):124–129.

Ing TS, et al. Treatment of refractory hemodialysis ascites with maintenance peritoneal dialysis. *Clin Nephrol* 1981;15:198–202.

Ishikawa I, et al. High incidence of common bile duct dilatation in autosomal dominant polycystic kidney disease patients. *Am J Kidney Dis* 1996;27(3):321–326.

Lauritsen K, et al. Clinical pharmacokinetics of drugs used in the treatment of gastrointestinal diseases (Part I). *Clin Pharmocokinet* 1990;19(1):11–31.

Lillemoe KD, et al. Intestinal necrosis due to sodium polystyrene (Kayexalate) in sorbitol enemas: clinical and experimental support for the hypothesis. *Surgery* 1987;101(3):267–272.

Mak SK, et al. A retrospective study on efficacy of proton-pump inhibitor-based triple therapy for eradication of *Helicobacter pylori* in patients with chronic renal failure. *Singapore Med J* 2003; 44(2):74–78.

Marcuard SP, Weinstock JV. Gastrointestinal angiodysplasia in renal failure. *J Clin Gastroenterol* 1988;10(5):482–484.

Matsuo H, et al. A case of hypermagnesemia accompanied by hypercalcemia induced by a magnesium laxative in a hemodialysis patient. *Nephron* 1995;71:477–478.

Melero M, et al. Idiopathic dialysis ascites in the nineties: resolution after renal transplantation. *Am J Kidney Dis* 1995;26(4):668–670.

Negri AL, et al. Upper gastrointestinal bleeding in patients in chronic hemodialysis. *Nephron* 1994(1);67:130.

Padilla B, et al. Pancreatitis in patients with end-stage renal disease. *Medicine* 1994(1);73:8–20.

Patterson D, et al. A double-blind multicenter comparison of dom-peridone and metoclopramide in the treatment of diabetic patients with symptoms of gastroparesis. *Am J Gastroenterol* 1999;94(5): 1230–1234.

Richardson JD, Lordon RE. Gastrointestinal bleeding caused by an-giodysplasia: a difficult problem in patients with chronic renal fail-ure receiving hemodialysis therapy. *Am Surg* 1993;59(10):636–638.

Robertson JA, et al. Sucralfate, intestinal aluminum absorption, and aluminum toxicity in a patient on dialysis. *Ann Intern Med* 1989;111(2):179–181.

Ross EA, Koo LC. Improved nutrition after the detection and treat-ment of occult gastroparesis in nondiabetic dialysis patients. *Am J Kidney Dis* 1998;31(1):62–66.

Rutsky EA, et al. Acute pancreatitis in patients with end-stage renal disease without transplantation. *Arch Intern Med* 1986;146(9):1741–1745.

Sotoudehmanesh R, et al. Endoscopic findings in end-stage renal dis-ease. *Endoscopy* 2003;35(6):502–505.

Stefanidis I, et al. Gastric antral vascular ectasia (watermelon stom-ach) in patients with ESRD. *Am J Kidney Dis* 2006;47(6):e77–82.

Tamura H, et al. Eradication of *Helicobacter pylori* in patients with end-stage renal disease under dialysis treatment. *Am J Kidney Dis* 1997;29(1):86–90.

Vreman HJ, et al. Taste, smell and zinc metabolism in patients with chronic renal failure. *Nephron* 1980;26(4):163–170.

Wasse H, et al. Risk factors for upper gastrointestinal bleeding among end stage renal disease patients. *Kidney Int* 2003;64(4):1455–1461.

Wu MJ, et al. Colonic transit time in long-term dialysis patients. *Am J Kidney Dis* 2004;44(2):322–327.

Genitourinary Tract and Male Reproductive Organs

Kar Neng Lai, Petras V. Kisielius,
and Biff F. Palmer

Although the kidneys in dialysis patients have, to a greater or lesser degree, "failed," they remain present and can be the source of stones, infection, and malignancy with their associated complications. Dialysis patients have many risk factors associated with erectile dysfunction along with pituitary–gonadal dysfunction. The substantial diagnostic and treatment experience in this population is reviewed.

I. Flank pain
A. Etiology and workup. Flank pain occurs in up to 36% of hemodialysis patients with adult polycystic kidney disease as opposed to 2% of hemodialysis patients with end-stage renal disease (ESRD) due to other causes. In general, the diagnostic workup of flank pain proceeds in a similar fashion as for nonuremic patients. The differential diagnoses are listed in Table 39-1.

B. Management

    1. Analgesic treatment. Morphine is the drug of choice but should be used with caution. Although morphine is metabolized mostly by the liver, the clearance of morphine metabolites is reduced in renal failure, resulting in a prolonged sedative effect. Codeine's half-life is prolonged in dialysis patients; therefore, the dosing interval for the drug should be raised from 6 to 24 hours. Aspirin should be avoided because of its effects on the bleeding time. Acetaminophen can be used in the usual dosage. Meperidine and propoxyphene should be avoided because their toxic nor-derivatives have prolonged half-lives in dialysis patients.

    2. Specific treatment. Specific treatment for flank pain depends on the underlying cause and follows standard urologic principles.

II. Bleeding
A. Etiology and workup. Bleeding from the collecting system or renal parenchyma can manifest as microscopic or gross hematuria. Causal factors are listed in Table 39-2. Up to one third of hemodialysis patients with polycystic kidney disease (PKD) experience hemorrhage into cysts. Intracystic bleeding can manifest as dull flank or abdominal pain. Orthostatic hypotension or even shock may supervene if hemorrhage is severe. Dissection of a hemorrhagic cyst into the collecting system is a common cause of microscopic and gross hematuria in patients with PKD and is the cause of gross hematuria in 5% of patients with acquired renal cystic disease (ARCD) (ARCD

Table 39-1.   Approach to flank pain in dialysis patients

Etiology

Cyst related
- Subcapsular hemorrhage
- Perirenal hemorrhage
- Hemorrhage into a cyst
- Enlarging cyst
- Extrinsic ureteral obstruction by a cyst
- Cyst infection

Pyelonephritis
Renal cell carcinoma
Acute ureteral obstruction (colicky pain)
- Stone
- Blood clot
- Sloughed papilla

Diagnosis

- Computed tomography and/or ultrasonography
- Retrograde pyelography

Management

- Pain control
- Codeine (give q24h instead of q6h); beware of constipation
- Morphine can be used cautiously (initially 50% of the usual dosage) for severe pain
- Treat the underlying disorder

---

is described below in section V). Bleeding into cysts results from the underlying renal disease as well as the coagulopathy associated with uremia and anticoagulants given during hemodialysis.

B.   Management. Management of bleeding is contingent on the underlying cause. Heparin-free or regional citrate methods should be used to perform hemodialysis if bleeding is active.

III.   Urolithiasis. The incidence of symptomatic urolithiasis in hemodialysis and continuous ambulatory peritoneal dialysis (CAPD) patients is about 5%–13%, compared with 3% in the general population (Viterbo and Mydlo, 2002). The incidence of asymptomatic urolithiasis is higher and many will have recurring stone disease; one study reported an 83% recurrence rate. The incidence is even higher in patients with PKD. Most stones are composed of protein matrix, amyloid material, calcium oxalate, or a combination of the three. Patients previously on long-term therapy with aluminum-containing phosphate binders may have formed aluminum–magnesium urate stones. Since dialysis patients have a wide range of urine output, the clinician should be alert to the possibility of stone formation.

In general, the symptoms of urolithiasis in hemodialysis patients are similar to those in nonuremic patients. Occasionally,

Table 39-2.   Approach to bleeding in dialysis patients (into the genitourinary system or retroperitoneum)

Etiology

- Urinary tract infection
- Nephrolithiasis
- Subcapsular or perinephric hematoma from a hemorrhagic cyst
- Renal cell carcinoma
- Transitional cell carcinoma
- Renal papillary necrosis
- Hematologic derangement
- Flank or retroperitoneal bleeding
- Cyst hemorrhage
- Spontaneous rupture of the kidney

Diagnosis

- Complete peripheral blood count
- Coagulation profile, bleeding time
- Urine culture
- Ultrasonography or computed tomography
- Urine cytology, cystoscopy, retrograde pyelography if hematuria present
- Angiographic localization of brisk bleeding site

Management

- Correction of any associated coagulopathy
- Treatment of hemorrhage or shock if present
- Correction of bleeding time if abnormal, using desmopressin (intravenous 0.3 mcg/kg in 50 mL normal saline over 30 minutes for three doses every 4 hours), cryoprecipitate, or conjugated estrogens (Premarin) (intravenous 0.6 mg/kg per day for 5 days)
- Angiographic embolization of a bleeding vessel for persistent or severe bleeding
- Endoscopic coagulation of bleeding sites in the calyces of the renal pelvis if possible
- Surgical nephrectomy if failed above-mentioned treatment

flank pain from a renal stone may be confused with early peritonitis in patients on CAPD.

Standard urologic management of symptomatic urolithiasis (with the exception of high fluid volume ingestion) is employed. The use of extracorporeal shock wave lithotripsy to pulverize upper tract stones and other current modalities may be used in dialysis patients with no greater morbidity than in their nondialysis counterparts. Hemodialysis patients with recurrent calcium oxalate stones secondary to primary hyperoxaluria type I should be treated with high-flux dialysis. Combined renal and hepatic transplantation may be required to reverse ongoing systemic complications of oxalosis. Patients with severe recurring intractable stone disease who are candidates for renal transplantation may be assessed critically for bilateral nephrectomies (Viterbo and Mydlo, 2002).

IV. Urinary tract infections (UTIs). The immune status of patients with ESRD is compromised, and coexisting malnutrition, diabetes, and peripheral vascular disease may further lower the resistance to infection. Patients on maintenance hemodialysis, especially those with underlying APKD, have an increased risk of developing nosocomial infections, especially UTIs. UTIs are more common in female dialysis patients, and the incidence increases with age in both sexes. Gram-negative organisms, notably *Escherichia coli,* and *Candida* species predominate.

A. Cystitis

  1. Clinical presentation. In oliguric patients, the symptoms of cystitis are similar to those in nonuremic individuals, although gross hematuria is unusually common and occurs in up to one third of cases. Anuric patients may present with suprapubic discomfort or foul-smelling urethral discharge and progress to pyocystis (see below).

  2. Diagnosis. Voided urine samples from oliguric patients, even from those voiding only a few milliliters per day, are usually sufficient for diagnosis. Urethral catheterization and bladder lavage may cause infection and should be reserved for the symptomatic anuric patient. The presence of pyuria is not a useful finding to rule in or rule out infection (Eisinger et al., 1997; Vera et al., 2002). Absence of visible bacteria does not rule out UTI. A urine culture is essential to make the diagnosis. As in nonuremic patients, a colony count greater than 10^3 in a properly collected urine specimen is considered to be suggestive of infection but there are no good studies in dialysis patients.

  3. Treatment

    a. Antimicrobials to use. Optimally, antimicrobial therapy should be based on sensitivity testing of the organism involved. If empirical therapy is warranted, penicillin, ampicillin, cephalexin, a fluoroquinolone, or trimethoprim should be used because they are safe and may attain adequate urine levels in ESRD patients. Male patients from susceptible populations (Asian and Mediterranean) should be tested for glucose-6-phosphatase deficiency before receiving trimethoprim–sulfamethoxazole. In female dialysis patients, trimethoprim–sulfamethoxazole is generally chosen over ampicillin for treatment of recurrent UTIs; trimethoprim–sulfamethoxazole is less likely to be associated with the emergence of resistant organisms in the fecal flora, the source of most urinary pathogens in women. The dosing of various antimicrobials is discussed in Chapter 33.

    b. Treatment duration. The most appropriate treatment schedule for dialysis patients with cystitis has not been well studied. A urine culture should be repeated on the third or fourth day of treatment documenting that the urine shows no growth, and therapy should be continued for a total of 5–7 days. Ten days of antimicrobial therapy is warranted in patients with adult polycystic kidney disease because of their increased susceptibility to pyogenic complications of UTIs. A follow-up urine culture should be obtained 7–10 days after completing therapy.

   c. Choice of antimicrobial. It is difficult to achieve adequate urinary drug levels of ticarcillin, doxycycline, sulfisoxazole, and the aminoglycosides in dialysis patients; hence, these agents are not recommended for treatment of cystitis. However, when the responsible urinary pathogen is resistant to trimethoprim–sulfamethoxazole, cephalexin, fluoroquinolones, and the penicillins, one of these alternative drugs can be employed if its use is supported by the results of bacterial sensitivity. The use of nalidixic acid, nitrofurantoin, tetracycline, and methenamine mandelate is generally contraindicated in anuric patients due to the prolonged half-lives of these agents and the accumulation of toxic metabolites.

  4. Problems

   a. Unresolved infection occurs when urine cultures remain positive despite antimicrobial treatment. Causes include:

    (1) Bacterial resistance

    (2) Selection of a resistant mutant while on therapy

    (3) Presence of a second unsuspected resistant bacterial species with resulting overgrowth

    (4) Inability of the diseased kidney to achieve bacteriostatic or bactericidal antimicrobial concentrations in the urine

    (5) Excessive bacterial load, such as with a staghorn calculus, an infected communicating renal cyst, or a bladder stone

    If repeated culture and sensitivity testing show bacterial resistance, then the antimicrobial therapy should be adjusted. If the original infecting organism is still sensitive to the initial therapy, the dosage should be increased if possible or intravesical antimicrobial therapy should be administered. If a source of bacteria, such as a staghorn calculus, is identified, it must be removed to cure the UTI permanently.

   b. Bacterial persistence is a recurrent infection from a source within the urinary tract. It is suspected if infections with the same bacteria return immediately after treatment is completed. Causes include:

    (1) Infected cysts

    (2) Infection stones (e.g., staghorn calculus)

    (3) Bacterial prostatitis

   c. Reinfection is a recurrent infection caused by the same or different species of bacteria entering the urinary tract at varied intervals. Reinfection is not usually due to an identifiable anatomic lesion but rather to reintroduction of bacteria from a source outside the urinary tract, most frequently the rectal flora. Vesicoenteric and vaginal fistulas are rare causes of reinfection.

   d. Diagnostic procedures. All patients with recurrent infection should be evaluated for residual urine and urethral stenosis, urethral stricture, or bladder outlet obstruction. A renal ultrasonographic study and plain film tomograms of the kidney should be obtained in dialysis patients with possible bacterial persistence. Computed tomography (CT) with and without contrast infusion may be used if ultrasonographic findings are indeterminate. Cystoscopy is recommended if hematuria occurs or to help rule out enterovesical fistula in patients with pneumaturia. Ureteral catheter localization studies should also be performed if bacterial persistence is suspected. Patients found to have a congenital or acquired anatomic abnormality responsible for their infections should have the defect removed surgically.

5. Antimicrobial prophylaxis. The safety of long-term antimicrobial prophylaxis in dialysis patients with frequent reinfections is not known. Low-dose trimethoprim–sulfamethoxazole and cephalexin would probably be the safest drugs to use.

B. Pyocystis

1. Definition. Pyocystis, the accumulation of pus in a nonfunctioning bladder, occurs with increased frequency in hemodialysis patients.

2. Presentation. Pyocystis should always be suspected in an anuric dialysis patient with fever of unknown origin. Symptoms can include suprapubic or abdominal pain, foul-smelling urethral discharge, or sepsis. Suprapubic tenderness and a distended bladder may be found on careful examination.

3. Diagnosis. A complete peripheral blood count often shows leukocytosis. Blood cultures may or may not be positive. Bladder catheterization reveals pus, culture of which usually grows a mixed flora.

4. Management. Treatment consists of adequate drainage via an indwelling urethral catheter, followed by intermittent catheterization and bladder irrigations with antimicrobial solutions until the infection clears. Parenteral antimicrobials, chosen according to culture and sensitivity reports, should be administered if systemic manifestations are present. Cystourethroscopy and possibly cystometrography should be performed to rule out a bladder outlet obstruction, a large bladder diverticulum, or a neurogenic bladder. Rarely, surgical drainage procedures or even simple cystectomy may be needed in refractory cases.

C. Prostatic abscess. Hemodialysis has been reported to be a risk factor for the development of prostatic abscess. Diagnosis should be suspected in a male patient with a febrile UTI associated with irritative and obstructive voiding symptoms, as well as perineal discomfort. Rectal examination will reveal a tender and boggy prostate that often harbors a fluctuant mass. Transrectal ultrasonography or CT should be used to confirm the diagnosis. Standard urologic management should be employed.

D. Upper urinary tract infections and pyogenic complications

1. Etiology and incidence. Upper tract infections in dialysis patients occur most commonly as a result of retrograde ascent of urinary pathogens in the urinary tract. Rarely, acute pyelonephritis occurs in dialysis patients from a hematogenic route. Patients with cystic kidneys and especially those with adult polycystic disease are particularly susceptible to upper tract infection and its complications. Infected cysts, pyonephrosis, and renal and perirenal abscesses may develop.

2.   Clinical presentation. A patient with an infected cyst or renal or perirenal abscess usually presents with dysuria, recurrent UTIs, fever, night sweats, abdominal or flank pain, or sepsis. Occasionally, the patient may be asymptomatic. A tender, tense mass may be palpable in the flank or abdomen. With systemic symptoms, these patients may develop dehydration due to poor fluid and food intake, sweating, and fever.

3.   Diagnosis. Leukocytosis is commonly present. Urine culture will identify the responsible organism if the parenchymal infection communicates with the collecting system. However, culture results can be negative when the infected cyst does not communicate with the urinary tract, or with pyonephrosis due to a cyst or stone that completely obstructs the ureter. Ultrasonography or CT may identify infected cysts and provide a point of reference for determining response to antimicrobial therapy. The use of indium-111 (^{111}In) leukocyte imaging and gallium-67 (^{67}Ga) citrate single photon emission computed tomography (SPECT) transaxial imaging in localizing infected cysts has been described and may be considered when findings from ultrasonography or CT are inconclusive.

4.   Antimicrobial therapy. In patients with cystic kidneys, antimicrobial therapy of upper tract infection should be continued for at least 3 weeks. Many antimicrobials penetrate renal cysts poorly, and the degree of antimicrobial penetration depends on whether the cysts are derived from the proximal tubule or the distal nephron. Lipid-soluble trimethoprim, ciprofloxacin, metronidazole, clindamycin, erythromycin, and doxycycline have been shown to achieve good bactericidal levels in the fluids of both types of cysts, and should be good treatment selections, depending on the suspected organism. Ciprofloxacin has been shown to sterilize infected cysts in some patients. Non–lipid-soluble antimicrobials, such as the aminoglycosides, the third-generation cephalosporins, and the penicillins, have generally failed to cure infections in polycystic kidneys, presumably because of their poor penetration into cysts derived from the distal nephron.

5.   Treatment of recurrent upper tract infection. Patients with adult polycystic kidneys with bacterial persistence localizing to one side (as documented by ureteral catheter localization studies) should have the source of infection removed surgically. Pyonephrosis and renal and perirenal abscesses cannot be cured by antimicrobial therapy alone and require immediate and definitive surgical intervention. Percutaneous drainage of an infected cyst under radiographic imaging may be appropriate in medically unstable patients, but surgical intervention currently remains the procedure of choice for most localized abscesses. Laparoscopic unroofing of a clearly identifiable infected cyst may be considered. Nephrectomy is indicated only when an infected cyst is unresponsive to antimicrobial therapy or cyst drainage. Delay in nephrectomy is associated with increased morbidity and mortality.

V. Acquired renal cystic disease (ARCD)

A. Etiology and incidence. Acquired renal cystic disease is characterized by the development of bilateral cortical and medullary cysts in previously noncystic kidneys in patients on hemodialysis or peritoneal dialysis. ARCD has been described in uremic patients before the commencement of dialysis. In recipients with chronic rejection, ARCD can develop within the transplant itself. The exact pathogenesis remains unknown.

Within the first 3 years of dialysis, approximately 10%–20% develop ARCD. By 5 years, 40%–60% have it, and by 10 years, more than 90% will have it. Men appear to have a more severe form of ARCD than women, although women are by no means spared. Neither are children. After successful transplantation, the cystic disease associated with ARCD regresses and the kidneys return to their baseline atrophic size; however, tumors associated with ARCD may become more aggressive after transplantation.

B. Symptoms and complications. Usually, ARCD is asymptomatic and diagnosed incidentally on ultrasonography, CT, or magnetic resonance imaging. However, patients with ARCD may develop secondary erythrocytosis (due to production of erythropoietin by the cysts), cyst infections, spontaneous rupture of the kidney, nephrolithiasis, and renal cell carcinoma. Many ARCD patients develop hemorrhagic renal cysts, and perinephric hematomas are not uncommon. Associated symptoms, such as flank or abdominal pain, hematuria, fever, weight loss, or an unexplained drop in hematocrit, warrant investigation with imaging studies. Occasionally, ARCD kidneys will increase markedly in size, such that inherited polycystic kidney disease is simulated (Bakir et al., 1999).

C. Management. Pain, bleeding, and infection are treated as described above. Asymptomatic patients with ARCD need to be screened periodically for renal cell carcinoma as described immediately below.

VI. Screening for malignancy

A. Renal cell carcinoma (with or without ARCD)

1. Incidence. The incidence of renal cell carcinoma in dialysis patients is increased, especially in those with ARCD. Transplantation may lower the malignant potential of native kidneys with ARCD but does not prevent the development of cancer in all.

2. Presentation. The manifestations of renal cell carcinoma include anorexia, weight loss, unexplained fever, hematuria, flank pain, and palpable mass.

3. Screening. Ultrasonography or CT is required to establish the diagnosis. Because of the possibility of malignancy, a baseline renal ultrasound or CT is recommended at the onset of maintenance hemodialysis or peritoneal dialysis.

Ultrasound should also be performed in all patients with any suggestive symptoms or with unexplained erythrocytosis. The presence of enlarged kidneys (in which the risk of malignant transformation is higher) mandates more frequent ultrasound scanning (e.g., every 4–6 months). CT is required to confirm the finding of a mass on ultrasound or to investigate inconclusive ultrasonographic findings.

    a.   Cost–benefit issues. Advocates of screening for ARCD suggest that a baseline study, preferably a CT, be obtained at the onset of dialysis and after 3 years on dialysis (Gulanikar et al., 1998). Depending on what is seen on this baseline, it is recommended that annual or semiannual studies, preferably CT, be obtained. However, all screening comes at a cost that must at least balance the benefits. Using a decision analysis model, screening is shown to provide significant benefits only to those patients with a life expectancy of 25 years or more (Sarasin et al., 1995).

4.   Treatment. Solid masses >3 cm in diameter or with CT attenuation numbers >20 Hounsfield units should be considered to be malignant and treated by radical nephrectomy. Though solid lesions <3 cm were traditionally considered to be benign adenomas in the past, 5% of such tumors have been known to metastasize. Since presently there are no reliable histopathologic, ultrastructural, or immunohistochemical criteria to differentiate benign renal adenoma from renal cell carcinoma, and since renal cell carcinoma can be found in otherwise benign oncocytomas, fine needle aspirations or biopsies of solid renal lesions are not viable diagnostic options at this time. Current management of small solid renal masses is very controversial; these should be managed by radical nephrectomy, partial nephrectomy, ablative therapies, or very careful follow-up with serial ultrasound or CT.

    In addition to the tumor criteria described above, radical nephrectomy should be considered for any tumor with unexplained liver function abnormalities, erythrocytosis, or hypercalcemia. Nephrectomy should also be considered in patients with rapidly enlarging kidneys and possibly in candidates for renal transplantation. Whereas in the past prophylactic nephrectomy for ARCD was rarely considered, the idea is more attractive today with the availability of erythropoietin.

B.   Carcinoma of the renal pelvis. Up to 40% of dialysis patients with analgesic nephropathy ultimately develop cancer of the renal pelvis; although transitional cell carcinoma is more common, squamous cell carcinoma may occur. Hematuria is the most frequent presenting complaint. Screening is described in Table 39-2. In patients with renal failure due to Chinese herb nephropathy, the prevalence of urothelial carcinoma is quite high. Some clinicians have proposed prophylactic removal of native kidneys and ureters (Nortier et al., 2000); annual screening for abnormal urine cytology and radiologic imaging of the urinary tract is a more conservative approach.

C. Adenocarcinoma of the prostate. The incidence is increased in hemodialysis patients. An annual prostate-specific antigen (PSA) blood level and digital rectal examination should be obtained in male patients 50 years of age or older, and in those 40 years of age or older who have a family history of prostate cancer or who are of African American descent. Annual PSA screening is appropriate in patients with a life expectancy of 10 years or more. The accuracy of total PSA as a marker of prostatic disease appears to be the same in hemodialysis and peritoneal dialysis patients as in nonuremics, but the ratio of free PSA to total PSA is nonspecifically increased (Sasagawa et al., 1998; Passadakis et al., 2004).

D. Other. An increased incidence of bladder cancer in younger dialysis patients and in female dialysis patients has been suggested (Stewart et al., 2003).

VII. Sexual dysfunction

A. Incidence and etiology. Erectile dysfunction is one of the most common manifestations of sexual dysfunction in men with chronic kidney disease. Prevalence has been reported to be as high as 70%–80% and is similar between patients on hemodialysis and peritoneal dialysis. This high prevalence is not surprising given that many of the diseases such as atherosclerosis, diabetes, and hypertension that are associated with erectile dysfunction are commonly found in patients with chronic kidney disease. Normal male sexual function is achieved through the integrative response of the vascular, neurologic, endocrine, and psychological systems. Men with chronic kidney disease can exhibit abnormalities in any one or all of these systems.

B. Evaluation

1. History. First, one must distinguish organic from functional impotence. Aspects from the history suggesting an organic cause include the absence of erections upon awakening or with masturbation; the use of cimetidine or antihypertensive, antipsychotic, antidepressant, or anticholinergic medication; diabetes; atherosclerotic vascular disease (claudication, angina); and a history of alcohol abuse, myocardial infarct or stroke, smoking, pelvic trauma, surgery, exposure to radiation, or long-distance bicycling (which may cause penile vascular compromise). Functional impotence is suggested by the presence of erections upon awakening, complaints of premature ejaculation, successful sexual activity with other partners or in other situations, abrupt onset of the dysfunction, and temporally related social stresses. Interview of the sexual partner is usually helpful in assessing the problem.

2. Physical examination. The examiner should note the presence or absence of secondary male sexual characteristics and gynecomastia; the presence, size, and consistency of the testes and prostate; whether the plaques of the Peyronie disease of the penis are present; the quality of femoral pulses; and the presence or absence of femoral bruits. The integrity of the somatic afferents of the erection reflex arc is assessed by testing of the bulbocavernosus reflex. The integrity of the sacral dermatomes is checked by assessing sensation to pin prick in the perineal region. Penile biothesiometry is a good screening test to rule out somatic afferent neuropathies of the penis.

3. Review of medications. Antihypertensive medications are common offenders, with centrally acting agents and beta-blockers being the most commonly implicated. The angiotensin-converting enzyme inhibitors or angiotensin receptor blockers are associated with a lower incidence of erectile dysfunction and represent a useful alternative. Other drugs commonly implicated include cimetidine, phenothiazines, tricyclic antidepressants, and metoclopramide.

4. Distinguishing psychological versus organic causes. If the history and physical examination reveal no obvious cause, then a psychological cause of erectile dysfunction may need to be considered. Testing for the presence of nocturnal penile tumescence can help discriminate between psychological and organic causes. During the rapid eye movement stage of sleep, males normally have an erection. If erectile dysfunction is psychogenic in origin, then nocturnal erections should still be present, whereas the absence of nocturnal erections makes an organic cause more likely. If a patient is found to have normal nocturnal erections, then psychological testing and evaluation are indicated. The effectiveness of antidepressant medications and/or psychiatric counseling in chronic kidney disease patients with sexual dysfunction has not been well studied. Use of antidepressant medications can be problematic since many of these agents can themselves cause sexual dysfunction.

5. Additional testing. With the availability of sildenafil and other phosphodiesterase inhibitors (see below) to use as a therapeutic trial, additional testing is generally reserved for nonresponders who are being considered for placement of a penile prosthesis. In sildenafil nonresponders, a vascular cause can be screened for with Doppler studies to measure penile blood flow and pressure. Neurogenic erectile dysfunction is suggested by detecting a prolonged latency time of the bulbocavernous reflex or confirming the presence of a neurogenic bladder. Penile biothesiometry is a good screening test to rule out somatic afferent neuropathies of the penis. The initial evaluation of an endocrine cause of erectile dysfunction should include measurement of plasma luteinizing hormone (LH), follicle-stimulating hormone (FSH), prolactin, and testosterone.

C. Treatment

1. General. The treatment of sexual dysfunction in the uremic man is initially of a general nature (Fig. 39-1). One needs to ensure optimal delivery of dialysis and adequate nutritional intake. Administration of recombinant human erythropoietin has been shown to enhance sexual function in chronic kidney disease, a benefit that is likely due to the improvement in well-being associated with correction of anemia. Correction of anemia with erythropoietin has also been associated with increases in plasma testosterone

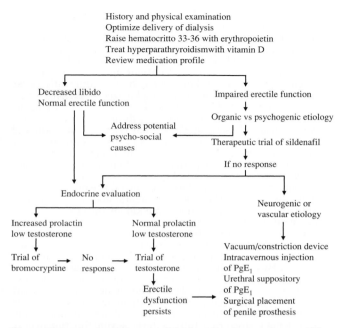

History and physical examination
Optimize delivery of dialysis
Raise hematocritto 33-36 with erythropoietin
Treat hyperparathryoidismwith vitamin D
Review medication profile

Decreased libido
Normal erectile function

Impaired erectile function

Organic vs psychogenic etiology

Address potential
psycho-social
causes

Therapeutic trial of sildenafil

If no response

Endocrine evaluation

Neurogenic or
vascular etiology

Increased prolactin
low testosterone

Normal prolactin
low testosterone

Trial of
bromocryptine → No → Trial of
response testosterone

Vacuum/constriction device
Intracavernous injection
of PgE₁
Urethral suppository
of PgE₁

Erectile
dysfunction →
persists

Surgical placement
of penile prosthesis

Figure 39-1. Approach to sexual dysfunction in uremic men. PG, prostaglandin.

levels, reductions in elevated prolactin levels, and normalization of the pituitary gonadal feedback mechanism. It is not clear whether these endocrinologic changes are solely the result of correction of the anemia or a direct effect of erythropoietin. Controlling the degree of secondary hyperparathyroidism with 1,25-$(OH)_2$-vitamin D has also been associated with an improvement in sexual function in some patients.

2. Phosphodiesterase type 5 inhibitors. The physiologic mechanism responsible for erection of the penis involves release of nitric oxide from nerve endings in the corpus cavernosum in response to sexual stimuli. Nitric oxide activates the enzyme guanylyl cyclase, which results in localized increased levels of cyclic guanosine monophosphate (cGMP), causing a cascade of events ultimately producing penile arteriole and corpus cavernosum smooth muscle relaxation. Phosphodiesterase type 5 is the predominant isoenzyme metabolizing cGMP in the smooth muscle cells of the corpus cavernosum. Sildenafil, vardenafil, and tadalafil prevent the breakdown of cGMP by inhibiting this enzyme, thus facilitating blood flow into the penis.

Published trials on the use of phosphodiesterase type 5 inhibitors in patients with ESRD have been confined to sildenafil. The response rate ranges from 60% to 80%, which is similar to that noted in nonuremic subjects. Sildenafil has similar efficacy in patients treated with hemodialysis or peritoneal dialysis. There is no correlation between patients who fail to respond to therapy and cause of erectile dysfunction, including blood levels of testosterone and prolactin, cause of kidney failure, and patient age. Patients not responding to sildenafil therapy may have significantly lower penile blood flow. It should be emphasized that these drugs are contraindicated in patients who are currently taking organic nitrates, because significant drops in blood pressure can occur in this setting. For similar reasons, sildenafil and similar drugs may only be taken 4 or more hours after any alpha-blocker. Caution should also be exercised when prescribing these drugs to patients with known coronary artery disease. To limit the possibility of hypotension among dialysis patients, some clinicians recommend use of sildenafil on nondialysis days. The dose of sildenafil does not need to be adjusted in patients with chronic kidney disease.

3.   **Endocrine treatment**

    a.   Testosterone therapy. Testosterone therapy is generally effective in states of low circulating levels of testosterone when due to causes other than chronic kidney disease. By contrast, administration of testosterone to uremic men usually fails to restore libido or potency, despite increased testosterone levels and reduced release of LH and FSH. In a recent report of 27 male dialysis patients with biochemically proven hypogonadism, administration of depot testosterone fully restored sexual function in only three patients (Lawrence et al., 1998). In two of the patients the benefit was short lived. The beneficial effects of testosterone therapy may be more apparent in those patients whose primary complaint is decreased libido. Transdermal delivery systems may prove to be the most effective way to administer the drug. Prior to starting hormonal replacement therapy, a digital rectal prostate examination and PSA determination to screen for adenocarcinoma of the prostate should be performed in males over the age of 40, and every 6–12 months thereafter as long as such therapy is continued.

    b.   Dopaminergic agonists. Patients with low circulating levels of testosterone in the setting of increased circulating levels of prolactin may benefit from a trial of bromocriptine. This agent is a dopaminergic agonist that has shown some efficacy in improving sexual function presumably by reducing elevated prolactin levels. However, its usefulness has been limited by a relatively high frequency of side effects. Other dopaminergic agonists, such as Parlodel and lisuride, seem to be better tolerated but have only been used in small, short-term studies.

4.   **Zinc therapy.** Zinc deficiency has been suggested as a cause of gonadal failure. Although in one controlled trial, supplemental zinc resulted in improved potency, libido, and frequency of intercourse, this initial report was not confirmed by subsequent studies, and zinc supplementation is no longer commonly used.

5. Vacuum tumescence device. There are additional options for those patients with a neurogenic or vascular cause of erectile dysfunction who have failed medical therapy. A vacuum tumescence device creates a vacuum over the shaft of the penis after a constricting band has been placed at the base of the penis. This causes pooling of blood in the penis distal to the band and an erection. This device has proven to be useful in dialysis patients with erectile dysfunction (Lawrence et al., 1998). Side effects include blocked ejaculation, temporary changes in penile sensation, blue discoloration of the penis, and a cool-feeling penis. The band should not be left on for more than 30 minutes.

6. Intraurethral prostaglandin E_1 (alprostadil). Intraurethral administration of prostaglandin E_1 provides the delivery of a vasodilator to the corpus cavernosum, resulting in an erection sufficient for intercourse. The drug is supplied in an applicator that is inserted in the urethra. The major side effect of intraurethral alprostadil therapy is urethral pain.

7. Penile prosthesis. Surgical placement of a penile prosthesis is typically considered in patients who fail the less invasive treatments. The success rate, operative mortality, and morbidity in the dialysis population have not been reported; however, among nonuremic patients the satisfaction rate has been high. Potential complications include infection, erosion, and mechanical failure.

VIII. Male subfertility

A. Incidence and etiology. Subfertility is a common problem in male hemodialysis patients. Fifty percent have diminished sperm counts, impaired sperm motility, and abnormal sperm forms. Hemodialysis patients have an increased incidence of testicular atrophy, interstitial fibrosis, and Leydig cell dysfunction. The pathogenesis is not fully known; hypothalamopituitary dysfunction/gonadotropin deficiency or resistance, discussed in Chapter 34, may play a role.

The diagnostic workup of subfertility is the same as that in nonuremic patients. Readily treatable causes, such as varicocele, retrograde ejaculation, hyperprolactinemia, hypogonadotropic hypogonadism, vas deferens obstruction, infection, and presence of antisperm antibodies, should be ruled out. Specific therapy depends on causal factors. The use of zinc, clomiphene, chronic human chorionic gonadotropin treatment, or recombinant erythropoietin treatment to restore fertility in dialysis patients is controversial. Transplantation appears to offer the best chance for cure.

IX. Priapism. Priapism has been reported to occur in patients on maintenance hemodialysis. The cause is unknown. The development of priapism for more than 4–6 hours requires prompt aspiration of blood from the corpora cavernosa. If the penis remains rigid, α-adrenergic agonists such as phenylephrine should be administered intracavernosally. Immediate surgical intervention is mandatory if the above measures fail. The successful use of 1–5 mg of metaraminol injected intracavernosally and a single incident involving use of continuous bupivacaine–fentanyl epidural anesthesia to reverse

spontaneous priapism have been described in hemodialysis patients. Cardiovascular monitoring should be conducted while
these agents are administered.

SELECTED READINGS

Bakir AA, et al. Dialysis-associated renal cystic disease resembling
autosomal dominant polycystic kidney disease: a report of two
cases. *Am J Nephrol* 1999;19:519–522.

Bellinghieri G, Savica V, Santoro D. Vascular erectile dysfunction in
chronic renal failure. *Semin Nephrol* 2006;26(1):42–45.

Bisceglia M, et al. Renal cystic diseases: a review [Review]. *Adv Anat
Pathol* 2006;13(1):26–56.

Chaudhry A, et al. Occurrence of pyuria and bacteriuria in asymptomatic hemodialysis patients. *Am J Kidney Dis* 1993;21:180–183.

Choyke PL. Acquired cystic kidney disease. *Eur Radiol* 2000;10:
1716–1721.

Cowie A. Renal imaging in patients requiring renal replacement therapy. *Semin Dial* 2002;15:237–249.

Daudon M, et al. Urolithiasis in patients with end stage renal failure.
J Urol 1992;147:977–980.

Denton MD, et al. Prevalence of renal cell carcinoma in patients
with ESRD pre-transplantation: a pathologic analysis. *Kidney Int*
2002;61:2201–2209.

Eisinger RP, et al. Does pyuria indicate infection in asymptomatic
dialysis patients?. *Clin Nephrol* 1997;47:50–51.

Gibson P, Watson ML. Cyst infection in polycystic kidney disease: a
clinical challenge. *Nephrol Dial Transplant* 1998;13:2455–2457.

Grossman EB, et al. The pharmacokinetics and hemodynamics
of sildenafil citrate in male hemodialysis patients. *Kidney Int*
2004;66:367–374.

Gulanikar AC, et al. Prospective pretransplant ultrasound screening
in 206 patients for acquired renal cysts and renal cell carcinoma.
Transplantation 1998;66:1669–1672.

Ishikawa I, et al. Twenty-year follow-up of acquired renal cystic disease. *Clin Nephrol* 2003;59:153–159.

Lawrence IG, et al. Correcting erectile dysfunction in male dialysis
patients: experience with testosterone replacement and vacuum
tumescence therapy. *Am J Kidney Dis* 1998;31:313–319.

Maisonneuve P, et al. Cancer in patients on dialysis for end-
stage renal disease: an international collaborative study. *Lancet*
1999;354:93–99.

Nortier JL, et al. Urothelial carcinoma associated with the use of a
Chinese herb. *N Engl J Med* 2000;342:1686–1692.

Ou JH, et al. Transitional cell carcinoma in dialysis patients. *Eur
Urol* 2000;37:90–94.

Palmer BF. Outcomes associated with hypogonadism in men
with chronic kidney disease. *Adv Chronic Kidney Dis* 2004;11:
342–347.

Palmer BF. Sexual dysfunction in men and women with chronic kidney disease and end-stage renal disease. *Adv Ren Replace Ther*
2003;10:48–60.

Passadakis P, et al. Serum levels of prostate-specific antigen and vitamin D in peritoneal dialysis patients. *Adv Perit Dial* 2004;20:203–
208.

Rosas SE, et al. Prevalence and determinants of erectile dysfunction in hemodialysis patients. *Kidney Int* 2001;59:2259–2266.

Sam R, Patel P. Sildenafil in dialysis patients. *Int J Artif Organs* 2006;29(3):264–268.

Sarasin FP, Wong JB, Levey AS. Screening for acquired cystic kidney disease: a decision analytic prospective. *Kidney Int* 1995;48:207–219.

Sasagawa I, et al. Serum levels of total and free prostate specific antigen in men on hemodialysis. *J Urol* 1998;160:83–85.

Seibel I, et al. Efficacy of oral sildenafil in hemodialysis patients with erectile dysfunction. *J Am Soc Nephrol* 2002;13:2770–2775.

Stewart JH, et al. Cancers of the kidney and urinary tract in patients on dialysis for end-stage renal disease: analysis of data from the United States, Europe, and Australia and New Zealand. *J Am Soc Nephrol* 2003;14:197–207.

Sumura M, et al. Diagnostic value of serum prostate-specific antigen in hemodialysis patients. *Int J Urol* 2003;10:247–250.

Terasawa Y, et al. Ultrasonic diagnosis of renal cell carcinoma in hemodialysis patients. *J Urol* 1994;152:846–851.

Truong LD, et al. Renal neoplasm in acquired cystic kidney disease. *Am J Kidney Dis* 1995;26:1–12.

Turk S, et al. Erectile dysfunction and the effects of sildenafil treatment in patients on haemodialysis and continuous ambulatory peritoneal dialysis. *Nephrol Dial Transplant* 2001;16:1818–1822.

Vera EM, et al. Urinalysis in the diagnosis of urinary tract infections in hemodialysis patients. *J Am Soc Nephrol* 2002;21:639A.

Viterbo R, Mydlo JH. Incidence and management of dialysis patients with renal calculi. *Urol Int* 2002;69:306–308.

Watanabe K, et al. Amyloid urinary-tract calculi in patients on chronic dialysis. *Nephron* 1989;52:334–337.

Obstetric and Gynecologic Issues

Susan Hou and Susan Grossman

In women with end-stage renal disease (ESRD), the possibility of pregnancy is substantial and needs to be prevented if not desired and managed appropriately if it occurs. The hypothalamic–pituitary–ovarian axis is deranged (see Chapter 34), giving rise to decreased fertility, loss of libido, and dysfunctional uterine bleeding.

I. Birth control

A. Indications. Forty percent of women under the age of 55 treated with dialysis menstruate, but anovulatory periods and infertility are the rule. There is some suggestion that the use of erythropoietin and the increasing dialysis dose may have changed some of the hormonal abnormalities previously described in dialysis patients and that the frequency of pregnancy may have increased. Dialysis patients may have occasional ovulatory periods and when pregnancies occur, patient management is enormously complicated. Birth control is advisable for women who do not wish to conceive. It is difficult to identify women at higher risk for pregnancy. Women who become pregnant once on dialysis frequently conceive again. Women who have become pregnant with renal insufficiency prior to starting dialysis and women with regular menses are at increased risk, but pregnancies have occurred in women following years of amenorrhea while treated with dialysis.

B. Methods of contraception. Diaphragms and condoms can be used as in individuals with normal renal function. Oral contraceptives can be used but are contraindicated in women with a history of thrombophlebitis and relatively contraindicated in women whose underlying renal disease is lupus. The provision of estrogen offers the theoretical benefit of protecting bones from the effects of hypoestrogenemia seen in dialysis patients.

Many women on dialysis have prolonged periods of anovulatory bleeding, associated with the unopposed effect of estrogen on the endometrium. Estrogen–progesterone cycling might reduce the risk of endometrial cancer, which is associated with unopposed estrogen. Use of intrauterine devices is discouraged, as they are associated with increased bleeding during hemodialysis as a result of heparinization and a risk of peritonitis in continuous ambulatory peritoneal dialysis (CAPD). Treatment of infertility has generally not been attempted because pregnancy is dangerous for the mother and the outcome is still poor.

II. Pregnancy

A. Frequency and outcome. The frequency of pregnancy in American women on dialysis is about 0.5% per year. For reasons that are unclear, conception occurs two to three times more frequently in hemodialysis patients than in CAPD patients. The likelihood of pregnancy resulting in a surviving infant, excluding elective abortions, approaches 60%–70% if the pregnant mother reaches the second trimester. For women who start dialysis after conception, the likelihood of having a surviving infant is 75%–80%. Seventy-two percent of unsuccessful pregnancies result in spontaneous abortion, about 10% end in stillbirth, 15% in neonatal death, and 3% in therapeutic abortion for life-threatening maternal problems. Approximately 40% of spontaneous abortions occur in the second trimester.

B. Diagnosis. The average gestational age at which diagnosis of pregnancy is made is 16.5 weeks. Amenorrhea is common and symptoms of early pregnancy such as nausea are often attributed to metabolic or gastrointestinal problems. A blood-based pregnancy test (serum levels of the β subunit of human chorionic gonadotropin [HCG]) should be done prior to gastrointestinal (GI) radiographs for abdominal complaints. Urine pregnancy tests are not reliable even if the patient is not anuric. Even with blood tests, false positives and false negatives occur. The small amounts of HCG produced by somatic cells in nonpregnant women may be excreted slowly enough in renal failure for blood levels to be borderline positive for pregnancy. Occasionally such borderline test results have led to cancellation of elective surgery. During pregnancy, HCG levels are more elevated than expected for gestational age, so this is best determined by ultrasound. The reasons for falsely negative tests are unclear. Similarly, serum tests of α-fetoprotein done to screen for Down syndrome may be falsely elevated in pregnant dialysis patients, so amniocentesis with karyotyping should be done.

C. Management

1. Hypertension during pregnancy. The major maternal risk associated with pregnancy in dialysis patients is severe hypertension. Eighty percent of pregnant dialysis patients have some degree of hypertension (blood pressure >140/90 mm Hg). Forty percent have severe hypertension with diastolic blood pressures >110 mm Hg or systolic blood pressures >200 mm Hg. Seventy-five percent of severe hypertension occurs before the third trimester. Intensive care unit admissions for control of accelerated hypertension are required in 2%–5% of pregnant dialysis patients. Patients should be taught to take their blood pressure daily and report any increases in blood pressure promptly. Hypertension, even when severe, may not require the termination of pregnancy.

a. Control of volume. The first step toward blood pressure control, as in the nonpregnant patient, is to make sure that the woman is euvolemic. Monitoring weight gain is problematic in pregnant dialysis patients. Recommended weight gain for women who become pregnant at their ideal body weight is 12–16 kg. Only 1.6 kg of this weight gain occurs in the first trimester. In early pregnancy, the change in dry weight should be only

0.9–2.3 kg, depending on the prepregnancy body mass index (BMI). Recommended weight gain in the second and third trimesters is between 0.3 and 0.5 kg per week, again depending on the prepregnancy BMI. While the nutritionist in a dialysis unit can provide dietary guidelines for appropriate weight gain during pregnancy, the most pressing question for the dialysis unit staff is determining how much of the weight change between treatments is excess fluid and how much is part of the desired pregnancy-associated weight gain. With daily dialysis, fluid gain between treatments should be small, but the majority of the change in weight is usually fluid. The woman should have a careful weekly examination to look for signs of fluid overload. With daily dialysis, volume-related hypertension should be minimized, and if there is any increase in blood pressure, particularly during dialysis, the patient should be evaluated for pre-eclampsia.

b.   Antihypertensive drugs. If the blood pressure remains >140/90 mm Hg when the patient is euvolemic, there are several first-line drugs than can be used safely, including α-methyldopa and labetalol. Calcium channel blockers also are widely used. There is less experience with beta-blockers, clonidine, and alpha-blockers, but these probably are safe. Hydralazine can be added to any of these first-line drugs, but it does not work as a single agent when given orally. Angiotensin-converting enzyme inhibitors and angiotensin receptor blockers are contraindicated in pregnancy. In animal studies they have been associated with a fetal loss rate of 80%–93%. In humans, their use has been associated with an ossification defect in the skull, dysplastic kidneys, neonatal anuria, and death from hypoplastic lungs.

c.   Superimposed pre-eclampsia and hypertensive crisis. Women treated with chronic dialysis are at increased risk for superimposed pre-eclampsia, but the diagnosis is almost impossible to make in the absence of findings of the HELLP syndrome (**H**emolysis, **E**levated **L**iver enzymes, **L**ow **P**latelet count), such as microangiopathic hemolytic anemia, elevated liver enzymes, or thrombocytopenia.

Intravenous hydralazine is the drug of first choice for hypertensive crisis in pregnant women and should be given in doses of 5–10 mg every 20–30 minutes. Labetalol is a good alternative. Magnesium is superior to other anticonvulsants for seizure prophylaxis in women with pre-eclampsia, but it must be used with extreme caution in dialysis patients. A loading dose can be given safely. Additional magnesium should not be given until after dialysis or until after a drop in serum magnesium level has been demonstrated. Magnesium potentiates the hypotensive effects of calcium channel blockers, and the calcium channel blocker should be stopped if magnesium is required.

2.   Dialysis regimen

a.   Modality. Although the previous edition of this handbook suggested that there is no difference in outcome of pregnancy between hemodialysis patients and peritoneal dialysis patients, either as measured by infant survival or mean gestational age of live born infants, it is easier to increase the amount of dialysis delivered with hemodialysis. The higher success rates reported in more recent studies have been achieved in hemodialysis patients. Although dialysis modality should not be changed because of pregnancy, it may be easier to start hemodialysis in a pregnant woman than peritoneal dialysis. If peritoneal dialysis is elected, placement of a peritoneal catheter is possible at any stage of pregnancy. Some nephrologists have elected to supplement peritoneal dialysis with hemodialysis when pregnancy nears term.

b. Intensive dialysis. There is growing evidence that the likelihood of a surviving infant is increased if the patient is dialyzed at least 20 hours per week. The frequency of severe prematurity is also decreased in intensively dialyzed women. One study reports successful pregnancy in a group of 12 patients dialyzed with short daily treatments, although 7 started dialysis after conception. Daily dialysis decreases the fluid removal at each treatment, decreasing the risk of hypotension during dialysis. Daily dialysis also allows the patient to eat a high-protein diet to ensure that the needs of pregnancy are met. Intensive six times per week hemodiafiltration is another option that has been successfully used (Haase et al., 2005). Increasing the intensity of dialysis in peritoneal dialysis patients is difficult. Late in pregnancy, women have difficulty with severe abdominal distension and exchange volume may have to be decreased. It becomes necessary to increase the frequency of exchanges even to maintain the same level of dialysis. A combination of daytime exchanges and nighttime cycler is often necessary.

Some have raised the question of whether increased dialysis might have a detrimental effect by removing progesterone. Progesterone withdrawal plays a role in the initiation of labor. Measurements of serum progesterone levels during dialysis in pregnant dialysis patients are variable. Brost et al. measured pre- and postdialysis progesterone levels in seven pregnant dialysis patients. Changes in serum progesterone ranged from a 52% decrease in levels to a 9% increase. Changes in serum progesterone were not associated with changes in home uterine activity monitoring.

c. Dialysis solution. With the recognition of the risk of soft tissue calcification in long-term dialysis patients, a 2.5 mEq/L (1.25 mM) calcium concentration has replaced 3.5 mEq/L (1.75 mM) as standard. When a bath containing 2.5 mEq/L (1.25 mM) is used, the patient is usually in slightly positive calcium balance. There is some production of calcitriol by the placenta, which may increase serum calcium. Predialysis serum calcium levels should be checked weekly. The fetus needs 25–30 g of calcium for calcification of the fetal skeleton. Orally, the patient will require 2 g per day if a 2.5 mEq/L

(1.25 mM) dialysis solution is used; calcium-containing phosphate binders should provide enough calcium if the patient requires them with daily dialysis. For women who need phosphate binders, calcium-containing binders are the only group known to be safe in pregnancy. There is no experience with sevelamer or lanthanum carbonate in pregnancy. Some women become hypophosphatemic. Often phosphate binders are no longer required, and it may be necessary to add phosphorus to the bath (e.g., 4 mg/dL [1.3 mM] phosphorus or higher).

With a standard bath, daily dialysis carries a risk of alkalosis. Metabolic alkalosis carries an increased risk in pregnant women who have a concurrent respiratory alkalosis; however, in the few instances where arterial blood gases have been done, compensatory hypercapnia has occurred in women with severe metabolic alkalosis. A dialysis bath containing 25 mM of bicarbonate may be necessary. When this is not available, bicarbonate can be removed by increasing ultrafiltration and replacing the losses with saline.

Normal serum sodium is decreased during pregnancy to approximately 134 mmol/L. Since thirst is normal, the pregnant woman will take in enough water to normalize serum sodium if it is high at the end of dialysis.

d. Heparinization. Clotting of the extracorporeal circuit and the dialysis access occurs frequently during pregnancy. Heparin does not cross the placenta, and unless there is vaginal bleeding, it is not necessary to lower the dose.

3. Anemia. Dialysis patients who become pregnant usually experience worsening anemia. The hematocrit usually has dropped by the time the pregnancy is recognized. It has become usual practice to continue erythropoietin during pregnancy. Congenital anomalies have not been reported in the infants of the small number of women who took erythropoietin during organogenesis. In animals, congenital anomalies have been seen only at dosages of 500 units/kg. There is little information on whether or not the drug crosses the placenta in humans. Erythropoietin has been associated with hypertension in nonpregnant patients, but it is difficult to determine what factors influence hypertension during pregnancy. Women treated with erythropoietin prior to pregnancy require markedly increased doses during pregnancy. We recommend doubling the dose. Pregnancy in normal women requires 700–1150 mg of iron. We have found an increase in iron requirements during pregnancy and have given intravenous iron. The Food and Drug Administration has labeled ferric gluconate as category B for pregnancy. Folate requirements are increased in normal pregnant women. Folate deficiency is associated with an increase in neural tube defects. Folate losses increase with intensive dialysis and folate supplementation should be doubled (4 mg per day).

III. Labor and delivery. Eighty percent of infants born to dialysis patients are premature. Reasons for prematurity include premature labor, maternal hypertension, and fetal distress. Home contraction monitoring can be used so that premature labor can be identified promptly. Premature labor has been successfully treated with terbutaline, magnesium, nifedipine, and indomethacin. Magnesium has been given intravenously in hemodialysis patients and has been added to the peritoneal dialysis solution in peritoneal dialysis patients. Magnesium must be used with extreme care in women with renal failure, as discussed above. Blood levels should be monitored frequently. A loading dose can be given, but additional doses should only be given after dialysis and when the level is low. The use of magnesium in combination with nifedipine should be avoided because the combination can cause profound hypotension. Indomethacin has also been used with success, but patients must be monitored for oligohydramnios and the fetus must be monitored for right heart dilation. In women with residual renal function, indomethacin may result in further deterioration in glomerular filtration rate and the need for increased dialysis.

Infants of dialysis patients are frequently small for gestational age, but it is not clear whether their growth restriction is the result of azotemia per se or of maternal hypertension. There is an increased risk of stillbirth in dialysis patients and antenatal monitoring should be started as soon as there is a chance of survival outside the mother (26 weeks). Biophysical profiles, Doppler of cord vessels, and amniotic fluid assessment are generally used. Contraction stress tests using oxytocin (now used infrequently) should be avoided because of the risk of precipitating premature labor.

In CAPD patients, cesarean section can be done extraperitoneally, leaving the catheter in place, and CAPD can be resumed 24 hours after delivery, starting with small exchange volumes and increasing over a 48-hour period. If there is leaking from the incision, the patient can be hemodialyzed for 2–4 weeks.

Even a normal-appearing infant should be monitored in a high-risk nursery. At birth, the infant, whose kidneys are normal, has a blood urea nitrogen and serum creatinine similar to the mother's, and the infant experiences a solute diuresis requiring careful monitoring of electrolytes and volume status.

There does not appear to be any increased risk of congenital anomalies, but the information on growth and development is sketchy.

IV. Dyspareunia. Some women dialysis patients may experience dyspareunia because of estrogen deficiency and resulting vaginal dryness. Dyspareunia resulting from atrophic vaginitis from low estrogen levels can be corrected by intravaginal conjugated estrogens (Premarin) 2–4 g daily or oral estrogen progesterone compounds. A daily dose of 0.3 mg of conjugated estrogen and 2.5 mg of medroxyprogesterone provides enough estrogen to prevent dyspareunia since estrogen is metabolized more slowly in dialysis patients. If there is breakthrough bleeding on this combination, progesterone can be increased to 5 mg. Since substantial amounts of estrogen are absorbed from intravaginal estrogens, these women should receive progesterone as well.

V. Sexual dysfunction

A. Incidence and etiology. Fifty percent of female dialysis patients under the age of 55 are sexually active. A majority of women on dialysis experience some sexual dysfunction. They suffer both decreased libido and decreased ability to achieve orgasm. Treatment with erythropoietin appears to be associated with an improvement in sexual function, but most of the data collected have been in men. Various reasons for sexual dysfunction have been proposed, including hyperprolactinemia, gonadal dysfunction, depression, hyperparathyroidism, and change in body image.

B. Hyperprolactinemia. Seventy-five percent to ninety percent of female dialysis patients are hyperprolactinemic. The mean serum levels in women with sexual dysfunction are higher than in patients with normal sexual function. Treatment of hyperprolactinemia with the dopamine agonist bromocryptine has been reported (in limited uncontrolled studies) to improve sexual function in both men and women on dialysis. It has not come into widespread use because hemodialysis patients may be particularly susceptible to the hypotensive effects of this drug. Bromocriptine can be started at a dose of 1.25 mg, and the first dose should be taken at night. Subsequent doses can be gradually increased. Doses of 2.5 mg twice daily should be adequate to suppress prolactin secretion. There is little experience with newer, better tolerated dopamine agonists in this population. When correctable physical problems cannot be found, dialysis patients should be referred for sex therapy, as would patients without renal failure.

VI. Dysfunctional uterine bleeding

A. Incidence. Many women develop amenorrhea when the glomerular filtration rate falls to <10 mL per minute. Menstruation often returns once dialysis is started, in as many as 60% of patients. Recently regular menstruation has become more common in premenopausal women with ESRD; however, over half of women with ESRD who menstruate report hypermenorrhea. Women on both hemodialysis and CAPD report similar menstrual abnormalities. Since many women on dialysis (~60% of those who menstruate) have irregular cycles, dysfunctional uterine bleeding is common, and is of concern because it may be an early sign of endometrial cancer. Blood loss may lead to severe anemia even in women treated with erythropoietin, although the introduction of erythropoietin has made the management of dysfunctional uterine bleeding substantially easier.

B. Management

  1. Screening for malignancy. Management depends on age and whether menses have ceased.

   a. Women older than 40 years of age with no menses for 1 year prior to the bleeding episode. Cancer risk is high and dilation and curettage should be performed.

b. Women older than 40 years in whom menstruation has not ceased for 1 year prior to bleeding. The cancer risk is moderate. Dilation and curettage is not routinely necessary, and performance of several endometrial biopsies is probably sufficient to screen for malignancy.

c. Women younger than 40 years. The cancer risk is relatively small, and a yearly Papanicolaou smear is usually sufficient screen for tumor.

2. Anticoagulation. The lowest possible dosage of heparin should be used to perform hemodialysis when a woman is menstruating. Heparin-free techniques and citrate anticoagulation also are good options.

3. Bloody peritoneal fluid during peritoneal dialysis. During menstruation or ovulation, the peritoneal fluid can become bloody. There is no specific management, except perhaps to avoid addition of heparin to the peritoneal dialysis solution. In some cases, frank hemoperitoneum may occur, requiring suppression of ovulation (Harnett et al., 1987). An aseptic peritonitis picture during menstruation or ovulation has also been reported (Poole et al., 1987). Bloody peritoneal fluid frequently occurs after gynecologic procedures.

4. Management of anemia. Anemia should be managed with erythropoietin, as in other dialysis patients. Heavy uterine bleeding will result in increased iron requirements, and additional intravenous iron may have to be given.

5. Hormonal therapy. Recent advances in therapy have facilitated the management of dysfunctional uterine bleeding in women with ESRD.

a. Oral contraceptives remain the safest therapy and the first-line treatment, although they should not be used if blood pressure control is a problem. The theoretical benefits of using estrogen–progesterone combinations to prevent uterine cancer and osteoporosis have been discussed above.

b. Medroxyprogesterone acetate (Depo Provera). Progesterone can be given either intramuscularly as Depo-Provera 100 mg once a week for 4 weeks or orally as 10 mg daily for the first 10 days of the menstrual cycle; this drug is best reserved for patients with chronic hypermenorrhea who do not respond to more conservative oral contraceptive therapy. Progestins work best in the setting of anovulatory bleeding. Because many patients on dialysis have a bleeding tendency, intramuscular injections on a regular basis are undesirable. Moreover, the half-life of intramuscular medroxyprogesterone acetate is unpredictable. Progestin-impregnated intrauterine devices are available to treat dysfunctional uterine bleeding but are relatively contraindicated in women on peritoneal dialysis because of the increased risk of infections.

c. Gonadotropin-releasing hormone agonists. These can be given as an intramuscular injection once a month (leuprolide acetate) or a daily intranasal dose. These drugs are extremely expensive and should be reserved for patients who continue to have excessive menstrual bleeding and do not respond to oral contraceptives or progestins. There is one report of ovarian hyperstimulation in a patient on chronic dialysis who received two doses of leuprolide acetate (Hampton et al., 1991).

    d. High-dosage intravenous estrogens. In the case of acute excessive blood loss, high-dosage estrogen therapy can be used, giving 25 mg of conjugated estrogens intravenously every 6 hours. Bleeding usually subsides within 12 hours.

    e. Deamino arginine vasopressin (DDAVP). In the setting of acute blood loss when bleeding time is prolonged, DDAVP, in a dosage of 0.3 pg/kg in 50 mL of saline, should be given every 4–8 hours for three to four doses.

  6. Nonsteroidal anti-inflammatory agents have been shown to be effective in women who ovulate. These agents may be less effective in the setting of ESRD because of the increased incidence of anovulatory cycles women. Also, women with ESRD are at increased risk of gastrointestinal complications.

  7. Endometrial ablation. Endometrial ablation can be performed by several surgical techniques: Hysteroscopic endometrial ablation with laser, photocoagulation, roller ball, or loop resection. Patients are pretreated with either danazol or gonadotropin-releasing hormone for 3–4 weeks before the procedure to thin the endometrium. The procedure leads to permanent infertility.

  8. Hysterectomy. For postmenopausal women with significant dysfunctional uterine bleeding, hysterectomy may be the approach of choice. Laparoscopic hysterectomy is now an option for leiomyomata too large for laparoscopic surgery. Hysterectomy is a less attractive option for premenopausal women who are candidates for renal transplantation because the latter will frequently restore fertility.

VII. Hormone replacement therapy (HRT). The role of HRT in dialysis patients has never been clear. About 10% of postmenopausal women on dialysis take HRT. In most of these cases HRT had been started before initiation of dialysis. Of women not on HRT, a majority say they would not take HRT, even if advised to do so by their doctors. Recent evidence of the risk of HRT raises concern about its use in ESRD patients. The Women's Health Initiative Study demonstrated an increased risk of breast cancer, pulmonary embolism, deep vein thrombophlebitis, and coronary and cerebrovascular disease after long-term replacement of estrogen and progesterone in nonuremic postmenopausal women. Women with ESRD have more than a 20-fold increased incidence of cardiovascular disease compared to women without ESRD, so for them the increased cardiovascular risk of HRT may be magnified.

  Bone disease, the cause of which is multifactorial but which often includes a component of osteoporosis, is common in dialysis patients. The risk of hip fracture is higher in dialysis patients than in healthy people of the same age and sex. When young women on dialysis who have regular menses are compared to young women with amenorrhea, the group with amenorrhea has a significantly lower bone mineral density.

The Women's Health Initiative Study did show reduced fractures in those nonuremic postmenopausal women treated with HRT, so this might be a justification for use of HRT in dialysis patients; however, raloxifene 60 mg daily has been used successfully to prevent bone loss in postmenopausal estrogen-deficient dialysis patients, and this drug provides a safe alternative to HRT.

The use of HRT should be limited to the relief of symptoms of estrogen deficiency that cannot be relieved by other treatments. Only the patient can decide the importance of relieving these symptoms after understanding the risks. The increased risk of cardiovascular disease and breast cancer in healthy women taking HRT was small enough that many women have continued it. Unfortunately, the specific risk of HRT in hemodialysis patients has not been determined, and we can only extrapolate from the data in healthy women and women with pre-existing heart disease in advising patients of the risk.

It is still the general practice to treat women with premature ovarian failure or early surgical menopause with HRT. Postmenopausal women can be distinguished from women with secondary amenorrhea due to renal failure (those who can be expected to have a return of menses posttransplant) by high follicle-stimulating hormone (FSH) and leuteinizing hormone (LH) levels similar to the levels in healthy postmenopausal women. A very small study (13 patients) found an improvement in sexual function and general well-being as well as an improvement in L2–L4 bone density in premenopausal dialysis patients taking HRT.

HRT is contraindicated in women with active liver disease and deep vein thrombophlebitis. Estrogen may make lupus flares more likely and may worsen hepatic cystic disease in women with polycystic kidney disease.

If HRT is prescribed, the dose should be adjusted in women on dialysis. Estrogen levels increase more in dialysis patients than in normal controls when estrogen is administered. If oral HRT is given to dialysis patients, the dose used should be about half what would be given to a woman without renal failure. Transdermal estrogen may have less effect on clotting factors than oral estrogen.

VIII.   Gynecologic neoplasms. Although it was previously believed that the incidence of endometrial carcinoma was elevated in women dialysis patients, several recent studies suggest that breast, endometrial, and ovarian cancers may in fact not be increased in this population.

A.   Screening. Several recent studies suggest that screening for malignancies in women with ESRD results in a negligible increase in life expectancy because of the shortened survival of women with ESRD. Such an outlook does not allow for the possibility that great strides will be made in the care of ESRD patients leading to prolonged survival. Young women, those taking HRT, those awaiting transplantation, and those with increased risk for breast, ovarian, or cervical cancer should be screened. Women with a high risk for cervical cancer include women who have been treated with immunosuppressive therapy or who are currently on immunosuppressive therapy, either for previous transplant or for their underlying disease, or women with acquired immunodeficiency syndrome (AIDS). These women should have Pap smears performed every 6 months.

B. Evaluation of cancer for women who are symptomatic. Endometrial cancer usually presents as dysfunctional uterine bleeding, the investigation and management of which have been discussed above. Ovarian cancer usually presents with vague abdominal symptoms and later as an ovarian mass. Abdominal discomfort, nausea, and weight loss induced by ovarian cancer may initially be misinterpreted as symptoms of uremia or underdialysis. In patients on peritoneal dialysis, ovarian cancer may present as bloody peritoneal fluid, an abnormal peritoneal cell count, or a change in the color of the fluid. A high index of suspicion is necessary to detect ovarian cancer at an early and potentially curable stage.

C. Diagnostic procedures

   1. Lower gastrointestinal series. Use of laxatives and purgatives to prepare the bowel for x-ray examinations is discussed in Chapter 38. When actually performing the lower gastrointestinal examination, the amount of water used to dilute the contrast material can be reduced to one-fourth the normal amount.

   2. Computed tomography (CT). Intravenous contrast infusion, if needed to perform a CT scan or angiography, is not contraindicated in a dialysis patient. Although the administration of contrast involves increasing intravascular volume and osmolality, immediate dialysis following the study can be performed if deemed necessary. Dialysis can be done the following day if the patient is asymptomatic. A patient on peritoneal dialysis requiring an abdominal CT scan should present for the examination with dialysis fluid in the abdomen.

   3. Ultrasonography. The patient on peritoneal dialysis with a suspected pelvic or ovarian lesion should undergo ultrasound scanning of the involved area. In those instances where pelvic pathologic changes cannot be visualized without distending the bladder, the latter can be filled via a Foley catheter.

   Unlike transabdominal pelvic ultrasound, it is best for the patient to have the transvaginal ultrasound study done while her bladder is empty. Since many patients on dialysis are not able to fill their bladders unless a Foley catheter is placed and fluid instilled into the bladder, it makes sense to first perform a transvaginal ultrasound if pelvic pathology is suspected and proceed to transabdominal pelvic sonogram if the information needed cannot be obtained with the transvaginal approach. CAPD patients should have the abdomen full for transabdominal ultrasound and empty for transvaginal ultrasound.

D. Gynecologic surgery in peritoneal dialysis patients. In patients with peritoneal catheters undergoing pelvic or abdominal operations, we leave the catheter in place unless there is bacterial contamination of the peritoneal cavity. When there is a low but measurable risk of peritoneal contamination, as in a vaginal hysterectomy, we administer 1.0 g of vancomycin hydrochloride and 1.0 g cefoxitin prophylactically intravenously just prior to surgery. If the patient is known to be colonized with *Pseudomonas,* tobramycin 2.0 mg/kg intravenously should be added to the prophylactic regimen. Postoperatively, the catheter is irrigated with 500 mL of peritoneal dialysis solution three times daily to maintain patency. Irrigations are decreased to once daily when the fluid is no longer bloody. We wait 10 days to 2 weeks before using the catheter again, maintaining the patient by hemodialysis during the interim.

E. Chemotherapy. Use of chemotherapeutic agents in dialysis patients is beyond the scope of this *Handbook.*

SELECTED READINGS

Brost BC, et al. Effect of hemodialysis on serum progesterone levels in pregnant women. *Am J Kidney Dis* 1999;33:917–919.

Buccianti G, et al. Cancer among patients on renal replacement therapy: a population based survey in Lombardy, Italy. *Int J Cancer* 1996;66:591–593.

Chertow GM, et al. Cost effectiveness of cancer screening in end stage renal disease. *Arch Intern Med* 1996;156:1345–1349.

Haase M, et al. A systematic approach to managing pregnant dialysis patients—the importance of an intensified haemodiafiltration protocol. *Nephrol Dial Transplant* 2005;20(11):2537–2542.

Hampton HL, Whitworth NS, Cowan BD. Gonadotropin-releasing hormone agonist (leuprolide acetate) induced ovarian hyperstimulation syndrome in a woman undergoing intermittent hemodialysis. *Fertil Steril* 1991;55:429.

Harnett JD, et al. Recurrent hemoperitoneum in women receiving continuous ambulatory peritoneal dialysis. *Ann Intern Med* 1987;107:341.

Hernandez E, et al. Effects of raloxifene on bone metabolism and serum lipids in postmenopausal women on chronic hemodialysis. *Kidney Int* 2003;63(6):2269–2274.

Holley JL, et al. Gynecologic and reproductive issues in women on dialysis. *Am J Kidney Dis* 1997;29:685–690.

Hou S. Daily dialysis in pregnancy. *Hemodial Int* 2004;8:167–171.

Hou SH. Pregnancy in chronic renal insufficiency and end stage renal disease. *Am J Kidney Dis* 1999;33:235–252.

Kramer HM, Curhan GC, Singh A. Permanent cessation of menses and postmenopausal hormone use in dialysis dependent women. *Am J Kidney Dis* 2003;41:643–650.

Mattix H, Singh AK. Estrogen replacement therapy: implications for postmenopausal women with end-stage renal disease. *Curr Opin Nephrol* 2000;9:207–214.

Okundaye IBAbrinko P, Hou S. A registry for pregnancy in dialysis patients. *Am J Kidney Dis* 1998;31:766–773.

Poole CL, et al. Aseptic peritonitis associated with menstruation and ovulation in a peritoneal dialysis patient. In: Khanna R, et al., eds.

Advances in continuous ambulatory peritoneal dialysis. Toronto: Peritoneal Dialysis Bulletin, 1987.

Smith WT, et al. Pregnancy in peritoneal dialysis: a case report and review of adequacy and outcomes. *Int Urol Nephrol* 2005;37(1): 145–151.

Tan LK, et al. Obstetric outcomes in women with end-stage renal failure requiring renal dialysis. *Int J Gynaecol Obstet* 2006;94:17–22.

Weisinger JR, Bellorin-Font E. Postmenopausal osteoporosis in the dialysis patient [Review]. *Curr Opin Nephrol Hypertens* 2003;12(4): 381–386.

Musculoskeletal and Rheumatic Diseases

Jonathan Kay

More than 70% of patients receiving hemodialysis report joint symptoms. Prevalence increases with number of years on dialysis. β_2-Microglobulin amyloid deposition causes joint pain and limitation of motion, as well as carpal tunnel syndrome and a destructive spondyloarthropathy. Several different intra-articular crystals may induce joint inflammation. Tendons may rupture spontaneously. Severe muscle weakness can develop. Autoimmune and inflammatory diseases may remain active or recur after dialysis has been initiated, causing joint pain and other symptoms.

I. β_2-Microglobulin amyloidosis

A. Pathophysiology. β_2-Microglobulin is the subunit protein in the amyloid associated with long-term dialysis. This nonglycosylated, 11,800 dalton protein is normally present in most biologic fluids, including serum, urine, and synovial fluid. It is filtered by glomeruli and catabolized after proximal tubular reabsorption.

Serum levels range up to 2.7 mg/L (0.23 mcmol/L) in healthy individuals. Because the rate of β_2-microglobulin synthesis exceeds the rate of its removal by dialysis, serum levels are often elevated; the degree of residual renal function appears to be the most important factor in determining the extent of this elevation. When residual renal clearance is minimal, serum β_2-microglobulin levels depend substantially on the type of dialysis being given; levels are then lower in patients treated with high-flux dialysis or hemodiafiltration than in those being treated with low-flux cellulose-based dialyzers.

Nonenzymatic glycation of β_2-microglobulin may be important. Advanced glycation end product (AGE) modification of proteins confers resistance to proteolysis, increased affinity for collagen, and the ability to stimulate activated mononuclear leukocytes to release proinflammatory cytokines. AGE-modified proteins are poorly cleared by dialysis. AGE-modified β_2-microglobulin has been identified in amyloid deposits; the propensity for β_2-microglobulin amyloid to deposit in osteoarticular tissue may be due to the enhanced binding of AGE-modified proteins to collagen.

B. Clinical manifestations. Signs and symptoms of β_2-microglobulin amyloidosis are rare in chronic kidney disease (CKD) patients who are not yet on dialysis. Most symptomatic patients have undergone dialysis for several years. Prevalence increases with number of years on dialysis. Shoulder pain, carpal tunnel syndrome, and flexion contractures of the fingers are common musculoskeletal manifestations (Table 41-1).

Table 41-1.   Musculoskeletal manifestations of
β_2**-microglobulin amyloidosis**

Upper extremities
   Scapulohumeral periarthritis
   Carpal tunnel syndrome
   Flexor tenosynovitis
Spine
   Destructive spondyloarthropathy
   Periodontoid pseudotumor
   Extradural amyloid deposits
Bone cysts
Pathologic fractures

1.   Shoulder pain. Shoulder pain, often bilateral, occurs in up to 84% of patients receiving hemodialysis for 10 years or longer. Patients often report anterolateral shoulder pain that is worse when supine, especially during dialysis treatments and at night, although it may improve when sitting or standing. The coracoacromial ligament and the bicipital groove are sometimes tender to palpation. Range of shoulder motion may be limited, especially in abduction, and adhesive capsulitis of the shoulder may be present.

2.   Carpal tunnel syndrome. This results from compression of the median nerve at the wrist where it passes through a narrowed carpal tunnel. Prevalence also increases with years on dialysis and is as high as 73% in patients who have been receiving hemodialysis for 10 years or longer.

The pathogenesis appears to be multifactorial. Deposits of β_2-microglobulin amyloid may compress the median nerve as it passes through the carpal tunnel. However, amyloid is not present in all biopsy specimens. Some patients report exacerbation of symptoms during hemodialysis, perhaps due to a fistula-induced arterial steal phenomenon causing median nerve ischemia. Also, the increase in extracellular fluid volume between dialysis treatments may lead to edema and median nerve compression.

   a.   Symptoms. Most often, patients complain of numbness, tingling, burning, or a sensation of "pins and needles" in the fingers of the affected hand. The hand may feel stiff or swollen. Although symptoms usually are present in the distribution of the median nerve (over the thumb, index and middle fingers, and radial aspect of the ring finger), patients sometimes complain of sensory disturbance over the entire hand. Aching pain may be referred to the forearm. Symptoms often are worse at night or during hemodialysis and are exacerbated by activities involving repeated flexion and extension at the wrist. They occur more frequently on the side of the longest functioning vascular access. However, some patients have developed symptoms in an arm that never had been used for a graft or fistula.

b. Examination. In early cases there may be no objective loss of sensation or muscle strength. Symptoms often can be provoked by tapping over the palmar aspect of the carpal tunnel (Tinel sign) or by having the patient hold his or her wrists in a flexed position for 1 minute (Phalen sign). In more advanced cases, perception of light touch, pinprick, temperature, or two-point discrimination may be diminished in the distribution of the median nerve. The abductor pollicis brevis muscle may be weak and, in longstanding cases, there may be atrophy of the thenar eminence.

c. Diagnosis. The differential diagnoses of carpal tunnel syndrome include spondylosis of the lower cervical spine, thoracic outlet syndrome, sensorimotor polyneuropathy or mononeuropathy, and radial arterial steal syndrome in patients with an arteriovenous fistula. Except in early cases, the diagnosis usually can be established definitively by electromyography (EMG) and nerve conduction velocity studies.

d. Treatment. Splinting the affected wrist in a neutral resting position, especially at night and during dialysis treatments, may relieve symptoms temporarily. If splinting is unsuccessful or poorly tolerated, injection of the carpal tunnel with microcrystalline corticosteroid esters will provide about 30% of patients with permanent relief. If symptoms improve inadequately after injection or if there is significant objective loss of motor or sensory function, surgical decompression of the carpal tunnel yields improvement in more than 90%, but symptoms often recur within 2 years.

3. Finger flexion contractures. β_2-Microglobulin amyloid can deposit along the flexor tendons of the hands. These deposits may make the digital flexor tendons of the hand adhere to one another, creating a subcutaneous soft tissue mass in the palm and irreducible flexion contractures of the fingers. Surgical debridement of amyloid deposits from the flexor tendon sheaths may allow greater finger extension, but these deposits frequently recur within several years.

4. Destructive spondyloarthropathy. β_2-Microglobulin amyloidosis affects the axial skeleton in about 10% of patients undergoing long-term hemodialysis, presenting as a destructive spondyloarthropathy. Radiographic features include narrowing of the intervertebral disk spaces and erosion of the vertebral end plates without appreciable formation of osteophyte. The lower cervical spine is most often affected, but similar changes may also occur in the dorsal and lumbar spine. Cystic deposits of β_2-microglobulin amyloid can be seen within the odontoid process and the vertebral bodies of the upper cervical spine. Also, peri-odontoid soft tissue masses of β_2-microglobulin amyloid, termed "pseudotumors," may be present.

The initial symptom of destructive spondyloarthropathy is pain, typically in the neck when the cervical spine is involved. However, most patients with radiographic abnormalities have no neck pain. Although neurologic compromise occurs infrequently, significant myelopathy has been reported, especially in patients who have received hemodialysis for 20 years or longer. Severe destructive spondyloarthropathy must be differentiated from vertebral osteomyelitis by magnetic resonance imaging.

5.   Bone cysts. Cystic bone lesions may develop in the appendicular skeleton. Subchondral amyloid cysts, most commonly found in the carpal bones, may also occur in the acetabulum and in long bones, such as the femoral head or neck, the humeral head, the distal radius, and the tibial plateau. Unlike brown tumors of hyperparathyroidism, these bone cysts typically occur adjacent to joints. On plain radiographs, they appear as well-defined radiolucencies, with occasional disruption of the bony cortex but no periosteal reaction. Cysts vary in size, ranging from 2 to 3 mm diameter in the carpal bones to as large as 40 mm in the acetabulum. These cysts increase in number and enlarge with time.

6.   Pathologic fractures, especially of the femoral neck, may occur through areas of bone weakened by amyloid deposits.

7.   Systemic manifestations of β_2-microglobulin amyloidosis. In contrast to osteoarticular β_2-microglobulin amyloid, which is deposited predominantly in the interstitium, visceral β_2-microglobulin amyloid is deposited predominantly in blood vessels. Although gastrointestinal tract and cardiovascular complications have been reported, visceral β_2-microglobulin amyloid deposits usually do not cause symptoms. Most such patients have undergone hemodialysis for 10 years or longer and also have carpal tunnel syndrome or arthropathy.

C.   Diagnosis. This is suggested primarily by clinical appearance. Radiographic findings, such as bone cysts, narrowing of the intervertebral disk space, and vertebral end-plate erosion, serve to corroborate the diagnosis. Diagnostic ultrasonography detects changes characteristic of β_2-microglobulin amyloidosis in articular and periarticular soft tissue structures, such as in the shoulder, thickening of the rotator cuff to larger than 8 mm and interposition of echogenic pads between muscle groups of the rotator cuff. Histologic identification of β_2-microglobulin amyloid by Congo red and immunohistochemical staining in biopsy specimens remains the "gold standard" for diagnosis.

D.   Treatment. The treatment of shoulder and other joint pain is symptomatic. Heat and range-of-motion exercises for the shoulder increase mobility. The intra-articular injection of corticosteroids or the application of 10% hydrocortisone cream to the shoulder using phonophoresis (enhancing the transcutaneous drug delivery through the use of ultrasound) may greatly decrease pain and increase function. Nonsteroidal anti-inflammatory drugs (NSAIDs) are useful in treating symptoms of pain involving multiple joints. Joint pain and restriction of motion may improve with oral prednisone, given in doses of up to 8 mg per day, although symptoms can recur within 48 hours upon discontinuation. Potential risks of corticosteroid-induced bone loss and atherosclerosis limit the use of low-dose prednisone. Patients with β_2-microglobulin amyloidosis who undergo successful renal transplantation experience a marked reduction in joint pain and stiffness.

E. Prevention. Hemodialysis with high-flux dialysis membranes or hemodiafiltration appears to postpone onset of carpal tunnel syndrome and bone cysts and reduce the incidence of amyloidosis. Early renal transplantation in appropriate candidates, before significant β_2-microglobulin amyloid deposition has occurred, may be the most effective preventive measure. After transplantation, β_2-microglobulin amyloid deposits do not progress and may regress, and the size and number of subchondral bone cysts stabilizes. Because AGEs appear to play a pivotal role in the pathogenesis of this condition, future treatment strategies directed toward inhibition of AGE formation (e.g., use of low-AGE diets or drugs that block AGE formation) might help prevent this condition or slow its progress.

II. Other forms of arthritis

A. Crystal-induced arthritis may be caused by any one of several different intra-articular crystals: Calcium pyrophosphate dihydrate, monosodium urate, carbonate apatite, or calcium oxalate. The clinical presentations of these entities are often similar, requiring synovial fluid examination for crystals to distinguish among these conditions.

1. Pseudogout. Attacks of pseudogout occur when calcium pyrophosphate dihydrate (CPPD) crystals are shed from cartilage into joints or periarticular tissues, inducing a sterile inflammatory response. CPPD crystals are more likely to cause painful joint inflammation in the dialysis patient than monosodium urate crystals, especially when hyperparathyroidism is poorly controlled. Pseudogout usually affects large or medium-sized joints, most commonly the knees, although small joints such as the first metatarsophalangeal joint may also be involved. Acute attacks of pseudogout present with the sudden onset of severe joint pain with swelling, erythema, and warmth of the overlying soft tissues. Joint aspiration reveals an exudative synovial fluid containing many neutrophils. The finding of weakly positively birefringent rod-shaped crystals in a joint fluid aspirate makes the diagnosis. Radiography of involved joints may demonstrate chondrocalcinosis.

Although episodes of arthritis associated with CPPD crystals may resolve spontaneously without treatment, joint aspiration (with or without injection of microcrystalline corticosteroid esters) or NSAID therapy may be helpful.

2. Gout. Gouty arthritis occurs when monosodium urate crystals induce a sterile inflammatory response in joints. Although common in patients with renal insufficiency before the initiation of dialysis treatment, acute attacks of gouty arthritis are uncommon among hyperuricemic individuals with uremia. The inflammatory response to monosodium urate crystals is diminished in patients receiving chronic hemodialysis, with decreased monocyte release of interleukin (IL)-1β, IL-6, and tumor necrosis factor (TNF)-α

when compared to individuals with normal renal function. In patients in whom acute gouty arthritis antedated renal failure, symptoms are typically milder once dialysis has been initiated.

The clinical presentation of gout is similar to that of pseudogout, although small joints, such as the first metatarsophalangeal joint, are most commonly affected. Finding needle- or rod-shaped crystals that are strongly negatively birefringent when viewed under compensated polarized light in a joint fluid aspirate makes the diagnosis.

Patients respond rapidly to treatment with NSAIDs, oral or intra-articular corticosteroids, intramuscular adrenocorticotropic hormone gel (40–80 IU), or intramuscular triamcinolone hexacetonide (60 mg). Both prophylactic and therapeutic use of colchicine should be avoided in dialysis patients for reasons described below in Section VI. Allopurinol may be used as prophylaxis but should be given in a markedly reduced dosage (see Section VI and Table 41-3).

3. Arthropathy associated with carbonate apatite crystals. Carbonate apatite crystals may also cause joint pain and swelling in patients undergoing dialysis, especially when the serum calcium–phosphorus product exceeds 75 mg^2/dL^2 (6.0 $mmol/L^2$). The inciting event is presumed to be precipitation of calcium–phosphorus salts under conditions of high calcium and phosphate concentrations. With better control of hyperphosphatemia and hyperparathyroidism in recent years, calcific periarthritis is no longer as prevalent as it was earlier.

The shoulder is the joint most commonly involved; deposits also may occur around the small joints of the hand, the hip, the wrist, the ankle, and the elbow. These deposits, which appear on radiographs of the shoulder as "multiloculated," nodular, periarticular calcifications, may enlarge to become palpable and visible masses (called "tumoral calcinosis"). Limited calcification in tendons, ligaments, and the joint capsule may be associated with acute attacks of painful periarticular inflammation. Although crystals usually are not seen when synovial fluid is examined by compensated polarizing light microscopy, they may be visualized when the fluid is stained with alizarin red S.

Treatment involves immobilization of the involved area and short-term administration of NSAIDs. Injection of microcrystalline corticosteroid esters and local anesthetic, with or without aspiration of carbonate apatite, may provide symptomatic relief and hasten recovery. Reduction of serum phosphorus levels as discussed in Chapter 35 is key. Tumoral calcinosis was improved markedly in several patients who were changed to a daily nocturnal hemodialysis schedule.

4. Arthropathy associated with calcium oxalate crystals. Calcium oxalate crystals can cause acute and chronic synovitis. Although the small joints of the distal extremities are more commonly affected, large joints also may become inflamed. Chondrocalcinosis may be evident on radiographs of involved joints. Characteristic strongly birefringent bipyramidal crystals are seen with compensated polarized light microscopy on examination of synovial fluid. Positive staining with alizarin red S confirms the presence of calcium in the crystals. Calcium oxalate crystals also may deposit in vascular smooth muscle, resulting in acrocyanosis and livedo reticularis.

Patients with calcium oxalate–associated arthritis have responded poorly or not at all to treatment with NSAIDs, intra-articular microcrystalline corticosteroid ester injections, colchicine, or increased frequency of hemodialysis. Because ascorbic acid (vitamin C) is metabolized to oxalate, caution should be observed in prescribing vitamin C supplementation for these patients.

B. **Septic arthritis.** Bacterial infections of joint spaces and bursae occur not infrequently among individuals undergoing hemodialysis, in whom percutaneous vascular access is established several times each week. The most common pathogenic organism is *Staphylococcus aureus.* Diagnosis and treatment are as for nonuremic patients.

C. **Osteonecrosis.** The prevalence of osteonecrosis among patients receiving chronic hemodialysis is increased. The femoral head is the most commonly affected site.

III. **Tendinitis/bursitis in dialysis patients**

A. **Spontaneous tendon rupture.** The quadriceps femoris tendon is the tendon most commonly involved, although ruptures of the Achilles, triceps brachii, patellar, and extensor tendons of the fingers all have been reported. The presence of bone erosion at the site of tendon insertion, weakening the tendon insertion, and relatively high levels of serum alkaline phosphatase suggest that hyperparathyroid bone disease is a predisposing cause. Ruptured tendons should undergo prompt surgical repair. Medical therapy should be directed to control secondary hyperparathyroidism, if present.

B. **Olecranon bursitis.** The bursa overlying the extensor surface of the elbow may become inflamed in patients receiving chronic hemodialysis, usually on the same side as the vascular access. Sustained pressure on the elbow exerted by the arm rest during repeated dialysis treatments is the most likely cause of this "dialysis elbow." The swollen bursa may be aspirated to relieve symptoms, and the fluid should be cultured to exclude an infectious cause. Recurrence should be treated by altering the position of the patient's arm during dialysis to avoid applying pressure to the elbow; intrabursal steroid injection may be performed. Surgical excision should be reserved for cases refractory to medical therapy.

IV. **Nephrogenic fibrosing dermopathy (nephrogenic systemic fibrosis).** Patients with renal failure can develop nephrogenic fibrosing dermopathy (NFD) (also called nephrogenic systemic fibrosis), a scleromyxedema-like condition that had not been reported prior to 1997. Although most individuals were receiving hemodialysis or peritoneal dialysis, NFD also has been reported in patients with acute renal failure, as well as in patients with functioning renal allografts. The development of NFD following magnetic resonance angiography (MRA) with gadodiamide (Omniscan) has suggested a potential causal relationship. Thus, gadodiamide use should be avoided in patients with underlying renal disease.

A. Clinical manifestations. NFD is characterized by brawny hyperpigmentation with thickening and tethering of the skin, predominantly on the extremities and, less commonly, on the torso. This condition can also present as indurated cutaneous plaques or papules. Patients with NFD often experience severe pain and, occasionally, pruritus. They frequently develop flexion contractures of the fingers, elbows, and knees that impair physical function. Yellowish scleral plaques have been observed in the eyes. Muscle and visceral involvement are occasionally seen.

B. Diagnosis. The diagnosis is suggested by clinical appearance. Histologic features vary with duration of disease. Fibroblasts are distributed diffusely in the dermis throughout the course of NFD. Capillary proliferation is observed in early skin biopsies; more established lesions show thickened collagen bundles separated from one another by clefts, elastic fibers oriented parallel to these collagen bundles, mucin deposition, and CD34-positive dendritic cells. Deeper biopsies demonstrate small clusters of factor XIIIa–positive cells and CD68-positive mononuclear and multinucleated giant cells.

C. Treatment. No consistently effective treatment has yet been reported. Several patients experienced resolution of their fibrosing skin lesions upon return of normal renal function following acute tubular necrosis. Oral thalidomide (50–150 mg daily) has been administered to several patients, with results ranging from mild improvement to complete resolution of skin tethering, thickening, and hyperpigmentation. Mild to marked improvement was reported following plasmapheresis in three patients who developed NFD after liver transplantation. Three other patients experienced improvement after receiving a series of extracorporeal photopheresis treatments. Erythropoietin (EPO) has been hypothesized to be a cause, and some patients appeared to improve when the EPO dose was lowered or when EPO was discontinued.

V. Systemic rheumatic diseases

A. Laboratory measures of the acute-phase response

    1. Erythrocyte sedimentation rate (ESR). The ESR is elevated (>25 mm per hour) slightly in many patients receiving dialysis (median 30 mm per hour). Part of the increase in ESR in uremia is due to anemia; the predictive value of a markedly elevated ESR in patients whose anemia is adequately controlled (Hct 33%–36%) has not been well studied.

    2. C-reactive protein (CRP). Levels of CRP are moderately elevated (10–50 mg/L) in up to 50% of patients undergoing dialysis who do not have active infection or inflammation. Marked elevation of the CRP level (>50 mg/L) is a more accurate indicator of active inflammation than the ESR in patients receiving dialysis. CRP levels may be elevated in the setting of a failed arteriovenous graft with occult infection or a retained failed allograft. High serum CRP levels are an independent predictor of mortality.

B. Systemic lupus erythematosus (SLE). The overall activity of nonrenal manifestations of SLE decreases after the initiation of dialysis treatments, even as immunosuppressive drug therapy is withdrawn, but does not disappear completely. Hydroxychloroquine (200–400 mg per day) should be given to patients with active SLE. Minor flares, which typically manifest as arthritis, rash, or serositis, usually can be controlled with the addition of NSAIDs or low doses of prednisone (5–15 mg per day). Infrequently, higher doses of prednisone, alone or with azathioprine, mycophenolate mofetil, or cyclophosphamide, are required to control more severe manifestations of SLE such as cerebritis or vasculitis.

C. Rheumatoid arthritis (RA). Joint inflammation occurring in dialysis patients with RA is treated initially with NSAIDs or small doses of prednisone (5–15 mg per day). Gold compounds and methotrexate (which is not dialyzable) should be avoided (see Table 41-3). Disease-modifying antirheumatic drugs (DMARDs), such as hydroxychloroquine (200–400 mg per day) or azathioprine (50–100 mg per day), may be administered in combination with anti-inflammatory drugs to reduce disease activity. The biologic response modifiers (the TNF-α inhibitors adalimumab, etanercept, and infliximab; the IL-1 receptor antagonist anakinra; the selective T-cell modulator abatacept; and the selective B-cell–depleting monoclonal antibody rituximab) have not been studied adequately in this population to determine their safety.

D. Antineutrophil cytoplasmic antibody (ANCA)-associated vasculitis. Vasculitis relapses in up to 50% of patients with Wegener granulomatosis (WG) while they are receiving chronic dialysis. Vasculitis activity also may relapse in patients with microscopic polyangiitis (MP). Relapses of WG or MP may involve the upper and lower respiratory tract, eyes, skin, joints, and intestinal tract. Prednisone and cyclophosphamide therapy, with substitution of azathioprine for cyclophosphamide after 3 months, may be necessary for treatment.

E. Mixed cryoglobulinemia. Mixed cryoglobulins are detectable in the serum of more than 30% of dialysis patients with hepatitis C viral infection, although levels usually are below 1%. Arthralgias and weakness have been reported in 38% of such patients, but vasculitis manifesting as palpable purpura is seen infrequently. If symptomatic, such patients may be treated with α-interferon 3 million units and ribavirin 200 mg subcutaneously three times weekly for 6–12 months (see Chapter 33 regarding issues of ribavirin use in renal failure), until the cryoglobulin no longer is present.

VI. Muscle weakness. Patients with chronic renal failure undergoing dialysis may develop diffuse muscle weakness, predominantly affecting the lower extremities and involving

Table 41-2.   Causes of muscle weakness in dialysis patients

Peripheral neuropathy
Vitamin D deficiency
Hyperparathyroidism
Carnitine deficiency
Aluminum intoxication
Hyperkalemia or hypokalemia
Acidosis
Iron overload
Severe hypophosphatemia
Drug toxicity (glucocorticoids, colchicine, clofibrate)
Muscle ischemia due to vascular calcification
Inactivity
Underlying systemic rheumatic disease

---

proximal muscles. Serum muscle enzyme levels are usually within the normal range. EMG reveals an abnormal increase in nonspecific polyphasic motor unit potentials. On muscle biopsy, type II fiber atrophy predominates. The cause of muscle weakness is often multifactorial (Table 41-2).

A.   Vitamin D deficiency is the most common non-neuropathic cause. Vitamin D seems to be important for preservation of normal muscle fiber architecture and function. Myopathy caused by vitamin D deficiency is suggested by the presence of diffuse proximal weakness, commonly manifesting as difficulty in arising from a seated position, asthenia, and coexisting osteopenia.

Muscle strength, EMG findings, and histologic changes usually improve after 6 weeks of oral therapy with 1,25-dihydroxyvitamin D_3 (0.5–1.5 mcg per day) or with ergocalciferol (50,000 units weekly). In most patients, the myopathy remits completely after a few months of vitamin D therapy; however, some patients may require 1–2 years of treatment. Hypercalcemia is a common complication of vitamin D therapy.

B.   Hyperparathyroidism may be associated with proximal muscle weakness and impaired respiratory muscle strength. Some patients may regain muscle strength after subtotal parathyroidectomy.

C.   Carnitine deficiency. L-Carnitine is involved in the transfer of long-chain fatty acids into mitochondria for oxidation, producing energy for muscle and other cells. In patients with chronic renal failure, carnitine production by the nonfunctioning kidneys is reduced and dietary carnitine intake is decreased. Additionally, hemodialysis removes L-carnitine. Thus, muscle carnitine concentrations are low in dialysis patients. Intravenous L-carnitine supplementation may improve muscle strength, function, and mass in dialysis patients.

D.   Aluminum intoxication. Muscle weakness in patients with aluminum intoxication has improved following chelation therapy with deferoxamine. The exact mechanism by which aluminum poisoning causes muscle weakness is unknown.

VII. Use of antirheumatic drugs in dialysis patients
(Table 41-3).
A. NSAIDs. Traditional NSAIDs, including aspirin, ibuprofen, naproxen, indomethacin, sulindac, oxaprozin, and nabumetone, inhibit both cyclooxygenase (COX)-1 and COX-2. At therapeutic concentrations, the selective COX-2 inhibitor celecoxib does not inhibit COX-1 and thus spares inhibition of thromboxane production by platelets and prostaglandin biosynthesis in the gastrointestinal tract. Accordingly, selective COX-2 inhibitors have no appreciable effect on bleeding and may have a lower risk of inducing gastric ulcers than traditional NSAIDs. However, several selective COX-2 inhibitors are associated with an increased risk of cardiovascular complications, such as myocardial infarction or stroke. All NSAIDs (including selective COX-2 inhibitors) inhibit prostaglandin production in the kidney and thus have the potential to cause reduced glomerular filtration, salt retention, and hyperkalemia (side effects that may be important in dialysis patients with residual renal function). Because dialysis patients are especially susceptible to gastrointestinal bleeding, consideration should be given to the concurrent use of a proton pump inhibitor or of a prostaglandin analog, such as misoprostol, along with traditional NSAIDs.

Little has been published about the chronic use of NSAIDs in dialysis patients. The liver primarily metabolizes all NSAIDs; very little (<10%) parent compound is excreted unchanged in the urine. An exception is indomethacin, 15%–25% of which is excreted unchanged in the urine. However, 40%–95% of NSAID metabolites are excreted in the urine as glucuronide conjugates or other compounds. Few data are available regarding the bioactivity and toxicity of these metabolites. Consequently, manufacturer product labeling suggests that NSAIDs be used with caution and at reduced doses in patients with renal failure. Because they are highly bound to proteins, NSAIDs are removed poorly by dialysis; postdialysis supplemental doses are unnecessary.

B. Drugs for gout
  1. Allopurinol. Both allopurinol and its active metabolite oxypurinol are cleared by dialysis. Because oxypurinol excretion is primarily renal, the dose of allopurinol should be markedly reduced in patients undergoing dialysis (e.g., to 100 mg daily), with dialysis-day doses given after the treatment.
  2. Colchicine. The half-life of colchicine is prolonged and toxicity occurs more frequently in individuals with compromised renal function. Because its bioavailability is extremely variable in renal failure and it is not cleared by dialysis, use of colchicine should be avoided. Prolonged administration of colchicine to patients with renal insufficiency has caused a severe lysosomal, vacuolar myopathy with marked elevation of serum creatine kinase levels. Severe heart failure also has been reported.
C. Corticosteroids. Purely pharmacokinetic considerations do not contraindicate the treatment of dialysis patients with corticosteroids. However, use of these drugs can result

Table 41-3. Use of antirheumatic drugs in dialysis patients

Drug	Unique Toxicity	Renal Excretion (%)	Dosage Adjustment for Dialysis Patients
Allopurinol	Exfoliative dermatitis	50–75[a]	Decrease dose and lengthen dosing interval; administer dose after HD or administer 50% supplemental dose
Colchicine	Rare xanthine stones Myopathy/neuropathy	10–20	Avoid use (not dialyzable)
Hydroxychloroquine	Myopathy/neuropathy; retinopathy	15–20	No dose modification
Sulfasalazine	Dizziness/headache; reversible oligospermia	50–70	
Auranofin	Diarrhea; stomatitis	60–90	Avoid use
Gold sodium thiomalate	Stomatitis; thrombocytopenia	60–90	Avoid use
Methotrexate	Hepatic cirrhosis and fibrosis; myelosuppression; pneumonitis	45–100	Avoid use (not dialyzable)
Leflunomide	Diarrhea; hypertension	40	No dose modification
Penicillamine	Aplastic anemia; myasthenia gravis	30–60	Avoid use in CAPD
Azathioprine	Myelosuppression; increased risk of neoplasia	2–10	Slightly dialyzable (5%–20%) by HD; CAPD effects unknown; supplement 0.25 mg/kg after HD
Cyclophosphamide	Myelosuppression; hemorrhagic cystitis	40[b]–80[b]	Administer pulse intravenous doses on day before HD; administer oral doses after HD

Cyclosporine	Hypertension; seizures and tremors	6	No dose modification
Mycophenolate mofetil	Diarrhea; myelosuppression	90^c–95^c	Decrease dose to 250–500 mg PO b.i.d. (active drug is dialyzable, but clearance of a metabolite that may cause side effects is reduced)
Corticosteroids			
Prednisone	Cushingoid features	20–35	No dose modification
Methylprednisolone		5	No dose modification (but administer supplemental dose after HD)
Hydrocortisone		5	No dose modification
Dexamethasone		3	No dose modification

HD, hemodialysis; CAPD, continuous ambulatory peritoneal dialysis; PO, by mouth; b.i.d., two times per day.

[a] Of allopurinol and its principal active metabolite, oxypurinol.

[b] Anecdotal evidence suggests that a 50% dose reduction, initially, may be prudent.

[c] Of mycophenolic acid and its principal metabolite, mycophenolic acid glucuronide.

in sodium and fluid retention, hypertension, glucose intolerance, osteoporosis, osteonecrosis, increased susceptibility to infection, and worsened azotemia (due to catabolic effects). Thus, every effort should be made to avoid their use or to administer the lowest dose for the shortest duration possible.

SELECTED READINGS

Allen A, Pusey C, Gaskin G. Outcome for renal replacement therapy in antineutrophil cytoplasmic antibody-associated vasculitis. *J Am Soc Nephrol* 1998;9:1258–1263.

Anderson-Haag T, Patel B. Safety of colchicine in dialysis patients. *Semin Dial* 2003;16:412–413.

Bardin T. Low dose prednisone in dialysis-related amyloid arthropathy. *Rev Rheum (Engl Ed)* 1994;61(9 Suppl):97S–100S.

Boulanger H, et al. Severe methotrexate intoxication in a hemodialysis patient treated for rheumatoid arthritis [letter]. *Nephrol Dial Transplant* 2001;16:1087.

Brouillard M, et al. Erythrocyte sedimentation rate, an underestimated tool in chronic renal failure. *Nephrol Dial Transplant* 1996;11:2244–2247.

Cowper SE, et al. Nephrogenic fibrosing dermopathy. *Am J Dermatopathol* 2001;23:383–393.

Dember LM, Jaber BL. Dialysis-related amyloidosis: late finding or hidden epidemic? *Semin Dial* 2006;19:105–109.

Gilliet M, et al. Successful treatment of three cases of nephrogenic fibrosing dermopathy with extracorporeal photopheresis. *Br J Dermatol* 2005;152:531–536.

Gómez-Fernández P, et al. Effect of parathyroidectomy on respiratory muscle strength in uremic myopathy. *Am J Nephrol* 1987;7:466–469.

Grobner T. Gadolinium—a specific trigger for the development of nephrogenic fibrosing dermopathy and nephrogenic systemic fibrosis? *Nephrol Dial Transplant* 2006;21:1104–1108.

Hamada J, et al. Uremic tumoral calcinosis in hemodialysis patients: clinicopathological findings and identification of calcific deposits. *J Rheumatol* 2006;33:119–126.

Hammoudeh M. Infliximab treatment in a patient with rheumatoid arthritis on haemodialysis [letter]. *Rheumatology (Oxford)* 2006;45:357–359.

Hande KR, Noone RM, Stone WJ. Severe allopurinol toxicity: description and guidelines for prevention in patients with renal insufficiency. *Am J Med* 1984;76:47–56.

Haubitz M, Koch KM, Brunkhorst R. Survival and vasculitis activity in patients with end-stage renal disease due to Wegener's granulomatosis. *Nephrol Dial Transplant* 1998;13:1713–1718.

Jimenez RE, et al. Development of gastrointestinal β_2-microglobulin amyloidosis correlates with time on dialysis. *Am J Surg Pathol* 1998;22:729–735.

Jones M, Kjellstrand CM. Spontaneous tendon ruptures in patients on chronic dialysis. *Am J Kidney Dis* 1996;28:861–866.

Kay J. β_2-Microglobulin amyloidosis. *Amyloid Int J Exp Clin Invest* 1997;4:187–211.

Kay J, et al. Utility of high resolution ultrasound for the diagnosis of dialysis-related amyloidosis. *Arthritis Rheum* 1992;35:926–932.

Krane NK, et al. Persistent lupus activity in end-stage renal disease. *Am J Kidney Dis* 1999;33:872–876.

Kim SJ, et al. Resolution of massive uremic tumoral calcinosis with daily nocturnal home hemodialysis. *Am J Kidney Dis* 2003;41: E12.

López-Gómez JM, et al. Presence of a failed kidney transplant in patients who are on hemodialysis is associated with chronic inflammatory state and erythropoietin resistance. *J Am Soc Nephrol* 2004;2494–2501.

Mendoza FA, et al. Description of 12 cases of nephrogenic fibrosing dermopathy and review of the literature. *Semin Arthritis Rheum* 2006;35:238–249.

Miyata T, et al. β_2-Microglobulin modified with advanced glycation end products is a major component of hemodialysis-associated amyloidosis. *J Clin Invest* 1993;92:1243–1252.

Prabhala A, et al. Severe myopathy associated with vitamin D deficiency in western New York. *Arch Int Med* 2000;160:1199–1203.

Schreiner O, et al. Reduced secretion of proinflammatory cytokines of monosodium urate crystal-stimulated monocytes in chronic renal failure: an explanation for infrequent gout episodes in chronic renal failure patients?. *Nephrol Dial Transplant* 2000;15:644–649.

Siami G, et al. Evaluation of the effect of intravenous L-carnitine therapy on function, structure and fatty acid metabolism of skeletal muscle in patients receiving chronic hemodialysis. *Nephron* 1991;57:306–313.

Swartz RD, et al. Nephrogenic fibrosing dermopathy: a novel cutaneous fibrosing disorder in patients with renal failure. *Am J Med* 2003;114:563–572.

Ward MM. Cardiovascular and cerebrovascular morbidity and mortality among women with end-stage renal disease attributable to lupus nephritis. *Am J Kidney Dis* 2000;36:516–525.

Wilbur K, Makowsky M. Colchicine myotoxicity: case reports and literature review. *Pharmacotherapy* 2004;24:1784–1792.

Word-Sims WS, Hall CD. Carpal tunnel syndrome in the dialysis patient. *Semin Dial* 1990;3:47–51.

Wu M-J, et al. Prevalence of subclinical cryoglobulinemia in maintenance hemodialysis patients and kidney transplant recipients. *Am J Kidney Dis* 2000;35:52–57.

Nervous System and Sleep Disorders

Anthony J. Nicholls, Robert L. Benz, and Mark R. Pressman

Uremia is accompanied by disordered functioning of both the central and peripheral nervous systems. The extent of neurologic dysfunction in apparently well-dialyzed patients is often only fully apparent after restoration of normal biochemistry by transplantation. Typically the patient reports rapid improvement in cognitive functioning, sleep, and sensorimotor function that was often unreported previously. Neurologic problems arise in dialyzed patients as a complication of treatment, from metabolic derangements, or from disordered homeostasis. This chapter is limited to cerebral disorders, sleep disorders, neuropathy, pain management, and seizures.

I. **Central nervous system abnormalities.** Cerebral symptoms occur in four main settings in the dialysis patient: (a) acute obtundation unassociated with dialysis itself, encountered either as a feature of advanced uremia or occurring in a previously stable dialysis patient; (b) disordered brain function during or immediately after dialysis; (c) chronic dementia; and (d) subclinical disturbances of cognitive function in apparently adequately treated patients.

A. **Acute obtundation not associated with the dialysis procedure**

1. **Uremic encephalopathy.** Encephalopathy is a cardinal feature of untreated uremia. Initial manifestations are subtle: flattened affect, irritability, and poor rapport with others. Formal evaluation at this stage may reveal patchy cognitive or psychomotor behavior. Event-related brain potentials (stimulus-evoked averaged electroencephalogram [EEG] waveforms) may be abnormal. As uremia advances, lassitude gives way to disorientation, confusion, delirium, stupor, and, preterminally, coma. There are accompanying motor disturbances: tremulousness, myoclonus, and asterixis (flapping tremor). These major signs of uremic encephalopathy will reliably regress within a week or so of initiation of regular dialysis; failure to do so should lead to an alternative or additional diagnosis.

2. **Acute aluminum intoxication.** In patients taking aluminum along with citrate in any form (Shohl solution, calcium citrate, or effervescent analgesics such as Alka-Seltzer), an acute neurotoxicity syndrome has been described characterized by agitation, confusion, seizures, myoclonic jerks, and coma. The acute syndrome also can be seen when dialysis solution is highly contaminated with aluminum or in the course of deferoxamine (DFO) therapy (see

Table 42-1. Partial differential diagnoses of acute obtundation not associated with dialysis

Uremic encephalopathy

Acute aluminum toxicity (coingestion of citrate, highly contaminated dialysate)

Central nervous system infection
  Meningitis
  Encephalitis
  Endocarditis

Hypertensive encephalopathy

Hemorrhage
  Subarachnoid
  Subdural
  Intracranial

Drug intoxication (by drugs renally excreted)
  Penicillin
  Cefazolin

Wernicke's encephalopathy (in patients with vomiting, poor food intake)

Chapter 43). The plasma aluminum level usually is more than 500 mcg/L (19 mcmol/L), and typical EEG changes (multifocal bursts of slow or delta wave activity, often accompanied by spikes) are present. Most of the reported patients died despite being treated with DFO.

3. Other causes of acute obtundation. Table 42-1 lists the main conditions to be considered in such cases. Appropriate history, examination, and special investigations (including computed brain tomography) usually reveal the diagnosis.

B. Acute cerebral dysfunction during or immediately after dialysis

1. Disequilibrium syndrome. Rapid correction of advanced uremia is sometimes complicated by a characteristic syndrome of neurologic dysfunction appearing in the last part of dialysis or shortly afterward. Hemodialysis is usually involved, but disequilibrium can also occur with peritoneal dialysis. In its mildest form, the syndrome is limited to restlessness, headache, nausea, and vomiting; more severe manifestations include confusion and major seizures. The syndrome is believed to be caused by brain swelling due to a lag in osmolar shifts between blood and brain during dialysis, but changes in brain pH may also play a role. Disequilibrium occurs in a major form in previously undialyzed patients, but minor features may complicate chronic therapy. Disequilibrium is more likely to occur when patients with advanced states of uremia are dialyzed for excessive lengths of time during their first treatment sessions. The initial dialyses should be relatively short, so as to reduce elevated serum urea levels slowly over the course of several days (see Chapter 8).

2. Intracranial bleeding. The most important differential diagnosis of dialysis disequilibrium syndrome is intracranial bleeding, precipitated or aggravated by anticoagulation during hemodialysis. Spontaneous subdural hemorrhage is typical, but intracranial or subarachnoid bleeds are not uncommon. This is a particular problem in patients with polycystic kidneys who may have intracranial aneurysms. Headache occurs in both disequilibrium and early cerebral hemorrhage, but the pattern of recovery is different. Thus, the patient whose clinical course is atypical for disequilibrium should be evaluated for possible intracranial hemorrhage by computed tomography (CT). Management is similar to that for nonuremic patients. Heparin-free dialysis should be used.

3. Other causes. Metabolic disorders and hypotension also can mimic disequilibrium (Table 42-2). These may be excluded by blood pressure measurement and simple laboratory tests. Aluminum intoxication, in addition to the acute manifestations described above and the chronic syndrome discussed below, can give rise to subacute central nervous system symptoms similar to disequilibrium syndrome, which sometimes appear to be worse just after dialysis.

C. Chronic dementia. Aluminum poisoning in dialysis patients causes a highly characteristic progressive myoclonic dementia. Typical early signs are stuttering and stammering. Signs and symptoms may be exacerbated by dialysis and by DFO administration. The diagnosis of aluminum-related dementia should be pursued by performing an EEG, which may show the characteristic multifocal bursts of delta or theta activity, measuring serum aluminum levels, and performing a DFO infusion test to help assess the body aluminum burden. These are described in Chapter 43.

Table 42-2. Conditions that may mimic dialysis disequilibrium syndrome

Intracranial bleeding
  Subdural
  Subarachnoid
  Intracranial

Metabolic disorders
  Hyperosmolar states
  Hypercalcemia
  Hypoglycemia
  Hyponatremia

Cerebral infarction

Hypotension
  Excessive ultrafiltration
  Cardiac arrhythmia
  Myocardial infarction
  Anaphylaxis

Aluminum intoxication (subacute)

Dialysis patients with progressive dementia in whom aluminum poisoning has been excluded are likely to suffer from some form of progressive cerebrovascular disease. Table 42-3 lists a brief differential diagnosis of chronic dementia in this population. Widespread atheromatous plaques commonly found in dialysis patients predispose them to develop multi-infarct dementia. At autopsy, the brains of these patients are seen to contain multiple lacunar infarcts in the basal ganglia, thalamus, internal capsule, pons, and cerebellum. Clinically, these patients present with a progressive stepwise decline in intellectual and neurologic functioning, and may have a variety of neurologic signs according to the site of the infarcts. The diagnosis of chronic subdural hematoma as a complication of anticoagulant treatment should always be borne in mind as the disease may present with pseudodementia, drowsiness, and confusion. The diagnosis is made by CT scanning. Metabolic disorders, including drug intoxication, are excluded by simple laboratory tests and a careful drug ingestion history. Lastly, thiamine deficiency has been described in a group of patients from Taiwan (Hung, 2001).

D. Subclinical cognitive dysfunction. Subclinical uremic encephalopathy may be present in chronic dialysis patients if inadequate dialysis is delivered. Reasons include noncompliance, vascular access recirculation, and impaired peritoneal transport. In elderly patients with vascular instability, the prescribed dialysis dose may often fail to be achieved as the patient may request termination of the dialysis session prematurely. This may not be fully apparent from scrutiny of a monthly *Kt/V* record if measurement of *Kt/V* is only made after a full dialysis treatment. Severe depression (and sometimes anxiety) can impair cognitive function, but these may be detected only if detailed and regular neuropsychological assessment is undertaken. Unrecognized alterations in cerebral function due to aluminum accumulation can rarely occur

Table 42-3. Partial differential diagnoses of chronic dementia in dialysis patients

Aluminum encephalopathy (dialysis dementia)
Multiinfarct dementia
Chronic subdural hematoma
Hydrocephalus (possibly secondary to subarachnoid hemorrhage)
Metabolic disorders
    Hypercalcemia (autonomous hyperparathyroidism or iatrogenic)
    Hypoglycemic brain damage
    Demyelination syndrome secondary to hyponatremia
    Uremia (underdialysis)
    Thiamine deficiency (chronic Wernicke-Korsakoff syndrome)
Drug intoxication
Anemia
Presenile dementias
Depressive pseudodementia
Chronic infection

as a result of therapy with aluminum-containing phosphorus binders.

Some of the chronic cerebral disturbances of dialysis patients are attributable to anemia. Both event-related potentials and neuropsychological test scores improve after treatment of anemia with erythropoietin (EPO).

E. Visual/auditory disturbances. A syndrome of acute visual or, more rarely, auditory loss has been described as a complication of DFO therapy, especially when higher dosages are used. Acute sight loss also has occurred due to retinal artery leukoembolization.

F. Atlanto-cervical spondylopathy. Progressive neck instability and cord compression due to destructive β_2-microglobulin–derived amyloidosis has been described in long-term dialysis patients. The condition can be diagnosed by magnetic resonance imaging (MRI). Early decompression is vital to avoid major disability. See Chapter 41 for a more complete discussion of amyloidosis and its complications.

II. Sleep disorders. Recent surveys of dialysis patients report that 41%–52% have one or more sleep complaints, and more than 50% studied in a sleep disorders laboratory have a sleep disorder objectively documented by polysomnography. Dialysis patients complain frequently of "insomnia" independent of anxiety or depression. They may have difficulty falling asleep or staying asleep. Patients often complain of awakening frequently during the night without apparent cause. Excessive daytime sleepiness (EDS) is a frequent complaint. It is common to enter a dialysis unit during the daytime and find many patients fast asleep while undergoing dialysis. Chronic daytime sleepiness may affect cognitive functioning, interfere with activities of daily living, and decrease quality-of-life. Daytime sleepiness may also interfere with the patient's ability to work and place him or her in danger while driving or operating heavy equipment.

A. Sleep apnea. Studies have found sleep apnea in 53%–75% of dialysis patients with sleep-related complaints. Sleep apnea can be classified as obstructive, central, or mixed. **Obstructive sleep apnea** is a very common medical disorder resulting from a collapse of the upper airway during sleep in the presence of continuing respiratory effort. It is often associated with loud snoring, gasping, and snorting sounds during sleep. It is reported to occur in 4% of normal men and 2% of women 30–60 years of age. As many as 81% of elderly nursing home patients are reported to have sleep apnea. Obstructive sleep apnea has been reported to be associated with increased morbidity and mortality. This morbidity is most often related to cardiovascular and cerebrovascular pathophysiologic processes, as well as accidents due to sleepiness. While dialysis patients may have obstructive sleep apnea, they also commonly have **central sleep apnea.** In central apnea, neither respiratory effort nor airflow is present, suggesting a malfunction in the respiratory centers of the brain. **Mixed apneas**, which refers to central sleep apnea with an obstructive component, are not uncommon in the dialysis population.

B. Restless legs syndrome (RLS) and periodic leg movements in sleep (PLMS).

1. Restless legs. One of the most common complaints among ESRD patients is RLS. RLS is a subjective complaint for which there is no objective test. Patients often describe an irritating sensation deep in the muscles of the lower leg, particularly in the calf muscle. Patients can relieve this sensation only by moving their legs and feet. The irritating sensation typically appears when patients are at rest, often in the hours prior to the patient's usual bedtime. RLS may significantly delay sleep onset.

2. PLMS is a common sleep disorder occurring with increased incidence with age and is common in the elderly of the general population. It generally consists of a dorsiflexion of the foot or movement of the lower limb lasting 2–4 seconds and repeating every 20–40 seconds numerous times. It occurs primarily in the first third of the sleep period during non–rapid eye movement sleep. Each movement may result in a brief arousal from sleep and can be the source of complaints about unrefreshing sleep and daytime fatigue. PLMS occurs in approximately 80% of patients who complain of RLS. PLMS is found in a very high percentage of ESRD patients. Dialysis patients with PLMS have a much higher number of movements per hour of sleep than patients in the general population with PLMS. In one case series of 45 dialysis patients, 71% had significant PLMS, with several patients having more than 1,500 leg movements in a single night. Many of the PLMS incidents were associated with repetitive arousals, resulting in very poor-quality sleep, daytime complaints of fatigue, and increased mortality.

C. Diagnosis

1. History. A sleep history can easily be obtained using a questionnaire or brief interview. Patients or bed partners should be questioned regarding quantity and quality of nocturnal sleep, number of awakenings from sleep, whether sleep is restorative, snoring, gasping, breathing pauses during sleep, lower limb movements (kicking) while awake or asleep, daytime fatigue, or inappropriate napping. A review of medications or social habits (e.g., excess caffeine) associated with excess irritability should be reviewed.

2. Polysomnography. Sleep disorders such as sleep apnea and periodic leg movements in sleep are easily identifiable via standard diagnostic polysomnography (sleep studies). These studies are usually performed in specially equipped laboratories found in many hospitals.

Polysomnography generally encompasses simultaneous electroencephalography, electrooculography, electromyography, and electrocardiography, as well as monitoring of breathing sounds, respiratory effort and airflow, arterial oxygen saturation, and leg movements during the patient's usual sleep period.

D. Treatment

1. Sleep apnea

a. Medication has not been shown to be effective in the treatment of obstructive sleep apnea. Benzodiazepines are contraindicated for obstructive sleep apnea, as are other central nervous system depressants, because they may result in longer apneas, greater O_2 desaturation, and more severe sleep fragmentation with consequently greater daytime fatigue.

b. Nocturnal dialysis. Both nocturnal HD (Hanly, 2003) and, recently, nocturnal cycler-assisted PD (Tang, 2006) have reported improvement in sleep apnea. The responsible mechanisms have not been established.

c. Continuous positive airway pressure (CPAP). CPAP consists of the administration of positive air pressure via the mouth or nares. The positive air pressure splints the upper airway open, effectively preventing obstruction. This has been shown to be an effective treatment for sleep apneas in the dialysis population, whether the cause is obstructive, central, or mixed. Noncompliance is a problem, however, in patients who use CPAP treatment for obstructive sleep apnea.

d. Surgery. Various surgical approaches have been used for the treatment of obstructive sleep apnea. These usually involve the surgical reduction or removal of the uvula and tissues of the soft palate. Surgeries for obstructive sleep apnea have been reported to have an overall success rate of 50%.

e. O_2. Administration of low-flow supplemental O_2 has been reported to be a successful treatment for central sleep apnea in some recent studies. However, if obstructive sleep apnea is also present, low-flow O_2 may result in a lengthening of apnea duration.

2. **RLS/PLMS**

a. Conservative measures. Iron repletion is helpful in the general population but is very rarely a problem in dialysis patients owing to continual monitoring of iron status. Nonetheless, iron deficiency should be avoided. General advice about caffeine, alcohol and nicotine avoidance is sometimes helpful. Regular exercise, massage, and either hot or cold baths may ameliorate symptoms. Chronic insomnia from restless legs adds to the burden of mood disturbance which may perpetuate a cycle of poor sleep.

b. Medication. Dopamine precursors or agonists such as L-dopa (e.g., Sinemet) have been shown to reduce the number and severity of both disorders and are considered the treatment of choice by many (Montplaisir and Godbout, 1989). Benzodiazepines, such as clonazepam, have been used for many years. Controversy exists as to whether benzodiazepines actually reduce the number of movements or simply suppress arousal. Longer acting dopamine agonists such as Requip (ropinirole) are now available but should be used cautiously in ESRD patients.

E. Effects of transplantation. Complete resolution of both sleep apnea and RLS/PLMS has been reported following kidney transplantation.

F. Mortality. Both presence of sleep apnea and a high PLMS index (e.g., more than 35 leg movements per hour of sleep) are associated with elevated mortality rates. It is not known if this is causal or merely associative, and whether treatment will improve survival in such patients also has not been determined.

III. Neuropathy

A. Uremic neuropathy. Uremic neuropathy is a distal, symmetric, mixed motor and sensory polyneuropathy. It typically involves the legs more than the arms. Clinical manifestations include paresthesia in the feet, painful dysesthesia, ataxia, and weakness. The sense of position and the vibratory threshold are often impaired. Physiologic studies show slowing of motor nerve conduction and sensory action potentials. The condition is due to one or more toxins retained in uremia and inadequately removed by dialysis. In patients with coexisting diabetes, the development of disabling neuropathy can be rapid, and unraveling the contribution of each cause may be difficult.

With effective dialysis, clinical uremic neuropathy is unusual, but subclinical manifestations can be detected in over 50% of patients. Serial electrophysiologic monitoring has been used to assess the adequacy of dialysis schedules, but is not routinely employed. If clinical signs of peripheral neuropathy appear, then the adequacy of the dialysis treatment should be carefully evaluated using urea kinetic modeling. A switch to a high-flux membrane or hemodiafiltration to increase the removal of middle molecules may be of benefit. More frequent hemodialysis, and especially six times per week nocturnal hemodialysis, may improve neuropathy, but solid data on neuropathy are not yet available. Neuropathy is most reliably reversed by successful renal transplantation.

B. Differential diagnosis. Uremic neuropathy has to be distinguished from disturbed peripheral nerve function due to an underlying systemic disease (e.g., amyloidosis or diabetes mellitus). Table 42-4 gives an abbreviated list of disorders to be considered in the differential diagnosis. Pyridoxine supplementation has been reported to improve peripheral polyneuropathy in a group of elderly Japanese dialysis patients; however, this was not a controlled study, and baseline pyridoxal 5'-phosphate levels were not decreased (Okada et al., 2000).

C. Mononeuropathies. Paresthesia in the extremities may also be due to a mononeuropathy, most commonly involving the median nerve at the wrist (carpal tunnel syndrome). This

Table 42-4. Principal differential diagnoses of uremic polyneuropathy

Diabetes mellitus
Ethanol abuse
Amyloidosis
Malnutrition
Polyarteritis
Lupus erythematosus
Multiple myeloma
Thiamine deficiency

commonly involves the fistula arm first, but usually becomes bilateral. The pathogenesis and management of the carpal tunnel syndrome are discussed in Chapter 41. Occasionally, prolonged recumbency during the hemodialysis procedure leads to ulnar and peroneal nerve palsies.

IV. Seizures

A. Etiology. Seizures are not uncommon in dialysis patients. Generalized seizures are an integral feature of advanced uremic encephalopathy. Seizures can also be a manifestation of severe disequilibrium syndrome, as discussed above. Table 42-5 lists the most common associated conditions. Intracranial hemorrhage commonly leads to focal seizures, while most of the other causes lead to generalized seizures.

B. Predisposing factors. Seizures characterize both aluminum-induced encephalopathy and severe hypertension. In children with renal failure, the incidence of seizures is higher than in adults. Predialysis hypocalcemia can result in seizures during or soon after dialysis due to the fall in serum ionized calcium level associated with rapid correction of acidosis. As in any patient with hypocalcemia, associated (and often causal) hypomagnesemia should be excluded. Hypoglycemia can occur if glucose-free dialysis solution is used.

The incidence of seizures in patients treated with EPO has come under close scrutiny; the risk appears to be 1 seizure per 13 patient-years of therapy, with the highest risk during the early months of treatment. There is little evidence of an excess of seizures in normotensive patients on EPO; however, when hematocrit rises, there is a tendency for a concomitant rise in blood pressure. This may provoke hypertensive encephalopathy and seizures if the rate of rise in blood pressure exceeds the capacity of the cerebral circulation to alter its autoregulatory thresholds.

Seizures tend to be more common in patients taking a variety of "epileptogenic" drugs. Penicillins and cephalosporins are common offenders, especially if high doses are given. A selection of other epileptogenic drugs is given in Table 42-5. A variety of poisonings in dialysis patients can present with seizures, including star fruit ingestion (numbness, weakness, obtundation, seizures; see Chang et al., 2000).

C. Diagnosis. Electroencephalography is of limited value in the evaluation of seizures in dialysis patients. Patients with renal failure rarely have a normal EEG, the most common abnormal findings being reduced voltage, loss of alpha activity, and the appearance of periodic, symmetric, and usually frontal delta wave slowing. In any case the EEG is unlikely to distinguish between the various causes of seizures listed in Table 42-5, and a search for aluminum poisoning, an underlying metabolic cause, a complication of the dialysis procedure, or a structural intracranial lesion is more appropriate.

D. Prevention. Susceptible patients can often be identified (see Table 42-5). The prevention of dialysis disequilibrium is discussed above. Patients with low serum ionized calcium levels can be given IV calcium at the start of dialysis, and a dialysis solution with a high calcium concentration can be used. Blood pressure needs to be monitored closely during

Table 42-5. Seizures in dialysis patients

Etiology

Uremic encephalopathy (unlikely in dialysis patients)
Disequilibrium syndrome
Aluminum encephalopathy
Hypertensive encephalopathy
Intracranial hemorrhage
Alcohol withdrawal
Toxins (star fruit ingestion)
Other (metabolic)
   Hypocalcemia
   Hyperosmolality due to peritoneal dialysis
   Hypernatremia (accidental due to hemodialysis machine
     malfunction) or hyponatremia
   Anoxia
     Arrhythmia
     Anaphylaxis
     Severe hypotension
     Air embolism

Prevention

   Identification of susceptible subgroups
   Predialysis serum urea nitrogen level >130 mg/dL (46 mmol/L)
   Severe hypertension
   Children
   Patients receiving erythropoietin (EPO)
   Previous seizure disorder
   Alcoholism
   Predialysis hypocalcemia (<6 mg/dL, 1.5 mmol/L) with acidosis
Limiting initial dialysis session length and blood flow rate
Maintenance of dialysis solution sodium concentration at or above
   plasma level
Use of 3.5 mEq/L (1.75 mM) or 4.0 mEq/L (2.0 mM) calcium bath in
   hypocalcemic patients; administration of IV calcium during
   dialysis if necessary
Scrupulous attention to blood pressure control during EPO therapy
Limiting exposure to ethanol and to "epileptogenic" drugs
   Penicillins
   Fluoroquinolones
   Cyclosporine
   Meperidine (Demerol)
   Theophylline
   Metoclopramide
   Lithium

Therapy

Stopping dialysis
Maintenance of airway patency
Drawing blood for glucose, calcium, and other electrolytes
If hypoglycemia is suspected, administration of IV glucose
Administration of IV diazepam or lorazepam, and also phenytoin
   if required
Treatment of metabolic disturbance if present

initiation of EPO therapy, and the dosage of antihypertensive medication may need to be raised.

E.   Management. The emergency treatment of convulsions should begin by stopping dialysis and ensuring patency of the airway. Blood should be sampled immediately and serum glucose, calcium, and other electrolyte values determined. IV glucose should be administered if hypoglycemia is suspected. If seizures persist, then 5–10 mg of diazepam can be infused slowly IV. Infusion can be repeated at 5-minute intervals to a maximum total dosage of 30 mg. Diazepam therapy can be followed by a loading dosage of phenytoin in a dose of 10–15 mg/kg given by slow IV infusion, at a rate no greater than 50 mg per minute, during constant electrocardiographic monitoring to guard against phenytoin-induced bradycardia, atrioventricular conduction block, or other arrhythmias.

F.   Drug prophylaxis. The prophylaxis of recurrent convulsions is usually effective with administration of phenytoin, carbamazepine, or sodium valproate. Fits of dialysis encephalopathy respond best to benzodiazepines, particularly clonazepam. Table 42-6 lists dosage schedules and other pharmacokinetic data for anticonvulsants in dialysis patients.

> **1.   Phenytoin**
>
> **a.   Reduced plasma half-life.** The half-life of phenytoin is reduced in dialysis patients, resulting in lower plasma levels at the usual therapeutic dosage.
>
> **b.   Increased free fraction in uremia.** Phenytoin is normally 90% protein bound, and drug effect is proportional to the free (unbound) drug level. Normal therapeutic blood levels of total (bound plus unbound) phenytoin are usually 10–20 mg/L, corresponding to about 1.0–2.0 mg/L of free phenytoin. In uremia, and also with low serum albumin, the unbound phenytoin fraction can increase from 10% to 30%, resulting in more marked drug effect for any given blood level of total phenytoin.
>
> **c.   Falsely high levels with immunoassay methods in uremia.** In uremic patients, a number of inactive metabolites of phenytoin can accumulate that are picked up rather indiscriminately by the usual immunoassay methods (e.g., the enzyme multiplied immunoassay, or EMIT, procedure), resulting in inaccurately high readings. Chromatographic methods (e.g., gas-liquid chromatography) are not subject to this error. The amount of overestimation by the EMIT procedure, initially considerable, is now less due to improvements in the immunoassay procedure.
>
> **d.   Therapeutic recommendations.** The usual loading and maintenance dosages of phenytoin should be given (see Table 42-6); one should give a divided daily maintenance dosage because of the reduced plasma half-life. Although the amount of drug given will depend on clinical response, a target blood level for total phenytoin measured by a chromatographic procedure should be in the range of about 4–10 mg/L.

G.   Other anticonvulsant drugs. Carbamazepine, ethosuximide, and valproic acid can be given in 75%–100% of the

Table 42-6. Pharmacokinetics of anticonvulsants in dialysis patients

Drug	Renal Excretion (%)	Nonuremic Dosage Range (mg per day)	Usual Dosage for ESRD Patients (% of nonuremic dose)	Nonuremic Patients	ESRD Patients	Removed by Hemodialysis	Notes
						Plasma Half-life (hours)	
Carbamazepine	3	600–1,600	100	10–20	Same[a]	No	NU-TPL = 4–12 mg/L
Clonazepam	<1	0.5–20.0	100	17–28	Same[a]	No	
Diazepam	<1	5–10 (IV)[b]	?50	20–70	Same[a]	No	Active metabolites may accumulate in renal failure
Ethosuximide	>30	750–2,000	100	50–60	Same[a]	Yes	NU-TPL = 40–100 mg/L
Phenobarbital	10–40	60–200	75	100	120–160	Yes	
Phenytoin	<5	300–600	100	10–30	Same[a]	±	NU-TPL = 10–20 mg/L ESRD-TPL = 4–10 mg/L due to decreased protein binding
Primidone	40[c]	500–2,000	Caution	5–15	Same[a]	Yes	Avoid in ESRD patients NU-TPL = 50–120 mg/L
Valproic acid	<4	750–2,000	75–100	6–16	Same[a]	±	
Vigabatrin	50	2000–4,000	25	7	14	Unknown	New drug; little experience in dialysis patients

ESRD, end-stage renal disease; NU-TPL, therapeutic plasma concentration in nonuremic subjects; ESRD-TPL, therapeutic plasma concentration in dialysis patients

[a]Inferred (estimated) from pharmacokinetic considerations.

[b]Initial dose.

[c]Extensive metabolism to phenylethylmalonamide (PEMA) and phenobarbital. Primidone and PEMA are excreted unchanged, and 10%–40% of phenobarbital is excreted by the kidneys.

usual dosage to dialysis patients. Protein binding of valproic acid may be reduced in uremia. Carbamazepine is not well removed by dialysis. Valproic acid is dialyzable when high-flux dialyzers are used (Kane et al., 2000). Ethosuximide is substantially dialyzable, and a posthemodialysis supplement may be required. Primidone is 40% renally excreted and is moderately dialyzable. Primidone should be used with extreme caution in dialysis patients; the need for a substantially reduced dosage should be anticipated, and a posthemodialysis supplement may be required. Phenobarbital can be given in 75%–100% of the usual dosage. Phenobarbital is dialyzable, and a dose should be scheduled after the dialysis treatment. Vigabatrin, a γ-aminobutyric acid-transaminase inhibitor, is eliminated by the kidney; major dosage reduction is necessary in dialysis patients (see Table 42-6).

SELECTED READINGS

Apostolou T, Gokal R. Neuropathy and quality-of-life in diabetic continuous ambulatory peritoneal dialysis patients. *Perit Dial Int* 1999;19(Suppl 2):S242–S247.

Bazzi C, et al. Uremic polyneuropathy: a clinical and electrophysiological study in 135 short- and long-term hemodialyzed patients. *Clin Nephrol* 1991;35:176.

Benz RL, et al. A preliminary study of the effects of correction of anemia with recombinant human erythropoietin therapy on sleep, sleep disorders, and daytime sleepiness in hemodialysis patients (the SLEEPO study). *Am J Kidney Dis* 1999;34:1089–1095.

Benz RL, et al. Potential novel predictors of mortality in end-stage renal disease patients with sleep disorders. *Am J Kidney Dis* 2000;35:1052–1060.

Chang JM, et al. Fatal outcome after ingestion of star fruit (Averrhoa carambola) in uremic patients. *Am J Kidney Dis* 2000;35:189–193.

Davison SN. Pain in hemodialysis patients: prevalence, cause, severity, and management. *Am J Kidney Dis* 2003;42:1239–1247.

Edmunds ME, Walls J. Pathogenesis of seizures during recombinant human erythropoietin therapy. *Semin Dial* 1991;4:163.

Glenn CM, et al. Dialysis-associated seizures in children and adolescents. *Pediatr Nephrol* 1992;6:182.

Hanly PJ, et al. Daytime sleepiness in patients with CRF: impact of nocturnal hemodialysis. *Am J Kidney Dis* 2003;41:403–410.

Hung SC, et al. Thiamine deficiency and unexplained encephalopathy in hemodialysis and peritoneal dialysis patients. *Am J Kidney Dis* 2001;38:941–947.

Jungers P, et al. Incidence and risk factors of atherosclerotic cardiovascular accidents in predialysis chronic renal failure patients: a prospective study. *Nephrol Dial Transplant* 1997;12:2597–2602.

Jungers P, et al. Incidence of atherosclerotic arterial occlusive accidents in predialysis and dialysis patients: a multicentric study in the Ile de France district. *Nephrol Dial Transplant* 1999;14:898–902.

Kane SL, et al. High-flex hemodialysis without hemoperfusion is effective in acute valproic acid overdose. *Ann Pharmacother* 2000;34:1146–1151.

Kavanagh D, et al. Restless legs syndrome in patients on dialysis. *Am J Kidney Dis* 2004;43:763–771.

Kawamura M, et al. Incidence, outcome, and risk factors of cerebrovascular events in patients undergoing maintenance hemodialysis. *Am J Kidney Dis* 1998;31:991–996.

Kiley JE. Residual renal and dialyser clearance, EEG slowing, and nerve conduction velocity. *ASAIO J* 1981;4:1.

Lass P, et al. Cognitive impairment in patients with renal failure is associated with multiple-infarct dementia. *Clin Nucl Med* 1999;24:561–565.

Mandayam S, et al. Subdural hematoma in dialysis patients. *J Am Soc Nephrol* 2004;14:616A.

Marsh JT, et al. rHuEPO treatment improves brain and cognitive function of anemic dialysis patients. *Kidney Int* 1991;39:155.

Molnar MZ, Novak M, Mucsi I. Management of restless legs syndrome in patients on dialysis. *Drugs* 2006;66(5):607–624.

Montplaisir J, Godbout R. Restless legs syndrome and periodic leg movements in sleep. In: Kryger MH, et al (eds). *Principles and practice of sleep medicine*. Philadelphia: WB Saunders 1989;402–409.

Novak M, et al. Diagnosis and management of sleep apnea syndrome and restless legs syndrome in dialysis patients. *Semin Dial* 2006;19(3):210–216.

Novak M, et al. Diagnosis and management of insomnia in dialysis patients. *Semin Dial* 2006;19(1):25–31.

Novak M, et al. Diagnosis and management of sleep apnea syndrome and restless legs syndrome in dialysis patients. *Semin Dial* 2006;19:210–216.

Okada H, et al. Vitamin B_6 supplementation can improve peripheral neuropathy in patients with chronic renal failure on high-flux hemodialysis and human recombinant erythropoietin. *Nephrol Dial Transplant* 2000;16:1410–1413.

Pressman MR, Benz RL. Sleep disordered breathing in ESRD: acute beneficial effects of treatment with nasal continuous positive airway pressure. *Kidney Int* 1993;43:1134–1139.

Silver SM. Cerebral edema after hemodialysis: the "reverse urea effect" lives. *Int J Artif Organs* 1998;21:247–250.

Tang S, et al. Alleviation of sleep apnea in patients with chronic renal failure by nocturnal cycler-assisted peritoneal dialysis compared with conventional continuous ambulatory peritoneal dialysis. *J Am Soc Nephrol* 2006;17:2607–2616.

Tattersall JE, et al. Rapid high-flux dialysis can cure uremic peripheral neuropathy. *Nephrol Dial Transplant* 1992;7:539.

Toepfer M, et al. Inflammatory demyelinating neuropathy in patients with end-stage renal disease receiving continuous ambulatory peritoneal dialysis. *Perit Dial Int* 1998;18:172–176.

Tucker KL, et al. High homocysteine and low B vitamin predict cognitive decline in aging men: The Veterans Affairs Normative Aging Study. *Am J Clin Nutr* 2005;82:627–635.

Winkelmayer W, et al. Optic neuropathy in uremia: an interdisciplinary emergency. *Am J Kidney Dis* 2001;37:E23.

Aluminum, Lanthanum, and Strontium

Patrick C. D'Haese and Marc E. De Broe

I. Aluminum (MW 27 daltons). In dialysis patients, the protective mechanisms against aluminum accumulation (renal excretion and the gastrointestinal barrier) are either absent or highly challenged by ingestion of pharmacologic doses of aluminum salts for the purpose of enteral phosphate binding. The clinical consequences of aluminum poisoning in dialysis patients include a neurologic syndrome, aluminum-induced bone disease, and anemia. At the present time, due to the availability of adequate procedures for water treatment and the almost universal use of aluminum-free phosphate binders such as calcium carbonate/acetate, lanthanum carbonate, or sevelamer, frank aluminum overload is rarely seen. Notwithstanding this, acute intoxications occasionally are reported in centers from various parts of the world. Furthermore, low-level accumulation of aluminum in some patients may lead to subtle disorders at the level of the parathyroid gland, osteoblast function, and hematopoiesis.

Hence, knowledge of patient risk factors, recognition of early signs and symptoms, and regular monitoring of serum aluminum levels (at least twice a year) are still recommended to limit the occurrence of aluminum toxicity in dialysis patients.

A. Risk factors. All dialysis patients who are ingesting aluminum-containing phosphate binders (e.g., aluminum hydroxide or carbonate) are at risk for aluminum poisoning. Frequent administration of certain aluminum-containing intravenous preparations (e.g., albumin, hyperalimentation solutions, and some medications) may exacerbate aluminum overload in dialysis patients. In the past, aluminum intoxication was also caused by aluminum absorption from dialysis solutions.

1. Hyperparathyroidism protects against aluminum overload. Patients with secondary hyperparathyroidism appear to be relatively resistant to aluminum-associated bone disease, possibly because aluminum accumulation in bone is inhibited in the presence of osteoclast activity. Conversely, after parathyroidectomy, patients are unusually susceptible to aluminum-induced osteomalacia and should be protected vigorously from aluminum exposure. Because aluminum poisoning of the parathyroid glands may suppress the release of parathyroid hormone (PTH), aluminum-related bone disease can occur eventually, even in initially hyperparathyroid patients.

2. Iron depletion. With iron depletion, there is increased binding of aluminum to transferrin together with an

Table 43-1. Symptoms and signs of aluminum-related neurologic toxicity

Early

Intermittent disturbances (stuttering, stammering)
Dyspraxia

Late

Constant speech disturbances
Apraxia[a]
Asterixis
Myoclonic jerks
Seizures
Personality changes
Global dementia

[a]Apraxia is the inability to perform learned movements on demand.

up-regulation of transferrin receptors in tissues such as the parathyroid gland, which results in an increased uptake of aluminum.

3. Diabetes. Diabetic patients also appear to be sensitive to aluminum-induced bone disease as a result of a low rate of bone formation and an increased rate of whole-body aluminum accumulation.

4. Children. Children are believed to have an increased gut absorptive capacity for aluminum and should not be treated with aluminum-containing phosphate binders if at all possible.

5. Citrate. Ingestion of citrate (e.g., as Shohl solution or even with citrate-containing juices) along with aluminum in any form can greatly increase gut aluminum absorption and lead to acute aluminum-induced encephalopathy.

B. Signs and symptoms. Signs and symptoms of brain, bone, and blood involvement may or may not occur concurrently, and absence of findings in one organ system does not preclude severe involvement in the others.

1. Neurologic syndrome. Although encephalopathy is now rare, it is the most dramatic and severe manifestation of aluminum toxicity. Symptoms and signs are listed in Table 43-1. The electroencephalographic findings consist of multifocal bursts of slow or delta waves, often accompanied by spikes. Onset or exacerbation of neurologic symptoms has been observed during deferoxamine (DFO) therapy, presumably because of redistribution of mobilized aluminum into the brain. As noted above, the neurologic syndrome may be precipitated by concomitant ingestion of aluminum-containing antacids or phosphorus binders and citrate.

2. Bone disease. The manifestations of aluminum-related bone disease are summarized in Table 43-2. The definitive diagnosis is established by bone biopsy. Overt

Table 43-2.   Manifestations of aluminum-related bone disease

Symptoms and signs

Severe and diffuse bone pain
Muscle weakness (especially upper legs)
Spontaneous fractures

Laboratory findings

Slightly elevated serum calcium value, which may rise dramatically
   after vitamin D administration
Normal or slightly elevated serum PTH level (i.e., low for the degree
   of renal failure)
Normal serum alkaline phosphatase concentration
Persistence of hypercalcemia after parathyroidectomy
Elevated serum aluminum levels and/or positive DFO test

Bone biopsy findings (see Chapter 35)

Either adynamic lesions or increased amount of unmineralized bone
   (osteomalacia)
Reduced bone formation rate by double tetracycline labeling
Positive aluminum staining at the trabecular surface (however,
   there may be falsely positive staining if iron is in excess)
Elevated bone aluminum content (not as good an indicator as
   aluminum staining)

PTH, parathyroid hormone; DFO, deferoxamine.

bone aluminum accumulation has disappeared over the past few years, but in some patients aluminum may be present in amounts sufficient to interfere with parathyroid gland function and bone turnover.

   3.   Anemia. The signs and symptoms of aluminum-related anemia at the patient level are the same as those of any other anemia. The anemia is typically microcytic, and the presence of microcytosis with normal serum ferritin levels suggests that aluminum intoxication may be the causative factor. Aluminum might induce a defect in iron utilization or interfere with the bioavailability of stored iron for erythropoiesis. Aluminum accumulation has also been associated with a resistance to erythropoietin therapy.

C.   Diagnosis of aluminum overload

   1.   Serum aluminum levels

      a.   Measurement. Because aluminum is ubiquitous in nature, special attention should be paid to avoid contamination of the serum sample during handling and preparation for aluminum determination (Table 43-3).

      b.   Indications. The serum aluminum concentration is no longer checked routinely in many parts of the world where oral aluminum-containing salts are no longer used as phosphorus binders. However, the possibility of inadvertent contamination of dialysis solution concentrate or

Table 43-3. Serum aluminum levels: prevention of contamination during sampling and aluminum determination

Sampling

Sample should be obtained before heparinization.

Use syringes and needles without detectable aluminum release.

Use no glassware.

Samples must be stored in stoppered plastic tubes pretested for the amount of aluminum that they release.

Determination

Use only double-distilled water with aluminum level of <1.0 mcg/L (37 nmol/L).

Ensure minimal number of manipulations.

Ensure minimal number of reagents.

Use pretested plastic sample tubes and sample cups.

Do not use pipettes with metallic bodies.

Work in a dust-free environment.

feed water must always be remembered. Some units continue to routinely check serum aluminum levels every 6–12 months. Of course, serum aluminum levels should be checked promptly in any patient suspected of suffering from aluminum-related involvement of brain, bone, or blood. Also, unexplained hypercalcemia, especially with a low serum PTH, should lead to consideration of possible aluminum toxicity. Determination of aluminum is difficult and should be performed by a qualified laboratory.

    c. Interpretation and normal values. In nonuremic patients, the serum aluminum concentration is normally less than 2 mcg/L (74 nmol/L). In most dialysis patients who have been receiving oral aluminum compounds, serum aluminum concentrations being monitored regularly will range between 5 and 30 mcg/L (180 and 1,100 nmol/L). Within this general range, the relationship between the serum aluminum value and the extent of aluminum accumulation is poorly predictable (Table 43-4). Evidence has been presented that in the current dialysis population a threshold serum aluminum level of 30 mcg/L (1,100 nmol/L) is a reliable index for the detection of aluminum overload (defined as a bone aluminum level >15 mcg [550 nmol/g] wet weight and/or a positive [>0%] aluminon staining). It has recently been shown that cessation of ingestion of aluminum-containing phosphate binders can quickly (over several days) reduce the serum aluminum concentration.

  2. DFO test

    a. Rationale. In some patients, particularly those with iron depletion or iron overload or in whom aluminum hydroxide has recently been withdrawn, the serum

Table 43-4. Serum aluminum levels: diagnostic value[a]

Serum Aluminum Level		Implication
mcg/L	nmol/L	
<2	<74	This is the normal range (subjects with normal renal function).
<30	<1,100	Aluminum-related bone disease is unlikely but possible, particularly when patients are iron-overloaded. In these subjects DFO testing is recommended.
30–60	1,100–2,200	Aluminum-related bone disease is quite possible, especially if serum PTH levels are low or low-normal. A DFO test is recommended.
>60	>2,200	Aluminum-related bone disease is probable, but not invariably present, especially if serum PTH levels are high, iron transferrin saturation is low, or the DFO test is negative.
>100	>3,700	Aluminum-related bone disease is most probable unless patient is iron deficient and/or the DFO test is negative. Neurologic disorders should be checked for by taking the patient's electroencephalogram.

DFO, deferoxamine; PTH, parathyroid hormone.
[a] Serum aluminum levels are a useful indicator of toxicity when determined at regular intervals (every 6 months).

aluminum level poorly predicts the bone/tissue aluminum deposition. The diagnostic value of serum aluminum monitoring can be enhanced when used in combination with a DFO test.

DFO is a chelating compound that liberates aluminum from its body stores (e.g., in bone, liver), causing DFO–aluminum (i.e., aluminoxamine) to enter the blood from these sites.

b. Method. A DFO dose of 5 mg/kg should be used. The DFO test should be performed under strictly standardized conditions as listed in Table 43-5.

c. Interpretation. An increment in the serum aluminum level (ΔSAl) of 50 mcg/L (~1,800 nmol/L) as determined 44 hours after DFO (5 mg/kg given intravenously during the last hour of a dialysis session) points to the presence of aluminum overload (bone aluminum >15 mcg [550 nmol/L] per g and/or a positive [>0%] aluminon

Table 43-5. The deferoxamine test

Hemodialysis patients

1. Obtain a baseline serum aluminum value prior to a hemodialysis session.
2. Infuse 5 mg/kg DFO in 150 mL of 5% glucose water into the venous blood line during the last 60 minutes of the same hemodialysis session; closely monitor vital signs during DFO infusion.
3. At the start of the next hemodialysis session (44 hours after DFO administration), determine a second serum aluminum level.

Peritoneal dialysis patients

1. Measure a baseline serum aluminum concentration at any time during the day.
2. Give 5 mg/kg DFO in 150 mL of 5% glucose water intravenously during the last 60 minutes of a CAPD exchange. Alternatively, add the same amount of DFO to the nocturnal exchange for CAPD patients or to the long daytime exchange for CCPD patients.
3. Determine the serum aluminum value in a second sample drawn 44 hours after termination of the DFO infusion or the DFO-containing exchange.

Side effects

Hypotension can occur during DFO infusion; treat by temporarily stopping the infusion, and administering a volume expander if required.

Continuation of aluminum-containing phosphate binders throughout the test

This is controversial. If these medications are stopped, then an acute decrease in the serum aluminum level can be expected.

DFO, deferoxamine; CAPD, continuous ambulatory peritoneal dialysis; CCPD, continuous cycling peritoneal dialysis.

staining). Moreover, in combination with a serum immunoreactive PTH (iPTH) measurement, a ΔSAl threshold of 50 mcg/L (1,800 nmol/L) will allow one to differentiate between (a) aluminum overload, (b) increased risk for toxicity (aluminon staining >0%), and (c) aluminum-related bone disease (>15% aluminon positivity and a bone formation rate below 220 mcm^2/mm^2 per day) (Table 43-6).

(1) **How serum iPTH levels affect interpretation of a positive DFO test.** Using the 5 mg/kg DFO test, patients with a ΔSAl >50 mcg/L (1,800 nmol/L) have a positive test and may have aluminum overload. However, if the serum iPTH is >650 pg/mL (70 pmol/L), then the high PTH levels may protect them against the

Table 43-6. Serum aluminum increment after 5 mg/kg deferoxamine diagnostic value[a]

Serum Aluminum Increment (ΔSAI) and Serum PTH level[b]		
mcg/L and ng/mL	SI units	Implications
<50 mcg/L	<1,800	Aluminum *overload* is unlikely to be present.
>50 mcg/L and iPTH >650 pg/mL	>1,800 nmol/L and iPTH >70 pmol/L	Aluminum *overload* is likely to be present; however, the risk for aluminum *toxicity* is minimal.
>50 mcg/L and iPTH 150–650 pg/mL	>1,800 nmol/L and iPTH 16–70 pmol/L	Aluminum-related bone disease most probable. PTH levels should be followed closely.
>50 mcg/L and iPTH <150 pg/mL	>1,800 nmol/L and iPTH <16 pmol/L	Aluminum-related bone disease is most probable. Confirm by bone biopsy and consider 5 mg/kg DFO treatment.
>300 mcg/L	>11 mcmol/L	Neurologic disorders and side effects are most probable. Check by taking the patient's electroencephalogram. Use the alternative schedule for DFO therapy.

DFO, deferoxamine; iPTH, intact parathyroid hormone.
[a]Using a 5 mg/kg DFO dose.
[b]Intact PTH values are listed. For biointact values, multiply by 0.55.

deleterious effects of the element at the bone mineralization front. Aluminum toxicity is more likely when a positive DFO test is accompanied by a serum iPTH lower than 650 pg/mL (70 pmol/L). There is a great chance for aluminum-related bone disease to be present in patients with a positive DFO test when the serum iPTH has decreased to below 150 pg/mL (16 pmol/L) (Table 43-6).

d. Indications. The DFO test should be performed in all dialysis patients who have signs or symptoms (related to bone, brain, or blood) suggestive of aluminum toxicity.

In patients with a normal iron status and a basal serum aluminum level below 30 mcg/L (1,100 nmol/L), the DFO test in general will not add much information to regular serum aluminum monitoring. In iron-overloaded patients, however, DFO testing will correct for false negatives because in these subjects low basal serum aluminum levels may be accompanied by an increased body burden. In patients treated for hyperparathyroidism with vitamin D and/or parathyroidectomy, the aluminum status should be re-evaluated since hypoparathyroidism holds an increased risk for aluminum toxicity.

D. **Treatment of aluminum overload.** Once aluminum overload has been identified, treatment should be initiated, especially in symptomatic patients.

   1. **Discontinuation of aluminum-containing medications**

      a. **General.** In all patients, the first line of therapy is to discontinue the use of aluminum-containing phosphate binders. These can be replaced with calcium-containing preparations or with lanthanum carbonate (see below) or sevelamer if hypercalcemia is present. Control of the serum phosphate level can often be improved by reducing dietary phosphate intake and by augmenting removal of phosphate by use of a large-surface-area dialyzer and a longer dialysis session length. In asymptomatic patients, there is preliminary evidence to suggest that simply stopping aluminum-containing medications can result in improved bone histology and an increased bone formation rate.

      b. **Hypercalcemia on switching to calcium-containing phosphate binders.** A common problem encountered when attempting to partially or completely change a patient's phosphate-binding regimen from aluminum- to calcium-based medication is the prompt induction of hypercalcemia. Because of the risk of hypercalcemia, vitamin D analogs should initially be withheld. Calcium must be given with meals to maximize the amount of phosphate binding and to limit the amount of calcium absorption. Use of a low-calcium dialysis solution may also be of benefit. Lanthanum carbonate and sevelamer hydrochloride (Renagel) are effective alternatives that contain neither calcium nor aluminum and where available obviate the problem of both hypercalcemia and aluminum toxicity.

   2. **DFO therapy**

      a. **Rationale.** Aluminum in the blood is about 80%–90% protein bound; protein binding is the primary reason for aluminum being poorly removed during dialysis, even when serum values are high. After DFO administration, the absolute serum aluminum concentration is increased, and most of the increase is in the form of a dialyzable DFO–aluminum complex, aluminoxamine (MW 583 daltons). The latter complex is removable by hemodialysis (with or without concomitant hemoperfusion) or by peritoneal dialysis. DFO administration may also increase markedly the fecal excretion of aluminum.

      b. **Indications.** DFO therapy should be considered for patients with clinically suspected or biopsy-proven aluminum-related bone disease. If bone aluminum staining is negative and the bone formation rate is not reduced, but the DFO test is positive (or baseline serum aluminum values are high), then DFO therapy should be deferred and the patient treated conservatively by stopping aluminum-containing phosphate binders and using calcium salts, lanthanum carbonate, or sevelamer instead. High PTH levels are protective, and as long as they are high, chelation therapy should be deferred.

c. **Risks of precipitating or exacerbating aluminum-related encephalopathy.** During DFO therapy, a neurologic syndrome similar to aluminum-related encephalopathy has been reported. The exact mechanism is unknown but is theorized to be due to redistribution of aluminum mobilized by DFO into the brain. The risk of encephalopathy will be lessened if low DFO doses are used to limit the rise in the serum aluminum levels as described in Table 43-7.

In severely intoxicated patients in whom the serum aluminum level after DFO may rise to above 300 mcg/L (11 mcmol/L), worsening of patients' neurologic state has been observed even when doses as low as 5 mg/kg were administered in the conventional fashion (i.e., during the last hour of dialysis followed by removal of the chelates 44 hours later). These side effects were not found when the chelator was given via an alternative schedule (4–5 hours before the start of the dialysis session). Patients with central nervous system manifestations of aluminum toxicity should undergo DFO therapy because there is no other method for removal of aluminum from the body.

d. **Other DFO side effects.** A number of side effects, including retinal and auditory toxicity, have been reported when DFO is used. These are listed in Table 43-8. Even though the risk for these side effects is greatly reduced by using a 5 mg/kg dose, it may be wise to obtain a baseline audiogram and funduscopic examination in all patients scheduled to undergo DFO treatment and to repeat these examinations periodically while therapy is in progress. The use of DFO has been associated with the development of often fatal sepsis with *Rhizopus*, particularly in patients with hemosiderosis. This is most likely due to the fact that the complex of iron and DFO (i.e., feroxamine) is used as a source of iron by these non–siderophore-producing germs. As the amount of feroxamine that is formed after DFO is highly dose dependent, the risk for this side effect should be reduced by using the 5 mg/kg dose.

e. **Method of DFO therapy.** One method of DFO administration is described in Table 43-7. Dose-finding studies have offered a growing body of evidence that sufficient aluminum chelation is obtained with lower DFO doses, thus providing a rationale for the use of a 5 mg dose per kg body weight in the treatment of aluminum overload. Recent clinical studies have demonstrated the latter dose to be efficient in the removal of aluminum, as well as in the

Table 43-7.   Deferoxamine treatment in hemodialyzed patients

Hemodialysis patients

A. Starting dose: 5 mg/kg DFO (dissolved in 150 mL of 5% glucose water) is administered IV (into the venous blood line) during the last 60 minutes of a hemodialysis session; vital signs are monitored closely during DFO infusion.

  1. If the baseline serum aluminum level is >300 mcg/L (11 mcmol/L), then initial therapy should consist of discontinuation of aluminum-containing phosphate binders. DFO should not be given until the baseline concentration falls below 300 mcg/L (11 mcmol/L).

  2. If the post-DFO serum aluminum level increases to above 300 mcg/L (11 mcmol/L), then the chelator should be administered 4–5 hours before the start of the dialysis session (alternative method).

B. Frequency of administration: DFO should be administered once a week.

C. The DFO test is repeated every 3 months after a 4-week washout period. If the serum aluminum increment 48 hours after DFO administration is <50 mcg/L (1,800 nmol/L) at two successive tests (1-month interval), further DFO treatment is not recommended.

Peritoneal dialysis patients

In general, the strategy is as for hemodialysis patients. DFO is given once a week. It may be given intraperitoneally in the same dose as listed for hemodialysis patients, added to the longest dwelling exchange of the day (nocturnal exchange in CAPD patients, daytime exchange in CCPD patients). The long-term safety of intraperitoneal DFO administration has not been established.

Duration of therapy and follow-up

DFO treatment may be continued for 6–12 months. Expect serum calcium levels to fall, alkaline phosphatase and PTH levels to rise, signs of hyperparathyroidism to increase, and erythrocyte mean corpuscular volume and hematocrit to rise slightly.

DFO, deferoxamine; CAPD, continuous ambulatory peritoneal dialysis; CCPD, continuous cycling peritoneal dialysis; PTH, parathyroid hormone.

Table 43-8.   Hazards of chronic deferoxamine administration[a]

Susceptibility to *Yersinia* sepsis and to mucormycosis
High-frequency sensorineural hearing loss
Decrease in visual acuity
Loss of color vision
Maculopathy
Acute mental changes?

[a] Acute side effects (e.g., hypotension) can occur during deferoxamine infusion.

reduction of side effects. DFO should be given once weekly. In subjects with post-DFO serum aluminum levels above 300 mcg/L (11 mcmol/L), the DFO should be given 4–5 hours before the dialysis session. This will ensure maximal aluminum chelation while limiting exposure to circulating aluminoxamine, feroxamine, and unchelated DFO. Intradialytic removal of the DFO–aluminum complex can be accelerated by using high-flux dialyzers or a charcoal cartridge inserted proximal to a conventional dialyzer.

f. Follow-up and response to DFO therapy. In most cases, clinical improvement of aluminum-related bone disease begins several weeks after initiation of DFO therapy. The rapid response can be explained by the preferential removal of aluminum from critical sites. As therapy is continued for a 6- to 12-month period, the following laboratory changes can be expected:

(1) Serum PTH concentrations may increase; this is probably due to the fact that secretion of PTH is no longer inhibited by aluminum. Concomitantly, the serum alkaline phosphatase values may rise.

(2) The serum calcium levels may fall due to increased mineralization of bone. The amount of calcium supplement may be increased and vitamin D may be restarted to keep the serum calcium concentrations at physiologic levels and prevent hyperparathyroidism.

(3) The serum ferritin levels may decrease as a result of concomitant removal of DFO-chelated iron. The decrease is usually to the normal range only; ordinarily, iron supplementation is not needed.

(4) The erythrocyte mean corpuscular volume and hematocrit may both increase.

A repeat bone biopsy after 6 months of DFO therapy should reveal decreased aluminum staining, an increased bone formation rate, and evidence of increased osteoblast and osteoblast activity.

E. Prevention. Water used for making dialysis solution should be analyzed periodically for its aluminum concentration to ensure that the water treatment system in use is functioning properly.

Administration of aluminum in any form to the patient groups identified at the outset of this chapter as being at increased risk for aluminum toxicity should be avoided whenever possible. Use of aluminum-free phosphorus binders is now the universal standard of care. For patients with gastrointestinal intolerance or hypercalcemia associated with calcium-containing agents, use of lanthanum carbonate or sevelamer hydrochloride (Renagel) should be the alternatives of choice.

II. Lanthanum. Lanthanum carbonate has recently been introduced as an effective, well-tolerated aluminum- and calcium-free phosphate binder. Efficacy and safety have been evaluated in various long-term studies, and no aluminum-like effects on bone have been observed so far in experimental and clinical studies. Available bone biopsy data in dialysis patients treated for up to 4 years with lanthanum carbonate indicate low-level bone deposition, the highest concentration in any patient being 9 mcg (65 nmol) per gram. This represents a low molar lanthanum:calcium ratio that is unlikely to cause physicochemical interactions of the metal with hydroxyapatite nucleation/development and structure in bone. Furthermore, no adverse cell biologic effects of lanthanum on osteoblasts have been observed in animals or humans. In contrast to aluminum, lanthanum is heterogeneously deposited in the bone, independent of the type of renal osteodystrophy.

Compared with aluminum, lanthanum accumulates to a lesser extent in the body of dialysis patients, mainly because of its ultralow gastrointestinal absorption and biliary elimination of the small absorbed fraction. Studies have shown that the absolute bioavailability in patients is below 0.002%, with the majority of an oral dose being excreted in the feces. Biliary elimination (80%) and direct transport across the gut wall into the lumen (13%) represent the main routes of elimination. Therefore, the elimination of lanthanum is not dependent on renal function; of a lanthanum dose of 1 g per day in healthy volunteers, only 0.00003% was excreted in the urine, indicating that, compared with individuals with normal renal function, chronic renal insufficiency patients are not at an increased risk for accumulation of the element. This has been confirmed in several phase 1 clinical studies, which have indicated similar plasma exposure and pharmacokinetics of lanthanum in dialysis patients and healthy individuals. Citrate does not influence gastrointestinal absorption of lanthanum. Even after long-term treatment, serum lanthanum levels rarely exceed 1 mcg/L (7 nmol/L).

III. Strontium (MW 88)

A. Increased strontium concentrations in bone and serum of dialysis patients.

The kidney plays an important role in the excretion of strontium from the body. For example, in one study strontium concentration in skeletal muscle of dialysis patients was increased five- to eightfold when untreated tap water used to prepare the dialysis solution (Rudolph, 1973). Strontium may play a role in renal osteodystrophy; bone strontium levels and strontium:calcium ratios are increased in dialysis patients with osteomalacia. Bone strontium levels were elevated not only compared to individuals with normal renal function, but also in comparison to dialysis patients with other types of renal osteodystrophy.

Serum strontium concentrations in subjects with normal renal function are around 25 mcg/L (280 nmol/L). Dialysis centers can be roughly categorized in two groups: Those with mean serum strontium levels below 100 mcg/L (1,150 nmol/L) and those with levels above this threshold. Only a small overlap between these two categories can be noted, and "high strontium" centers are mainly found in developing countries. A strong correlation exists between dialysis solution concentrate and serum strontium levels. Some concentrates (mostly acetate based) may have strontium concentrations up to 16 mg/L (0.180 mmol/L). Such concentrates should not be used.

SELECTED READINGS

Barata JD, et al. Low-dose (5 mg/kg) desferrioxamine treatment in acutely intoxicated haemodialysis patients using two drug administration schedules. *Nephrol Dial Transplant* 1996;11:125–132.

Behets GJ, et al. Lanthanum carbonate: a new phosphate binder. *Curr Opin Nephrol Hypertens* 2004;13:403–409.

De Broe ME, et al. Consensus conference: diagnosis and treatment of aluminium overload in end-stage renal failure patients. *Nephrol Dial Transplant* 1993;8(Suppl 1):1.

D'Haese PC, et al. A multicenter study on the effects of lanthanum carbonate (Fosrenol) and calcium carbonate on renal bone disease in dialysis patients. *Kidney Int* 2003;63(Suppl 85):73–78.

D'Haese PC, Couttenye MM, DeBroe ME. Diagnosis and treatment of aluminium bone disease. *Nephrol Dial Transplant* 1996; 11(Suppl 3):74–79.

D'Haese PC, et al. Increased bone strontium levels in hemodialysis patients with osteomalacia. *Kidney Int* 2000;57:1107–1114.

D'Haese PC, et al. Use of the low-dose desferrioxamine test to diagnose and differentiate between patients with aluminum-related bone disease, increased risk for aluminum toxicity, or aluminum overload. *Nephrol Dial Transplant* 1995;10:1874–1884.

Froment DP, et al. Site and mechanism of enhanced gastrointestinal absorption of aluminum by citrate. *Kidney Int* 1989;36:978–984.

Hutchison AJ, et al. Long-term efficacy and tolerability of lanthanum carbonate: results from a 3-year study. *Nephron Clin Pract* 2006;102(2):61–71.

Mazzaferro S, et al. Relative roles of intestinal absorption and dialysis-fluid–related exposure in the accumulation of aluminum in haemodialysis patients. *Nephrol Dial Transplant* 1997;12:2679–2682.

Olivieri NF, et al. Visual and auditory neurotoxicity in patients receiving subcutaneous deferoxamine infusions. *N Engl J Med* 1986;314:869–873.

Rosenlöf K, Fyhrquist F, Tenhunen R. Erythropoietin, aluminium, and anaemia in patients on haemodialysis. *Lancet* 1990;335:247–249.

Rudolph H, et al. Muscle and serum trace element profile in uremia. *Trans Am Soc Artif Intern Organs* 1973;19:456–465.

Schrooten I, et al. Increased serum strontium levels in dialysis patients. An epidemiological survey. *Kidney Int* 1999;56:1886–1892.

Smans KA, et al. Transferrin; mediated uptake of aluminum by human parathyroid cells results in a reduced parathyroid hormone secretion. *Nephrol Dial Transplant* 2000;15:1328–1336.

Van Landeghem GF, et al. Competition of iron and aluminum for transferrin: the molecular basis for aluminum deposition in iron-overloaded dialysis patients?. *Exp Nephrol* 1997;5:239–245.

Vasilakakis DM, et al. Removal of aluminoxamine and ferrioxamine by charcoal hemoperfusion and hemodialysis. *Kidney Int* 1992;41:1400–1407.

Urea Kinetic Modeling: Tables and Figures

Table A-1. Estimating dialyzer blood water clearance from K_0A, Q_B, and Q_D

Step 1: Reduce industry-reported K_0A by 10%.[a]

Step 2: Adjust resultant K_0A upward by 2% for each 100 mL per minute of dialysate flow rate >500 mL per minute (e.g., multiply by 1.00 when $Q_D = 500$ mL per minute, 1.02 when $Q_D = 600$ mL per minute, and 1.06 when $Q_D = 800$ mL per minute).

Step 3: Adjust blood flow to compensate for prepump negative pressure (the tubing in the pump segment becomes more oval as prepump negative pressure increases, reducing its stroke volume) and other factors.

Adjustment factor $F = 1.0 - (Q_B - 200)/2{,}000$

Adjusted Q_B (Q_{badj}) = Q_B F

(no adjustment when Q_B <200 mL per minute)

Example: $Q_B = 400$ mL per minute

$F = 1 - (400 - 200)/2{,}000 = 0.90$

$Q_{badj} = 360$ mL per minute

(This blood flow correction step can be skipped if the unit is using blood lines that have been strengthened to prevent this problem.)

Step 4: Compute diffusive blood water clearance (K_{difw}) from adjusted K_0A and adjusted Q_B. K_{difw} depends on K_0A_{adj}, Q_B (Q_{badj}), and the dialysate flow rate Q_D, according to a fairly complicated equation.

To simplify writing it, we define an intermediate variable called Z. Then:

$Z = \exp [K_0A_{adj}/Q_{badj} * (1 - Q_{badj}/Q_D)]$

$K_{difw} = 0.894 * Q_{badj} * (Z - 1)/(Z - Q_{badj}/Q_D)$

The 0.894 multiplier is to correct clearance for blood water, as discussed in the text.

Step 5: Add convective clearance to diffusive clearance. First, we compute the ultrafiltration rate in milliliters per minute (Q_f), and then compute the total blood water clearance (K_{totw}) from the diffusive clearance (K_{difw}), the blood flow rate (Q_{badj}), and Q_f.

$Q_f = W_{tlosskg} * 1{,}000/(t_{min})$

$K_{totw} = [1 - Q_f/(0.894 * Q_{badj})] * K_{difw} + Q_f$

---

*Denotes multiplication; $\exp (x) = e^x$.

[a]Actually, industry reported K_0A should be reduced by 20%–30% for a true in vivo clearance, but this will vary by manufacturer, and then the urea distribution volume (V) will be 15%–20% lower than anthropometrically estimated total body water.

Table A-2.   Anthropometric estimates for total body water

Watson estimate of anthropometric volume:

For men: V (L) = 2.447 + 0.3362 * W (kg) + 0.1074 * H (cm)
  − 0.09516 * Age (years)

For women: V = −2.097 + 0.2466 * W + 0.1069 * H

Hume-Weyers method:

For men: V = −14.012934 + 0.296785 * W + 0.192786 * H

For women: V = −35.270121 + 0.183809 * W + 0.344547 * H

For a nomogram of the Hume-Weyers methods, see Figs. A-6 and A-7.

Mellits-Cheek method for children:

For boys:

V (L) = −1.927 + 0.465 * W (kg) + 0.045 * H (cm), when H <132.7 cm

V = −21.993 + 0.406 * W + 0.209 * H, when H >132.7 cm

For girls:

V = 0.076 + 0.507 * W + 0.013 * H, when H <110.8 cm

V = −10.313 + 0.252 * W + 0.154 * H, when H >110.8 cm

---

*Denotes multiplication.

References: Watson PE, Watson ID, Batt RD. Total body water volumes for adult males and females estimated from simple anthropometric measurements. *Am J Clin Nutr* 1980;33:27–39; Hume R, Weyers E. Relationship between total body water and surface area in normal and obese subjects. *J Clin Pathol* 1971;24:234–238; Mellits ED, Cheek DB. The assessment of body water and fatness from infancy to adulthood. *Monogr Soc Res Child Dev* (Serial 140) 1970;35:12–26; Du Bois D, Du Bois EF. A formula to estimate the approximate surface area if height and weight are known. *Arch Intern Med* 1916;17:863–971.

Caveat: Watson underestimates V in African Americans; Hume-Weyers overestimates V in older men (Daugirdas JT, et al. [Abstract]. *J Am Soc Nephrol* 1996;7:1510).

Table A-3. Equations for dialyzer K_0A from In vitro clearances

Step 1: Compute the ultrafiltration rate (Q_f in mL per minute) at which the clearances were done.

Ignore this step if clearances were done at TMP = 0.

If not, find the ultrafiltration coefficient of the dialyzer in question. Compute Q_f as follows:

Q_f (mL per minute) = (1/60) $*$ K_{Uf} (mL per hour per mm Hg) $*$ TMP (mm Hg)

Example: Assume K_{Uf} = 20, and the clearance was done at TMP 40 mm Hg. Q_f (mL per hour) = 20 $*$ 40 = 800 mL per hour = 800/60 = 13.3 mL per minute.

Step 2: Read the clearance of the dialyzer specification sheet or clearance graph. Take at least two different blood flow rates, preferably >200 mL per minute. This clearance is K_{totw}. Now subtract the ultrafiltration component of clearance from this as follows, to get the diffusive clearance:

$K_{dif} = (K_{totw} - Q_f)/(1 - Q_f/Q_B)$

Example: Assume clearance at Q_B = 300 mL per minute is 240 mL per minute from a spec sheet, but this was done using Q_f of 13 mL per minute. K_{totw} = 240 mL per minute.

$K_{dif} = (240 - 13)/(1 - 13/300) = 227/0.957 = 237$ mL per minute

Step 3: Compute in vitro K_0A from K_{dif}, Q_B, and Q_D, using the uncorrected values for Q_B and Q_D on the dialyzer specification sheet based on the following equations:

N = log $((K_{dif}/Q_D - 1)/(K_{dif}/Q_B - 1))$
D = $(1 - Q_B/Q_D)$
$K_0A = 200 * $ N/D

$*$Denotes multiplication in equations; log (x) denotes natural logarithm of x; N and D stand for intermediate variables (numerator, denominator) to make the overall equation simpler to write. Note that when reported clearances are obtained at a nonzero TMP, the values for K_0A computed by these equations will be somewhat lower than by using the nomogram in Fig. A-5, which does not make the ultrafiltration correction.

Table A-4. Tattersall equation for postdialysis rebound for short daily dialysis*

$eKt/V = spKt/V \, (t/(t + 35))$ (t in minutes)

Example: $spKt/V = 0.8$, 90 minute dialysis session length

$eKt/V = 0.8 \times (90/125) = 0.58$

*More accurate than standard rate equation when dialysis session length is <2.5 hours. The 35 minute time constant applies to arteriovenous access. Use 22 minutes for a venous access.

Reference: Tattersall JE, et al. The post-hemodialysis rebound: predicting and quantifying its effect on *Kt/V*. *Kidney Int* 1996;50(6):2094–2102.

Table A-5. Leypoldt equation to estimate standard *Kt/V* based on single-pool *Kt/V* (sp*Kt/V*) and equilibrated *Kt/V* (e*Kt/V*)

$$\text{std}Kt/V = \frac{10080 \frac{1-e^{-eKt/V}}{t}}{\frac{1-e^{-eKt/V}}{spKt/V} + \frac{10080}{N*t} - 1}$$

eKt/V = equilibrated Kt/V (from Table A-4); $spKt/V$ = single-pool Kt/V; N = sessions per week; t = session length in minutes.

For more information see Leypoldt JK, Jaber BL, Zimmerman DL. Predicting treatment dose for novel therapies using urea standard *Kt/V*. *Semin Dial* 2004;17(2):142–145; Gotch FA. The current place of urea kinetic modelling with respect to different dialysis modalities. *Nephrol Dial Transplant* 1998; 13(Suppl 6):10–14. For a std*Kt/V* calculator see hdcn.com/calcf/ley.htm. Accessed 09/25/06.

Table A-6.   Surface-area-normalized (SAN) values for single-pool Kt/V (spKt/V) and standard Kt/V (stdKt/V)

SAN-Kt/V = Kt/V (spKt/V or stdKt/V calculated in the usual manner) multiplied by $V_{ant}/(3.271 \times V_{ant}^{2/3})$, and in females, multiplied again by 0.91.

The 3.271 term is simply $35/35^{2/3}$ and is designed to make the correction neutral when $V_{ant} = 35$ L for males. The 0.91 multiplier was derived from studying average values of $3.271 \times V_{ant}^{2/3}/BSA$ (body surface area) in women versus men from 1,696 baseline patients enrolled in the HEMO trial. If we consider the National Kidney Foundation's (NKF) Kidney Disease Outcome Quality Initiative (KDOQI) requirements for spKt/V and stdKt/V of at least 1.2/dialysis three times per week and 2.0/week, respectively, then the minimum spKt/V and stdKt/V needed to achieve these new adequacy measures based on SAN-spKt/V $\geq$1.2 and SAN-stdKt/V $\geq$2.0 are shown below.

spKt/V required to achieve a SAN-spKt/V of 1.2/dialysis three times per week)

V_{ant}	25	30	35	40	50
Men	1.34	1.26	**1.20**	1.15	1.06
Women	1.48	1.39	1.32	1.26	1.17

stdKt/V target required to achieve a SAN-std Kt/V of 2.0/week)

Men	2.24	2.10	**2.0**	1.91	1.78
Women	2.47	2.31	2.20	2.10	1.96

spKt/V target (3 $\times$ week) required to achieve a SAN-stdKt/V of 2.0/week[a]

Men	1.46	1.34	1.24	1.16	1.06
Women	1.76	1.56	1.44	1.34	1.21

[a]Based on a K/V of 0.4 per hour. Calculations were done using the equations in Tables A-4 and A-5. Note that for smaller patients, these spKt/V values are HIGHER than those required to achieve a SAN-spKt/V of 1.2.

Note: This is a hypothetical way of expressing dialysis dose, and its superiority over the usual Kt/V targets has not been validated by outcomes data.

Reference: Daugirdas JT, et al. SAN (surface area normalized) values for single-pool and standard Kt/V [Abstract F-FC111]. *J Am Soc Nephrol* 2006; 17:p60A.

Table A-7. Approximate standard *Kt/V* values for various single-pool *Kt/V* values with different dialysis schedules

| | | Standard *Kt/V* | | | | | |
| | | Sessions/week | | | | | |
Sp*Kt/V*	Min	2	3	4	5	6	7
0.4	120	0.54	0.81	1.08	1.36	1.64	1.92
0.5	120	0.65	0.98	1.31	1.64	1.98	2.32
0.6	120	0.75	1.13	1.51	1.90	2.29	2.69
0.7	120	0.85	1.27	1.71	2.14	2.58	3.03
0.8	120	0.93	1.41	1.88	2.37	2.86	3.35
0.9	135	1.03	1.56	2.09	2.63	3.17	3.73
1.0	150	1.13	1.70	2.28	2.87	3.47	4.08
1.1	165	1.21	1.83	2.46	3.10	3.75	4.41
1.2	180	1.29	1.95	2.62	3.31	4.00	4.71
1.3	195	1.36	2.06	2.78	3.50	4.25	5.00
1.4	210	1.43	2.16	2.92	3.69	4.47	5.28
1.5	225	1.49	2.26	3.05	3.86	4.69	5.53
1.6	240	1.54	2.35	3.17	4.02	4.89	5.78
1.7	255	1.60	2.43	3.28	4.16	5.07	6.01
1.8	270	1.64	2.50	3.39	4.30	5.25	6.23
1.9	285	1.69	2.57	3.49	4.44	5.42	6.44
2.0	300	1.73	2.64	3.58	4.57	5.58	6.64
2.1	315	1.76	2.70	3.67	4.68	5.73	6.83
2.2	330	1.80	2.75	3.75	4.79	5.88	7.02
2.3	345	1.83	2.81	3.83	4.90	6.02	7.20
2.4	360	1.86	2.86	3.90	5.00	6.16	7.38
2.5	375	1.89	2.90	3.97	5.10	6.29	7.55

Assumption made is that 0.4 sp*Kt/V* units are being delivered per hour except for values of 0.4 to 0.7, where a minimum session length of 120 min is used in the calculations. Sp*Kt/V* = single-pool *Kt/V*; min = session length in minutes. Calculated using the methods described in Tables A-4 (Tattersall) and A-5 (Leypoldt). The minimum std-*Kt/V* should always be at least 2.0 and this minimum target should be set higher in women and small patients (see Table A-6 for one experimental way to do this). For patients with $K_{ru} > 2$, the minimum std-*Kt/V* target (excluding renal clearance) can be set to 1.6 for 3 to 7 time per week schedules, and 1.7 for twice-a-week schedules. The residual urea clearance in L/week can NOT simply be subtracted from the std-*Kt/V*. But using minimum targets of 1.6 and 1.7 for std-*Kt/V* in patients with $K_{ru} > 2$ will give results consistent with 2006 KDOQI guidelines. The results are sensitive to session length; a more detailed calculator is available on the HDCN website at hdcn.com/calcf/ley.htm.

Table A-8. Frame size as determined from elbow breadth

Age (yr)	Frame Size		
	Small	Medium	Large
Men			
18–24	≤ 6.6	>6.6 and <7.7	≥ 7.7
25–34	≤ 6.7	>6.7 and <7.9	≥ 7.9
35–44	≤ 6.7	>6.7 and <8.0	≥ 8.0
45–74	≤ 6.7	>6.7 and <8.1	≥ 8.1
Women			
18–24	≤ 5.6	>5.6 and <6.5	≥ 6.5
25–34	≤ 5.7	>5.7 and <6.8	≥ 6.8
35–44	≤ 5.7	>5.7 and <7.1	≥ 7.1
45–54	≤ 5.7	>5.7 and <7.2	≥ 7.2
55–74	≤ 5.8	>5.8 and <7.2	≥ 7.2

Frame size by elbow breadth (cm) of U.S. male and female adults derived from the combined NHANES I and II datasets.
Data from Frisancho AR. New standards of weight and body composition by frame size and height for assessment of nutritional status of adults and the elderly. *Am J Clin Nutr* 1984;40:808–819.

Table A-9. Median weights for men and women in the United States by age, height, and frame size

Height		25–54			55–74		
in.	cm	S	M	L	S	M	L
Men							
62	157	64	68	82	61	68	77
63	160	61	71	83	62	70	80
64	163	66	71	84	63	71	77
65	165	66	74	79	70	72	79
66	168	67	75	84	68	74	80
67	170	71	77	84	69	78	85
68	173	71	78	86	70	78	83
69	175	74	78	89	75	77	84
70	178	75	81	87	76	80	87
71	180	76	81	91	69	84	84
72	183	74	84	91	76	81	90
73	185	79	85	93	78	88	88
74	188	80	88	92	77	95	89
Women							
58	147	52	63	86	54	57	78
59	150	53	66	78	55	62	78
60	152	53	60	87	54	65	78
61	155	54	61	81	56	64	79
62	157	55	61	81	58	64	82
63	160	55	62	83	58	65	80
64	163	57	62	79	60	66	77
65	165	60	63	81	60	67	80
66	168	58	63	75	68	66	82
67	170	59	65	80	61	72	80
68	173	62	67	76	61	70	79
69	175	63	68	79	62	72	85
70	178	64	70	76	63	73	85

[a]Frame size as defined in Table A-8.

Data derived from the combined NHANES I and II datasets. *Data source*: Frisancho AR. New standards of weight and body composition by frame size and height for assessment of nutritional status of adults and the elderly. *Am J Clin Nutr* 1984;40:808–819.

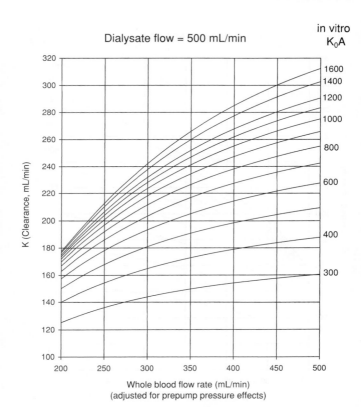

Figure A-1a.   Relationship between nominal blood flow rate (Q_B) and blood water urea clearance (K) as a function of dialyzer efficiency (K_0A). $K = K_{totw}$ was computed as per the equations in Table A-1. These dialyzer clearance values still overestimate true in vivo values. To use, start with blood flow rate on the horizontal axis. Go up to intersect with the proper dialyzer K_0A line, and then go left for the dialyzer clearance, K. The x-axis shows the nominal blood flow rate, but the prepump pressure adjustment has been applied to lower the blood flow rate used in the calculations per Table A-1.

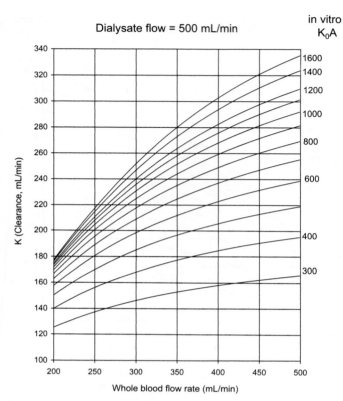

Figure A-1b.   Same nomogram as Fig. A-1a, except that the prepump blood flow rate adjustment has not been applied. Use this nomogram if you are using the new blood lines that do not reduce output at high prepump pressures. Because this prepump correction has not been made, clearances at higher blood flow rates are slightly greater than those shown in Fig. A-1a.

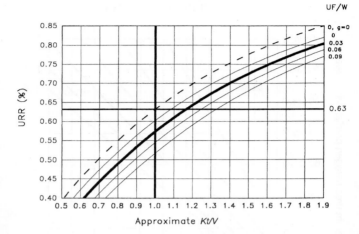

Figure A-2.   Relationship between fractional urea clearance (*Kt/V*) and urea reduction ratio (URR), taking into account urea generation and the effects of volume contraction. To use, start with the URR on the vertical axis. Move right until you intersect with the proper UF/W line (e.g., for a 4.2-kg weight loss in a 70-kg patient, UF/W = 4.2/70 = 0.06). Then drop down to the horizontal axis for the *Kt/V*. (Reproduced with permission from Daugirdas JT. Urea kinetic modeling. *Hypertens Dial Clin Nephrol* Available at: http://www.hdcn.com. Accessed 9/25/06.)

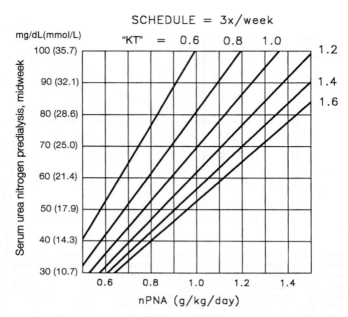

Figure A-3. The relationship between normalized protein nitrogen appearance (nPNA), the midweek predialysis serum urea nitrogen (SUN), and *Kt/V* for patients undergoing thrice-weekly dialysis. A similar nomogram designed for first-of-the-week predialysis SUN sampling is given in Chapter 3. To use, find the predialysis SUN on the vertical axis, move right to the proper "KT" diagonal, and then drop down to read nPNA on the horizontal axis. "KT" is the treatment *Kt/V* adjusted for Kru, using the equation "KT" = Kt/V + 4.5 × Kru/V, where Kru is the residual renal urea clearance in mL per minute and *V* is the urea distribution volume in L. If Kru = 0, then "KT" = Kt/V. (Reproduced with permission from Daugirdas JT. Urea kinetic modeling. *Hypertens Dial Clin Nephrol* Available at: http://www.hdcn.com. Accessed 9/25/06.)

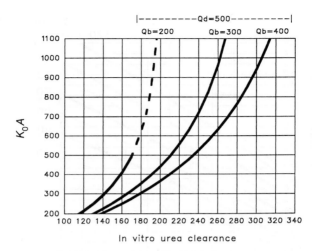

Figure A-4.   **Estimating the in vitro K_0A-urea from a dialyzer specification sheet. In most cases, the in vitro urea clearance reported at 300 mL of "blood" flow, and preferably that reported at 400 mL per minute, should be used. To find the K_0A, first find the urea clearance on the horizontal axis, rise vertically to the blood flow rate used, and read the K_0A off the vertical axis. The 200 mL per minute blood flow line has been dotted deliberately in the range of high-K_0A dialyzers; use clearances at 300 or 400 mL per minute blood flow rate only. (From Daugirdas JT, Depner TA. A nomogram approach to hemodialysis urea modeling. _Am J Kidney Dis_ 1994;23:33–40.)**

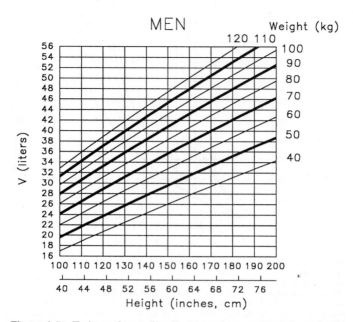

Figure A-5.   Estimated urea distribution volume (*V*) in male dialysis patients. These data are based on the assumption that *V* = total-body water (TBW) as measured by tritium (actually *V* is somewhat lower than tritium TBW). The TBW was computed based on body surface area according to Hume and Weyers (*J Clin Pathol* 1971;24:234–238), with body surface area derived according to Du Bois and Du Bois (*Arch Intern Med* 1916;17:863–871). To use, find the height on the horizontal axis, rise until the appropriate weight (postdialysis) line has been reached, and read *V* off the vertical axis. (From Daugirdas JT, Depner TA. A nomogram approach to hemodialysis urea modeling. *Am J Kidney Dis* 1994;23:33–40.)

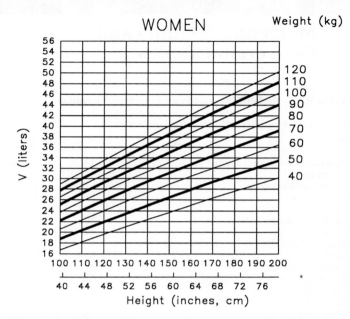

Figure A-6. Estimated *V* in female dialysis patients. The data are based on the same assumptions as noted for Fig. A-6. To use, follow the instructions in Fig. A-5. (From Daugirdas JT, Depner TA. A nomogram approach to hemodialysis urea modeling. *Am J Kidney Dis* 1994;23:33–40.)

Appendix B

Molecular Weights and Conversion Tables

Table B-1. Molecular weights and conversion tables

I. Molecular weights (MW) of some substances

Substance	MW
Acetylsalicylic acid (aspirin)	180
Albumin	68,000
β_2-microglobulin	11,600
Cholesterol	386
Creatinine	113
Dextrose (glucose monohydrate)	198
Ethanol	46
Ethylene glycol	62
Glucose	180
Hemoglobin	68,800
Isopropyl alcohol (isopropanol)	60
Light chains	23,000
Lithium	7
Methanol	32
Myoglobin	17,800
Parathyroid hormone	9,500
Phenobarbital	232
Theophylline	180
Triglycerides	886
Urea	60
"Urea nitrogen" (blood urea nitrogen [BUN] or serum urea nitrogen [SUN])	28
Vancomycin	1,486
Vitamin B_{12}	1,355
Vitamin D_3 (25-D_3)	402

II. Converting between weight, valency, and molarity
A. Number of milligrams in 1 mEq or 1 mmol of substance

Substance	1 mEq	1 mmol
Na^+	23	23
K^+	39	39
Ca^{2+}	20	40
Mg^{2+}	12	24
Li^+	7	7
$HCO3^-$	61	61
Cl^-	35.5	35.5
N (nitrogen)		14
P (phosphorus)		31
C (carbon)		12

continued

Table B-1. *Continued.*

B. Changing milligrams to milliequivalents or millimoles
   1. Sodium, potassium, chloride, bicarbonate

1 g NaCl	$= 1{,}000$ mg$/(23 + 35.5)$ mg
	$= 17$ mEq or mmol of Na^+
1 g Na^+	$= 1{,}000$ mg$/23$ mg
	$= 43$ mEq or mmol of Na^+
1 g KCl	$= 1{,}000$ mg$/74.5$ mg
	$= 14$ mEq or mmol of K^+
1 g K^+	$= 1{,}000$ mg$/39$ mg
	$= 26$ mEq or mmol of K^+
1 g $NaHCO_8$	$= 1{,}000$ mg$/84$ mg
	$= 12$ mEq or mmol of Na^+
	$= 12$ mEq or mmol of $HCO3^-$

   2. Calcium Normal serum Ca level
   $= 10$ mg/dL
   $= 100$ mg/L
   $= 100/20$ mmol/L, since 20 mg $= 1$ mEq
   $= 5$ mEq/L
   $= 5/2$ mmol/L since 2 mEq $= 1$ mmol
   $= 2.5$ mmol/L

   3. Magnesium Normal serum Mg level
   $= 2.4$ mg/dL
   $= 24$ mg/L
   $= 24/12$ mEq/L, since 12 mg $= 1$ mEq
   $= 2$ mEq/L
   $= 2/2$ mmol/L, since 2 mEq $= 1$ mmol
   $= 1$ mmol/L

   4. Phosphorus (P) Normal serum inorganic P level
   $= 2.5$ to 4 mg/dL
   $= 25$ to 40 mg/L
   $= (25/31$ to $40/31)$ mmol/L,
      since 1 mmol of P $= 31$ mg
   $= 0.8$ to 1.3 mmol/L

As P values when expressed in mEq/L change with alterations in pH, the mEq/L unit is not ordinarily used in clinical practice.

Subject Index

NOTE: Page numbers followed by *f* indicate figure; those followed by *t* indicate table.